ACLS

QUICK REVIEW STUDY GUIDE

Second Edition

Barbara Aehlert, RN, BSPA

President/CEO
Southwest EMS Education, Inc.

with 378 illustrations

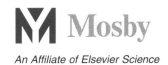
Mosby

An Affiliate of Elsevier Science

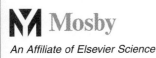

Mosby

An Affiliate of Elsevier Science

Publishing Director: Andrew Allen
Executive Editor: Claire Merrick
Developmental Editor: Kelly Trakalo
Project Manager: John Rogers
Project Specialist: Kathleen L. Teal
Designer: Kathi Gosche

Second Edition 2002

Previous edition copyrighted 1994

Printed in the United States

Mosby, Inc.
An Affiliate of Elsevier Science
11830 Westline Industrial Drive
St. Louis, Missouri 63146

International Standard Book Number 0-323-00892-5

03 04 05 WB/RRD-R 9 8 7 6 5 4 3 2

PREFACE

This book is designed for use by paramedic, nursing and medical students, ECG monitor technicians, nurses, and other allied health personnel working in emergency departments, critical care units, post-anesthesia care units, operating rooms, or telemetry units, who are preparing for an Advanced Cardiac Life Support Provider Course.

This second edition has been designed for use with the American Safety and Health Institute Advanced Cardiac Life Support Provider Course and may be used as supplemental material by participants of ACLS courses offered by other organizations.

The ten "core" cases presented in an ACLS Provider course include:

Case   1: Respiratory Arrest
Case   2: Ventricular Tachycardia/Ventricular Fibrillation with an AED
Case   3: Pulseless Ventricular Tachycardia/Ventricular Fibrillation
Case   4: Asystole
Case   5: Pulseless Electrical Activity (PEA)
Case   6: Acute Coronary Syndromes
Case   7: Symptomatic Bradycardia
Cases 8-9: Stable and Unstable Tachycardias
Case   10: Acute Ischemic Stroke

The second edition of this book consists of two primary divisions. Chapters 1 through 9 comprise the "preparatory" section of the text. These chapters are designed to provide the foundation for the case presentations in the second portion. A sample case presentation has been provided for each of the standard "core" cases presented in an ACLS course. The case presentations provided were not intended to cover every possible dysrhythmia that may be presented in an actual ACLS course. Rather, they are provided as examples to help you assimilate the information presented in the preparatory section of the text.

Each chapter contains instructional objectives followed by a review of the critical elements related to the subject. A 50-question pretest and posttest are provided in addition to quizzes at the conclusion of each chapter. Answers and rationales are provided for all questions in this text.

Every effort has been made to provide information that is consistent with current research and resuscitation guidelines; however, the reader is advised to consult expert opinion articles/guidelines for more authoritative advice. In clinical practice it is essential to confirm all medication doses, indications, and contraindications before use. The author and publisher assume no responsibility or liability for loss or damage resulting from the use of information contained within.

Barbara Aehlert, RN, BSPA
http://www.swemsed.com

ILLUSTRATION CREDITS

Pretest
All illustrations from Aehlert: ECGs Made Easy, 2e. St. Louis, 2002. Mosby.

Chapter 1
1-1 with permission from American Safety and Health Institute.
1-2, 1-4, 1-5, 1-6, 1-7, 1-8, 1-9 Henry and Stapleton: EMT Prehospital Care, 2e. Philadelphia, 1997. WB Saunders.
1-3, 1-13 Sanders: Mosby's Paramedic Textbook, 2e. St. Louis, 2000. Mosby.
1-10 Cummins: ACLS Scenarios: Core Concepts for Case-Based Learning. St. Louis, 1996. Mosby-Year Book.
1-11, 1-12 Shade: Mosby's EMT-Intermediate Textbook. St. Louis, 1997. Mosby-Year Book.

Chapter 2
2-1, 2-2, 2-3, 2-4, 2-5 Thibodeau: Anatomy & Physiology, 4e. St. Louis, 1999. Mosby.
2-6, 2-7 Herlihy: The Human Body in Health and Illness. Philadelphia, 2000. WB Saunders.
2-8, 2-14, 2-36 Stoy: Mosby's EMT-Basic Textbook. St. Louis, 1996. Mosby.
2-9, 2-11, 2-12, 2-13, 2-15, 2-16, 2-18, 2-19, 2-20, 2-23, 2-28, 2-33, 2-34, 2-35, 2-37, 2-44, 2-45, 2-50, 2-55, 2-57, 2-60, 2-61, 2-62, 2-65, 2-66, 2-67, 2-68, 2-69, 2-70, 2-71, 2-72, 2-73 Sanders: Mosby's Paramedic Textbook, 2e. St. Louis, 2000. Mosby.
2-10, 2-42, 2-43, 2-46, 2-47 Cummins: ACLS Scenarios: Core Concepts for Case-Based Learning. St. Louis, 1996. Mosby-Year Book.
2-17, 2-21, 2-25, 2-26, 2-27, 2-29, 2-30, 2-31, 2-32, 2-38, 2-39, 2-40, 2-41, 2-48, 2-49, 2-54, 2-56, 2-58, 2-59, 2-63, 2-64, 2-74 Shade: Mosby's EMT-Intermediate Textbook. St. Louis, 1997. Mosby-Year Book.
2-22, McSwain: The Basic EMT: Comprehensive Prehospital Care. 2e. St. Louis, 2001. Mosby.
2-24, 2-51, 2-52, 2-53 Henry and Stapleton: EMT Prehospital Care, 2e. Philadelphia. 1997. WB Saunders.

Chapter 3
3-1, 3-2, 3-3 Shade: Mosby's EMT-Intermediate Textbook. St. Louis, 1997. Mosby-Year Book.
3-4, 3-5, 3-6, 3-7, 3-8, 3-9 Sanders: Mosby's Paramedic Textbook, 2e. St. Louis, 2000. Mosby.
3-10, 3-11, 3-12, 3-13, 3-14 Reprinted with permission fom Johnson & Johnson Medical.

Chapter 4
4-1, 4-2, 4-12, 4-13 Thibodeau: Anatomy & Physiology, 4e. St. Louis, 1999. Mosby.
4-3, 4-4, 4-5 Herlihy: The Human Body in Health and Illness. Philadelphia, 2000. WB Saunders.
4-6, 4-18, 4-31,4-66, 4-69, 4-70, 4-72, 4-73 Crawford: Common Sense Approach to Coronary Care, 6e. St. Louis, 1994. Mosby.
4-7 Guyton and Hall: Textbook of Medical Physiology. 9e. Philadelphia 1996. WB Saunders.
4-8, 4-60, 4-61,4-62, 4-63 Phalen: The 12-Lead ECG in the Acute Myocardial Infarction. St. Louis, 1996. Mosby-Year Book.
4-9, 4-14, 4-17, 4-28 Thelan: Critical Care Nursing, 2e. St. Louis, 1994. Mosby.
4-10 Clochesy: Critical Care Nursing, 2e. Philadelphia. 1996. WB Saunders.
4-11, 4-19, 4-20, 4-21, 4-22, 4-23, 4-24, 4-25, 4-27, 4-29, 4-33, 4-34, 4-35, 4-36, 4-37, 4-38, 4-39, 4-40, 4-41, 4-42, 4-43, 4-45, 4-46, 4-47, 4-48, 4-49, 4-50, 4-51, 4-52, 4-53, 4-54, 4-55, 4-56, 4-57, 4-58, 4-59, 4-64, 4-65, 4-75 Aehlert: ECGs Made Easy, 2e. St. Louis, 2002. Mosby.
4-15 Grauer: A Practical Guide to ECG Interpretation, 2e. St. Louis, 1998. Mosby-Year Book.
4-16, 4-26 Goldberger: Clinical Electrocardiography: A Simplified Approach, 6e. St. Louis. 1999. Mosby.
4-30 Braunwald: (ed) Atlas of Heart Diseases, Arrhythmias: Electrophysiologic Principles, Vol. 9. St. Louis. 1995.
4-32, 4-44 Chou: Electrocardiography in Clinical Practice: Adult and Pediatric, 4e. Philadelphia. 1996. WB Saunders.
4-67, 4-68, 4-71, 4-74 Kinney: Andreoli's Comprehensive Cardiac Care, 8e. St. Louis, 1995. Mosby.

Chapter 5
5-1, 5-14 Cummins: ACLS Scenarios: Core Concepts for Case-Based Learning. St. Louis, 1996. Mosby-Year Book.
5-2, 5-3, 5-8, 5-9, 5-10, 5-11 Shade: Mosby's EMT-Intermediate Textbook. St. Louis, 1997. Mosby-Year Book.
5-4 Sanders: Mosby's Paramedic Textbook, 2e. St. Louis, 2000. Mosby.
5-5, 5-6 Tilkian and Daily: Cardiovascular Procedures, St. Louis. 1986. Mosby-Year Book.
5-7 Well and Tang: CPR Resuscitation of the Arrested Heart. Philadelphia. 1999. WB Saunders.
5-12, 5-13, 5-15, 5-16, 5-17 Henry and Stapleton: EMT Prehospital Care, 2e. Philadelphia. 1997. WB Saunders.
5-18 reprinted with permission from Cardiac Pacemakers, Inc., St. Paul, MN.
5-19 reprinted with permission from Medtronic, Inc. Minneapolis, MN.
5-20 Braunwald (ed) Atlas of Heart Diseases, Arrhythmias: Electrophysiologic Principles, Vol. IX. St. Louis. 1995.

5-21, 5-22, 5-23, 5-24, 5-25, 5-26, 5-27, 5-28 Aehlert: ECGs Made Easy, 2e. St. Louis, 2002. Mosby.
5-29 Guzetta and Dossey: Cardiovascular Nursing: Bodymind Tapestry, St. Louis, 1994. Mosby-Year Book.

Chapter 6
6-1, 6-8, 6-9 Herlihy: The Human Body in Health and Illness. Philadelphia, 2000. WB Saunders.
6-2, 6-10, 6-11, 6-14, 6-16, 6-23 Thelan: Critical Care Nursing, 2e. St. Louis, 1994. Mosby.
6-3 Goldman and Braunwald: Primary Cardiology. Philadelphia, 1998. WB Saunders.
6-4 Falk and Anderson: Pathology of Atherosclerotic Plaque: Stable, Unstable, and Infarctional. In *Interventional cardiovascular medicine: principles and practice*. Roubin, Califf, O'Neill et al (ed). New York: Churchill Livingstone 1994: 57-68.
6-5 Mandel: Cardiac Arrhythmias. Philadelphia: JB Lippincott, 1980: 21, 214.
6-6, 6-13 Friedman and Van den Bovenkamp: The Pathogenesis of a Coronary Thrombus. *Am J Path* 1966, 48:19-44.
6-7, 6-19, 6-24, 6-26, 6-28, 6-30, 6-32 Phalen: The 12-Lead ECG in the Acute Myocardial Infarction. St. Louis, 1996. Mosby-Year Book.
6-12 Grauer: A Practical Guide to ECG Interpretation, 2e. St. Louis, 1998. Mosby-Year Book.
6-15 reprinted with permission from American Health Consultants. Emergency Medical Reports, November 2000.
6-17 Crawford: Common Sense Approach to Coronary Care, 6e. St. Louis, 1994. Mosby.
6-18 Henry and Stapleton: EMT Prehospital Care, 2e. Philadelphia. 1997. WB Saunders.
6-20 Sanders: Mosby's Paramedic Textbook, 2e. St. Louis, 2000. Mosby.
6-21 Clochesy: Critical Care Nursing, 2e. Philadelphia. 1996. WB Saunders.
6-22 Lounsbury: Cardiac Rhythm Disorders, 2e.
6-25 Goldberger: Clinical Electrocardiography: A Simplified Approach, 6e. St. Louis. 1999. Mosby.
6-27, 6-29, 6-31 Kinney: Andreoli's Comprehensive Cardiac Care, 8e. St. Louis, 1995. Mosby.

Chapter 7
7-1, 7-3, 7-4, 7-8 Sanders: Mosby's Paramedic Textbook, 2e. St. Louis, 2000. Mosby.
7-2 Herlihy: The Human Body in Health and Illness. Philadelphia, 2000. WB Saunders.
7-5, 7-7 Thibodeau: Anatomy & Physiology, 4e. St. Louis, 1999. Mosby.
7-6, 7-9 Weiderhold: Electrocardiography: The Monitoring & Diagnostic Leads, 2e. Philadelphia. 1999. WB Saunders.

Chapter 8
(all unnumbered figures in order of appearance)
8-1, 8-2, 8-3, 8-4, 8-5 Henry and Stapleton: EMT Prehospital Care, 2e. Philadelphia. 1997. WB Saunders.
8-6, 8-8, 8-11, 8-12, 8-18 Cummins: ACLS Scenarios: Core Concepts for Case-Based Learning. St. Louis, 1996. Mosby-Year Book.
8-7, 8-10, 8-13 Shade: Mosby's EMT-Intermediate Textbook. St. Louis, 1997. Mosby-Year Book.
8-9, 8-24, 8-32, 8-33, 8-34, 8-35, 8-36, 8-37, 8-38, 8-40, 8-44 Goldberger: Clinical Electrocardiography: A Simplified Approach, 6e. St. Louis. 1999. Mosby.
8-14, 8-15, 8-16, 8-17, 8-22, 8-25, 8-29, 8-31, 8-45 Sanders: Mosby's Paramedic Textbook, 2e. St. Louis, 2000. Mosby.
8-19, 8-20, 8-21, 8-26, 8-42, 8-43 Grauer: A Practical Guide to ECG Interpretation, 2e. St. Louis, 1998. Mosby-Year Book.
8-23, 8-28 Aehlert: ECGs Made Easy, 2e. St. Louis, 2002. Mosby.
8-27 Paul and Hebra: Nurse's Guide to Cardiac Rhythm Interpretation: Implications for Patient Care. Philadelphia, 1998. WB Saunders.
8-30, 8-41 Crawford: Common Sense Approach to Coronary Care, 6e. St. Louis, 1994. Mosby.
8-39 Khan: Rapid ECG Interpretation. Philadelphia, 1997. WB Saunders.

Chapter 9
9-1 Henry and Stapleton: EMT Prehospital Care, 2e. Philadelphia. 1997. WB Saunders.
9-2 Seidel: Mosby's Guide to Physical Examination, 3e. St. Louis, 1995. Mosby.
9-3, 9-4 McCance and Huether: Pathophysiology: The Biologic Basis for Disease in Adults and Children, 3e. St Louis, 1998. Mosby.
9-5 Shade: Mosby's EMT-Intermediate Textbook. St. Louis, 1997. Mosby-Year Book.
9-6 Courtesy of National Institute of Neurological Disorders and Stroke. National Institute of Health.
9-7 Courtesy of Chelsea Kidwell, MD. Department of Neurology. UCLA Medical Center.

Chapter 10
(unnumbered figures in order of appearance)
10-1, 10-2, 10-3, 10-4, 10-5, 10-6, 10-10, 10-11, 10-12 Sanders: Mosby's Paramedic Textbook, 2e. St. Louis, 2000. Mosby.
10-7, 10-8, 10-9 Cummins: ACLS Scenarios: Core Concepts for Case-Based Learning. St. Louis, 1996. Mosby-Year Book.

Posttest
(unnumbered figures in order of appearance)
11-1, 11-2 Aehlert: ECGs Made Easy, 2e. St. Louis, 2002. Mosby.
11-3 Goldberger: Clinical Electrocardiography: A Simplified Approach, 6e. St. Louis. 1999. Mosby.
11-4 Crawford: Common Sense Approach to Coronary Care, 6e. St. Louis, 1994. Mosby.

DEDICATION

To

My father, Bobby R. Mahoney

For your inspiration, guidance, love, and support

My husband, Dean
For your love, patience, and understanding for more than 20 years

and

In loving memory of:

My grandfather, John Dallas Mahoney

and uncles

William Jarrell Mahoney and Donald C. Mahoney

ABOUT THE AUTHOR

Barbara Aehlert, R.N., is the President/CEO of Southwest EMS Education, Inc. in Phoenix, Arizona and EMS Coordinator with the City of Mesa Fire Department. She has been a registered nurse for more than 25 years with clinical experience in medical/surgical and critical care nursing and, for the past 15 years, in prehospital education. As an active instructor Barbara regularly teaches courses related to the care of the adult cardiac patient.

ACKNOWLEDGMENTS

I would like to thank:

- Claire Merrick and her team for their support, advice, encouragement, humor, and the resources necessary to complete this project.
- My family—Dean, Andrea, Sherri, and Tony. Thanks for your words of encouragement, laughter, and attention to all of the "little things" for the months it took to write this book.
- The Southwest EMS Education "team"—James Bratcher, CEP; Lynn Browne-Wagner, RN; Ken Bruck, CEP; Randy Budd, CEP; Thomas Cole, CEP; Bill Loughran, RN; Captain Garret Olson, CEP; Jeff Pennington, CEP; Captain Greg Ruiz, CEP; and Maryalice Witzel, RN. I sincerely appreciate the hours you spent teaching on my behalf while I completed this project. A special thanks to Lynn for her ACLS "pearls" and to Bill and Maryalice for providing words of encouragement when I needed it most.
- Gregg Rich and Tim Eiman of the American Safety and Health Institute (ASHI) and Lou Jordan of emsbooks.com. Thank you for your words of encouragement and advice.
- Those who have attended ACLS courses in which I have taught. Your questions continue to provide me with an endless opportunity to learn and grow.

PUBLISHERS ACKNOWLEDGMENTS

The editors wish to acknowledge and thank the many reviewers of this book, who devoted countless hours to intensive review. Their comments were invaluable in helping develop and fine-tune the manuscript.

Becky Scott Devoss, RN, EMT-P, MSHA
Fairfield Medical Center
Lancaster, OH

Peter H. Goldman, MD
Medical Director
American Safety and Health Institute
Allentown, PA

Karen Jackson, RN, EMT-P
St. Petersburg Junior College, Clearwater Fire Rescue
Clearwater, FL

Sharon S. Kelly, BS
Associates In Emergency Medical Education, Inc.
Tampa, FL

Eric Niegelberg, EMT-P, BBA, MS
EMS Director
State University of New York at Stony Brook
Stony Brook University Hospital
Stony Brook, NY

Keith Wesley, M.D. FACEP
Director of EMS Education
Sacred Heart Hospital
Eau Claire, WI

CONTENTS

Pretest

1. Which of the following describes the proper method for insertion of an oropharyngeal airway in the adult patient?
   a. Gently inserted into the nares and slid along the floor of the nostril into the posterior pharynx
   b. Inserted with the curved side up and rotated 90 degrees when the distal tip reaches the posterior wall of the pharynx
   c. Inserted sideways and rotated 180 degrees when the distal tip reaches the hard palate
   d. Inserted upside down into the mouth and rotated 180 degrees when the distal tip reaches the posterior wall of the pharynx

2. The QT interval represents:
   a. Atrial depolarization
   b. Total atrial activity
   c. Ventricular depolarization
   d. Total ventricular activity

3. Which of the following patient medications is correctly paired with its recommended use?
   a. Procainamide—symptomatic bradycardia
   b. Beta-blockers—pulseless ventricular tachycardia/ventricular fibrillation
   c. Glycoprotein IIb/IIIa inhibitors—chest pain patients with ST-segment depression or T wave changes
   d. Amiodarone—chest pain patients with ST-segment elevation myocardial infarction (MI)

4. How does stimulation of the parasympathetic division of the autonomic nervous system affect the heart?
   a. Heart rate increases
   b. The rate of conduction through the AV node decreases
   c. The rate of discharge of the SA node increases
   d. The force of myocardial contraction increases

5. The recommended dose for atropine administration via an endotracheal tube is:
   a. 0.5 to 1.0 mg
   b. 1 to 1.5 mg/kg
   c. 2 to 3 mg
   d. 0.03 to 0.04 mg/kg

6. Select the INCORRECT statement regarding fibrinolytic therapy in acute coronary syndromes.
   a. Fibrinolytics should be used in conjunction with aspirin therapy
   b. Patients with chest pain and nondiagnostic/normal ECGs are those most likely to benefit from fibrinolytic therapy
   c. Fibrinolytics may lead to significant complications, including intracranial bleeding
   d. When indicated, fibrinolytics should be administered as soon as possible after the onset of symptoms

7. The recommended initial adult dosage of furosemide is:
   a. 0.2 to 0.5 mg/kg IV push
   b. 0.5 to 1.0 mg/kg IV push
   c. 1.0 to 1.5 mg/kg IV push
   d. 5 to 10 mg/kg IV push

8. A junctional escape rhythm occurs as a result of:
   a. Multiple irritable sites firing within the AV junction
   b. Slowing of the rate of the heart's primary pacemaker
   c. Severe chronic obstructive pulmonary disease
   d. Intrathoracic pressure changes associated with the normal respiratory cycle

9. Synchronized cardioversion is indicated in the management of the hemodynamically unstable patient in _____. The energy levels that should be used for this dysrhythmia are _____.
   a. Sinus tachycardia; 50, 100, 200, 300, 360 joules or equivalent biphasic energy
   b. Ventricular fibrillation; 200, 200 to 300, 360 joules or equivalent biphasic energy
   c. Pulseless electrical activity; 100, 200, 300, 360 joules or equivalent biphasic energy
   d. Paroxysmal supraventricular tachycardia; 50, 100, 200, 300, 360 joules or equivalent biphasic energy

10. *True* or *False*. Side effects associated with transcutaneous pacing are most often related to muscle contraction, pain, and patient intolerance of the pacing stimulus.

11. You are caring for a patient with a possible stroke. Which of the following statements is true regarding the use of the Glasgow Coma Scale (GCS)?
    a. The GCS is used to assess the patient's verbal response, motor response, and pupillary reactivity
    b. When assigning a score using the GCS, the maximum possible score is 13
    c. When using the GCS, the minimum possible score is 3
    d. The GCS is used to assess the patient's verbal response, motor response, and capillary refill

12. Which of the following dysrhythmias is most easily confused with multifocal atrial tachycardia?
    a. Atrial flutter
    b. Atrial fibrillation
    c. Sinus tachycardia
    d. Ventricular tachycardia

13. *True* or *False*. Endotracheal intubation eliminates the risk of aspiration.

14. End points of procainamide administration include all of the following EXCEPT:
    a. Suppression of the dysrhythmia
    b. Development of respiratory depression
    c. Maximum of 17 mg/kg is administered
    d. QRS complex widens more than 50% of its original width

15. Which of the following approaches is recommended during an *initial* patient evaluation?
    a. Oxygen, IV, monitor
    b. Level of responsiveness, airway, breathing, circulation, defibrillation if necessary
    c. Temperature, pulse, respirations, blood pressure
    d. Oxygen, IV fluid challenge, vital signs, level of responsiveness

16. *True* or *False*. Vasopressin is the first medication administered in a cardiac arrest caused by pulseless VT/VF, asystole, or pulseless electrical activity.

17. Angiotensin-converting enzyme (ACE) inhibitors:
    a. Increase blood pressure
    b. Increase myocardial workload
    c. May be used in the management of ST-segment elevation MI
    d. Include medications such as metoprolol, atenolol, and propranolol

18. *True* or *False*. The laryngeal mask airway (LMA) protects the lower airway from aspiration.

19. A 62-year-old male is complaining of chest pain. Assessment now reveals the patient's level of responsiveness is rapidly decreasing, BP 50/P, P 188, R 6. The cardiac monitor reveals ventricular tachycardia. Your interventions should include:
    a. Immediate transcutaneous pacing
    b. Synchronized cardioversion with 25 joules
    c. Defibrillation with 100 joules
    d. Defibrillation with 200 joules

20. You are ventilating a patient with a bag-valve-mask. The patient does not have an endotracheal tube in place. Supplemental oxygen has been connected to the bag at 15 L/min. The recommended tidal volume that should be delivered to this patient is:
    a. 2 to 4 mL/kg given over 1 to 2 seconds until the chest rises
    b. 6 to 7 mL/kg given over 1 to 2 seconds until the chest rises
    c. 10 mL/kg delivered over 2 seconds and sufficient to make the chest rise
    d. 12 to 15 mL/kg delivered over 2 seconds and sufficient to make the chest rise

21. The effects of dopamine administration at an infusion rate greater than 20 mcg/kg/min include:
    a. Arterial vasoconstriction only
    b. Venous vasoconstriction only
    c. Both arterial and venous peripheral vasoconstriction
    d. Effects similar to that of nitroglycerin administration

22. ST-segment elevation viewed in leads II, III, and aVF in a patient presenting with an acute coronary syndrome suggests:
    a. Inferior wall myocardial infarction
    b. Anterior wall myocardial infarction
    c. Lateral wall myocardial infarction
    d. Ischemia of the anterior wall

23. Which of the following statements is correct regarding the automated external defibrillator (AED)?
    a. More training is required to operate an AED and maintain skill proficiency than with a conventional defibrillator
    b. An AED may be used for an apneic, pulseless patient
    c. An AED may be used for continuous ECG monitoring if the patient is more than 12 years of age
    d. AEDs currently available are capable of defibrillation, synchronized cardioversion, and pacing

24. Early defibrillation is considered the delivery of a shock within _____ of the time EMS receives the call.
    a. 5 minutes
    b. 10 minutes
    c. 15 minutes
    d. 30 minutes

25. A 75-year-old man is exhibiting signs suggestive of a stroke. The patient is awake, but his speech is garbled. You note he appears malnourished and prepare to check his blood sugar. Which of the following should you consider administering to this patient?
    a. Morphine, 2 to 4 mg IV
    b. Furosemide, 40 mg IV
    c. Naloxone, 0.4 to 2.0 mg IV
    d. Thiamine, 100 mg IV

26. Which of the following statements is *true* regarding polymorphic ventricular tachycardia?
    a. Polymorphic VT consists of QRS complexes that are of similar shape and amplitude
    b. The unstable patient with polymorphic VT should be managed as if the rhythm were ventricular fibrillation
    c. Polymorphic VT associated with a normal QT interval is called torsades de pointes
    d. Polymorphic VT associated with a long QT interval should be treated with procainamide

27. *True* or *False*. A hemorrhagic stroke occurs when a cerebral artery is blocked by a blood clot that develops within the artery itself or a clot that develops in another part of the body and migrates to the brain.

28. A 65-year-old patient has suffered a respiratory arrest. A carotid pulse is present. This patient should be ventilated with a bag-valve-mask at a rate of:
    a. 6 to 7 ventilations/min
    b. 12 ventilations/min
    c. 20 ventilations/min
    d. 24 to 30 ventilations/min

29. *True* or *False*. Sodium bicarbonate forms a precipitate when mixed with calcium chloride or amiodarone.

30. Isoproterenol may be used in the management of:
    a. Ventricular tachycardia with a pulse and narrow QRS supraventricular tachycardia
    b. Atrial fibrillation and asystole
    c. Torsades de pointes and symptomatic bradycardia
    d. Ventricular fibrillation and atrial flutter

31. Atropine:
    a. Is the medication of choice for second-degree AV block, type II
    b. Is the first medication recommended in the management of asystole
    c. Should be used with caution in acute myocardial infarction
    d. Should be administered slowly IV push over 3 to 5 minutes

32. Assuming a patient was symptomatic in each of the following situations, in which of the situations might epinephrine be administered as a continuous IV infusion?
    a. Wide-complex tachycardia of unknown origin
    b. Complete (third-degree) AV block
    c. Atrial fibrillation
    d. Acute pulmonary edema

33. Control of chest pain in the patient experiencing an acute coronary syndrome is important for all of the following reasons EXCEPT:
    a. Relief of pain usually relieves anxiety
    b. Relief of pain may reduce the incidence of dysrhythmias
    c. Relief of pain results in a decrease in myocardial oxygen demand
    d. Relief of pain stimulates the release of catecholamines

34. Select the INCORRECT statement regarding digitalis.
    a. If it is necessary to defibrillate a patient taking digitalis, the lowest possible energy levels should be used
    b. Digitalis has a narrow toxic-to-therapeutic ratio
    c. Digitalis may be used in the management of symptomatic bradycardia
    d. Digitalis may worsen heart block if administered with calcium channel blockers

35. What is meant by the term *pulseless electrical activity (PEA)*?
    a. Refers to a slow rhythm with a wide QRS complex
    b. Refers to a flat line on the cardiac monitor (asystole)
    c. Refers to a chaotic dysrhythmia that is likely to result in cardiac arrest
    d. Refers to an organized rhythm on the cardiac monitor (other than VT), although a pulse is not present

36. An inferior wall myocardial infarction is usually the result of occlusion of the _____ coronary artery.
    a. Right
    b. Left

37. As myocardial cells die, intracellular substances pass through broken cell membranes and leak substances into the bloodstream. The presence of these substances in the blood can subsequently be measured by means of blood tests to verify the presence of an infarction. These substances are called:
    a. Electrolytes
    b. Serum cardiac markers
    c. Resuscitation indicators
    d. Serum-clotting factors

38. The recommended dose of vasopressin in cardiac arrest is:
    a. 1 mEq/kg IV bolus repeated once in 5 minutes
    b. A single IV bolus dose of 40 units
    c. 40 units IV bolus repeated once in 5 minutes at half the initial dose
    d. 2 to 4 mg IV bolus administered in 2 mg increments, titrated to desired response

39. Local complications common to all intravenous techniques include:
    a. Catheter-fragment embolism
    b. Thrombophlebitis
    c. Sepsis
    d. Pulmonary embolism

40. *True* or *False.* The purpose of cricoid pressure is to facilitate visualization of the vocal cords during intubation.

41. Identify the following rhythm strip.

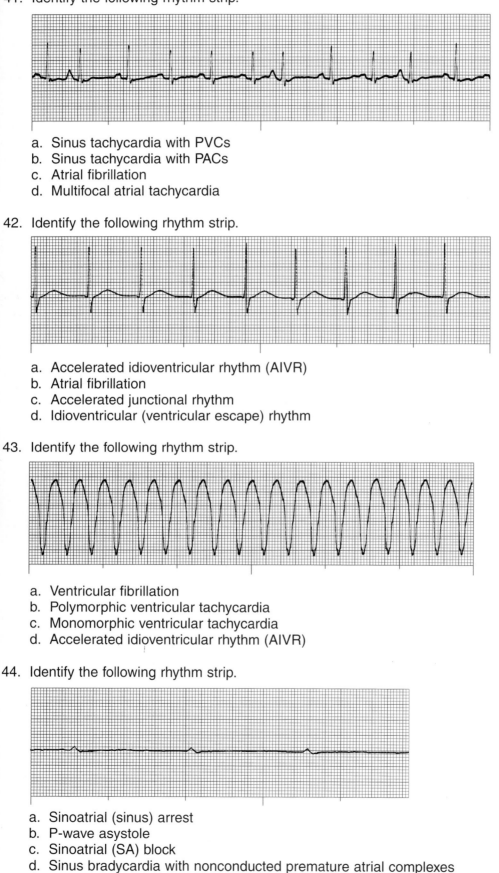

    a. Sinus tachycardia with PVCs
    b. Sinus tachycardia with PACs
    c. Atrial fibrillation
    d. Multifocal atrial tachycardia

42. Identify the following rhythm strip.

    a. Accelerated idioventricular rhythm (AIVR)
    b. Atrial fibrillation
    c. Accelerated junctional rhythm
    d. Idioventricular (ventricular escape) rhythm

43. Identify the following rhythm strip.

    a. Ventricular fibrillation
    b. Polymorphic ventricular tachycardia
    c. Monomorphic ventricular tachycardia
    d. Accelerated idioventricular rhythm (AIVR)

44. Identify the following rhythm strip.

    a. Sinoatrial (sinus) arrest
    b. P-wave asystole
    c. Sinoatrial (SA) block
    d. Sinus bradycardia with nonconducted premature atrial complexes

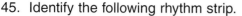

45. Identify the following rhythm strip.

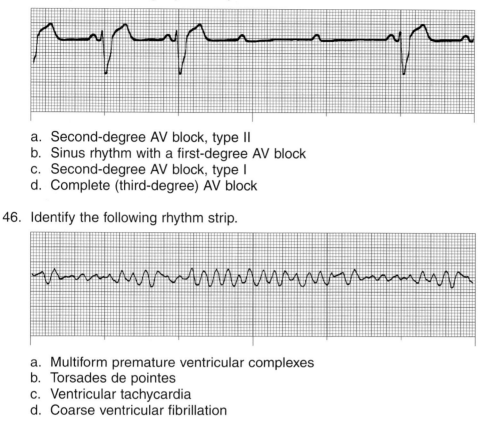

    a. Second-degree AV block, type II
    b. Sinus rhythm with a first-degree AV block
    c. Second-degree AV block, type I
    d. Complete (third-degree) AV block

46. Identify the following rhythm strip.

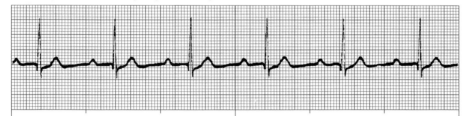

    a. Multiform premature ventricular complexes
    b. Torsades de pointes
    c. Ventricular tachycardia
    d. Coarse ventricular fibrillation

47. Identify the following rhythm strip.

    a. Second-degree AV block, type I
    b. Sinus rhythm with a first-degree AV block
    c. Second-degree AV block, type II
    d. Complete (third-degree) AV block

48. Identify the following rhythm strip.

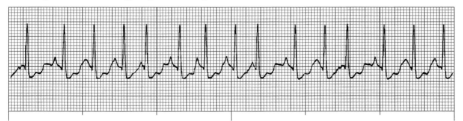

    a. Atrial fibrillation
    b. Multifocal atrial tachycardia
    c. Atrial flutter
    d. Sinus tachycardia

49. Identify the following rhythm strip.

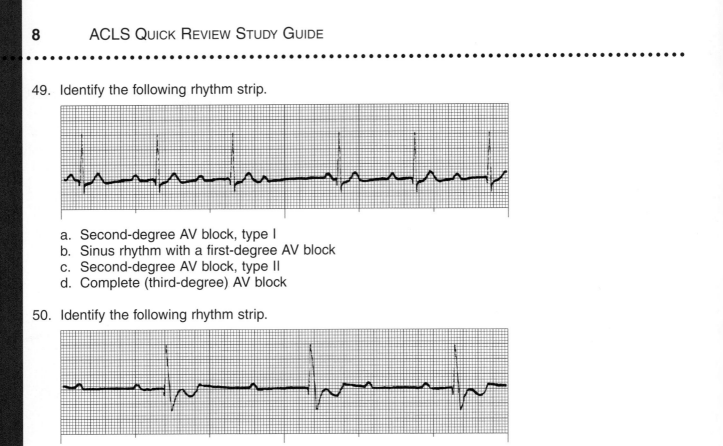

   a. Second-degree AV block, type I
   b. Sinus rhythm with a first-degree AV block
   c. Second-degree AV block, type II
   d. Complete (third-degree) AV block

50. Identify the following rhythm strip.

   a. Second-degree AV block, type I
   b. Sinus rhythm with a first-degree AV block
   c. Second-degree AV block, type II
   d. Complete (third-degree) AV block

PRETEST ANSWERS AND RATIONALES

1. d. The oropharyngeal airway is inserted upside down into the mouth and rotated 180 degrees when the distal tip reaches the posterior wall of the pharynx.

2. d. The QT interval represents total ventricular activity—the time from ventricular depolarization (activation) to repolarization (recovery). The QT interval is measured from the beginning of the QRS complex to the end of the T wave. The duration of the QT interval varies according to age, gender, and particularly heart rate. As the heart rate increases, the QT interval decreases. As the heart rate decreases, the QT interval increases. The patient with a prolonged QT interval is at risk for cardiac dysrhythmias, such as torsades de pointes.

3. c. Glycoprotein IIb/IIIa inhibitors are used in chest pain patients with non-ST-segment elevation (ST-segment depression/T wave changes) MI. Procainamide is used for many dysrhythmias including PSVT (with impaired heart function), stable wide-complex tachycardia of unknown origin, and atrial fibrillation with a rapid ventricular rate in Wolff-Parkinson-White (WPW) syndrome. Beta-blockers may be used in many situations, including suspected MI, unstable angina, and supraventricular dysrhythmias. Amiodarone also has multiple uses, including controlling tachycardias in patients with impaired heart function, junctional tachycardias that fail to respond to adenosine and vagal stimulation, narrow QRS ectopic or multifocal atrial tachycardia, pulseless VT/VF, and stable monomorphic VT with poor cardiac function.

4. b. Parasympathetic stimulation slows the rate of discharge of the SA node, slows conduction through the AV node, decreases the strength of atrial contraction, and can cause a small decrease in the force of ventricular contraction. The net effect of parasympathetic stimulation is slowing of the heart rate. Stimulation of sympathetic nerve fibers results in the release of norepinephrine, a neurotransmitter, which increases the force of ventricular contraction, heart rate, blood pressure, and cardiac output.

5. c. The recommended dose for atropine administration via the endotracheal tube is 2 to 3 mg. The IV dose of atropine, when used in the management of a symptomatic bradycardia, is 0.5 to 1.0 mg. In asystole or bradycardic pulseless electrical activity, the initial dose of atropine is 1.0 mg. Atropine may be repeated every 3 to 5 minutes to a maximum dose of 0.03 to 0.04 mg/kg.

6. b. Patients with ST-segment elevation of 1 or more mm in two anatomically contiguous leads or new or presumably new left bundle branch block strongly suspicious for injury are those most likely to benefit from fibrinolytic therapy if the time from symptom onset is <12 hours. Fibrinolytics should be used in conjunction with aspirin therapy. The earlier the treatment with fibrinolytics in these patients, the more myocardium that can potentially be salvaged. Fibrinolytics may lead to significant complications, including intracranial bleeding.

7. b. The recommended initial adult dosage of furosemide is 0.5 to 1.0 mg/kg IV push.

8. b. A junctional escape beat and/or rhythm may occur when the SA node fails to discharge (e.g., sinus arrest), an impulse from the SA node is generated but blocked as it exits the SA node (e.g., SA block), the rate of discharge of the SA node is slower than that of the AV junction (e.g., sinus bradycardia or the slower phase of a sinus arrhythmia), or an impulse from the SA node is generated and conducted through the atria but is not conducted to the ventricles (e.g., AV block).

9. d. Synchronized cardioversion is indicated in the management of the hemodynamically unstable patient in PSVT. Energy levels that should be used for this dysrhythmia are 50, 100, 200, 300, and 360 joules. Synchronized cardioversion is also indicated in the management of:

   - Unstable atrial flutter: 50, 100, 200, 300, 360 joules or equivalent biphasic energy
   - Unstable atrial fibrillation: 100, 200, 300, 360 joules or equivalent biphasic energy
   - Unstable VT with a pulse: 100, 200, 300, 360 joules or equivalent biphasic energy

10. True.   Side effects associated with transcutaneous pacing are most often related to muscle contraction, pain, and patient intolerance of the pacing stimulus.

11. c. The Glasgow Coma Scale is used to assess a patient's level of responsiveness by evaluating best verbal response, best motor response, and eye opening. The minimum possible score is 3, maximum possible score 15.

12. b. Multifocal atrial tachycardia (MAT) may be confused with atrial fibrillation because both rhythms are irregular; however, P waves (although varying in size, shape, and direction) are clearly visible in MAT.

13. False. Endotracheal intubation *reduces*, but does not eliminate, the risk of aspiration.

14. b. End points of procainamide administration include the development of hypotension, suppression of the dysrhythmia, administration of a maximum dose of 17 mg/kg, widening of the QRS complex by more than 50% of its original width, and the onset of torsades de pointes.

15. b. The initial patient evaluation should consist of evaluation of the patient's level of responsiveness, airway, breathing, circulation, and the need for defibrillation.

16. False. Vasopressin is the first medication administered in a cardiac arrest caused by pulseless VT or VF; however, there is currently insufficient data to recommend its use in cardiac arrest resulting from asystole or pulseless electrical activity.

17. c. Angiotensin-converting enzyme (ACE) inhibitors prevent the conversion of angiotensin I to angiotensin II. As a result, blood vessels relax, reducing the pressure the heart must pump against and decreasing myocardial workload. Use of ACE inhibitors is a Class I intervention in patients within the first 24 hours of a suspected acute MI with ST-segment elevation in two or more anterior precordial leads or with clinical heart failure in the absence of hypotension (SBP <100 mm Hg) or known contraindications to the use of ACE inhibitors. Metoprolol, atenolol, and propranolol are beta-blockers.

18. False. The LMA may be used as an alternative to either an endotracheal tube or a face mask with either spontaneous or positive-pressure ventilation, however, the LMA does **not** provide protection against aspiration.

19. c. This patient's condition warrants immediate attention. The patient in unstable VT with a pulse who is hypotensive, unresponsive, or has pulmonary edema should receive unsynchronized shocks (defibrillation) beginning with 100 joules. If the patient's condition remains unchanged after the first shock, subsequent shocks should be delivered with 200, 300, and 360 joules (or equivalent biphasic energy). Defibrillation is used instead of synchronized shocks in the profoundly unstable patient to avoid possible delays with synchronization.

20. b. When ventilating with a bag-valve-mask, lower tidal volumes are recommended if oxygen *is* available. Deliver a tidal volume of approximately 6 to 7 mL/kg (400 to 600 mL) **over 1 to 2 seconds** until the chest rises (Class IIb). If oxygen *is not* available, tidal volumes and inspiratory times for bag-valve-mask ventilation should be approximately 10 mL/kg (700 to 1000 mL) delivered **over 2 seconds** and sufficient to make the chest rise (Class IIa).

21. c. At doses greater than 20 mcg/kg/min, dopamine causes arterial and venous constriction. Vasoconstriction may compromise the circulation of the limbs and may increase heart rate and oxygen demand to undesirable limits.

22. a. ST-segment elevation suggests myocardial injury. Leads II, III, and aVF view the inferior wall of the left ventricle. Thus ST-segment elevation viewed in leads II, III, and aVF in a patient presenting with an acute coronary syndrome suggests an inferior wall MI.

23. b. Less training is required to operate and maintain skill proficiency with an AED than with a conventional defibrillator. Currently available AEDs are able to defibrillate; however, they do not have synchronized cardioversion or pacing capability. AEDs should be used only on patients who are apneic and pulseless. AEDs are not currently recommended for continuous ECG monitoring.

24. a. The European Resuscitation Council, the American Heart Association, and the International Liaison Committee on Resuscitation have advocated the widespread dissemination of AEDs. The use of AEDs is part of the "early defibrillation" link in the chain of survival. Early defibrillation is the delivery of a shock within 5 minutes of the time EMS receives the call.

25. d. During your initial assessment of this patient, it is important to check his blood sugar to rule out hypoglycemia as a possible cause of his symptoms. If the patient is hypoglycemic, 50% dextrose should be administered IV. Because he appears malnourished, thiamine 100 mg IV should be administered slowly IV push over 5 minutes. Thiamine (vitamin B_1) is required for the production and use of glucose.

26. b. The unstable patient with sustained polymorphic VT should be managed as if the rhythm were ventricular fibrillation. Polymorphic VT consists of QRS complexes of varying shape and amplitude. When associated with a *long* QT interval, the rhythm is called *torsades de pointes*. Because procainamide lengthens the QT interval, use of this medication should be *avoided* in the management of the patient with polymorphic VT associated with a long QT interval (torsades).

27. False. A hemorrhagic stroke occurs because of the rupture of a cerebral artery, with bleeding either onto the surface of the brain (subarachnoid hemorrhage) or into the brain (intracerebral hemorrhage). An *ischemic* stroke occurs when a cerebral artery is blocked by a blood clot that develops within the artery itself (thrombus) or a clot that develops in another part of the body and migrates to the brain (embolus).

28. b. Ventilate the patient once every 5 seconds (12 ventilations/min). Ventilations should be delivered slowly, allowing the bag to refill completely between ventilations. Slow, gentle ventilation helps minimize the risk of gastric inflation.

29. True. Sodium bicarbonate forms a precipitate when mixed with calcium chloride or amiodarone and is incompatible with most medications.

30. c. Isoproterenol may be used as a temporizing measure before pacing for torsades de pointes (Class Indeterminate), for symptomatic bradycardia when atropine and dopamine have failed and transcutaneous/transvenous pacing is not available (Class IIb), for temporary bradycardia management in heart transplant patients (denervated heart unresponsive to atropine), or beta-adrenergic blocker poisoning.

31. c. Atropine increases heart rate and may exacerbate myocardial ischemia; thus it should be used with caution in acute myocardial infarction. It should be used with caution in second-degree AV block type II and third-degree AV block with a new wide QRS (may be ineffective or cause paradoxical slowing). Epinephrine (not atropine) is the first medication recommended in the management of asystole. Do not push atropine slowly or in smaller than recommended doses. Small doses (under 0.5 mg) produce modest paradoxical cardiac slowing that may last 2 minutes.

32. b. Epinephrine may be administered as a continuous IV infusion for symptomatic bradycardia at a rate of 2 to 10 mcg/min.

33. d. Pain causes a release of catecholamines, which increases heart rate and myocardial oxygen demand. Relief of pain is a high priority in the management of the patient experiencing an acute coronary syndrome. Pain relief may decrease the incidence of dysrhythmias, decrease anxiety, and decrease myocardial oxygen demand.

34. c. Digitalis is used to control the ventricular response rate in patients with atrial fibrillation or atrial flutter, to slow the ventricular response in PSVT, and to improve cardiac output in heart failure caused by poor left ventricular contractility. Because digitalis slows the heart rate, it should not be used in the management of a symptomatic bradycardia. If it is necessary to defibrillate a patient taking digitalis, the lowest possible energy levels should be used to avoid ventricular dysrhythmias. Digitalis has a narrow toxic-to-therapeutic ratio and may worsen heart block if administered with calcium channel blockers.

35. d. Pulseless electrical activity refers to an organized rhythm on the cardiac monitor (other than VT) although a pulse is not present.

36. a. An inferior wall myocardial infarction is usually the result of occlusion of the right coronary artery.

37. b. As myocardial cells die, intracellular substances pass through broken cell membranes and leak substances into the bloodstream. The presence of these substances in the blood can subsequently be measured by means of blood tests to verify the presence of an infarction. These substances (called *cardiac markers* or *serum cardiac markers*) include creatine kinase (CK) MB isoforms, troponin, and myoglobin.

38. b. Vasopressin may be used as an alternative pressor to epinephrine in the treatment of adult shock-refractory pulseless VT/VF (Class IIb). The recommended IV/IO dose is a single dose of 40 units. (If no response, epinephrine may be used after 10 to 20 minutes).

39. b. Thrombophlebitis is a local complication of IV therapy, Catheter-fragment embolism, sepsis, and pulmonary embolism are systemic complications.

40. False. Cricoid pressure (Sellick maneuver) compresses and occludes the esophagus between the cricoid cartilage and the fifth and sixth cervical vertebrae, minimizing gastric distention and aspiration during positive-pressure ventilation. Cricoid pressure is *not* intended to facilitate visualization of the vocal cords during intubation.

41. b. Sinus tachycardia with three PACs; from the left, beats 2, 7, and 10 are PACs

42. c. Accelerated junctional rhythm

43. c. Monomorphic ventricular tachycardia

44. b. P-wave asystole

45. a. Second-degree AV block, type II

46. d. Coarse ventricular fibrillation

47. b. Sinus rhythm at 60 beats/min with a first-degree AV block

48. b. Multifocal atrial tachycardia (MAT)

49. a. Second-degree AV block, type I

50. d. Complete AV block with a ventricular escape pacemaker (QRS 0.12–0.14 sec.)

PART I

Preparatory

The ABCDs of Emergency Cardiovascular Care

1

On completion of this chapter, you will be able to:

1. Identify the components of advanced cardiac life support.
2. Identify and describe the components of the sequence of survival.
3. Define *cardiac arrest* and *sudden cardiac death*.
4. Identify the primary mechanisms of cardiac arrest.
5. Describe risk factors for coronary artery disease.
6. Discuss the commonly accepted principles of medical ethics.
7. Explain *advance directives*, *do not resuscitate*, *do not attempt resuscitation*, and *no CPR* orders.
8. Discuss the medical-legal aspects of advanced cardiac life support, including when it is appropriate to begin, withhold, and discontinue resuscitation efforts.
9. List the purpose and components of the Primary ABCD Survey.
10. List the purpose and components of the Secondary ABCD Survey.
11. Describe the role of each member of the resuscitation team.
12. Discuss the *phased response* of code organization.
13. Describe the principles of cardiac arrest management.
14. Identify the current classification of therapeutic interventions.
15. Identify the physical, behavioral, mental, and emotional warning signs of stress
16. Define the terms *critical incident*, *critical incident stress debriefing*, and *defusing*.

WHAT IS EMERGENCY CARDIOVASCULAR CARE (ECC)?[1]

1. ECC includes all responses necessary to deal with sudden and often life-threatening events affecting the cardiovascular, cerebrovascular, and pulmonary systems.
2. ECC specifically includes:
   a. Recognition of early warning signs of heart attack and stroke
   b. Provision of immediate Basic Life Support (BLS) at the scene when needed
   c. Rapid provision of Advanced Cardiac Life Support (ACLS) at the scene as needed
   d. Transfer of the stabilized victim to a hospital where definitive cardiac care can be provided
3. Basic Life Support (BLS)
   a. Assess/Alert/Attend
      (1) **Assess**
         (a) Scene safety

(b) Patient for life-threatening conditions

(c) Nature of the emergency

(2) **Alert** emergency medical services (EMS) for medical assistance if necessary

(3) **Attend** to the patient and provide necessary care until advanced medical help arrives and assumes responsibility for the patient's care

b. Patient positioning

c. Rescue breathing for victims of respiratory arrest

d. Recognition and relief of foreign body airway obstruction (FBAO)

e. Chest compressions and rescue breathing for victims of cardiopulmonary arrest

f. Defibrillation of patients with VF or VT with an automated external defibrillator (AED)

It is important to note the inclusion of AED use in BLS skills.

4. The layperson is the most important link in the ECC system in the community. The success of ECC depends on the layperson's:

a. Understanding of the importance of early activation of the EMS system

b. Willingness and ability to promptly initiate effective CPR

c. Training in, and the safe use of, the AED

Components of Advanced Cardiac Life Support (ACLS)

1. Basic life support

2. Use of advanced equipment and techniques for oxygenation, ventilation, and circulation

3. ECG monitoring, 12-lead ECG interpretation, and dysrhythmia recognition

4. Vascular access (intravenous, intraosseous)

5. Guidelines for the treatment of patients with:

a. Cardiac or respiratory arrest

b. Suspected acute coronary syndromes

6. Rapid assessment and treatment of eligible stroke patients with fibrinolytics

Sequence of Survival (SOS)

1. **Sequence of Survival (SOS)** represents the ideal series of events that should take place immediately following the recognition of injury or the onset of sudden illness. The sequence consists of six crucial steps (Figure 1-1). Following these steps gives the victim the best chance of surviving sudden cardiac arrest

a. Recognition of an emergency

b. Rapid activation of EMS (9-1-1 or another designated emergency number)

c. Citizen providing life-sustaining care—CPR, rescue breathing, and/or first aid

d. AED and supplemental oxygen provided if available and/or necessary

(1) Defibrillation is the step in the sequence of survival most likely to improve the adult cardiac arrest victim's chances of survival. The likelihood of successful resuscitation is affected by the speed with which defibrillation is performed

(2) Defibrillation performed by laypersons at the scene is called *public access defibrillation* (Figure 1-2)

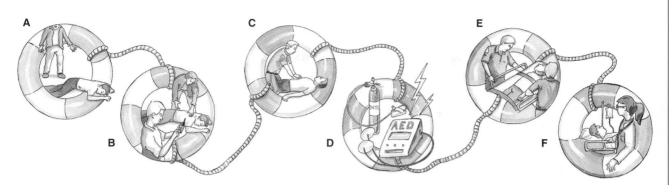

Figure 1-1   Sequence of Survival: **A,** recognition of an emergency; **B,** rapid activation of EMS (9-1-1); **C,** citizen providing life-sustaining care (CPR, rescue breathing, and/or first aid); **D,** AED and supplemental oxygen provided if available and/or necessary; **E,** arrival of EMS and provision of advanced care, and **F,** hospital care.

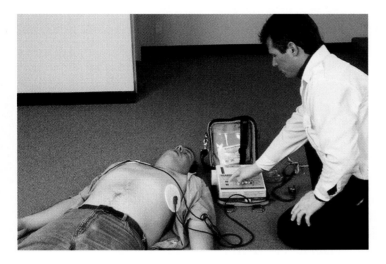

Figure 1-2   Early defibrillation is the step in the sequence of survival most likely to improve the adult cardiac arrest victim's chances of survival. Defibrillation may be performed by laypersons at the scene (public access defibrillation) and/or by emergency personnel that respond to the scene.

    e. Arrival of EMS and provision of advanced care
       (1) Involves providing advanced life support including advanced airway management, ECG/dysrhythmia recognition, vascular access, and administration of medications
    f. Hospital care—Emergency Department (ED) staff assume responsibility for the patient's care on arrival of the patient in the ED
  2. Because time is critical when dealing with a victim of sudden cardiac arrest, a break in any of the links in the chain can reduce the chance of survival

QUICK REVIEW

Can you name the components of the sequence of survival (SOS)?

The steps in the sequence of survival are (1) recognition of an emergency; (2) rapid activation of EMS (9-1-1); (3) citizen providing life-sustaining care (CPR, rescue breathing, and/or first aid); (4) AED and supplemental oxygen provided if available and/or necessary; (5) arrival of EMS and provision of advanced care, and (6) hospital care.

SUDDEN CARDIAC DEATH

1. Definitions
   a. **Cardiac arrest**
      (1) Defined by the Utstein II International Consensus Group as the "cessation of cardiac mechanical activity, confirmed by the absence of a detectable pulse, unresponsiveness, and apnea or agonal, gasping respiration."
      (2) "This definition emphasizes that cardiac arrest is a clinical syndrome that involves the sudden (not precisely defined but usually less than 1 hour from onset of first symptoms until death) loss of detectable pulse, quickly followed by cessation of spontaneous breathing."[2]
   b. **Sudden cardiac death** is an unexpected death of cardiac etiology, occurring either immediately or within 1 hour of onset of symptoms
2. Survival rates from cardiac arrest
   a. The national survival rate from cardiac arrest in the United States is not known but it is estimated that the overall survival rate may be between 3% and 5%, but some cities have survival rates as high as 18%. In many large urban areas, the survival rate has been observed to be less than 2%[3]
3. Causes of cardiac arrest
   a. Cardiac causes
      (1) Coronary artery disease (CAD) most common cause
         (a) CAD is believed to produce cardiac arrest when the transient effects of myocardial ischemia precipitate a lethal dysrhythmia
         (b) On autopsy, most victims of sudden cardiac death have underlying coronary artery disease; yet, only 25% of patients who survive a sudden cardiac arrest will have experienced an acute myocardial infarction (MI)[4]
         (c) Most patients who suffer sudden cardiac death have no warning symptoms immediately before collapse. In up to 25% of patients who experience cardiac arrest, cardiovascular collapse may be the first evidence of CAD
      (2) Other possible cardiac causes of sudden cardiac death include cardiac dysrhythmias, acute MI, valvular heart disease, cardiomyopathy or myocarditis, prolonged QT interval, congenital heart disease, intracardiac tumor, Wolff-Parkinson-White syndrome, and pericardial tamponade

b. Noncardiac causes of cardiac arrest (partial list)
   (1) Pulmonary embolism, choking and asphyxia, drug ingestion (prescribed or nonprescribed), substance abuse, stroke, hypoxia, hypoglycemia, alcoholism, allergic reactions, and electrical shock
4. Primary mechanisms of cardiac arrest
   a. It has been reported that the most common initial dysrhythmias encountered in cases of out-of-hospital sudden cardiac deaths are VT or VF[28] Pulseless electrical activity (PEA) and asystole are encountered in approximately 1/3 of out-of-hospital cardiac arrest victims.
   b. PEA and asystole are being reported with increasing frequency as the presenting rhythm in out-of-hospital sudden cardiac deaths. "This rhythm group now appears to represent the majority of patients in whom out-of-hospital resuscitation is attempted." [29]

A Canadian study evaluated EMS-witnessed cardiac arrest and attempted to determine predictors of survival in this group.[5] This study included all adults with an EMS-witnessed cardiac arrest in the 21 communities of the Ontario Prehospital Advanced Life Support (OPALS) study. The EMS systems provided basic life support with defibrillation (BLS-D) level of care. Over a 5-year period, there were 9072 cardiac arrest cases in the study communities. Of these, 610 (6.7%) were EMS-witnessed. The majority had preexisting cardiac or respiratory disease (81.5%) and experienced prodromal symptoms before the arrival of EMS personnel (91.4%). PEA was the initial rhythm in 50.1% of patients, pulseless VT/VF in 34.2%, and asystole in 15.7%. Survival to discharge was 12.6%. Patients with chest pain were more likely than dyspneic patients to experience pulseless VT/VF (62% vs. 17%), and were five times more likely to survive (30.6% vs. 6.3%). The authors concluded that EMS-witnessed cases are an important subset of out-of-hospital cardiac arrest cases, characterized by two distinct symptom groups: chest pain and dyspnea. These symptoms are important predictors of survival and may help determine underlying mechanisms before patient collapse.

In Italy, researchers reviewed 708 consecutive cardiac arrests in which 438 patients underwent CPR.[6] Of these, 344 arrests of cardiac etiology were identified. Asystole was the initial underlying rhythm in 166 patients (48.3%), VF in 104 (30.2%), and PEA in 74 (21.5%). EMS-witnessed cardiac arrests had the best outcome (49% return of spontaneous circulation [ROSC], 21% hospital discharge). When cardiac arrest was witnessed by lay people, 20.5% had ROSC and 4.4% were discharged alive from the hospital. When the arrest was unwitnessed, ROSC and hospital discharge were 8.6% and 1.7%, respectively. VF was highly predictive of outcome. Both ROSC and hospital discharge correlated inversely with the delay of the first defibrillation. Overall, the highest probability of survival was achieved when CPR interventions were started within the first minutes after collapse. Basic Life Support begun after 9 minutes of untreated cardiac arrest was still followed by a ROSC, but none of these patients survived.

QUICK REVIEW

1. _____ _____ is the cessation of cardiac mechanical activity, confirmed by the absence of a detectable pulse, unresponsiveness, and apnea or agonal, gasping respiration.
2. _____ _____ _____ is an unexpected death of cardiac etiology occurring either immediately or within 1 hour of onset of symptoms.
3. What is the most common cardiac cause of a cardiac arrest?

4. Can you name two dysrhythmias associated with cardiac arrest?

1. Cardiac arrest.   2. Sudden cardiac death.   3. Coronary artery disease.   4. Ventricular tachycardia, ventricular fibrillation, asystole, pulseless electrical activity (PEA).

RISK FACTORS FOR CORONARY ARTERY DISEASE

Nonmodifiable (Fixed) Factors

1. *Heredity:* Family history plays an important part in the development of cardiovascular disease and affects some of the modifiable risk factors.
2. *Gender:* Since 1984, the number of cardiovascular disease deaths for females has exceeded those for males. The 1997 mortality for cardiovascular disease was 502,938 for females compared with 450,172 for males.[7]
3. *Race:* The incidence of cardiac arrest is significantly higher in African-Americans than in Caucasians.
4. *Age:* The incidence of cardiac arrest increases with age.

Modifiable Factors

1. *Alcohol intake*
   a. Moderate alcohol intake (1 to 3 drinks/day on 5 to 6 days/week) has a favorable effect on vascular disease–related mortality and morbidity (particularly ischemic heart disease). This cardioprotective effect is thought to be the result of significant effects on cardiovascular risk factors such as high-density lipoprotein (HDL) concentration and an inhibition of platelet aggregation.[8-10]
   b. Excessive alcohol intake is associated with increased mortality.
2. *Hypertension*
   a. Systolic blood pressure of 160 mm Hg or more or a diastolic blood pressure of 95 mm Hg or more is associated with an increased risk of coronary artery disease
   b. Hypertension is a major risk factor for coronary heart disease and the major risk factor identified in the development of ventricular hypertrophy (which is thought to be an independent cause of dysrhythmias and sudden cardiac death). Control of hypertension dramatically decreases the incidence of stroke

     c. African-Americans and Caucasians in the southeastern United States have a greater prevalence of hypertension and higher death rates from stroke than those from other regions of the country[7]

3. *Lipids and cholesterol*
    a. Lipoproteins consist of lipids, such as cholesterol, and water-soluble proteins. Lipids are not soluble in water-based substances, such as the blood. Because of the presence of lipoproteins, water-insoluble materials can be transported in the bloodstream
      (1) High-density lipoproteins (HDLs)
        (a) Help remove cholesterol from the blood, preventing accumulation of cholesterol in the arterial walls
        (b) Often called "good cholesterol"
        (c) Increasing activity and exercise level and losing weight have been shown to increase the concentration of HDLs in the blood
      (2) Low-density lipoproteins (LDLs)
        (a) Transport cholesterol from the liver to other parts of the body where it can be used
        (b) LDLs carry most of the cholesterol in the blood. If these lipoproteins are not removed from the blood, cholesterol and fat can build up in arteries and contribute to atherosclerosis
        (c) Often called "bad cholesterol"
    b. Increased serum cholesterol and triglyceride levels are associated with an increased risk of coronary artery disease. Studies show that a higher percentage of women than men have a total blood cholesterol of 200 mg/dL or higher, beginning at age 50.

4. *Cigarettes and smoking tobacco*
    a. Most important single cause of preventable death in the United States
    b. Thought to produce sudden cardiac death and cardiovascular disease through catecholamine release

5. *Drug use:* For 1 hour after its use, cocaine has been associated with a large abrupt and transient increase in the risk of a myocardial infarction in patients who are otherwise at relatively low risk.[11]

6. *Stress:* Some studies suggest that individuals with a Type A personality may be at increased risk of sudden cardiac death.[12,13] Evidence exists indicating that psychosocial factors, particularly depression and social support, are independent etiological and prognostic factors for coronary heart disease[14]

Contributing Risk Factors

1. *Inactive lifestyle:* Regular physical activity decreases the risk of coronary artery disease
2. *Obesity:* Obesity is associated with an increased risk for coronary disease and mortality and contributes to other coronary disease risk factors, including high blood pressure, glucose intolerance, low levels of HDL cholesterol, and elevated triglyceride levels[15]
3. *Diabetes:* Hyperglycemia is associated with an increased risk of developing coronary artery disease. Diabetes is associated with other risk factors including obesity, increased cholesterol, and hypertension
    a. The risk of diabetes for Mexican-Americans and non-Hispanic blacks is almost twice that for non-Hispanic whites[7]
    b. Among Native Americans between the ages of 45 and 74, 43.5% of men and 52.4% of women have diabetes[7]

Transient Factors[3]

Proarrhythmia is a new or worsened rhythm disturbance paradoxically precipitated by treatment with antiarrhythmic medications.

1. Although risk factors for cardiac arrest have been identified, the reason an individual suddenly develops a cardiac arrest at a particular moment remains unclear. Cardiac arrest may be caused by some transient abnormality that occurs in a susceptible myocardium, triggering a lethal dysrhythmia

2. Transient factors include ischemia and reperfusion, systemic factors (e.g., hypoxia, hypotension, acidosis, electrolyte abnormalities) that can affect the heart's susceptibility to dysrhythmias and medications that produce proarrhythmic side effects (e.g., quinidine, psychotropic medications, cocaine)

QUICK REVIEW

1. Can you name four nonmodifiable risk factors for coronary artery disease?

2. Can you name four modifiable risk factors?

3. What is meant by the term, proarrhythmia?

1. Heredity, gender, race, age. 2. Modifiable risk factors include alcohol intake, hypertension, lipids and cholesterol, cigarettes and smoking tobacco, drug use, and stress. 3. A proarrhythmia is a new or worsened rhythm disturbance precipitated by treatment with an antiarrhythmic medication.

ETHICAL ASPECTS OF ECC

Medical Ethics

1. Autonomy, beneficence, nonmaleficence, and justice are commonly accepted principles of medical ethics
   a. **Autonomy**—addresses the concept of independence
      (1) Patient autonomy may be thought of as "control over one's destiny" and is the basis for the practice of "informed consent"
      (2) "The principle of autonomy dictates that the patient has the right to choose among offered therapies and the right to refuse any treatment (including CPR) even though this decision may result in the patient's death"[3]
   b. **Beneficence**—doing good to others
      (1) Dictates that medical personnel have an obligation to act in the best interests of their patients. This includes being proactive and preventing harm when possible
      (2) Hippocratic Oath, the physician's pledge to act for the good of the patient, embodies the principle of beneficence
   c. **Nonmaleficence**—ethical principle embodied by the phrase "Above all, do no harm"

(1) Harm is understood in terms of wrongfully injuring a patient, whether deliberately or negligently

(2) Some consider this principle the most critical of all the principles of medical ethics

d. **Justice**—in health care ethics, refers to fairness in the allocation of resources concerning the delivery of health care

(1) Considered when attempting to make decisions about competing interests, or when answering questions about who will receive what share of society's resources

(2) May be viewed as nondiscrimination and fair distribution

2. Clinical situations can cause conflict by pitting one of these principles against another

a. Conflict between the principles of autonomy and beneficence is the cause of most ethical dilemmas involving CPR[3]

b. For example, a situation in which an acutely ill patient with a treatable condition wishes to refuse treatment and be allowed to die may bring conflict between respect for the patient's right to choose among offered therapies (and the right to refuse any treatment), and the health care provider's duty to care for the patient's well-being (beneficence)

Advance Directives

1. In the United States, the patient's consent to the performance of CPR is presumed under the theory of implied consent. The presence of an advance directive is a recognized exception to this presumption

2. An **advance directive** is a written document recording an individual's decisions concerning medical treatment that is to be applied (or not applied) in the event of physical or mental inability to communicate these wishes

Types of Advance Directives

1. **Living will**

a. A type of advance directive in which the patient puts in writing his or her wishes about medical treatment should he or she become terminally ill and incapable of making decisions regarding his or her medical care

b. State law may define when the living will goes into effect and may limit the treatments to which the living will applies

Although a patient may have an advance directive, consent for medical treatment must be obtained from the patient as long as he or she remains able to make decisions regarding his or her healthcare.

2. **Durable power of attorney for health care**

a. A written document that identifies a legal guardian to make health care decisions for a patient when the patient can no longer make such decisions for him or herself

b. May also be called a *health care proxy* or *appointment of a health care agent*

c. The person appointed may be called the patient's *health care agent*, *surrogate*, *attorney-in-fact*, or *proxy*

d. In many states, a durable power of attorney applies to any medical situation in which the patient is unable to make his or her own medical decisions, not just terminal illness

3. **Combination document:** Combines elements of a living will and durable power of attorney for health care decisions into one document

> *All 50 states and the District of Columbia recognize both the living will and the durable power of attorney for health care–type advance directives. However, the laws of each state vary considerably in terminology, the scope of decision-making addressed, restrictions, and the formalities required for making an advance directive.*

Complications Associated with Advance Directives

1. Despite the existence of an advance directive, complications may arise when the health care team or facility is not aware of its existence
   a. It is essential that the patient and those close to him or her ensure that everyone who might need a copy of the directive in fact has a copy
2. Another complication may arise when the patient has not expressed his or her wishes clearly in the advance directive
   a. Use of vague language that requests "no heroic measures" or "no treatment measures that only prolong the process of dying" gives rise to problems with interpreting the patient's wishes
   b. Problems can be avoided if the patient and surrogate have previously discussed the patient's wishes
      (1) Unfortunately, the surrogate is sometimes unaware of what it is the patient would want done in a given situation
3. In the prehospital setting, challenges may arise when a dying patient with an advance directive (or the patient's family) calls 9-1-1
   a. In general, EMS personnel are required to resuscitate and stabilize patients and, when necessary, transport them to an appropriate facility
   b. States have begun to address this situation by developing protocols that allow EMS personnel to refrain from resuscitating terminally ill patients who possess a legal document or other approved identifier (e.g., special bracelet or form) verifying a "do not resuscitate" order (Figure 1-3)
   c. In the absence of such documentation (or other identifier), prehospital personnel will generally begin resuscitation procedures while simultaneously attempting to obtain orders from a physician medical director

> In the Study to Understand Prognoses and Preferences for Outcomes and Risks of Treatments (SUPPORT) project, less than 40% of 9000 seriously ill patients discussed their CPR preferences with their physician, and only 20% had prepared advance directives. In data obtained from the SUPPORT project, almost one quarter of patients hospitalized with severe heart failure expressed a preference not to be resuscitated. A substantial proportion of patients who did not want to be resuscitated changed their minds within 2 months of discharge.
>
> In another study, 90% of hospitalized patients expressed preference for resuscitation if their admission level of function could subsequently be restored.[16]
>
> Of patients more than 55 years of age who had been discharged after a stay in an intensive care unit, 74% expressed certainty that they would undergo another intensive care unit stay to prolong survival for 1 additional month of life.[17]

DO NOT RESUSCITATE (DNR) REQUEST

MISSOURI DEPARTMENT OF HEALTH
BUREAU OF EMERGENCY MEDICAL SERVICES

OUTSIDE THE HOSPITAL DO NOT RESUSCITATE (DNR) REQUEST

DNR # 13132

I, _____, request limited emergency care as herein described.
(name)

I understand DNR means that if my heart stops beating or if I stop breathing, no medical procedure to restart breathing or heart functioning will be instituted.

I understand this decision will <u>not</u> prevent me from obtaining other emergency medical care by outside the hospital care providers and/or medical care directed by a physician prior to my death.

I understand I may revoke this directive at any time.

I give permission for this information to be given to the outside the hospital care providers, doctors, nurses, or other health personnel as necessary to implement this directive.

I hereby agree to the "Do Not Resuscitate" (DNR) order.

Patient/Appropriate Surrogate Signature **(Mandatory)**	Date
▶	
Witness **(Mandatory)**	Date
▶	

REVOCATION PROVISION

I hereby revoke the above declaration.

Signature	Date

I AFFIRM THIS DIRECTIVE IS THE EXPRESSED WISH OF THE PATIENT/PATIENT'S APPROPRIATE SURROGATE, IS MEDICALLY APPROPRIATE, AND IS DOCUMENTED IN THE PATIENT'S PERMANENT MEDICAL RECORD.

In the event of a cardiac or respiratory arrest, no cardiopulmonary resuscitation will be initiated.

Physician's Signature **(Mandatory)**	Date
▶	
Physician - Printed Name	Physician's Telephone Number
Address	Facility or Agency Name

MO 580-1936 (8-94)   EMS-21

THIS DNR REQUEST FORM SHOULD BE KEPT WITH THE PATIENT IN A VISIBLE LOCATION AT ALL TIMES.
THIS FORM WILL NOT BE ACCEPTED IF IT HAS BEEN AMENDED OR ALTERED IN ANY WAY.

DO NOT RESUSCITATE (DNR) REQUEST

Figure 1-3 Example of a do-not-resuscitate order.

Do-Not-Resuscitate Orders

1. The phrases "do not resuscitate" (DNR), "do not attempt resuscitation" (DNAR), and "no CPR" are often used interchangeably
   a. "Do not resuscitate" may be misleading because it implies that resuscitation would be successful if performed
   b. "Do not attempt resuscitation" may more clearly reflect the chances of successful patient resuscitation
2. DNAR orders should not be confused with advance directives, including living wills.
   a. Existence of a living will does not necessarily indicate that a patient wishes CPR or other medical interventions withheld
   b. Although a no-CPR order may exist, other medical interventions may be appropriate (e.g., oxygen administration, parenteral fluid administration, or administration of medications for control of cardiac dysrhythmias, blood pressure, pain, or sedation)
   c. However, a living will may expressly state the patient does not wish any resuscitative measures, including CPR, defibrillation, parenteral medication administration, etc.
   d. To avoid confusion, resuscitation directives should be explicit—for example, "In the event of a cardiac arrest, do not provide chest compressions, mechanical ventilation support, defibrillation, or intravenous medications"

Some patients choose to have a DNAR order included as part of their advance directive.

Studies have demonstrated that the public has unrealistic expectations of the potential for successful recovery following administration of CPR. In a recent study, investigators concluded, "Regardless of the source, the public is not accurately informed about the effectiveness of CPR. This creates a situation in which people may elect CPR for themselves or for family members when survival, not to mention recovery, is unlikely. Without dissemination of realistic statistics regarding survival and recovery following CPR, the public will maintain unrealistic expectations of CPR, and be unable to make well-informed decisions concerning its use."[18]

QUICK REVIEW

1. A written document recording an individual's decisions concerning medical treatment that is to be applied (or not applied) in the event of physical or mental inability to communicate these wishes is called a(n) _____ _____.
2. True or False. A durable power of attorney for health care is a type of advance directive that identifies a legal guardian to make health care decisions for a patient when the patient can no longer make such decisions for himself or herself; also called a "health care proxy" or "appointment of a health care agent."
3. True or False. A do-not-attempt-resuscitation order is the same as a living will.

1. Advance directive. 2. True. 3. False.

Futility

1. The ethical principle of **futility** involves two major factors: length of life and quality of life.
   a. "Despite the evolution of the concept of medical futility that has occurred over the past 10 years in the United States, no clear consensus yet exists among physicians, ethicists, and lawyers about what constitutes medical futility or futile medical treatments. The most well-known and most often cited are the quantitative and qualitative definitions of futility put forth in 1990 by Schneiderman and colleagues, proponents of a patient-centered therapeutic approach meant to benefit the whole of the patient, not merely an organ system or a purely physiologic function"[19]
2. **Quantitatively futile** describes "an action with a desired outcome that is highly improbable and not systematically predictive" and that "if useless in the last one hundred cases . . . can be considered futile"[19]
   a. ". . . resuscitation should be offered to all patients who want it unless there is clear evidence of quantitative futility. Quantitative futility implies that survival is not expected after CPR under given circumstances. Several factors that predict a patient's prognosis after resuscitation have been investigated in well-designed studies from multiple institutions. Patient variables include comorbid diseases and medications. Cardiac arrest variables include witnessed arrest, initial rhythm, and system factors, including time to CPR, defibrillation, and ACLS. No single factor or combination of factors, such as morbidity scores or unwitnessed asystolic arrest, meets the criteria for quantitative futility"[20]
3. **Qualitatively futile** describes any treatment that "preserves permanent unconsciousness or fails to end total dependence on intensive medical care"[21]
   a. This definition implies the possibility of hidden value judgments
   b. "In resuscitation, a qualitative definition of futility must include low chance of survival and low quality of life afterward. Key factors are the underlying disease before cardiac arrest and expected state of health after resuscitation"[20]

> *"A careful balance of the patient's prognosis for both length of life and quality of life will determine whether CPR is appropriate. CPR is inappropriate when survival is not expected or if the patient is expected to survive without the ability to communicate."* [20]

4. The term **physiologic futility** has been proposed as a "value-free" definition
   a. Physiologic futility applies when a treatment cannot achieve its expected effect on physiologic function or, stated more simply, "there is a physiologic basis by which the intervention cannot possibly work."[3] For example, CPR would be physiologically futile in a patient with left ventricular rupture
5. Patients or families may ask physicians to provide inappropriate care
   a. Physicians are not obliged to provide such care when there is scientific and social consensus that such treatment is ineffective. Some examples are CPR for patients with signs of irreversible death such as:
   (1) Rigor mortis

(2) Decapitation

(3) Dependent lividity

(4) Decomposition

b. In addition, health care providers are not obliged to provide CPR if no benefit from CPR and ACLS can be expected.[20]

Recommendations

1. Criteria for not starting CPR
   a. The International Guidelines 2000 for CPR and ECC recommend that all patients in cardiac arrest receive resuscitation unless:
      (1) The patient has a valid DNAR order
      (2) The patient has signs of irreversible death: rigor mortis, decapitation, or dependent lividity
      (3) No physiological benefit can be expected because vital functions have deteriorated despite maximal therapy for such conditions as progressive septic or cardiogenic shock
2. Criteria for terminating resuscitation efforts
   a. Research has shown that "in the absence of mitigating factors, prolonged resuscitative efforts for adults and children are unlikely to be successful and can be discontinued if there is no return of spontaneous circulation at any time during 30 minutes of cumulative ACLS. If return of spontaneous circulation of any duration occurs at any time, however, it may be appropriate to consider extending the resuscitative effort"[20]
   b. Consider factors such as drug overdose and severe prearrest hypothermia (e.g., near-drowning in icy water) when determining whether to extend resuscitation efforts
3. Terminating attempted resuscitation in prehospital systems that lack ACLS providers
   a. The International Guidelines 2000 for CPR and ECC recommend that BLS rescuers who initiate resuscitation efforts should continue until one of the following occurs:
      (1) Restoration of effective, spontaneous circulation and ventilation
      (2) Care is transferred to a more senior level of emergency medical professional who may determine unresponsiveness to resuscitation
      (3) Recognition of reliable criteria indicating irreversible death
      (4) The rescuer is unable to continue resuscitation because of exhaustion, the presence of dangerous environmental hazards, or continuation of resuscitation places other lives in jeopardy
      (5) Presentation of a valid DNAR order to the rescuers

Criteria for *termination* of resuscitation efforts at the scene following unmonitored, out-of-hospital, adult, primary cardiac arrest:

1. Adult cardiopulmonary arrest (not associated with trauma, body temperature aberration, respiratory etiology, or drug overdose)
2. Standard ACLS for 25 minutes
3. No restoration of spontaneous circulation (spontaneous pulse rate of >60 beats/min for at least one 5-minute period)
4. Absence of persistently recurring or refractory ventricular fibrillation/tachycardia or any continued neurological activity (e.g., spontaneous respiration, eye opening, or motor response)

From Bonnin MJ, Pepe P, Kimball KT, Clark PS. Distinct criteria for termination of resuscitation in the out-of-hospital setting, *JAMA*; 270:1457-1462, 1993.

QUICK REVIEW

Complete the following. In general, all patients in cardiac arrest receive resuscitation unless:
- *The patient has a valid DNAR order.*
- *The patient has signs of irreversible death:*

_____

_____

- *No physiological benefit can be expected because vital functions have deteriorated despite maximal therapy for such conditions as progressive septic or cardiogenic shock.*

Rigor mortis, decapitation, dependent lividity (or decomposition)

CLASSIFICATION OF THERAPEUTIC INTERVENTIONS

The International Guidelines 2000 for CPR and ECC recommendations have been classified as follows:
1. Class I: Definitely recommended. Interventions are always acceptable, proven safe, and definitely useful
2. Class IIa: Acceptable and useful. Interventions are acceptable, safe, and useful. Considered intervention of choice by majority of experts
3. Class IIb: Acceptable and useful. Interventions are acceptable, safe, and useful. Considered optional or alternative interventions by majority of experts
4. Indeterminate: Promising, evidence lacking. Describes treatments of promise but limited evidence
5. Class III: May be harmful; no documented benefit. Describes interventions with no evidence of any benefit, or studies suggest or confirm harm

PATIENT ASSESSMENT

Assessment of the patient experiencing a cardiopulmonary emergency or cardiac arrest should be performed using a systematic approach. The *ABCs* have been a part of emergency care for many years and have been used consistently by health care professionals in the assessment of both trauma and medical patients. Similarly, the concept of performing a primary and secondary survey is not new. In ACLS, these memory aids and patient assessment sequences have simply been modified to reflect the essential parameters that must be assessed in a patient experiencing a respiratory arrest, cardiopulmonary arrest, or other cardiopulmonary emergency.

ACLS guidelines include suggestions for assessment and management of "periarrest" conditions
1. The "periarrest" period includes the interval preceding a cardiac arrest (also referred to as the *prearrest period*) and the immediate postresuscitation interval
   a. The periarrest period is considered to be 1 hour before and 1 hour after a cardiac arrest
2. Prompt recognition and proper treatment of critical conditions in the "prearrest" or "periarrest" period may prevent a full cardiac arrest

The term *cardiac arrest* is more commonly used than *cardiopulmonary arrest* when referring to a patient who is apneic and pulseless.

Primary ABCD Survey

1. Begins after the scene has been determined to be safe or has been made safe
2. Purpose is to detect the presence of life-threatening problems that require rapid intervention
3. Usually requires less than 30 seconds to complete but may take longer if intervention is needed at any point
4. The primary survey is performed quickly in the following order:
   a. Level of responsiveness
   b. *A = Airway*
   c. *B = Breathing*
   d. *C = Circulation*
   e. For the patient experiencing a cardiopulmonary emergency, the ABCs have been modified to include a fifth step that is noted as *D*, for defibrillation.
5. Uses the senses of sight, speech, hearing, and smell during the initial patient assessment to provide clues regarding the patient's condition[22]
   a. *Sight:* Flushed or pale skin, ill appearance
   b. *Speech and hearing:* Level of responsiveness, presence or absence of breathing, degree of breathing difficulty, degree of pain
   c. *Smell:* Odors of vomitus, loss of bowel control

> The primary ABCD survey focuses on basic life support (BLS) patient assessment and management.

The Primary ABCD Survey

Airway
Breathing
Circulation
Defibrillation, if necessary

Assess Responsiveness

1. After determining that the scene is safe, quickly determine the patient's level of responsiveness. If trauma to the head or neck is suspected, have someone maintain in-line stabilization of the cervical spine to minimize movement and avoid further injury.
   a. Use the *AVPU* acronym when evaluating level of responsiveness:
      (1) *A = A*lert
      (2) *V* = Responds to *v*erbal stimuli
      (3) *P* = Responds to *p*ainful stimuli
      (4) *U = U*nresponsive
   b. A patient oriented to person, place, time, and event is "alert and oriented times four"
2. If the patient is responsive, ask the patient questions to determine his or her level of responsiveness and the adequacy of his or her airway and breathing
3. If the patient appears unresponsive, questions such as "Are you okay?" or "Can you hear me?" may elicit a response
   a. If there is no response, attempt gentle tactile stimulation (e.g., rubbing the patient's shoulder or sternum, pinching the skin of the patient's earlobe or neck muscles) to elicit a response (Figure 1-4)
   b. Position the unresponsive victim supine on a firm, flat surface to aid assessment and treatment

> "Alert" does not necessarily mean "oriented." "Alert" only means the patient is spontaneously aware of his/her environment.

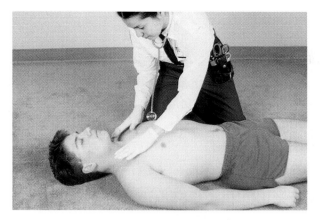

Figure 1-4   Assess responsiveness. If the patient appears unresponsive and does not respond to verbal stimuli, attempt gentle tactile stimulation to elicit a response.

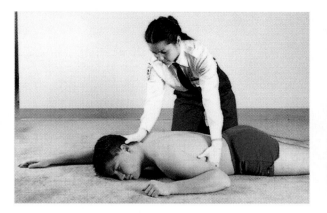

Figure 1-5   If the patient is found lying face down, roll the patient so that the head, shoulders, and torso move simultaneously as a unit without twisting.

   c. If the patient is found lying face down, roll the patient so that the head, shoulders, and torso move simultaneously as a unit **without** twisting (i.e., log-roll) (Figure 1-5)

     (1) Improper movement of the patient with an injury to the spine or spinal cord may cause paralysis

     (2) If the patient is unresponsive, activate EMS (call 9-1-1 or other emergency number), call for a defibrillator, and continue the Primary ABCD Survey

Airway

1. If the patient is responsive and the airway is open (patent), move on to evaluation of the patient's breathing. If the patient is responsive but cannot talk, cry, or cough forcefully, evaluate for possible airway obstruction

2. If the patient is unresponsive:

   a. Use manual airway maneuvers such as a head-tilt chin-lift or jaw thrust without head-tilt to open the airway (see Chapter 2). If trauma is suspected, use the jaw thrust without head-tilt maneuver to open the airway (Figure 1-6)

   b. Assess the patient's airway (Figure 1-7)

     (1) If the airway is open, move on to evaluate the patient's breathing

     (2) If the airway is not open, assess for sounds of airway compromise (snoring, gurgling, stridor)

       (a) Gurgling is an indication for immediate suctioning

     (3) Look in the mouth for blood, broken teeth or loose dentures, gastric contents, and foreign objects

       (a) If present, position the patient to facilitate drainage and suction the mouth

       (b) If solid material is visualized, remove it with a gloved finger covered in gauze

       (c) If a foreign body obstruction is suspected but not visualized, perform abdominal thrusts to clear the obstruction

If dentures are loose or broken, remove them. If they are intact and well fitting, leave them in place to help maintain the contour of the mouth and provide a firm surface when performing mouth-to-mask or bag-valve-mask ventilation.

(4) Insert an airway adjunct (e.g., oropharyngeal or nasopharyngeal airway) as needed to maintain an open airway

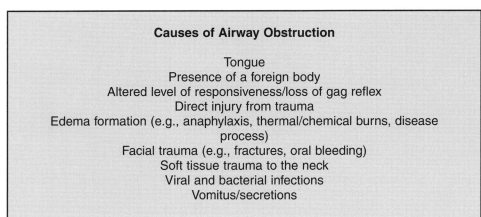

Causes of Airway Obstruction

Tongue
Presence of a foreign body
Altered level of responsiveness/loss of gag reflex
Direct injury from trauma
Edema formation (e.g., anaphylaxis, thermal/chemical burns, disease process)
Facial trauma (e.g., fractures, oral bleeding)
Soft tissue trauma to the neck
Viral and bacterial infections
Vomitus/secretions

Signs and symptoms of a partial airway obstruction with good air exchange:
• Forceful cough
• Can usually speak
• Wheezing may be heard between coughs

Signs and symptoms of a partial airway obstruction with poor air exchange:
• Weak, ineffective cough
• Cyanosis
• Restlessness, anxiety
• Difficult/labored breathing
• Noisy breathing (e.g., stridor, snoring, crowing, gurgling)

Signs and symptoms of a complete airway obstruction:
• No air movement
• Inability to speak, cry, cough, or make any other sound

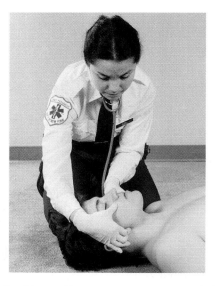

Figure 1-6 Airway. If necessary, use manual airway maneuvers to open the airway. If trauma is suspected, use the jaw-thrust without head-tilt maneuver.

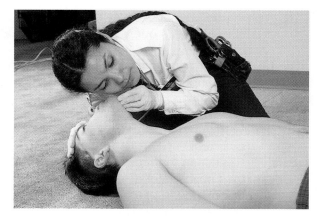

Figure 1-7 Breathing. Look, listen, and feel for breathing.

Breathing

1. An open airway does not ensure adequate ventilation. Adequate oxygenation requires an open airway *and* adequate air exchange
2. If the patient is breathing, determine if breathing is adequate or inadequate (Table 1-1). If breathing is adequate, move on to assessment of circulation

Table 1-1 Signs of Adequate and Inadequate Breathing

	Adequate Breathing	Inadequate Breathing
Rate	12 to 20 breaths/min (adult) at rest	Respiratory rate outside normal range for age and situation
Rhythm	Regular	Irregular
Quality	1. Breath sounds present and equal 2. Chest expansion adequate and equal with each breath 3. No excessive use of accessory muscles during inspiration or expiration	1. Breath sounds diminished or absent 2. Chest expansion unequal or inadequate 3. Increased effort (work) of breathing
Depth (tidal volume)	Adequate	Inadequate/shallow
Skin	Pink, warm, dry	Pale, cyanotic; cool, clammy

Look at the Rise and Fall of the Chest

1. Evaluate depth (tidal volume) and symmetry of movement with each breath
   a. Chest expansion should be:
      (1) Adequate with sufficient tidal volume to make the chest rise
      (2) Equal with no excessive use of accessory muscles during inspiration or expiration
   b. The patient with difficulty breathing often has inadequate or shallow respirations
      (1) Shallow respirations, even in the presence of an increased respiratory rate, may be inadequate to ventilate the patient
   c. The patient with inadequate breathing may require positive-pressure ventilation with 100% oxygen
2. Estimate the respiratory rate
   a. Normal respiratory rate for an adult at rest is 12 to 20 breaths/min
   b. The patient with breathing difficulty often has a respiratory rate outside the normal limits for his or her age
3. Note signs of increased work of breathing (respiratory effort)—nasal flaring, pursed-lip breathing, use of accessory muscles, leaning forward to inhale, and/or retractions
4. Note the rhythm of respirations
   a. Prolonged inspiration suggests upper airway obstruction
   b. Prolonged expiration suggests lower airway obstruction

An increase in the respiratory rate is an early sign of respiratory distress.

Listen for Air Movement

1. Note if respirations are quiet, absent, or noisy (e.g., stridor, wheezing, snoring, crowing, gurgling)

2. Wheezing may be heard throughout the lungs or, in the case of a foreign body obstruction, may be localized

Feel for Air Movement

1. Feel for air movement from the nose or mouth against your chin, face, or palm of your hand
2. If the unresponsive patient is breathing adequately and there are no signs of trauma, place the patient in the recovery position
3. If breathing is difficult and the rate is too slow or too fast, provide supplemental oxygen and, if necessary, positive-pressure ventilation
4. If breathing is absent, deliver two slow breaths and ensure the patient's chest rises with each breath. Insert an airway adjunct (if not previously done) and provide positive-pressure ventilation with a pocket mask or bag-valve-mask. Continue the Primary ABCD Survey

---

During the Primary ABCD survey, evaluation of breathing should take no more than 10 seconds.

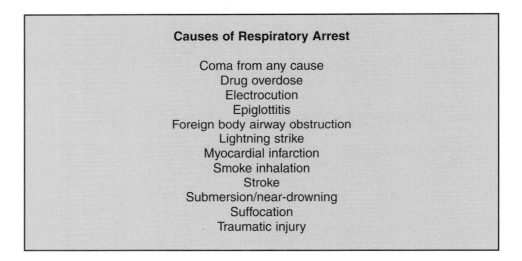

Causes of Respiratory Arrest

Coma from any cause
Drug overdose
Electrocution
Epiglottitis
Foreign body airway obstruction
Lightning strike
Myocardial infarction
Smoke inhalation
Stroke
Submersion/near-drowning
Suffocation
Traumatic injury

Circulation

Other signals of circulation include unresponsiveness, absence of coughing or movement, and blue or ashen skin.

1. Assess for the presence of a pulse and other signals of circulation for up to 10 seconds
   a. If the patient is unresponsive, assess the carotid pulse on the side of the patient's neck nearest you (Figure 1-8)
   b. If the patient is responsive, assess the radial pulse
2. If a pulse is present, quickly estimate the rate and determine the quality of the pulse (e.g., fast/slow, regular/irregular, weak/strong), then perform the Secondary ABCD Survey.
3. If there is no pulse, begin CPR until an AED or monitor/defibrillator is available.

Defibrillation

1. If there is no pulse, attach an AED or conventional monitor/defibrillator when available (Figure 1-9)

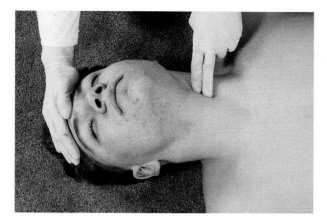

Figure 1-8 Circulation. Assess for the presence of a pulse. If the patient is unresponsive, assess the carotid pulse on the side of the patient's neck nearest you.

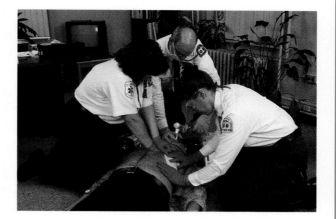

Figure 1-9 Defibrillation. If there is no pulse, attach an AED or conventional monitor/defibrillator when available.

2. If the cardiac rhythm is VF or pulseless VT:
   a. Defibrillate up to 3 times in rapid succession pausing only to analyze/verify rhythm ("serial shocks")
   b. Defibrillate with 200 joules (J), 200 to 300 J, 360 J (or equivalent biphasic energy) as necessary
3. If the cardiac rhythm is *not* VF/VT, perform the Secondary ABCD Survey

The success of defibrillation decreases by approximately 10% for each minute from arrest.[3]

QUICK REVIEW

1. What is the purpose of the primary survey?

2. Can you name the components of the primary survey?

3. During the primary survey, for what length of time should you assess for the presence of a pulse and other signals of circulation?

4. What is the normal respiratory rate for an adult at rest?

5. True or False. An open airway ensures adequate ventilation.

1. Detect the presence of life-threatening problems that require rapid intervention. 2. Airway, Breathing, Circulation, Defibrillation, if necessary. 3. Up to 10 seconds. 4. 12 to 20 breaths/min. 5. False.

Secondary ABCD Survey

1. Secondary ABCD Survey consists of ABCD components similar to that of the Primary ABCD Survey, but the focus of care is on *advanced* life support (ALS) interventions and management
2. Secondary ABCD Survey components are (Advanced) *A*irway, *B*reathing, *C*irculation, and differential *D*iagnosis

Secondary ABCD survey focuses on *advanced* life support (ALS) interventions and management.

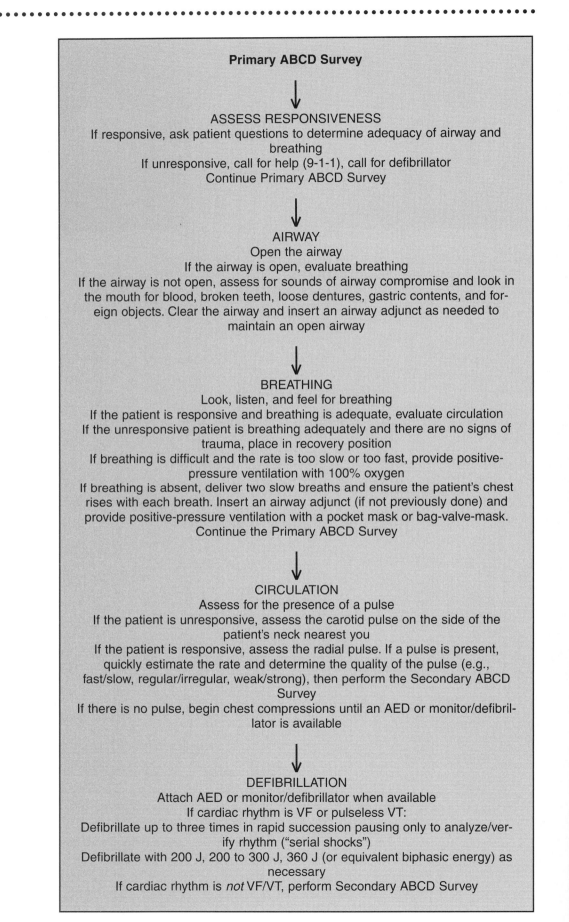

Primary ABCD Survey

↓

ASSESS RESPONSIVENESS
If responsive, ask patient questions to determine adequacy of airway and breathing
If unresponsive, call for help (9-1-1), call for defibrillator
Continue Primary ABCD Survey

↓

AIRWAY
Open the airway
If the airway is open, evaluate breathing
If the airway is not open, assess for sounds of airway compromise and look in the mouth for blood, broken teeth, loose dentures, gastric contents, and foreign objects. Clear the airway and insert an airway adjunct as needed to maintain an open airway

↓

BREATHING
Look, listen, and feel for breathing
If the patient is responsive and breathing is adequate, evaluate circulation
If the unresponsive patient is breathing adequately and there are no signs of trauma, place in recovery position
If breathing is difficult and the rate is too slow or too fast, provide positive-pressure ventilation with 100% oxygen
If breathing is absent, deliver two slow breaths and ensure the patient's chest rises with each breath. Insert an airway adjunct (if not previously done) and provide positive-pressure ventilation with a pocket mask or bag-valve-mask.
Continue the Primary ABCD Survey

↓

CIRCULATION
Assess for the presence of a pulse
If the patient is unresponsive, assess the carotid pulse on the side of the patient's neck nearest you
If the patient is responsive, assess the radial pulse. If a pulse is present, quickly estimate the rate and determine the quality of the pulse (e.g., fast/slow, regular/irregular, weak/strong), then perform the Secondary ABCD Survey
If there is no pulse, begin chest compressions until an AED or monitor/defibrillator is available

↓

DEFIBRILLATION
Attach AED or monitor/defibrillator when available
If cardiac rhythm is VF or pulseless VT:
Defibrillate up to three times in rapid succession pausing only to analyze/verify rhythm ("serial shocks")
Defibrillate with 200 J, 200 to 300 J, 360 J (or equivalent biphasic energy) as necessary
If cardiac rhythm is *not* VF/VT, perform Secondary ABCD Survey

---

Secondary ABCD Survey
(Advanced) Airway
Breathing
Circulation
Differential Diagnosis

(Advanced) Airway

Reassess the effectiveness of initial airway maneuvers and interventions. Perform endotracheal intubation if needed.

Breathing

1. Assess the adequacy of ventilations
2. Confirm endotracheal tube placement (or other airway device) by at least two methods
3. Provide positive-pressure ventilation with 100% oxygen and assess the effectiveness of ventilations

Circulation

1. Establish vascular access with normal saline (NS) or lactated Ringer's (LR) solution
   a. Peripheral IV infusion
   b. Intraosseous infusion
2. Attach ECG electrodes and connect the patient to an ECG monitor to allow continuous recording and reassessment of his or her cardiac rhythm
3. Administer medications appropriate for the cardiac rhythm/clinical situation

Differential Diagnosis

1. Search for, find, and treat reversible causes of the cardiac arrest, rhythm, or clinical situation

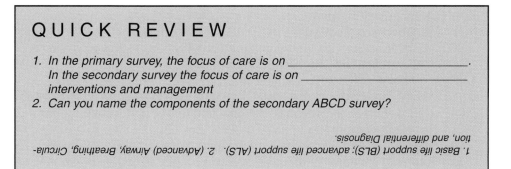

QUICK REVIEW

1. In the primary survey, the focus of care is on _____.
   In the secondary survey the focus of care is on _____
   interventions and management
2. Can you name the components of the secondary ABCD survey?

1. Basic life support (BLS); advanced life support (ALS). 2. (Advanced) Airway, Breathing, Circulation, and differential Diagnosis.

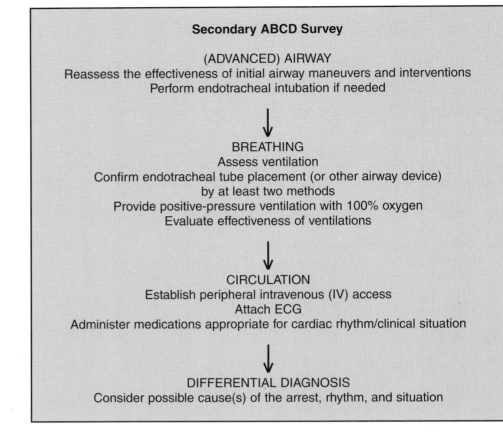

Secondary ABCD Survey

(ADVANCED) AIRWAY
Reassess the effectiveness of initial airway maneuvers and interventions
Perform endotracheal intubation if needed

↓

BREATHING
Assess ventilation
Confirm endotracheal tube placement (or other airway device)
by at least two methods
Provide positive-pressure ventilation with 100% oxygen
Evaluate effectiveness of ventilations

↓

CIRCULATION
Establish peripheral intravenous (IV) access
Attach ECG
Administer medications appropriate for cardiac rhythm/clinical situation

↓

DIFFERENTIAL DIAGNOSIS
Consider possible cause(s) of the arrest, rhythm, and situation

RESUSCITATION TEAM

1. Goals of the resuscitation team
   a. Reestablish spontaneous circulation and respiration
   b. Preserve function in vital organs during resuscitation
      (1) **Cerebral resuscitation** is a term used to emphasize the need to preserve the cerebral viability of the cardiac arrest victim
2. Critical tasks of resuscitation
   a. Airway management
   b. Chest compressions
   c. Monitoring and defibrillation
   d. Vascular access and medication administration (including endotracheal medication administration)
3. Configuration of the resuscitation team:
   a. Ideally, the leader of the resuscitation effort *(team leader)* should be in a position to "stand back" to view and direct resuscitation efforts instead of performing specific tasks. However, the size of a resuscitation team and the skills of each team member vary
   b. Some critical tasks of resuscitation can be performed by personnel with basic life support training, while others require advanced training
4. Team leader responsibilities:
   a. Directs team members and assigns the four critical resuscitation tasks (Figure 1-10)
      (1) Airway management
      (2) Chest compressions
      (3) Monitoring and defibrillation
      (4) Vascular access and medication administration

Applying the Information—Primary and Secondary ABCD Surveys

Time: 6:00 pm. You are a paramedic called to a private residence for a 67-year-old male complaining of chest pain. On arrival, you find the patient sitting in bed.

Patient History (AMPLE)
- *A*llergies: No known allergies
- *M*edications: The patient has taken 1 Advil. He takes an unknown medication for high cholesterol once daily
- *P*ast medical history: High cholesterol
- *L*ast oral intake: Lunch at noon today
- *E*vents prior: The patient states he was shopping earlier today when he experienced chest pain. The pain began in the center of his chest and radiated to both shoulders. On return home, the patient took 1 Advil and the pain subsided. Four hours later, the pain has returned and is radiating to his left hand

Primary Survey
- Level of responsiveness: The patient is awake and talking with you. He is alert and oriented to person, place, time, and event
- Airway: Patent
- Breathing: Respiratory rate 14, equal rise and fall of the chest, good tidal volume
- Circulation: Carotid and radial pulses present, rate approximately 80; strong and regular
- Defibrillation: Not indicated at this time

Secondary Survey
- Advanced airway: Oxygen is administered by nonrebreather mask at 15 L/min
- Breathing: Breath sounds are clear bilaterally
- Circulation: Establish an IV of normal saline, place patient on cardiac monitor
- Differential diagnosis: Obtain vital signs. Ask questions of this patient to determine if he may be experiencing an acute coronary syndrome (Chapter 7) including his age (already known), signs and symptoms including his pain presentation (location of pain, duration, quality, relation to effort, time of symptom onset), history of coronary artery disease, and the presence of coronary artery disease risk factors. Administer medications appropriate for the patient's cardiac rhythm/clinical situation.

Four Critical Tasks of Resuscitation

- *Airway management*
- *Chest compressions*
- *Monitoring and defibrillation*
- *Vascular access and medication administration*

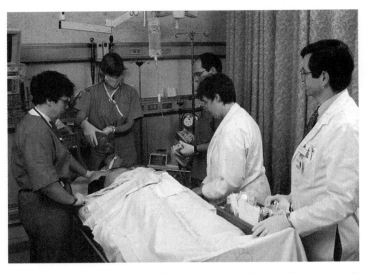

Figure 1-10 The team leader assigns the four critical resuscitation tasks: 1, Airway management; 2, chest compressions; 3, monitoring and defibrillation; and 4, IV access and medication administration.

b. Assesses the patient
c. Orders interventions according to protocols
d. Considers reasons for the cardiac arrest and possible reversible causes
e. Supervises team members, ensuring each member of the team performs his or her tasks safely and correctly
f. Evaluates the adequacy of chest compressions, including hand position, depth of cardiac compressions, proper rate, and ratio of compressions to ventilations
g. Ensures the patient is receiving 100% oxygen
h. Evaluates the adequacy of ventilation by assessing bilateral, symmetrical chest expansion with each ventilation
i. Ensures that defibrillation, when indicated, is performed safely and correctly
j. Calls for assessment of a pulse following defibrillation
k. Ensures the correct choice and placement of IV access
l. Confirms proper endotracheal tube position using at least two methods
m. Ensures medications administered are appropriate for the clinical situation/dysrhythmia and the correct dose, route, and concentration (if applicable)
n. Ensures IV bolus medications are followed with a 20-mL fluid flush
o. Ensures the safety of all members of the resuscitation team, especially when procedures such as defibrillation are performed
p. Problem solves, including reevaluating possible causes of the arrest and recognizing malfunctioning equipment and/or misplaced or displaced tubes or lines
q. Decides when to terminate resuscitation efforts

5. Team member responsibilities:
   a. Airway management team member
      (1) The ACLS team member responsible for airway management should:
         (a) Be able to perform manual airway maneuvers including the jaw-thrust without head-tilt maneuver and head-tilt/chin-lift maneuver
         (b) Be able to correctly size and insert an oropharyngeal airway and nasopharyngeal airway
         (c) Be able to correctly apply and understand the indications, contraindications, advantages, disadvantages, complications, liter flow range, and concentration of delivered oxygen for oxygen delivery devices, including the nasal cannula, simple face mask, pocket mask, nonrebreathing mask, and bag-valve-mask device (Figure 1-11)
         (d) Be able to suction the upper airway by selecting an appropriate suction device, catheter, and technique
         (e) Know how to correctly perform cricoid pressure during endotracheal intubation
         (f) Know the indications, contraindications, advantages, disadvantages, complications, equipment, and technique for (if within his or her scope of practice) endotracheal intubation
         (g) Know how to confirm placement of an endotracheal tube using at least two methods
   b. CPR team member
      (1) The ACLS or BLS team member responsible for CPR must know how to properly perform CPR and provide chest compressions of adequate rate, force, and depth in the correct location

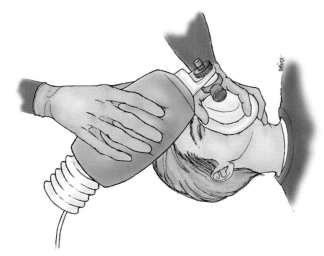

Figure 1-11   The resuscitation team member responsible for airway management has many responsibilities, including proper operation of the bag-valve-mask device.

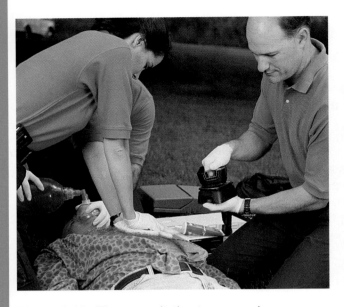

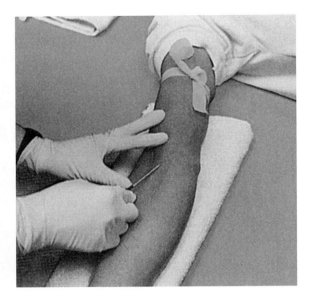

Figure 1-12 The resuscitation team member responsible for chest compressions must know how to properly perform CPR and provide chest compressions of adequate rate, force, and depth in the correct location. The team member responsible for defibrillation has many responsibilities, including safe operation of the defibrillator.

Figure 1-13 The ACLS team member responsible for IV access and medication administration must know the sites of first choice during a resuscitation effort and be able to anticipate the medications that will be ordered during the cardiac arrest.

c. Defibrillation team member
   (1) ACLS team member responsible for defibrillation (Figure 1-12) should know:
      (a) The difference between defibrillation and synchronized cardioversion, the indications for, and potential complications of these electrical interventions
      (b) The proper placement of conventional defibrillator paddles
      (c) How to perform a "quick-look"
      (d) The safety precautions that must be considered when performing electrical interventions
      (e) The primary clinical indications for and possible complications of transcutaneous pacing
      (f) How to problem solve equipment failure
d. Vascular access and medication administration team member
   (1) ACLS team member responsible for vascular access (Figure 1-13) and medication administration should know:
      (a) Site(s) of first choice for vascular access if no IV is in place at the time of cardiac arrest
      (b) IV fluids of first choice in cardiac arrest
      (c) Importance of following each medication administered in a cardiac arrest with a 20-mL IV fluid bolus
      (d) Routes of administration and appropriate dosages for IV, ET, and IO resuscitation medications
e. Support roles in a resuscitation effort include:
   (1) Management of supplies
   (2) Assistance with procedures
   (3) Documentation of the resuscitation effort
   (4) Liaison functions
   (5) Crowd control

QUICK REVIEW

Can you name the four critical tasks of resuscitation?

1. Airway management, chest compressions, monitoring and defibrillation, vascular access and medication administration.

Code Organization - "Phased Response"

1. Phase I: Anticipation
   a. During this phase, rescuers either move to the scene of a possible cardiac arrest or await the arrival of a possible cardiac arrest from outside the hospital
   b. Necessary steps include:
      (1) Analyzing initial data
      (2) Assembling the resuscitation team
      (3) Identifying the team leader
      (4) Assigning critical resuscitation tasks
      (5) Preparing and checking equipment
      (6) Positioning the team leader and resuscitation team members to begin (or continue) resuscitation efforts
2. Phase II: Entry
   a. During the entry phase, the team leader identifies himself or herself and begins to obtain information as the resuscitation effort begins or continues
   b. The team leader:
      (1) Ensures the patient is transferred in a safe and orderly manner from the stretcher/gurney to the resuscitation bed
      (2) Instructs team members to obtain baseline ABCD information and communicate this information to the team leader in the ABCD sequence
      (3) When applicable, the team leader of the previous setting (i.e., paramedic) provides a concise history of the event and interventions performed to the team leader accepting the patient (i.e., emergency department physician)
      (4) Considers baseline laboratory values and other relevant data if necessary
      (5) Evaluates the information at hand and acts on that information

Although not always available, information pertinent to the arrest should be sought, including:
- When and where did the arrest occur?
- Was the arrest witnessed?
- Was CPR performed? If yes, how long was the patient down before CPR was started?
- What was the patient's initial cardiac rhythm? If VF or pulseless VT, when was the first shock delivered?
- Are there any special circumstances to consider (e.g., hypothermia, trauma, drug overdose, do-not-attempt-resuscitation orders, etc.)?
- What interventions have been done?
- What information is available regarding the patient's past medical history?

3. Phase III: Resuscitation
   a. This phase focuses on the ABCDs of resuscitation. The team leader directs the resuscitation team through the various resuscitation protocols
   b. The team LEADER should:
      (1) Be decisive, professional, and speak in a firm, confident tone
      (2) Communicate his or her observations to team members
      (3) Be open to and actively seek suggestions from team members
      (4) Provide periodic observations necessary for cohesiveness of the resuscitation team
   c. Team MEMBERS should provide the following information to the team leader:
      (1) State vital signs every 3 to 5 minutes or with any change in the ABCDs of resuscitation
      (2) State when procedures and medications are completed (e.g., "IV started—left antecubital vein," "1 mg 1:10,000 epinephrine given IV")
      (3) Clarify orders as needed
      (4) Provide primary and secondary ABCD information

Reassess the ABCDs:
- *When interventions do not appear to be working*
- *When vital signs are unstable*
- *Before any procedures*
- *When a change in rhythm is observed on the cardiac monitor*

---

4. Phase IV: Maintenance
   a. In the maintenance phase of the resuscitation effort, a spontaneous pulse has returned or the patient's vital signs have stabilized
   b. Efforts of the resuscitation team should be focused on:
      (1) Anticipating and preventing deterioration of the patient's condition
      (2) Repeated reevaluation of the patient's airway, breathing, and circulation
      (3) Stabilizing vital signs
      (4) Securing tubes and lines
      (5) Troubleshooting any problem areas
      (6) Preparing the patient for transport/transfer
5. Phase V: Family Notification
   a. If family members are not present during the resuscitation effort, they should be told that resuscitation efforts have begun and should be periodically updated
   b. The result of the resuscitation effort, whether successful or unsuccessful, should be relayed to the family promptly with honesty and compassion
   c. Speak slowly in a quiet, calm voice and use simple terms, not medical terminology. Pause every few seconds to ask if they understand what is being said and realize that it may be necessary to repeat the information several times
   d. Enlist the assistance of a social worker or clergy as needed

6. Phase VI: Transfer
   a. The resuscitation team's responsibility to the patient continues until patient care is transferred to a health care team of equal or greater expertise
   b. When transferring care, provide information that is well organized, concise, and complete
7. Phase VII: Critique
   a. Regardless of the outcome of the resuscitation effort or its length, the team leader is responsible for ensuring that the resuscitation effort is critiqued by the team
   b. A critique of the resuscitation provides:
      (1) An opportunity to express grieving
      (2) An opportunity for education ("teachable moment")
      (3) Feedback to hospital and prehospital personnel regarding the efforts of the team

PRINCIPLES OF CARDIAC ARREST MANAGEMENT

1. On recognition of a cardiac arrest:
   a. Place patient on a firm surface (if not already done)
   b. Call for help
   c. Begin CPR with 100% oxygen, airway adjunct, and bag-valve-mask device until arrival of monitor/defibrillator
2. Upon arrival of the resuscitation team, emergency cart, monitor/defibrillator, begin interventions
   a. Identify the team leader who will:
      (1) Assess the patient
      (2) Direct and supervise team members
      (3) Solve problems
      (4) Obtain a history and information leading to arrest situation
   b. Identify the cardiac rhythm
      (1) If leads are not already attached, perform a "quick-look"
      (2) Connect limb leads
   c. If indicated, defibrillate promptly and then resume CPR
   d. Perform endotracheal intubation
      (1) Connect suction equipment
      (2) Intubate patient in less than 30 seconds
      (3) Confirm tube position using at least two methods
      (4) Oxygenate
   e. Establish vascular access
      (1) Intravenous
         (a) Large-bore catheter
         (b) Antecubital or external jugular vein if no IV in place at time of arrest
      (2) Intraosseous
      (3) IV solution: normal saline or lactated Ringer's
   f. Administer medications
      (1) Use correct algorithm
      (2) Follow each medication with a 20-mL fluid flush
3. On-going assessment of response to interventions
   a. Assess pulses with CPR
   b. Assess adequacy of ventilation
   c. Assess pulses after interventions and/or rhythm change
   d. If pulse returns, reassess ABCs

In animal studies, drug circulation times have been shown to be 40% shorter after administration of a 20-mL flush, than those without a saline flush.[2]

e. If a pulse is present, assess blood pressure

f. If no response to interventions, consider termination of efforts

4. Documentation—accurately record the events during the resuscitation effort

5. Draw blood for laboratory tests and treat as needed based on results

---

QUICK REVIEW

A 65-year-old male is in cardiac arrest. CPR is being performed. A "quick-look" reveals the patient's cardiac rhythm is ventricular fibrillation. Four capable ACLS providers are present to assist you. Emergency equipment is immediately available. The patient has received three serial shocks, and there has been no change in his cardiac rhythm. As the team leader of this resuscitation effort, what should you direct your team to do now?

Instruct team members to resume CPR. Instruct the airway management team member to intubate the patient (if trained to do so). Instruct the vascular access/medication team member to establish an IV (assuming no IV is in place) with normal saline or lactated Ringer's solution. Preferred sites are the antecubital or external jugular vein. Reassess the rhythm on the monitor. Continue interventions, including medication administration, using the algorithm appropriate for the dysrhythmia/ clinical situation.

ASSISTING THE FAMILY

Conveying the News of a Death to Concerned Survivors

1. Health care professionals may not receive sufficient training regarding how the death of a loved one should be conveyed to survivors

2. In one survey of family members of patients who had died,[23] the most important features of delivering bad news were determined to be:
   a. Attitude of the news-giver (ranked most important by 72%)
   b. Clarity of the message (70%)
   c. Privacy (65%)
   d. Knowledge/ability to answer questions (57%)

3. In this survey, the attire of the news-giver ranked as least important (3%). Sympathy, time for questions, and location of the conversation were ranked of intermediate importance. Touching was unwanted by 30% of the respondents but encouraged or acceptable in 24%

General Guidelines for Communicating with the Family

1. Call the family if they have not been notified. Explain that their loved one has been admitted to the hospital and that the situation is serious
   a. In most cases, survivors should not be told of the death over the telephone. However, circumstances may exist (e.g., travel distance) necessitating telephone notification

2. Obtain as much information as possible about the patient, the circumstances surrounding the death, and the events of the resuscitation effort
   a. Before meeting with the family, know in advance what happens next and who will sign the death certificate
   b. Consider tissue donation and the need for an autopsy
3. If not already present, enlist the assistance of a social worker or the clergy
   a. Find a quiet, private setting in which to talk with the family member(s)
   b. News of a sudden death should not be delivered in a hallway or with strangers listening
4. Introduce yourself as you assume a sitting position to speak with the family
   a. This position reflects that you are taking the time to have a conversation and allows you to speak at eye level
   b. Be aware of your nonverbal communication
5. Speak slowly in a quiet, calm voice
   a. Pause every few seconds and ask the family if they understand what is being said
   b. Generally, you should make eye contact with the family members—except where cultural differences may exist
6. Preface the bad news by saying, "This is hard to tell you, but . . ."
   a. Then, using simple terms (not medical jargon), briefly describe the circumstances leading to the death and the events that occurred during the resuscitation.
   b. Use the words "death," "dying," or "dead" instead of euphemisms such as "passed on," or "no longer with us."
7. Allow time for the shock to be absorbed and as much time as necessary for questions and discussion
   a. Assume nothing as to how the news is going to be received. The family's reaction to the disclosure of bad news may be anger, shock, sorrow, incomprehension, or even inappropriate
   b. An empathic response such as, "You have my (our) sincere sympathy" may be used to convey your feelings. However, there are times when silence is appropriate. Silence respects the family's feelings and allows them to regain composure at their own pace
8. Allow the family the opportunity to see their relative. If equipment is still connected to the patient, prepare the family for what they will see
9. Offer to contact the patient's attending or family physician and to be available if there are further questions. Arrange for follow-up and continued support during the grieving period

Family Presence During Invasive Procedures and Resuscitation

1. **Witnessed resuscitation** is a phrase used to describe the process of active "medical" resuscitation in the presence of family members
   a. Although acceptance of witnessed resuscitation programs is not universal among all groups of health care professionals and concerns exist about the ethics of witnessed resuscitation and its medical-legal implications,[24] some institutions have allowed family members to be present in these situations with positive results
2. Surveys have revealed that most relatives of patients requiring CPR would like to be offered the possibility of being in the resuscitation

room.[25,26] In follow-up surveys with family members that had witnessed a resuscitation effort, most felt their adjustment to the death or grieving was facilitated by their witnessing the resuscitation and that their presence was beneficial to the dying family member[27]

> *The Emergency Nurses Association (ENA) has resolved that family presence during invasive procedures and resuscitation is the right of the patient and is beneficial for both patients and family members.*

HELPING THE CAREGIVERS

Although a health care provider may regularly deal with stress, a critical incident is an event or circumstance that overwhelms the health care provider's usual coping skills.

1. Stress accompanies a career in health care. Although each health care professional may deal with stress differently, some situations will cause almost all health care workers to feel stress
2. **Critical incident:** Situation that causes a health care provider to experience unusually strong emotions and may interfere with the provider's ability to function immediately or in the future
   a. Because stressful situations may lead to stress long after the incident, it is important to recognize the warning signs of stress in yourself and others and know how to deal with it

Warning Signs of Stress

1. Physical signs: Chest pain/tightness, palpitations; exhaustion, fatigue; difficult/rapid breathing; nausea, vomiting; dry mouth; tremors of the lips or hands; profuse sweating, flushed skin; sleep disturbances; aching muscles and joints; headaches
2. Behavioral signs: Crying spells, hyperactivity or underactivity, withdrawal/desire to be isolated from others, changes in eating habits, increased substance use or abuse (e.g., smoking, alcohol consumption, medications, illegal substances), excessive humor or silence, violence
3. Mental (cognitive) signs of stress: Inability to make decisions; disorientation, decreased level of awareness; memory problems, inability to concentrate; lowered attention span; disruption in logical thinking
4. Emotional signs of stress: Panic reactions, denial, fear, guilt, anger; feelings of hopelessness, abandonment, numbness; general loss of control; depression

Critical Incident Stress Management

CISD sessions are non-threatening and confidential.

1. **Critical incident stress debriefing (CISD):** Group meeting led by a mental health professional (or other properly trained individuals) and peer support personnel to allow caregivers to share thoughts, emotions, and other reactions to a critical event
   a. Goals of CISD:
      (1) Reduce the impact of a critical event
      (2) Accelerate the normal recovery process after experiencing a critical incident
      (3) Help prevent development of post-traumatic stress disorder
   b. CISD provides an opportunity for:
      (1) Emergency workers to share feelings and emotions

(2) Receive stress reduction education, information regarding coping techniques, and emotional reassurance
   c. Ideally, a session should be held within 24 to 72 hours of a critical incident
2. **Defusing:** Shorter, less structured version of a debriefing for caregivers held shortly after a critical event
   a. Goal of a defusing session—stabilize emergency workers so they can return to work or, if they are at the end of their shift, return home without unusual stress
   b. Defusing:
      (1) Concentrates on the most seriously affected workers
      (2) Is usually held within 1 to 4 hours of a critical event
      (3) Session lasts about 30 to 45 minutes and is often led by peer counselors but may be led by a mental health professional
      (4) May eliminate the need for a formal debriefing
   c. The critique phase of a cardiac arrest may provide an opportunity for defusing. If such an opportunity exists, consider these guidelines:
      (1) Hold the defusing session as soon as possible after the event
      (2) If possible, all members of the resuscitation team should be present
      (3) Review the events of the resuscitation effort, including:
         (a) Relevant patient history and events preceding the arrest
         (b) Decisions made during the arrest and any variations from usual protocols
      (4) Discuss the elements of the resuscitation that went well, those areas that could be improved, and recommendations for future resuscitation efforts
      (5) Team members should be encouraged to discuss their feelings, reactions, and thoughts regarding the resuscitation effort
      (6) Team members unable to attend the defusing should be notified of the process followed, the discussion that occurred, and recommendations made.

Talking about the event often helps put things in perspective.

Warning Signs of Stress

Anxiety
Loss of appetite
Irritability with coworkers, friends, family
Inability to concentrate
Difficulty sleeping or nightmares
Guilt
Depression
Indecisiveness
Misuse of alcohol or drugs
Loss of interest in sexual activity
Loss of interest in work
Physical symptoms

STOP AND REVIEW

1. Which of the following memory aids may be used when evaluating a patient's level of responsiveness?
   a. ABCD
   b. AVPU
   c. OPQRST
   d. ALONE

2. The "D" in the Primary ABCD Survey stands for:
   a. Disability
   b. Decision
   c. Defibrillation
   d. Differential Diagnosis

3. *True* or *False*. The "periarrest" period includes the interval preceding a cardiac arrest and the immediate postresuscitation interval.

4. Establishing peripheral intravenous access is part of:
   a. "A" in the Primary ABCD Survey
   b. "B" in the Secondary ABCD Survey
   c. "C" in the Secondary ABCD Survey
   d. "D" in the Primary ABCD Survey

5. When an IV line is established during CPR:
   a. 5% dextrose in water is the preferred solution for use during cardiac arrest
   b. It is preferable to administer some medications by intracardiac injection rather than IV
   c. IV medications administered by bolus injection should be followed with a 20-mL flush of IV fluid
   d. Attempts should be focused on accessing the central venous circulation rather than peripheral veins

6. *True* or *False*. During a resuscitation effort, team members should frequently reassess the patient and keep the team leader informed of any changes in the patient's vital signs or ABCs.

7. List the four critical tasks performed in a resuscitation effort.

   1. _____

   2. _____

   3. _____

   4. _____

8. Which of the following is a non-modifiable risk factor?
   a. Obesity
   b. Heredity
   c. Lack of exercise
   d. Cigarette smoking

9. A therapeutic intervention that is "of no documented benefit; may be harmful" is categorized as:
   a. Class I
   b. Class IIa
   c. Class IIb
   d. Class III

10. Which of the following is NOT one of the steps in the sequence of survival (SOS)?
    a. Rapid activation of EMS
    b. Early warning
    c. Provision of advanced care
    d. Hospital care

11. Cerebral resuscitation is a term:
    a. Synonymous with acute ischemic stroke
    b. Used to emphasize the need to preserve the cerebral viability of the cardiac arrest victim
    c. Refers to gradual circulatory failure and collapse of circulation before loss of pulse
    d. Refers to an abrupt loss of consciousness and pulse without prior circulatory collapse

12. Which step in the sequence of survival is most likely to improve the adult cardiac arrest victim's chances of survival?

    _____

13. Sudden cardiac death is an unexpected death of cardiac etiology occurring _____ of onset of symptoms.
    a. Immediately or within 1 hour
    b. Within 2 hours
    c. Within 12 hours
    d. Within 24 hours

14. Which of the following dysrhythmias are most commonly associated with sudden cardiac death?
    a. Asystole, bradycardia
    b. Supraventricular tachycardia, ventricular tachycardia
    c. Pulseless electrical activity, asystole
    d. Ventricular fibrillation, ventricular tachycardia

15. A 78-year-old male is in cardiac arrest. CPR is in progress and an IV line has not yet been established. The preferred sites for IV cannulation while chest compressions are being performed are the:
    a. Antecubital or external jugular vein
    b. Subclavian or antecubital vein
    c. Internal or external jugular vein
    d. Femoral or internal jugular vein

STOP AND REVIEW ANSWERS

1. b. The AVPU acronym is used to quickly assess a patient's level of responsiveness. AVPU—Alert, responds to verbal stimuli, responds to painful stimuli, unresponsive. ABCD are components of the primary and secondary surveys. OPQRST is an acronym used when evaluating a patient's complaint of pain. ALONE is an acronym used to recall medications that may be administered via an endotracheal tube (atropine, lidocaine, oxygen, naloxone, epinephrine).

2. c. The "D" in the Primary ABCD Survey stands for defibrillation. If the Primary ABCD Survey reveals the patient has no pulse, an automated external defibrillator (AED) should be attached to the patient (or a monitor/defibrillator) when available.

3. True. The "periarrest" period includes the interval preceding a cardiac arrest (also referred to as the *prearrest period*) and the immediate postresuscitation interval.

4. c. The Primary ABCD Survey focuses on basic life support assessment and intervention. The Secondary ABCD Survey focuses on advanced life support assessment and interventions. Thus establishing peripheral intravenous access is part of "C" (Circulation) in the Secondary ABCD Survey.

5. c. IV medications administered by bolus injection in a cardiac arrest should be followed with a 20-mL flush of IV fluid.

6. True. During a resuscitation effort, team members should frequently reassess the patient and inform the team leader of any changes in the patient's vital signs or ABCs. Patient reassessment and communication with the team leader should occur at least every 3 to 5 minutes through the resuscitation effort.

7. The four critical tasks performed in a resuscitation effort are:
   - Airway management
   - Chest compressions
   - Monitoring and defibrillation
   - IV access and medication administration

8. b. Heredity is a nonmodifiable risk factor (as are age, gender, and race).

9. d. A Class III therapeutic intervention is one that is "of no documented benefit; may be harmful."

10. b. The steps in the sequence of survival are (1) recognition of an emergency, (2) rapid activation of EMS (9-1-1), (3) citizen providing life-sustaining care (CPR, rescue breathing, and/or first aid), (4) AED and supplemental oxygen provided if available and/or necessary, (5) arrival of EMS and provision of advanced care, and (6) hospital care.

11. b. *Cerebral resuscitation* is a term used to emphasize the need to preserve the cerebral viability of the cardiac arrest victim.

12. *Defibrillation* is the step in the sequence of survival most likely to improve the adult cardiac arrest victim's chances of survival.

13. a. Sudden cardiac death is an unexpected death of cardiac etiology occurring *immediately or within 1 hour* of onset of symptoms.

14. d. In the adult patient, the dysrhythmias most commonly associated with sudden cardiac death are ventricular tachycardia and ventricular fibrillation. Pulseless ventricular tachycardia quickly deteriorates to ventricular fibrillation.

15. a. If no IV line exists at the time of arrest, the antecubital or external jugular vein should be cannulated first because CPR often has to be interrupted to establish central venous access.

REFERENCES

1. The American Heart Association in Collaboration with the International Liaison Committee on Resuscitation (ILCOR): Introduction to the International Guidelines 2000 for CPR and ECC: a consensus on science, Part I, *Circulation* 102(suppl I):1-3, 2000.
2. Paradis NA, Halperin HR, Nowak RM, editors: *Cardiac arrest: the science and practice of resuscitation medicine*, Baltimore, 1996, Williams & Wilkins.
3. Weil MH, Tang W, editors: *CPR: resuscitation of the arrested heart*, Philadelphia, 1999, WB Saunders.
4. Gibler WB, Aufderheide TP: *Emergency cardiac care*, St Louis, 1994, Mosby.
5. De Maio VJ, Stiell IG, Wells GA, Spaite DW. Cardiac arrest witnessed by emergency medical services personnel: descriptive epidemiology, prodromal symptoms, and predictors of survival. OPALS study group, *Ann Emerg Med* 35(2):138-146, 2000.
6. Kette F, Sbrojavacca R, Rellini G, Tosolini G, Capasso M, Arcidiacono D, Bernardi G, Frittitta P. Epidemiology and survival rate of out-of-hospital cardiac arrest in north-east Italy: The FACS study, Friuli Venezia Giulia Cardiac Arrest Cooperative Study, *Resuscitation*; 36(3):153-159, 1998.
7. American Heart Association: *2000 heart and stroke statistical update*, Dallas, Texas, 1999, American Heart Association.
8. Papadakis JA, Ganotakis ES, Mikhailidis DP: Beneficial effect of moderate alcohol consumption on vascular disease: myth or reality? *J R Soc Health* 120(1):11-15, 2000.
9. Gronbaek M, Becker U, Johansen D, Gottschau A, Schnohr P, Hein HO, Jensen G, Sorensen TI: Type of alcohol consumed and mortality from all causes, coronary heart disease, and cancer, *Ann Intern Med* 133(6):411-419, 2000.
10. Klatsky AL: Moderate drinking and reduced risk of heart disease, *Alcohol Res Health* 23(1):15-23, 1999.
11. Mittleman MA, Mintzer D, Maclure M, Tofler GH, Sherwood JB, Muller JE: Triggering of myocardial infarction by cocaine. *Circulation* 99(21):2737-2741, 1999.
12. Coelho R, Ramos E, Prata J, Maciel MJ, Barros H: Acute myocardial infarction: psychosocial and cardiovascular risk factors in men, *J Cardiovasc Risk* 6(3):157-162, 1999.
13. Barrick CB: Sad, glad, or mad hearts? Epidemiological evidence for a causal relationship between mood disorders and coronary artery disease, *J Affect Disord* 53(2):193-201, 1999.
14. Hemingway H, Marmot M: Evidence-based cardiology: psychosocial factors in the aetiology and prognosis of coronary heart disease. Systematic review of prospective cohort studies, *BMJ* 318(7196):1460-1467, 1999.
15. Gibbons RJ, Chatterjee K, Daley J, et al: ACC/AHA/ACP–ASIM guidelines for the management of patients with chronic stable angina: executive summary and recommendations: a report of the American College of Cardiology/American Heart Association Task Force on Practice Guidelines (Committee on Management of Patients With Chronic Stable Angina), *Circulation* 99:2829-2848, 1999.
16. Frankl D, Oye RK, Bellamy PE: Attitudes of hospitalized patients toward life support: a survey of 200 medical inpatients, *Am J Med* 86:645-648, 1989.
17. Danis M, Patrick DL, Southerland LI, Green ML: Patients' and families' preferences for medical intensive care, *JAMA* 260:797-802, 1988.
18. Jones GK, Brewer KL, Garrison HG: Public expectations of survival following cardiopulmonary resuscitation, *Acad Emerg Med* 7(1):48-53, 2000.
19. Kettler PA: Medical futility: The need for precise definition and standardization of care practices, *Med J Allina*, Vol 7/No 2/Spring 1998, http://www.allina.com/Allina_Journal/Spring1998/ kettler.html.
20. The American Heart Association in Collaboration with the International Liaison Committee on Resuscitation (ILCOR): Ethical Aspects of CPR and ECC, Part II *Circulation* 102(suppl I):1-14, 2000.
21. Schneiderman LJ, Jecker NS, Jonsen AR. Medical futility: its meaning and ethical implications, *Ann Intern Med* 112(12):949-954, 1990.
22. Polsky SS, Fontanarosa P, Pons P, Cason D, editors: *In paramedic field care: a complaint-based approach*, 1997, American College of Surgeons.

23. Jurkovich GJ, Pierce B, Pananen L, Rivara FP, Krizek TJ. Giving bad news: the family perspective, *J Trauma* 48(5):865-870, 2000.
24. Boyd R: Witnessed resuscitation by relatives, *Resuscitation* 43(3):171-176, 2000.
25. Barratt F, Wallis DN: Relatives in the resuscitation room: their point of view [see comments], *J Accid Emerg Med* 15:109-111, 1998.
26. Meyers TA, Eichhorn DJ, Guzzetta CE. Do families want to be present during CPR? A retrospective survey, *J Emerg Nurs* 24:400-405, 1998.
27. Doyle CJ, Post H, Burney RE, Maino J, Keefe M, Rhee KJ. Family participation during resuscitation: an option, *Ann Emerg Med* 16:673-675, 1987.

BIBLIOGRAPHY

American Heart Association: *2000 heart and stroke statistical update*, Dallas, Texas, 1999, American Heart Association.

Beauchamp TL, Childress JF: *Principles of biomedical ethics*, ed 4, New York, 1994, Oxford University Press.

Buckman R, with contributions by Kason: *How to break bad news: a guide for health care professionals*, Baltimore, 1992, Johns Hopkins University Press.

Clochesy JM, Breu C, Cardin S, Whittaker AA, Rudy EB: *Critical care nursing*, ed 2, Philadelphia, 1996, WB Saunders.

Gibler WB, Aufderheide TP: *Emergency cardiac care*, St Louis, 1994, Mosby.

Mitchell J, Bray G: *Emergency services stress: guidelines for preserving the health and careers of emergency services personnel*, Englewood Cliffs, NJ, 1990, Prentice-Hall.

Paradis NA, Halperin HR, Nowak RM, editors: *Cardiac arrest: the science and practice of resuscitation medicine*, Baltimore, 1996, Williams & Wilkins.

Tamparo CT, Lindh WQ: *Therapeutic communications for health professionals*, ed 2, Canada, 2000, Delmar Thompson Learning.

The American Heart Association in Collaboration with the International Liaison Committee on Resuscitation (ILCOR): *International guidelines 2000 for CPR and ECC, Circulation*: 102 (suppl I): 1-3, 2000.

Weil MH, Tang W, editors: *CPR: resuscitation of the arrested heart*, Philadelphia, 1999, WB Saunders.

Airway Management: Oxygenation and Ventilation

2

OBJECTIVES

On completion of this chapter, you will be able to:

1. Name the major structures of the respiratory system.
2. Describe the steps in performing the head-tilt/chin-lift and jaw thrust without head tilt maneuvers for opening the airway.
3. Relate mechanism of injury to opening the airway.
4. Describe correct suctioning technique and complications associated with this procedure.
5. Describe the method of correct sizing, insertion technique, and possible complications associated with insertion of the oropharyngeal airway and nasopharyngeal airway.
6. Describe the use of alternative airways, including the esophageal-tracheal Combitube (ETC), pharyngotracheal lumen airway (PTL), laryngeal mask airway (LMA), and cuffed oropharyngeal airway (COPA).
7. Describe how to artificially ventilate a patient with a pocket mask.
8. Describe the steps in performing the skill of artificially ventilating a patient with a bag-valve-mask for one and two rescuers.
9. Identify the recommended tidal volume that should be delivered when using the bag-valve-mask device.
10. Describe the signs of adequate artificial ventilation using the bag-valve-mask.
11. Describe the signs of inadequate artificial ventilation using the bag-valve-mask.
12. Describe the oxygen liter flow/minute and estimated inspired oxygen concentration delivered for a pocket mask and bag-valve-mask device.
13. Describe advantages and disadvantages associated with the use of an automatic transport ventilator and a flow restricted, oxygen-powered ventilation device.
14. Describe the oxygen liter flow/minute and estimated oxygen percentage delivered for each of the following devices:
    a. Nasal cannula
    b. Simple face mask
    c. Partial nonrebreather mask
    d. Nonrebreather mask
    e. Venturi mask
15. Describe the indications, advantages, and technique for performing endotracheal intubation.

ANATOMY OF THE RESPIRATORY SYSTEM

Divisions of the Airway

For the purposes of this text, airway structures located above the glottis are considered upper airway structures. Structures located below the glottis are considered lower airway structures.

1. *Upper* airway
   a. Consists of structures located outside the chest cavity including the nose and nasal cavities, pharynx, and larynx
   b. Function—filter, warm, and humidify the air, protecting the surfaces of the lower respiratory tract
2. *Lower* airway
   a. Contains the organs located in the chest cavity, including the trachea, bronchi, bronchioles, alveoli, and the lungs (Figure 2-1)
   b. Functions in the exchange of oxygen and carbon dioxide

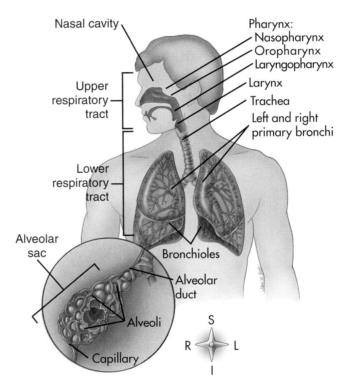

Figure 2-1 Structures of the upper and lower respiratory tract.

Upper Airway

The pharynx is a passageway common to both the respiratory and digestive systems.

1. The nasal cavity and the mouth meet at the pharynx (throat)
2. The pharynx extends from the nasal cavities to the larynx and includes three parts: the nasopharynx, oropharynx, and laryngopharynx (or hypopharynx) (Figure 2-2)
3. Nasopharynx
   a. Functions in respiration and is the portion of the pharynx immediately behind the nasal cavities and above the soft palate
   b. Its mucous lining filters, warms, and moistens the air
   c. Contains adenoid tissue and eustachian tube openings
   d. Tissues of the nasopharynx are extremely delicate and vascular. Improper or overly aggressive placement of tubes or airways may result in significant bleeding

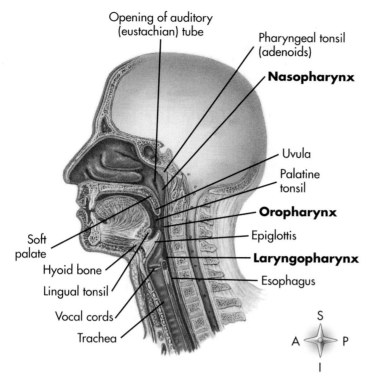

Figure 2-2   Pharynx. Midsagittal section illustrating the three divisions of the pharynx—nasopharynx, oropharynx, and laryngopharynx.

4. Oropharynx
   a. Functions in respiration and digestion and is the portion of the pharynx that is visible via the mouth
   b. Includes the teeth, tongue, palate, adenoids, epiglottis, and **vallecula** and extends from the soft palate superiorly to the vallecula inferiorly
      (1) *Vallecula* means "little valley" and is the space (or "pocket") between the base of the tongue and the epiglottis
   c. **Soft palate:** Composed of mucous membrane, muscular fibers, and mucous glands and is suspended from the posterior border of the hard palate, forming the roof of the mouth
   d. **Uvula:** a pendulous structure that hangs suspended from the midpoint of the posterior border of the soft palate
   e. **Hard palate:** Bony portion of the roof of the mouth that forms the floor of the nasal cavity. (Figure 2-3)
5. Laryngopharynx (hypopharynx)
   a. Functions in respiration and digestion and is the portion of the pharynx that lies inferior to the tip of epiglottis to the esophagus
   b. Larynx (voice box)
      (1) Connects the pharynx and trachea at the level of the cervical vertebrae and is a tubular structure composed of cartilage, muscles, and ligaments
      (2) Conducts air between the pharynx and the lungs, prevents food and foreign substances from entering the trachea, and houses the vocal cords (involved in speech production)
      (3) Most of the larynx is innervated with nerve endings from the vagus nerve
         a) Bradycardia can result from stimulation of the larynx by a laryngoscope blade or endotracheal (ET) tube

The vallecula is an important landmark when performing endotracheal intubation with a curved laryngoscope blade.

An airway obstruction may occur at the level of the pharynx due to displacement of the tongue, swelling of the epiglottis, secretions (e.g., blood or vomitus), or a foreign body.

An airway obstruction may occur at the level of the larynx because of trauma, presence of a foreign body, edema, or laryngospasm.

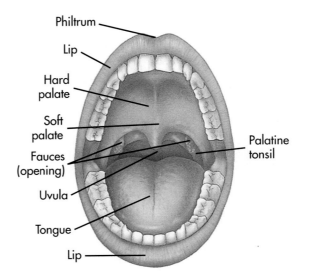

Figure 2-3 The oral cavity illustrating the hard and soft palate.

ET = endotracheal.
ETT = endotracheal tube

(4) Consists of connective tissue that contains nine cartilages. The three largest cartilages are the thyroid cartilage, the epiglottis, and the cricoid cartilage.
(5) Thyroid cartilage (Adam's apple)
    (a) Largest and most superior cartilage
    (b) Shaped like a shield (Figure 2-4)
    (c) More pronounced in adult males than adult females
    (d) The true vocal cords and the space between them are together designated the glottis. The glottic opening is located directly behind the thyroid cartilage and is the narrowest part of the adult larynx (Figure 2-5)

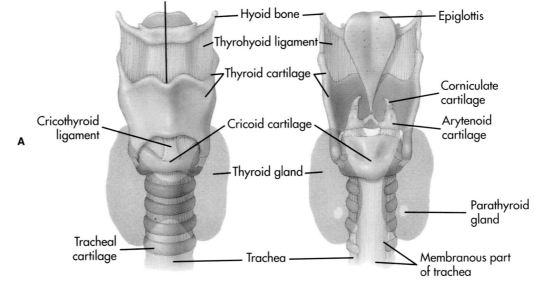

Figure 2-4 Anatomy of the larynx. **A,** Anterior view. **B,** Posterior view.

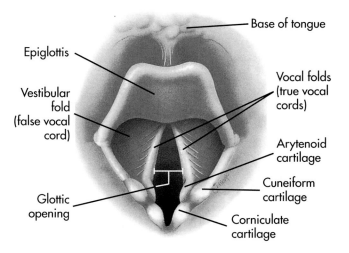

Figure 2-5 Vocal cords viewed from above.

(6) Cricoid cartilage
   (a) Shaped liked a signet ring
   (b) Most inferior of the nine laryngeal cartilages
      (i) First tracheal ring and the only completely cartilaginous ring in the larynx
      (ii) Narrowest diameter of the airway in infants and children less than 10 years of age is at the cricoid cartilage
      (iii) Compression of the cricoid cartilage occludes the esophagus, reducing the risk of aspiration. This technique is called *cricoid pressure* or the **Sellick maneuver**
   (c) Cricothyroid membrane: Fibrous membrane located between the cricoid and thyroid cartilages. This site may be used for surgical and alternative airway placement
(7) **Epiglottis:** a small, leaf-shaped cartilage located at the top of the larynx that prevents food from entering the respiratory tract during swallowing

Lower Airway

1. Consists of the trachea, bronchial tree (primary bronchi, secondary bronchi, and bronchioles), alveoli, and the lungs
   a. Functions in the exchange of oxygen and carbon dioxide
2. Trachea
   a. A rigid tube approximately 4 to 5 inches long and about 1 inch in diameter
   b. Conducts air to and from the lungs
   c. Extends from the larynx in the neck to the primary bronchi in the thoracic cavity, where it divides (bifurcates) into the right and left bronchi (Figure 2-6)
      (1) The point where the trachea bifurcates into the right and left mainstem bronchi is called the **carina** (approximately the level of the fifth or sixth thoracic vertebra)

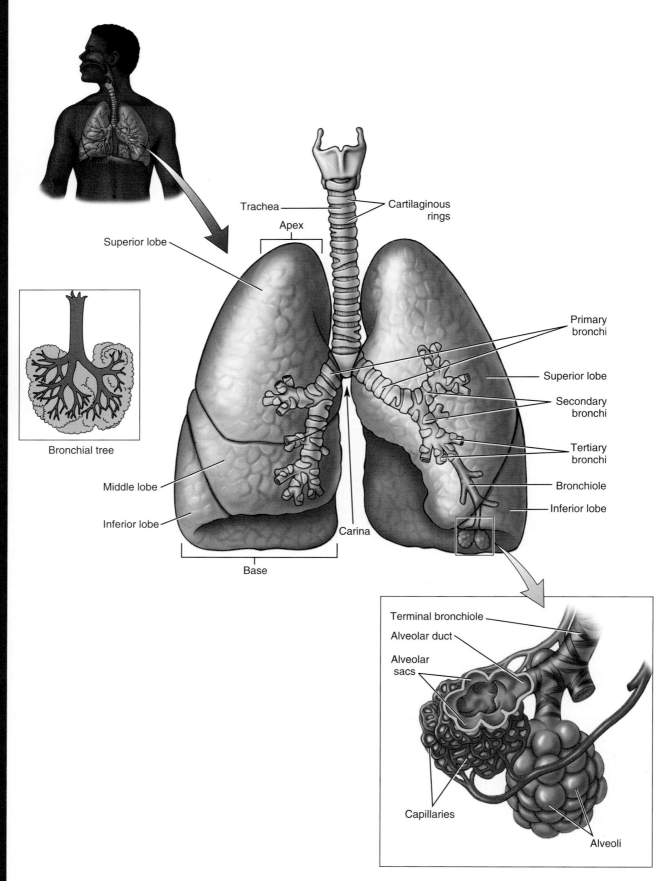

Figure 2-6 Trachea, bronchi, bronchioles, and alveoli.

d. Walls of the trachea are supported and held open by a series of C-shaped rings of cartilage that are open (incomplete) on the posterior surface
   (1) These rings are open to permit the esophagus, which lies behind the trachea, to bulge forward as food moves from the esophagus to the stomach
e. The area between the tracheal cartilages is made up of connective tissue and smooth muscle
   (1) Tracheal smooth muscle is innervated by the parasympathetic division of the autonomic nervous system
f. Trachea is lined with mucus-producing cells and cilia that filter the air before it enters the bronchi

3. Bronchi
   a. The trachea divides at the carina into the right and left mainstem bronchi, which have the same structure as the trachea
      (1) Primary (mainstem) bronchi branch into narrowing secondary and tertiary bronchi that branch into bronchioles

4. Bronchioles
   a. Composed entirely of smooth muscle supported by connective tissue
   b. Responsible for regulating the flow of air to the alveoli. The bronchioles subdivide into terminal bronchioles, which extend into the alveoli
   c. Right mainstem bronchus is shorter, wider, and straighter than the left
      (1) An endotracheal tube (ETT) that it inserted too far or foreign material that is aspirated is more likely to enter the right mainstem bronchus than the left

5. Alveoli
   a. Bronchioles subdivide into tiny tubes called *alveolar ducts*. These ducts end in alveoli, which are tiny, hollow air sacs
   b. Each alveolus is surrounded by a pulmonary capillary. Oxygen passes through the thin walls of the alveoli to capillaries and carbon dioxide passes from the capillaries to the alveoli
   c. Each lung of an average adult contains approximately 300 million alveoli

> Obstruction of the trachea will result in death if not corrected within minutes.

> Stimulation of beta-2 receptor sites in the bronchioles results in relaxation of bronchial smooth muscle.

LUNG VOLUMES

1. **Tidal volume:** Volume of air moved into or out of the lungs during a normal breath
   a. Average tidal volume for an adult male at rest is about 500 mL (5 to 7 mL/kg) (Figure 2-7)
   b. Tidal volume can be indirectly evaluated by observing the rise and fall of a patient's chest

2. **Minute volume:** Amount of air moved in and out of the lungs in 1 minute
   a. Determined by multiplying the tidal volume by the respiratory rate
   b. Thus a change in either the tidal volume *or* respiratory rate will affect the minute volume

---

Evaluation of a patient's respiratory status should include assessment of the patient's tidal volume (depth of respiration) and respiratory rate.

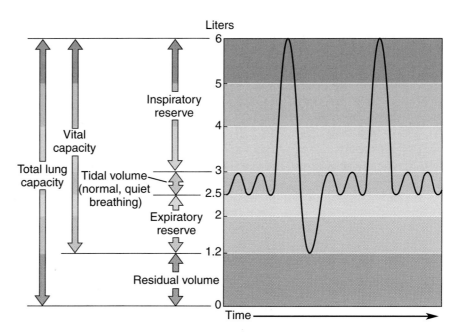

Figure 2-7 Lung volumes and capacities.

QUICK REVIEW

1. True or False. In adults, the narrowest diameter of the airway is at the cricoid cartilage.
2. What structure prevents food and liquids from entering the trachea during swallowing?

3. What is the name given to the space (or "pocket") between the base of the tongue and the epiglottis?

4. The _____ _____ is the bony portion of the roof of the mouth that forms the floor of the nasal cavity.
5. The true vocal cords and the space between them are together called the _____.

6. What is the carina?

7. Why is an endotracheal tube that is inserted too far or foreign material that is aspirated more likely to enter the right mainstem bronchus than the left?

1. False.   2. Epiglottis.   3. Vallecula.   4. Hard palate.   5. Glottis.   6. The point where the trachea bifurcates into the right and left mainstem bronchi.   7. The right mainstem bronchus is shorter, wider, and straighter than the left.

Personal Protective Equipment (PPE)

PPE must be worn when exposure to blood or other potentially infectious material can be reasonably anticipated. PPE includes eye protection, protective gloves, gowns, and masks.

Eye Protection
- Not required for routine patient care but should be worn when splashing of body fluids into the face or eyes of an emergency worker is likely
- If prescription eyeglasses are worn, removable side shields can be applied to them

Protective Gloves
- Disposable vinyl or latex gloves should be used for contact with blood or bloody body fluids
- Gloves should be changed between contact with different patients
- *Never* reuse vinyl or latex gloves
- Utility gloves are needed for cleaning equipment, vehicles
- Wearing gloves does NOT eliminate the need for handwashing after each patient contact

Gowns
- Gowns should be used in situations where large amounts of blood or body fluids are anticipated (e.g., during childbirth, major trauma)
- Disposable gowns should be used whenever possible
- After patient care activities are complete, appropriately discard the gown and, if possible, change uniforms
- In some situations, use of a gown may pose a risk to the emergency worker. For example, a gown may be hazardous during firefighting or extrication procedures. Check department/agency policy concerning gown use

Masks
- Surgical-type face masks should be worn to protect against possible blood or other body fluid splatter and/or in situations in which an airborne disease is suspected
- For patients with a known or suspected airborne disease, a disposable surgical-type mask should be worn by the patient
- In dealing with patients with known or suspected tuberculosis, a High Efficiency Particulate Air (HEPA) respirator should be worn by emergency workers and a disposable surgical-type mask should be worn by the patient

MANUAL AIRWAY MANEUVERS

1. In the unresponsive patient, a partial airway obstruction may occur if:
   a. The tongue falls back against the back of the throat because of a loss of muscle control (Figure 2-8)
   b. The epiglottis acts as a flap to obstruct the airway at the level of the larynx

The tongue is the most common cause of airway obstruction in the unresponsive patient.

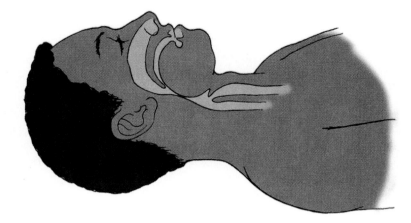

Figure 2-8 In the unresponsive patient, the tongue may fall back against the back of the throat due to a loss of muscle control, causing an airway obstruction

2. If the patient is breathing, snoring respirations are a characteristic sign of airway obstruction resulting from displacement of the tongue. In the apneic patient, airway obstruction caused by the tongue may go undetected until ventilation is attempted.
   a. Ventilating an apneic patient with an airway obstruction is difficult. If the airway obstruction is caused by the tongue, repositioning patient's head and jaw may be all that is needed to open the airway
3. Head-tilt/chin-lift
   a. Preferred technique for opening the airway of an unresponsive patient without suspected cervical spine injury
   b. Indications
      (1) Unresponsive patients who:
         (a) Do not have a mechanism for cervical spine injury
         (b) Are unable to protect their own airway
   c. Contraindications
      (1) Awake patients
      (2) Possible cervical spine injury
   d. Advantages
      (1) No equipment required
      (2) Simple
      (3) Noninvasive
   e. Disadvantages
      (1) Head tilt hazardous to patients with cervical spine injury
      (2) Does not protect the lower airway from aspiration
   f. Technique
      (1) Place the patient in a supine position
      (2) Place one of your hands on the patient's forehead and apply firm downward pressure with your palm to tilt the patient's head back (Figure 2-9)
      (3) Place the tips of the fingers of your other hand under the bony part of the patient's chin and gently lift the jaw forward

Positioning your fingers under the bony part of the patient's chin is important because compression of the soft tissue under the patient's chin can obstruct the airway.

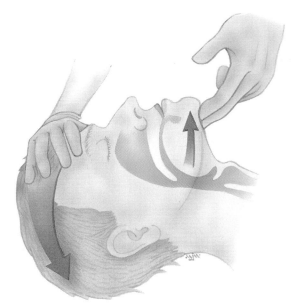

Figure 2-9 Head tilt/chin lift maneuver. Place one your hands on the patient's forehead and apply firm downward pressure with your palm to tilt the patient's head back. Place the tips of the fingers of your other hand under the bony part of the patient's chin and gently lift the jaw forward.

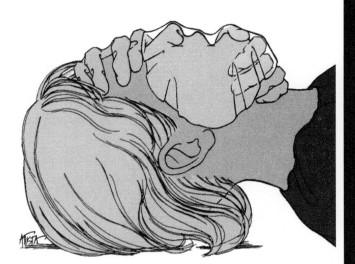

Figure 2-10 Using the thumb of the same hand used to lift the chin, open the patient's mouth by pulling down on the patient's lower lip.

(4) Using the thumb of the same hand used to lift the chin, open the patient's mouth by pulling down on the patient's lower lip (Figure 2-10)

4. Jaw thrust without head-tilt maneuver
   a. The jaw thrust without head-tilt maneuver should be used to open the airway when cervical spine injury is suspected
   b. Indications
      (1) Unresponsive patient with possible cervical spine injury
      (2) Unable to protect own airway
   c. Contraindications
      (1) Awake patient
   d. Advantages
      (1) Noninvasive
      (2) Requires no special equipment
      (3) May be used with cervical collar in place
   e. Disadvantages
      (1) Difficult to maintain
      (2) Requires second rescuer for bag-valve-mask ventilation
      (3) Does not protect against aspiration
   f. Technique
      (1) To perform a jaw thrust without head tilt maneuver, place the patient in a supine position (log-roll)
      (2) While stabilizing the patient's head in a neutral position, grasp the angles of the patient's lower jaw with both hands, one on each side, and displace the mandible forward (Figure 2-11)

The head tilt/chin lift maneuver should NOT be used if cervical spine injury is suspected.

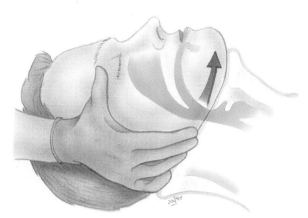

Figure 2-11 Jaw thrust without head-tilt maneuver. While stabilizing the patient's head in a neutral position, grasp the angles of the patient's lower jaw with both hands, one on each side, and displace the mandible forward.

(3) The combination of a head lift, forward displacement of the jaw and opening of the mouth is called the *triple airway maneuver*, or *jaw thrust maneuver*.[1] The manual maneuver described and recommended for opening the airway of a patient with suspected cervical spine injury is the *jaw thrust without head-tilt* maneuver.

SUCTIONING

1. Purpose of suctioning:
   a. Remove vomitus, saliva, blood, and other material from the patient's airway
   b. Improve gas exchange
   c. Prevent atelectasis
   d. Obtain secretions for diagnosis
2. Suction devices
   a. Fixed (stationary, installed) suction devices
      (1) Mounted in hospitals, extended care facilities, and in many emergency vehicles
      (2) Electrically operated by vacuum pumps or by the vacuum produced by a vehicle engine manifold (Figure 2-12)
      (3) Should be capable of generating a vacuum of >300 mm Hg when the distal end of the tube is occluded and provide an airflow of >40 L/min when the tube is open
      (4) Amount of suction should be adjustable for use in children and intubated patients
   b. Portable suction units (Figure 2-13):
      (1) May be hand-, foot-, or oxygen powered, electrically powered, or battery powered
      (2) Hand-operated suction devices are popular because they are lightweight, compact, reliable, and inexpensive (Figure 2-14)
      (3) Should provide a vacuum and airflow adequate for pharyngeal suction
      (4) Should be fitted with large-bore, nonkinking suction tubing and semi-rigid pharyngeal tips[2]

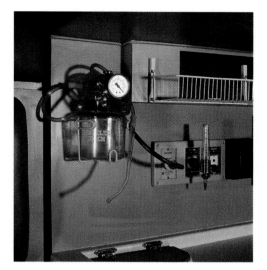

Figure 2-12 Fixed suction device.

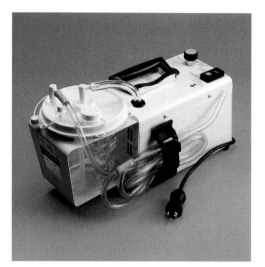

Figure 2-13 Portable suction device.

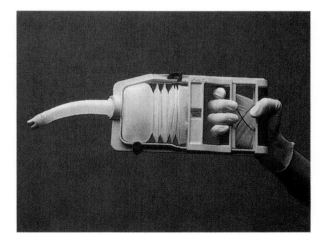

Figure 2-14 A hand-operated portable suction device.

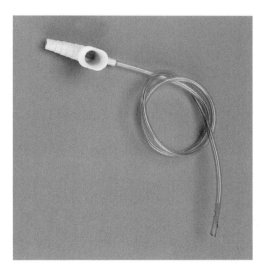

Figure 2-15 Soft suction catheter.

3. Suction catheters:
   a. Soft catheters
      (1) Also called "whistle-tip" or "French" catheters
      (2) Long, narrow, flexible pieces of plastic primarily used to clear blood or mucus from an ET or the nasopharynx (Figure 2-15)
      (3) A side opening present at the proximal end of most catheters is covered with the thumb to produce suction. (In some cases, suctioning is initiated when a button is pushed on the suction device itself)
      (4) Can be inserted into the nares, oropharynx, or nasopharynx, through an oropharyngeal or nasopharyngeal airway, or through an ET tube
      (5) To measure the correct length to insert the suction catheter for nasal (or oral) tracheal suctioning, measure the distance from the nose (or mouth) to the ear and add the distance from the ear to the sternal notch.

The primary difference between pharyngeal and tracheal suctioning is the depth suctioned and the potential for complications.[3]

   b. Rigid catheters
      (1) Also called *hard*, *tonsil tip*, or *Yankauer* catheters
      (2) Made of hard plastic and are angled to aid removal of sections from the mouth and oropharynx (Figure 2-16)
      (3) Typically, have one large and several small holes at the distal end through which particles may be suctioned
      (4) Because of its size, the rigid suction catheter is not used to suction the nares, except externally

4. Suctioning technique
   a. Using personal protective equipment, preoxygenate the patient with 100% oxygen to offset hypoxemia during interrupted oxygenation and ventilation
      (1) If using a soft catheter, measure the proper distance the catheter should be inserted.
      (2) If using a rigid catheter, place the catheter tip in the posterior pharynx.
   b. Insert the catheter WITHOUT applying suction
   c. Apply intermittent suction while withdrawing the catheter
   d. Suction should not be applied for more than 10 to 15 seconds (adults)
   e. Before repeating the procedure, ventilate the patient with 100% oxygen for approximately 30 seconds
   f. When possible, perform tracheal suction before suctioning the pharynx. The mouth and pharynx contain more bacteria than the trachea; therefore suctioning the trachea first will lead to less potential for bacterial contamination of the lungs

In adults, children, and infants older than 28 days, **hypoxemia** is defined as an arterial oxygen tension (PaO_2) of less than 60 torr or arterial oxygen saturation (SaO_2) of less than 90% in an individual breathing room air or with a PaO_2 and/or SaO_2 below the desirable range for a specific clinical situation.[4]

5. Possible complications of suctioning:
   a. Hypoxia
   b. Dysrhythmias
   c. Increased intracranial pressure
   d. Local edema
   e. Hemorrhage
   f. Tracheal ulceration
   g. Tracheal infection
   h. Bronchospasm
   i. Bradycardia and hypotension because of vagal stimulation

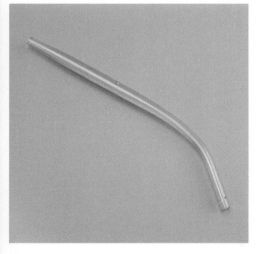

Figure 2-16 Rigid suction catheter.

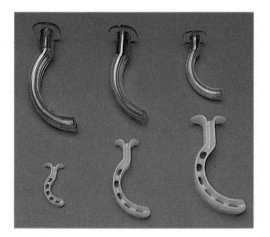

Figure 2-17 Types of oropharyngeal airways.

AIRWAY ADJUNCTS

Oropharyngeal Airway (OPA, Oral Airway)

1. Description and function
   a. J-shaped plastic device designed for use in unresponsive patients without a gag reflex
   b. When correctly positioned, the OPA extends from the patient's lips to the pharynx. The flange of the device rests on the patient's lips or teeth. The distal tip lies between the base of the tongue and the back of the throat, preventing the tongue from occluding the airway. Air passes around and through the device.
   c. Two main types of oropharyngeal airways (Figure 2-17)
      (1) Guedel—tubular design
      (2) Berman—airway channels along each side of the device
2. Indications
   a. To aid in maintaining an open airway in an unresponsive patient who is not intubated (Class IIa)
   b. To aid in maintaining an open airway in an unresponsive patient with no gag reflex who is being ventilated with a bag-valve-mask or other positive-pressure device
   c. May be used as a bite block after insertion of an ETT or oral gastric tube
3. Contraindications
   a. Responsive patient
4. Advantages
   a. Positions the tongue forward and away from the posterior pharynx
   b. Easily placed
5. Disadvantages
   a. Does not protect the lower airway from aspiration
   b. May produce vomiting if used in a responsive or semiresponsive patient with a gag reflex
6. Sizing
   a. Available in a variety of sizes (infant, child, adult)
   b. Size of the airway is based on the distance, in millimeters, from the flange to the distal tip
   c. Proper airway size is determined by holding the device against the side of the patient's face and selecting an airway that extends from the corner of the mouth to the tip of the earlobe or the angle of the jaw (Figure 2-18)

Note: The OPA does *not* protect the lower airway from aspiration.

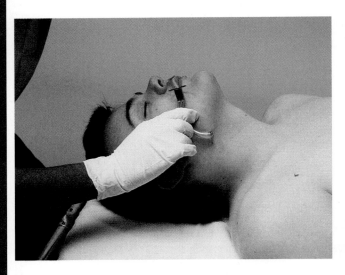

Figure 2-18 Proper airway size is determined by holding the device against the side of the patient's face. An OPA of correct size extends from the corner of the mouth to the tip of the earlobe or the angle of the jaw.

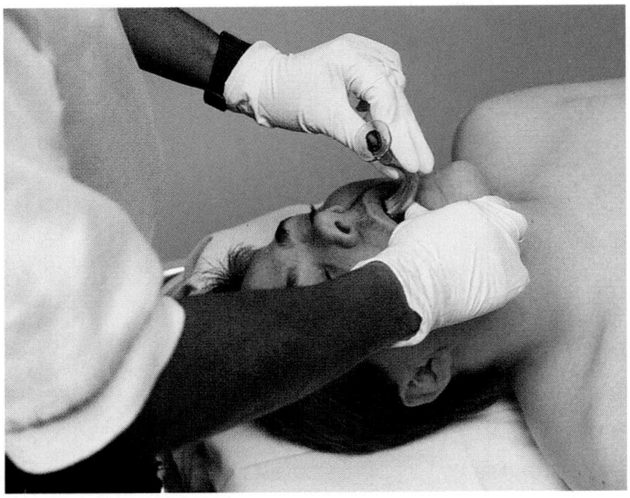

Figure 2-19 To insert the OPA, hold the device at its flange end and insert it into the mouth with the tip pointing toward the roof of the patient's mouth.

An OPA should only be inserted by persons properly trained in its use.

    d. Common sizes
      (1) Large adult   = 100 mm (length) (Guedel size 5)
      (2) Medium adult =   90 mm (Guedel size 4)
      (3) Small adult   =   80 mm (Guedel size 3)
  7. Insertion
    a. Before inserting an OPA, use personal protective equipment, open the airway using a head tilt/chin lift or jaw thrust without head-tilt maneuver, and ensure the mouth and pharynx are clear of secretions, blood, and vomitus
    b. After selecting an OPA of proper size, hold the device at its flange end and insert it into the mouth with the tip pointing toward the roof of the patient's mouth (Figure 2-19). Advance the airway along the roof of the mouth. When the distal end reaches the posterior wall of the pharynx, rotate the airway 180 degrees so that it is positioned over the tongue
    c. Another method of OPA insertion requires the use of a tongue blade to depress the tongue. If this method is used, the OPA is inserted with the tip of the OPA facing the floor of the patient's mouth (curved side down). Using the tongue blade to depress the tongue, the OPA is gently advanced into place over the tongue (Figure 2-20)
    d. Regardless of the insertion method used, when the OPA is properly inserted, the flange of the device should rest comfortably on the patient's lips or teeth
    e. Proper placement of the device is confirmed by ventilating the patient. If the OPA is correctly placed, chest rise should be visible and breath sounds should be present on auscultation of the lungs during ventilation
  8. Special considerations
    a. The OPA should only be used in the unresponsive patient. Use in responsive or semi-responsive patients may stimulate the gag reflex when the back of the tongue or posterior pharynx is touched, resulting in retching, vomiting, and/or laryngospasm
    b. If the OPA is improperly positioned, the tongue may be pushed back into the posterior pharynx, causing an airway obstruction

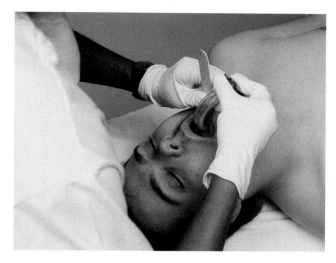

Figure 2-20   If a tongue blade is used, the OPA is inserted with the tip pointing toward the floor of the patient's mouth and advanced until the tip is positioned at the base of the tongue.

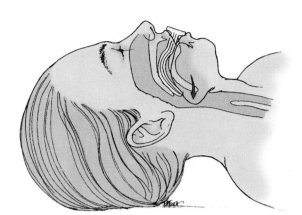

Figure 2-21   An improperly positioned OPA can cause an airway obstruction.

    c. Improper size.
       (1) If the airway is too long, it may press the epiglottis against the entrance of the larynx resulting in a complete airway obstruction (Figure 2-21)
       (2) If the airway is too short, it will not displace the tongue and may advance out of the mouth
    d. An OPA does not protect the lower airway from aspiration.
    e. Use of the OPA *does not* eliminate the need for maintaining proper head position

Nasopharyngeal Airway (NPA, NP Airway, Nasal Trumpet)

1. Description and function
    a. Soft, uncuffed rubber or plastic tube designed to keep the tongue away from the pharynx
       (1) The device is placed in one nostril and advanced until the distal tip lies in the posterior pharynx just below the base of the tongue, while the proximal tip rests on the external nares
       (2) Available in many sizes varying in length and internal diameter (ID) (Figure 2-22)
       (3) Usually well tolerated in the responsive or semi-responsive patient with an intact gag reflex
2. Indications
    a. To aid in maintaining an airway when use of an OPA is contraindicated or impossible (Class IIa), as in:
       (1) Trismus (spasm of the muscles used to grind, crush, and chew food)
       (2) Biting
       (3) Clenched jaws or teeth
3. Contraindications
    a. Patient intolerance
    b. Caution in presence of facial fracture or skull fracture
4. Advantages
    a. Provides a patent airway
    b. Tolerated by responsive patients
    c. Does not require mouth to be open

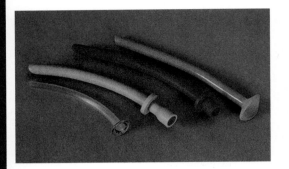

Figure 2-22 Nasopharyngeal airways are available in sizes of varying length and internal diameter.

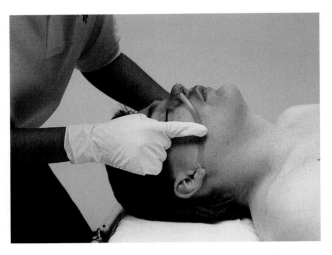

Figure 2-23 Proper airway size is determined by holding the device against the side of the patient's face and selecting an airway that extends from the tip of the nose to the angle of the jaw or the tip of the ear.

5. Disadvantages
   a. Improper technique may result in severe bleeding, resulting epistaxis may be difficult to control
   b. Does not protect the lower airway from aspiration
6. Sizing
   a. Proper airway size is determined by holding the device against the side of the patient's face and selecting an airway that extends from the tip of the nose to the angle of the jaw or the tip of the ear (Figure 2-23)
   b. An airway that is too long may stimulate the gag reflex. One that is too short may not be inserted far enough to keep the tongue away from the posterior pharynx

An NPA should only be inserted by persons properly trained in its use.

7. Insertion
   a. Before inserting an NPA, use personal protective equipment and open the airway using a head-tilt/chin lift or jaw thrust without head-tilt maneuver. Lubricate the distal tip of the device liberally with a water-soluble lubricant to minimize resistance and decrease irritation to the nasal passage
   b. After selecting an NPA of the proper size, hold the device at its flange-end like a pencil and slowly insert it into the patient's nostril with the bevel pointing toward the nasal septum (Figure 2-24)
   c. Advance the airway along the floor of the nostril, following the natural curvature of the nasal passage, until the flange is flush with the nostril
   d. The nasal cavity is very vascular. During insertion, do not force the airway as it may cause abrasions or lacerations of the nasal mucosa and result in significant bleeding, increasing the risk of aspiration
      (1) If resistance is encountered, a gentle back-and-forth rotation of the device between your fingers may ease insertion. If resistance continues, withdraw the NPA, reapply lubricant, and attempt insertion in the patient's other nostril

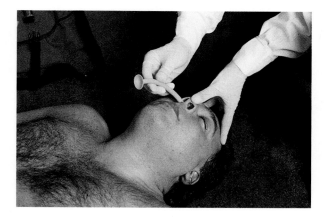 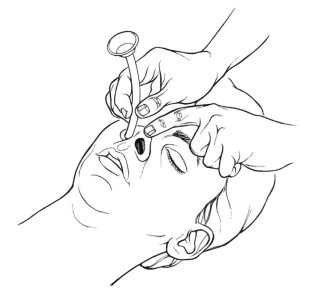

Figure 2-24   After selecting a NPA of the proper size, hold the device at its flange end and insert it into the patient's nostril with the bevel pointing toward the nasal septum.

    e. Proper placement of the device is confirmed by ventilating the patient. If the NPA is correctly placed, chest rise should be visible and breath sounds should be present on auscultation of the lungs during ventilation

> *Some nasopharyngeal airways have a slide at the flange end of the device to adjust for proper length. If present, this slide should NOT be removed. Incidents have occurred in which an NPA that was improperly sized (too small) and in which the adjustable slide had been removed was subsequently "sucked" into the patient's lower airway, necessitating removal by bronchoscopy.*

8. Special considerations
    a. NPA does not protect the lower airway from aspiration
    b. Suctioning through an NPA is difficult
    c. Use of the NPA *does not* eliminate the need for maintaining proper head position
    d. The NPA should not be used in patients with a known or suspected basilar skull fracture
    e. If the NPA is too long, it may enter the esophagus, causing gastric distention and hypoventilation, or it may stimulate the laryngeal or glossopharyngeal reflexes to produce laryngospasm, retching, or vomiting
    f. Although most responsive and semi-responsive patients can tolerate an NPA, the gag reflex may be stimulated in sensitive patients, precipitating laryngospasm and vomiting

Alternative Airways

The esophageal-tracheal Combitube and pharyngotracheal lumen airway are also called *multi-lumen* or *dual-lumen* airways.

Alternative airways include the esophageal-tracheal Combitube (ETC), the pharyngotracheal lumen airway (PTL), and the laryngeal mask airway (LMA). Alternative airways may be used in areas where tracheal intubation is not permitted, or communities in which health care providers have little opportunity to obtain experience with the technique of tracheal intubation because of few patients.

The Esophageal-Tracheal Combitube (ETC)

Class IIa

1. Description and function
   a. The esophageal-tracheal airway, or Combitube, allows ventilation of the lungs and reduces the risk of aspiration of gastric contents.
      (1) Blindly inserted (i.e., without visualization of the vocal cords) to ventilate the trachea, regardless of esophageal or tracheal placement
   b. Dual-lumen tube with two balloon cuffs
      (1) Proximal (pharyngeal) balloon is located near the halfway point of the tube and is considerably larger than the distal cuff
         (a) When inflated, the balloon fills the space between the base of the tongue and the soft palate, anchoring the ETC into position, and isolating the oropharynx from the hypopharynx
      (2) When both balloon cuffs are inflated, an airtight pocket is created in the pharynx between the upper portion of the esopha-

In 1993, researchers evaluated the safety and effectiveness of the Combitube as used by ICU nurses under medical supervision compared with an endotracheal airway established by ICU physicians during CPR.[5] Thirty-seven patients suffering from cardiac arrest in a medical ICU over a 7-month period had emergency intubation performed with either the Combitube by nurses or the endotracheal airway by physicians with subsequent mechanical ventilation. Blood gases were evaluated after 20 minutes of mechanical ventilation. This study found that intubation time was shorter for the Combitube and blood gases for each device showed comparable results; the PaO_2 was slightly higher during ventilation with the Combitube. This study concluded that the Combitube, as used by ICU nurses, was as effective as establishment of the endotracheal airway by intensivists during CPR.

In a 1997 study,[6] researchers compared three alternative airway devices and the oral airway for use by non-advanced life support emergency medical assistants. The pharyngeal tracheal lumen (PTL) airway, the laryngeal mask airway, and the esophageal tracheal Combitube were compared objectively for success of insertion, ventilation, and arterial blood gas and spirometry measurements performed on hospital arrival. Results revealed successful insertion and ventilation with the Combitube was 86%, 82% with the PTL airway, and 73% with the laryngeal mask airway. No significant difference was found for objective measurements of ventilatory effectiveness (ABGs and spirometry). The researchers concluded that the PTL, laryngeal mask airway, and Combitube appear to offer substantial advances over the oral airway/bag-valve-mask system. Although the most costly, the Combitube was associated with the least problems with ventilation and was the most preferred by a majority of emergency medical assistants.

  gus (blocked by a balloon) and the area behind the tongue and molars (blocked by the other balloon)

  (a) Air can escape only into the trachea and then to the lungs

 (3) When the Combitube is in place, a bag-valve-mask (or other ventilation device) is then used to blow air into the tube, with the outlet between the two balloons

 c. Available in 41 and 37 French (Fr) sizes

  (1) 37 Fr size is used for patients between 4 and 5 feet tall

  (2) 41 Fr size is used for patients over 5 feet tall

2. Indications

 a. Difficult face mask fit (beards, absence of teeth)

 b. Patient in whom intubation has been unsuccessful and ventilation is difficult

 c. Patient in whom airway management is necessary but the health care provider is untrained in the technique of visualized orotracheal intubation

 d. Whenever a direct view of the vocal cords is difficult or impossible (e.g., view obscured by edema, blood, tissue damage or anatomic distortion).

3. Contraindications

 a. Patient with an intact gag reflex

 b. Patient with known or suspected esophageal disease

 c. Patient known to have ingested a caustic substance

 d. Suspected upper airway obstruction because of laryngeal foreign body or pathology

 e. Patient less than 4 feet tall

4. Advantages

 a. Minimal training and retraining required

 b. Visualization of the upper airway or use of special equipment not required for insertion

The trachea is isolated from the esophagus when the pharyngeal and esophageal balloons are inflated. When inflated, the pharyngeal balloon holds the device in place and helps prevent the escape of air through the nose or mouth. Once inflated, the esophageal balloon seals the esophagus so that air does not enter the stomach, reducing the risk of aspiration of gastric contents.

Ventilation with the Combitube begins with the esophageal tube because of the high probability of esophageal placement after blind insertion.

The Combitube functions as a standard ETT when the device is placed in the trachea.

The Combitube should be used in conjunction with an end-tidal CO_2 or esophageal detector device (discussed later in this chapter).

c. Reasonable technique for use in suspected neck injury because the head does not need to be hyperextended

d. Because of the oropharyngeal balloon, the need for a face mask is eliminated

e. Can provide a patent airway with either esophageal or tracheal placement

f. If placed in the esophagus, allows suctioning of gastric contents without interruption of patient ventilation

g. Reduces risk of aspiration of gastric contents

5. Disadvantages
   a. Proximal port may be occluded with secretions
   b. Proper identification of tube location may be difficult, leading to ventilation through the wrong lumen
   c. Soft tissue trauma because of rigidity of tube
   d. Impossible to suction the trachea when the tube is in the esophagus
   e. Esophageal or tracheal trauma from poor insertion technique or use of wrong size device
   f. Damage to the cuffs by the patient's teeth during insertion
   g. Inability to insert because of limited mouth opening

6. Technique
   a. Using personal protective equipment, open the patient's mouth and clear the airway of any dentures, foreign objects, or debris. If an oropharyngeal airway was inserted, remove it
   b. Auscultate bilateral breath sounds to establish a baseline and instruct an assistant to preoxygenate the patient with 100% oxygen. Assemble the proper equipment and check the cuffs for leaks
   c. Insert the ETC in the same direction as the natural curvature of the pharynx. Insert the tip into the mouth in the midline and advance it gently along the base of the tongue and into the airway until the black rings (heavy black lines) on the tube are positioned at the level of the patient's teeth (or gums, if the patient lacks teeth). If the tube does not insert easily, do not use force—withdraw and retry
   d. Inflate the proximal (pharyngeal) cuff with 100 mL of air through the blue pilot tube marked #1. Inflate the distal (esophageal) cuff with 15 mL of air through the white pilot tube marked # 2
   e. Attach a bag-valve device to the longer (blue) connecting tube marked #1 (the esophageal tube) and begin ventilation. Confirm placement and ventilation by observing chest rise and auscultating over the epigastrium and bilaterally over each lung. If the chest rises, breath sounds are present bilaterally, and epigastric sounds are absent; therefore, the ETC is in the esophagus (Figure 2-25). Continue to ventilate through long (blue) tube. When esophageal tube placement has been verified, the short (clear) tube (marked #2) can be used for gastric suction with the suction catheter provided in the airway kit
      (1) If the chest does not rise or sounds are only heard over the epigastrium, attach the bag-valve device to the second (endotracheal) tube and begin ventilation to determine if the ETC has entered the trachea. If the device is in the trachea, the chest should rise when ventilating through the second (shorter, clear) tube (Figure 2-26). Confirm placement and ventilation by observing chest rise, auscultation over epigastrium, and bilaterally over each lung. If the ETC is in the trachea and placement has been confirmed, continue ventilation through the second tube.

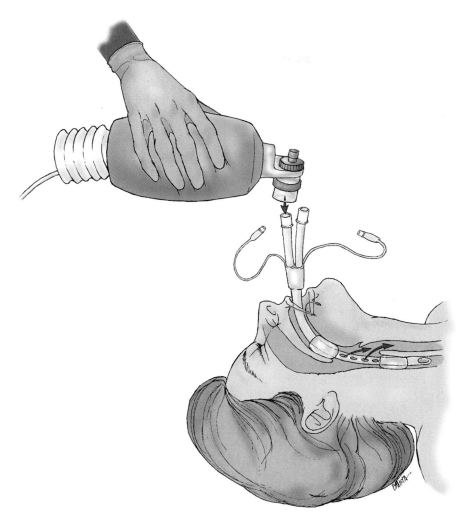

Figure 2-25   The Combitube inserted into the esophagus.

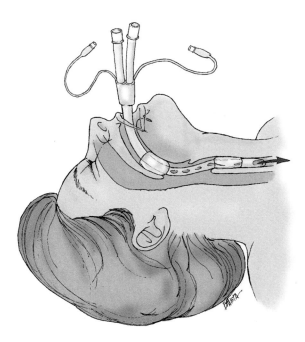

Figure 2-26   The Combitube inserted into the trachea.

(2) If breath sounds *and* epigastric sounds are absent, immediately deflate the cuffs (blue first). Slightly withdraw the tube and then reinflate the cuffs (blue first). Ventilate and reassess placement. If breath sounds and epigastric sounds are still absent, immediately deflate the cuffs and remove the tube. Suction as necessary, insert an oropharyngeal or nasopharyngeal airway, ventilate the patient with a bag-valve-mask, and reassess

The Pharyngotracheal Lumen Airway (PTL)

Class IIa

1. Description and function
    a. A dual-lumen tube that allows either tracheal or esophageal placement
        (1) Like the Combitube, the device is inserted blindly
    b. Consists of two parallel tubes of unequal length and two balloon cuffs that inflate simultaneously when air is blown into the inflation port with a bag-valve device
        (1) The first tube (green in color) is short (21 cm), wide, and has a balloon located at the lower portion of the tube. When inflated, the balloon inflates in the oropharynx, providing a seal to prevent air that is blown in during ventilations from escaping back out through the mouth and nose
        (2) The second tube is longer than the first (31 cm in overall length) and has a distal balloon cuff at its end. When inflated, the balloon at the distal end of the tube provides a seal around the tube and helps anchor it in either the trachea or esophagus (Figure 2-27)
        (3) When the long tube is in the esophagus, the patient is ventilated through the first (shorter/green) tube. When the long tube is positioned in the trachea, the patient is ventilated directly through it (functions as a standard ETT) (Figure 2-28)
    c. Requires no additional parts, syringes to inflate the balloons, or accessories, and has an integrated bite block to aid in keeping the airway patent. A slide clamp allows the oropharyngeal cuff to be deflated and the small, distal balloon to remain inflated when intubating around the PTL airway. An adjustable cloth neck strap holds the device in place

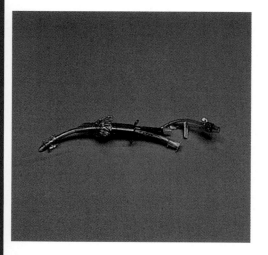

Figure 2-27 The pharyngotracheal lumen airway (PTL).

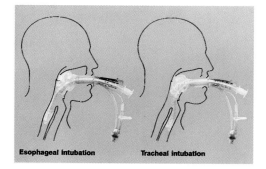

Esophageal intubation   Tracheal intubation

Figure 2-28 Esophageal and tracheal placement of the PTL airway.

2. Indications
   a. Difficult face mask fit (beards, absence of teeth)
   b. Patient in whom airway management is necessary but the health care provider is untrained in the technique of visualized orotracheal intubation
   c. Patient in whom intubation has been unsuccessful and ventilation is difficult
   d. When bag-valve-mask ventilation is inadequate or causing excessive gastric distention
3. Contraindications
   a. Patient with an intact gag reflex
   b. Patients less than 5 feet or more than 6 feet 7 inches tall
   c. Patients less than 14 years of age (height primary factor)
   d. Patient with known or suspected esophageal disease
   e. Patients known to have ingested a caustic substance
   f. Suspected upper airway obstruction because of laryngeal foreign body or pathology
4. Advantages
   a. Visualization of the upper airway or use of special equipment not required for insertion
   b. Reasonable technique for use in suspected neck injury because the head does not need to be hyperextended
   c. Because of the oropharyngeal balloon, the need for a face mask is eliminated
   d. Can provide a patent airway with either esophageal or tracheal placement
   e. Can protect the trachea from upper airway bleeding or secretions
5. Disadvantages
   a. Patient must be unresponsive without a gag reflex
   b. Must be removed when the patient becomes responsive or agitated
   c. Proper identification of tube location may be difficult, leading to ventilation through the wrong tube
   d. Impossible to suction trachea when tube is in esophagus
   e. Esophageal or pharyngeal trauma possible during insertion
   f. When the longer tube is in the esophagus, the device does not keep the patient from aspirating blood, vomitus, or other material present in the upper airway
6. Technique
   a. Using personal protective equipment, open the patient's mouth and, clear the airway of any dentures, foreign objects, or debris. If an oropharyngeal airway was inserted, remove it
   b. Auscultate bilateral breath sounds to establish a baseline and instruct an assistant to preoxygenate the patient with 100% oxygen
   c. Assemble the proper equipment and check the cuffs for leaks by blowing air into the inflation valve using your mouth (Figure 2-29), a bag-valve-device, or other ventilation device. In order for the cuffs to inflate, the relief port under the inflation valve must be closed with the small white cap and the slide clamp must be open. After checking the cuffs, remove the white cap, and simultaneously squeeze both cuffs to deflate them. Replace the white cap on the relief port and lubricate the distal end of the long tube with a water-soluble lubricant

Air may be blown into the inflation valve using your mouth (or other ventilation device) because the valve serves only the cuffs of the PTL and does not connect with the patient's esophagus or airway.

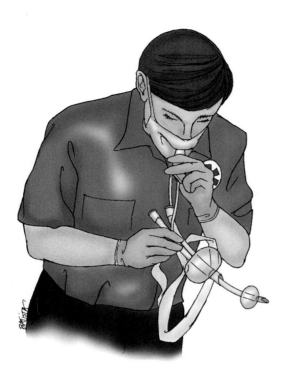

Figure 2-29 Check the cuffs of the PTL for leaks by blowing air into the inflation valve.

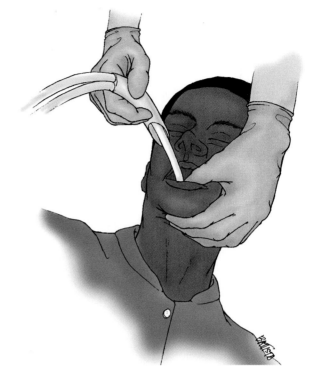

Figure 2-30 Position yourself at the patient's head and insert the PTL in the same direction as the natural curvature of the pharynx. Insert the tip into the mouth in the midline and advance it gently along the base of the tongue and into the airway until the flange of the plastic bite block rests against the patient's teeth.

d. Position yourself at the patient's head and insert the PTL in the same direction as the natural curvature of the pharynx. Insert the tip into the mouth in the midline (Figure 2-30). Advance it gently along the base of the tongue and into the airway until the flange of the plastic bite block rests against the patient's teeth. The tube should pass easily through the patient's mouth and pharynx. If resistance is encountered during insertion, slightly withdraw the tube, redirect it, and reinsert

e. Quickly loop the white strap around the patient's head and secure it in place. This helps prevent movement of the device out of the patient's mouth when the oropharyngeal balloon is inflated

f. Ventilate into the inflation valve to simultaneously inflate both distal cuffs

g. Attach a bag-valve device to the short (green) tube and begin ventilation. Confirm placement and ventilation by observing chest rise and auscultating over the epigastrium and bilaterally over each lung. It is probable that the longer tube of the PTL is in the esophagus when breath sounds are present bilaterally and epigastric sounds are absent (Figure 2-31). Continue to ventilate through the green tube. When esophageal tube placement has been verified by the presence of breath sounds, a gastric tube may be inserted through the long tube to evacuate stomach contents

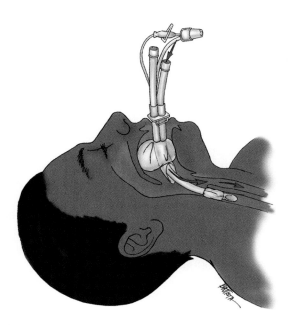

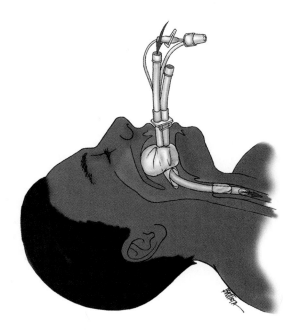

Figure 2-31 Ventilate the patient through the short (green) tube of the PTL to determine if the longer tube is in the esophagus. If the chest rises, continue ventilation through the short tube. A gastric tube may be inserted through the long tube to evacuate stomach contents.

Figure 2-32 If the long tube of the PTL is in the trachea, removal of the stylet will cause air to travel through the long tube into the trachea. Continue to ventilate through the long tube.

   h. If the chest does not rise, determine if the longer tube is in the trachea. Stop ventilation through the short (green) tube. Remove the stylet from the longer tube, attach a bag-valve device to that tube, and begin ventilation
   i. Confirm placement and ventilation by observing chest rise, auscultation over epigastrium, and bilaterally over each lung. If the long tube is in the trachea, removal of the stylet will cause air to travel through the long tube into the trachea (Figure 2-32). Continue to ventilate through the long tube

> The PTL functions as a standard ETT when the device is placed in the trachea. This device should be used in conjunction with an end-tidal CO_2 or esophageal detector.

Laryngeal Mask Airway (LMA)

Class IIa

1. The LMA may be used as an alternative to either the ETT or the face mask with either spontaneous or positive-pressure ventilation[7]
   a. Because of the relative ease of learning how to use the device, health care workers in an emergency setting who are not trained in endotracheal intubation can use the LMA
   b. LMA may be used as the primary airway, as a channel for an ET tube, or as an option in the management of a difficult airway where intubation is unsuccessful
2. Description and function
   a. Consists of a tube that is fused to an elliptical, spoon-shaped mask at a 30-degree angle
      (1) When inserted, the tube protrudes from the patient's mouth and is connected to a ventilation device via a standard 15-mm connector

(2) The mask resembles a miniature face mask and has an inflatable rim that is filled with air from a syringe using a pilot valve-balloon system

(3) The tube opens into the middle of the mask by means of three vertical slits that prevent the tip of the epiglottis from falling back and blocking the lumen of the tube (Figure 2-33)

b. The LMA is inserted through the mouth and into the pharynx. The device is advanced until resistance is felt. Then the mask is inflated, providing a low-pressure seal around the laryngeal inlet. The posterior aspect of the tube is marked with a longitudinal black line. When the LMA is correctly placed, the black line on the tube should rest in the midline against the patient's upper lip

c. Because masks are available in several sizes, the LMA can be used in patients of all ages, from neonates to adults

d. Different types of LMAs are available, including the original (reusable) LMA (LMA-Classic), a single-use LMA (LMA-Unique), a reinforced/flexible LMA (LMA-Flexible), and an LMA specifically designed for tracheal intubation (LMA-Fastrach)

3. Indications

a. Difficult face mask fit (beards, absence of teeth)

b. Patient in whom intubation has been unsuccessful and ventilation is difficult

c. Patient in whom airway management is necessary, but the health care provider is untrained in the technique of visualized orotracheal intubation

d. Many elective surgical procedures (i.e., minimal soft tissue trauma with less patient discomfort and relatively short periods of anesthesia)

4. Contraindications

a. Health care provider untrained in use of LMA

b. Contraindicated if a risk of aspiration exists (i.e., patients with full stomachs)

5. Advantages

a. Can be quickly inserted to provide ventilation when bag-valve-mask ventilation is not sufficient and endotracheal intubation cannot be readily accomplished

b. Tidal volume delivered may be greater when using the LMA than with face mask ventilation

> The disposable LMA is made of polyvinyl chloride and has dimensions identical to the reusable LMA, but the tube is stiffer and the cuff thicker.

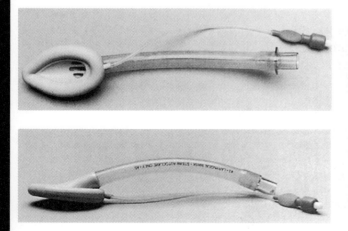

Figure 2-33 The Laryngeal Mask Airway (LMA).

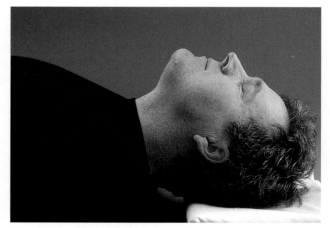

Figure 2-34 Sniffing position.

   c. Less gastric insufflation than with bag-valve-mask ventilation

   d. Provides equivalent ventilation to the tracheal tube

   e. Training simpler than with tracheal intubation

   f. Unaffected by anatomical factors (e.g., beard, absence of teeth)

   g. No risk of esophageal or bronchial intubation

   h. When compared to tracheal intubation, less potential for trauma from direct laryngoscopy and tracheal intubation

   i. Less coughing, laryngeal spasm, sore throat, and voice changes than with tracheal intubation

6. Disadvantages

   a. Does not provide protection against aspiration

   b. Cannot be used if the mouth cannot be opened more than 0.6 in (1.5 cm)

> During bag-valve-mask ventilation, excess pressure is forced down the esophagus. When using the LMA, gastric insufflation is minimized because excess pressure is vented upward around the LMA, rather than being forced down the esophagus.

A 1997 study compared the ease of insertion of the LMA using the standard uninflated cuff approach or insertion with a fully inflated cuff.[8] Two hundred consecutive patients 16 years of age and older undergoing anesthesia were randomized to receive an LMA with a standard deflated cuff or an inflated cuff. No muscle relaxants were used before LMA insertion. A satisfactory airway was achieved in 94% of the standard-technique (uninflated-cuff) patients vs. 97% of the inflated-cuff group, most in one or two attempts. Additional successful insertions were achieved in each group by changing to the other technique. Patients who received standard technique (uninflated-cuff) insertion had a higher rate of traumatic insertion as evidenced by blood on the removed mask (15% vs. 0%) and sore throat (21% vs. 4%). The authors concluded that insertion of the LMA with the cuff fully inflated is equally successful to the standard uninflated approach in experienced hands. The inflated technique was associated with less minor pharyngeal mucosal trauma and, consequently, a lower incidence of postoperative sore throat.

In a 1993 study,[9] researchers evaluated the emergency use of the LMA by nurses. The study compared the tidal volume achieved by nurses during hand ventilation using standard resuscitation equipment with a face mask, with or without a Guedel airway, and following placement of a laryngeal mask in the same patients. In this study, tidal volumes measured while using the LMA were significantly greater than those measured during face mask ventilation.

In another 1993 study, 10 volunteers with no previous experience of resuscitation were formally trained in the use of the LMA and the Guedel oropharyngeal airway and bag and face mask for manual ventilation of the lungs in 104 fit anesthetized adults. The volunteers then used both airways in turn. Success rates for the LMA and the Guedel airway and bag and face mask were 87% and 43%, respectively. "The laryngeal mask airway proved to be easier to use for manual ventilation than the Guedel airway and bag and mask for inexperienced personnel who had received a period of formal training in both techniques."[10]

Researchers from Britain compared the use of the LMA and Combitube in a 1999 study to determine which device was easiest for unskilled staff to use.[11] Twenty-six class I or II elective anesthesia patients (adults) were randomized to undergo insertion of both a Combitube and LMA in random order by a nurse not experienced with these devices or laryngoscopy. Nurses not previously trained in airway support were briefly trained on a mannequin and then had two practice attempts with each device before the study. Both devices were inserted in random order and the time to successful ventilation of the lungs recorded. Twenty-six patients were successfully ventilated with the LMA and 24 successfully ventilated with the Combitube. The two Combitube failures were the result of "faulty operator technique." The median times to insertion were 40 seconds and 45 seconds for the LMA and Combitube, respectively.

c. May not be effective when respiratory anatomy is abnormal (i.e., abnormal oropharyngeal anatomy or the presence of pathology is likely to result in a poor mask fit)

d. May be difficult to provide adequate ventilation if high airway pressures are required

7. Technique

a. Using personal protective equipment, open the patient's mouth and clear the airway of any foreign objects or debris. If an OPA was inserted, remove it

b. Auscultate bilateral breath sounds to establish a baseline and instruct an assistant to preoxygenate the patient with 100% oxygen

c. Assemble the proper equipment and check the cuff and valve for leaks. Deflate the cuff and apply water-soluble lubricant. (Avoid lubricating the anterior surface of the mask, because the lubricant may be aspirated). Position the rim of the mask so that it is facing away from the mask opening. There should be no folds near the tip

d. Position the patient in the "sniffing" position (neck flexed and head extended) (Figure 2-34). During the insertion procedure, maintain this position with your nondominant hand

---

In the "sniffing" position, the neck is flexed at the fifth and sixth cervical vertebrae, and the head is extended at the first and second cervical vertebrae. This position aligns the axes of the mouth, pharynx, and trachea. The sniffing position is not used in cases of suspected trauma.

When the LMA has been properly positioned, the cuff tip lies at the base of the laryngopharynx, the sides in the pyriform fossae, and the upper border of the mask at the base of the tongue, pushing it forward.

Failure to ensure that the black line on the LMA is correctly positioned may result in misplacement of the cuff and a partial airway obstruction.

e. With the distal opening of the LMA facing anteriorly, insert the tip of the LMA into the patient's mouth. Press the tip of the mask upward against the hard palate to flatten it out. Using your index or third finger, in one smooth movement advance the mask over the hard palate, the soft palate, and as far as possible into the laryngopharynx until resistance is felt

f. Ensure that the black line on the LMA is in the midline against the patient's upper lip. Without holding the tube, inflate the cuff with a volume of air appropriate for the mask size selected. As the cuff is inflated, there will be a slight outward movement of the tube as the cuff centers itself around the laryngeal inlet. This results in slight movement of the thyroid and cricoid cartilages

g. Confirm placement of the LMA with auscultation, observation of chest rise, and use of an end-tidal CO_2 detector.

h. Secure the LMA and a bite-block in place

Cuffed Oropharyngeal Airway (COPA)

Class Indeterminate

1. Description and function

a. COPA is a modified Guedel-type oropharyngeal airway with an inflatable cuff at its distal end

   (1) The cuff is inflated through a one-way valve attached to a pilot balloon that emerges from the device at the tooth-lip guard

   (2) Proximal end has a standard 15-mm connector, an integrated bite-block, and two posts for attaching the elastic fixation strap included with the device

(3) It is currently available in four sizes: 8, 9, 10, and 11. These numbers refer to the distance (in centimeters) between the tooth-lip guard and the distal tip of the device

b. After the COPA is inserted and the cuff is inflated, the device displaces the tongue anteriorly and provides a seal between the base of the tongue and the posterior wall of the pharynx

2. Indications
   a. For use in the spontaneously breathing patient with no risk of aspiration
   b. May be useful during cardiac and/or respiratory arrest

3. Contraindications
   a. Patient with an intact gag reflex
   b. Health care provider untrained in use of COPA
   c. Contraindicated if a risk of aspiration exists (i.e., patients with full stomachs)
   d. Not indicated for use as a replacement for an ETT

4. Advantages
   a. Inexpensive
   b. Quick and easy to use; inserts like an oropharyngeal airway
   c. Provides a clear airway; cuff properly positions tongue and epiglottis
   d. Connects to any ventilation device by means of a standard 15-mm connector
   e. No risk of esophageal or bronchial misplacement
   f. More secure than a face mask; semi-rigid anatomical shape and inflated cuff hold the device in place
   g. Inflated cuff guards against air leak
   h. Integral bite block ensures patent airway
   i. Single-use design eliminates chance of cross contamination
   j. Pharyngeal placement excludes trauma to trachea, vocal cords, or larynx
   k. High volume, low-pressure cuff improves seal, distributes forces, and reduces risk of tissue damage

5. Disadvantages
   a. Overinflation of the cuff increases the risk of complications as well as cuff distortion or rupture
   b. Trauma to the oropharynx
   c. Does not provide protection against aspiration
   d. May not be effective when respiratory anatomy is abnormal (i.e., abnormal oropharyngeal anatomy or the presence of pathology likely to result in a poor cuff fit)

6. Special considerations
   a. COPA should only be inserted by persons properly trained in its use. Insertion of a COPA is the same as that used for a conventional OPA
   b. COPA should not be used if the cuff does not inflate, leaks, or has poor continuity with the pilot balloon
   c. COPA should only be used in the unresponsive patient. Use in responsive or semi-responsive patients may stimulate the gag reflex when the back of the tongue or posterior pharynx is touched, resulting in retching, vomiting, and/or laryngospasm

Note: COPA does *not* provide protection against aspiration.

QUICK REVIEW

1. Why is an oropharyngeal airway not used in responsive or semi-responsive patients?

2. What is the purpose of suctioning?

3. What is the combination of a head lift, forward displacement of the jaw, and opening of the mouth called?

4. True or False. The laryngeal mask airway is available in only one size.
5. How do you determine the correct size nasopharyngeal airway?

6. List four contraindications for use of the Combitube.

1. Use in responsive or semi-responsive patients may stimulate the gag reflex when the back of the tongue or posterior pharynx is touched, resulting in retching, vomiting, and/or laryngospasm. 2. To remove vomitus, saliva, blood, and other material from the patient's airway. 3. Triple airway maneuver, or jaw thrust maneuver. 4. False. 5. Align the NPA on the side of the patient's face. Proper size is determined by selecting a device that extends from the tip of the nose to the angle of the jaw or the tip of the ear. 6. Patient with an intact gag reflex, patient with known or suspected esophageal disease, patient known to have ingested a caustic substance, suspected upper airway obstruction caused by laryngeal foreign body or pathology, patient less than 4 feet tall.

TECHNIQUES OF ARTIFICIAL VENTILATION

Adequate oxygenation requires an open airway (Table 2-1) *and* adequate air exchange. After the airway has been opened, determine if the patient's breathing is adequate or inadequate. If respiratory efforts are inadequate, the patient's breathing may be assisted by forcing air into the lungs (i.e., delivering positive-pressure ventilations).

1. Several methods may be used to deliver positive-pressure ventilation:
   a. Mouth-to-mask ventilation
   b. Bag-valve-mask ventilation, one-person, or two-person (preferred)
   c. Automatic transport ventilators
   d. Flow-restricted oxygen-powered ventilation devices

Table 2-1 Airway Adjuncts

Device	Indications	Sizing
Oropharyngeal airway (oral airway, OPA)	• Maintaining open airway in unresponsive patient • Bite block after insertion of ETT or oral gastric tube	Corner of mouth to tip of earlobe or angle of jaw
Nasopharyngeal airway (nasal airway, nasal trumpet, NPA)	• Maintaining open airway when use of an OPA is contra-indicated or impossible	From the tip of the nose to the angle of the jaw or the tip of the ear
Esophageal-tracheal combitube (ETC)	• Difficult face mask fit (beards, absence of teeth) • Deep unresponsiveness, cardiac and/or respiratory arrest • Patient in whom intubation has been unsuccessful and ventilation is difficult • Patient in whom airway management is necessary but health care provider is untrained in the technique of visualized orotracheal intubation • When bag-valve-mask ventilation is inadequate or is causing excessive gastric distention	Two sizes: 37 Fr size is used for patients between 4 and 5 feet; tall; 41 Fr size is used for patients over 5 feet tall
Pharyngotracheal lumen airway (PTL)	• Difficult face mask fit (beards, absence of teeth) • Deep unresponsiveness, cardiac and/or respiratory arrest • Patient in whom intubation has been unsuccessful and ventilation is difficult • Patient in whom airway management is necessary but the healthcare provider is untrained in the technique of visualized orotracheal intubation • When bag-valve-mask ventilation is inadequate or is causing excessive gastric distention	One size: Do not use in patients less than 5 feet or more than 6 feet 7 inches tall or patients less than 14 years of age
Laryngeal mask airway (LMA)	• Difficult face mask fit (beards, absence of teeth) • Patient in whom intubation has been unsuccessful and ventilation is difficult • Patient in whom airway management is necessary but health care provider is untrained in the technique of visualized orotracheal intubation • Many elective surgical procedures	Because masks are available in several sizes, the LMA can be used in patients of all ages, from neonates to adults.
Cuffed oropharyngeal airway (COPA)	• For use in the spontaneously breathing patient with no risk of aspiration • May be useful during cardiac and/or respiratory arrest	Insertion technique same as that for conventional OPA. Typically, correct size is one size larger than conventional OPA.

> *Regardless of the method used, effective positive-pressure ventilation requires the delivery of an adequate volume of air at an appropriate rate.*

Mouth-to-Mask Ventilation

1. Description and function
    a. The device used for mouth-to-mask ventilation is commonly called a **pocket mask** or pocket face mask. The pocket mask is a transparent semi-rigid mask that is sealed around the mouth and nose of an adult, child, or infant (Figure 2-35)

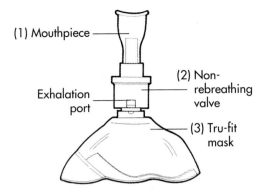

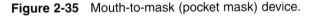

(1) Mouthpiece

Exhalation
port

(2) Non-
rebreathing
valve

(3) Tru-fit
mask

Figure 2-35   Mouth-to-mask (pocket mask) device.

    b. A pocket mask should be:
      (1) Made of transparent material to allow evaluation of the patient's lip color and detection of vomitus, secretions, or other substances
      (2) Capable of a tight seal on the face, covering the mouth and nose
      (3) Fitted with an oxygen inlet to allow the delivery of increased oxygen concentrations to the patient
      (4) Equipped with a standard 15- to 22-mm connector
      (5) Available in one average size for adults, with additional sizes for infants and children
      (6) (Ideally) equipped with a one-way valve that diverts the patient's exhaled gas, reducing the risk of infection

2. Tidal volumes and inspiratory times (adult patient)[12]
    a. If oxygen *is not* available, tidal volumes and inspiratory times for mouth-to-mask ventilation should be approximately 10 mL/kg (700 to 1000 mL) delivered **over 2 seconds** (Class IIa) and sufficient to make the chest rise
    b. If oxygen *is* provided, lower tidal volumes are recommended (Class IIb)—a tidal volume of approximately 6 to 7 mL/kg (400 to 600 mL) given **over 1 to 2 seconds** until the chest rises

3. Inspired oxygen concentrations
    a. Without supplemental oxygen—16% to 17% (exhaled air)
    b. Mouth-to-mask breathing combined with supplemental oxygen at a minimum flow rate of 10 L/min—50%

4. Advantages
    a. Aesthetically more acceptable than mouth-to-mouth ventilation
    b. Easy to teach and learn
    c. Provides physical barrier between the rescuer and the patient's nose, mouth, and secretions
    d. Reduces the risk of exposure to infectious disease
    e. Use of a one-way valve at the ventilation port eliminates exposure to patient's exhaled air
    f. If the patient resumes spontaneous breathing, the mask can be used as a simple face mask to deliver 40% to 60% oxygen by administering supplemental oxygen through the oxygen inlet on the mask (if so equipped)
    g. A greater tidal volume can be delivered with mouth-to-mask ventilation than with a bag-valve-mask device. (Both of the rescuer's hands can be used to secure the mask in place while simultaneously maintaining proper head position, and with the rescuer's vital capacity to compensate for leaks, the result is greater lung ventilation[13])

Some mouth-to-mask devices are disposable, others are reusable. Some have an oxygen inlet on the mask, allowing delivery of supplemental oxygen; others do not.

h. With mouth-to-mask ventilation, the rescuer can feel the **compliance** (resistance of the patient's lung tissue to ventilation) of the patient's lungs

5. Disadvantages
   a. Rescuer fatigue
6. Technique
   a. Cephalic technique
      (1) Rescuer is positioned directly above the victim's head, permitting the rescuer to observe the victim's chest while delivering ventilations
         (a) A single rescuer can use this technique when the patient is in respiratory arrest (but not cardiac arrest) or when two-rescuer CPR is being performed
      (2) If not already attached, connect a one-way valve to the ventilation port on the mask and connect oxygen tubing to the oxygen inlet on the mask (Figure 2-36). Set the oxygen flow rate at 10 to 15 L/min
      (3) Using personal protective equipment, position yourself at the top of the supine patient's head. Open the patient's airway with a head-tilt/chin-lift or, if trauma is suspected, perform the jaw thrust without head-tilt maneuver. If needed, clear the patient's airway of secretions or vomitus. If the patient is unresponsive, insert an OPA
      (4) Select a mask of appropriate size and place it on the patient's face.
         (a) Apply the narrow portion (apex) of the mask over the bridge of the patient's nose and stabilize it in place with your thumbs
         (b) Lower the mask over the patient's face and mouth
         (c) Use the remaining fingers of both hands to stabilize the wide end (base) of the mask over the groove between the lower lip and chin and maintain proper head position

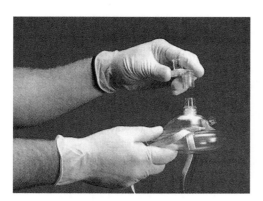

Figure 2-36 Mouth-to-mask ventilation. If not already attached, connect a one-way valve to the ventilation port on the mask and connect oxygen tubing to the oxygen inlet on the mask.

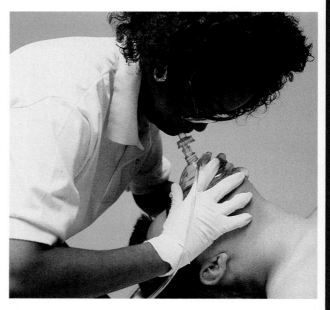

Figure 2-37 Apply the mask to the patient's face and stabilize it in place. Before each ventilation, take a deep breath to optimize the amount of oxygen in your exhaled air. Ventilate the patient through the one-way valve on the top of the mask, slowly delivering each breath. Observe for chest rise.

Selection of a mask of proper size is essential to ensuring a good seal. A mask of correct size should extend from the bridge of the nose to the groove between the lower lip and chin. If the mask is not properly positioned and a tight seal maintained, air will leak from between the mask and the patient's face, resulting in less tidal volume delivery to the patient.

If an assistant is available, cricoid pressure should be applied. This technique takes advantage of the rigid cartilaginous rings of the trachea to occlude the esophagus. Applying cricoid pressure helps minimize inflation of the stomach during ventilation, reducing the likelihood of vomiting and aspiration.

(5) Take a deep breath before each ventilation to optimize the amount of oxygen in your exhaled air. Ventilate the patient through the one-way valve on the top of the mask and deliver slow, steady breaths (Figure 2-37)
  (a) Stop ventilation when adequate chest rise is observed. Allow the patient to exhale between breaths
  (b) Adequate ventilation is being provided if you see the chest rise and fall with each breath and you hear and feel air escape during exhalation
b. Lateral technique
  (1) Rescuer is positioned at the victim's side
  (2) Used when performing one-rescuer CPR because the rescuer can maintain the same position for both rescue breathing and chest compressions

Bag-Valve-Mask (BVM) Ventilation

Ventilation of patients in cardiac arrest often requires higher than usual airway pressures. To effectively ventilate a patient during CPR, these pressures may exceed the limits of the pop-off valve. Thus a pop-off valve may prevent generation of sufficient tidal volume to overcome the increase in airway resistance. Disabling the pop-off valve, or using a BVM with no pop-off valve, helps ensure delivery of adequate tidal volumes to the patient during resuscitation. **Note:** higher than usual ventilation pressures may also be needed in situations involving near-drowning, pulmonary edema, and asthma.

1. Description and function
  a. BVM is the most common mechanical aid used to deliver positive-pressure ventilation in emergency care
  b. Consists of a self-inflating bag, a nonrebreathing valve with an adapter that can be attached to a mask, ET tube or other invasive airway device, and an oxygen inlet valve (Figure 2-38)
  c. A bag-valve-mask may also be referred to as a *bag-mask device* or *bag-mask resuscitator* (when the mask is used), or a *bag-valve device* (when the mask is not used; i.e., when ventilating a patient with an ETT in place)
  d. BVM should:
    (1) Consist of a self-refilling bag that is disposable (or easily cleaned and sterilized), and easy to grip and compress
    (2) Be made of transparent material to allow evaluation of the patient's lip color and detection of vomitus, secretions, or other substances
    (3) Capable of a tight seal on the face, covering the mouth and nose
    (4) Include a non-jam valve system that can accommodate a maximum oxygen inlet flow of 30 L/min
    (5) Have either no pop-off valve (pressure-release valve) or a pop-off valve that can be disabled during resuscitation
      (a) To disable a pop-off valve, depress the valve with a finger during ventilation or twist the pop-off valve into the closed position
    (6) Have standard 15- to 22-mm fittings to allow for attachment of the device to a standard mask, ETT, or other airway management device
    (7) Include a system for delivering high concentrations of oxygen with an oxygen reservoir and supplemental oxygen source

(8) Have a nonrebreathing valve that does not permit the patient's exhaled gases to escape into the bag

(9) Perform satisfactorily under all common environmental conditions and temperature extremes

e. BVMs are available in adult, child, and infant sizes. Most adult devices are capable of storing approximately 1600 mL of air.

2. Oxygen delivery

a. BVM used without supplemental oxygen will deliver 21% oxygen (room air) to the patient. (Figure 2-39)

b. BVM should be connected to an oxygen source

(1) Attach one end of a piece of oxygen connecting tubing to the oxygen inlet on the BVM and the other end to an oxygen regulator

(2) A BVM used with supplemental oxygen set at a flow rate of 15 L/min will deliver approximately 40% to 60% oxygen to the patient. (Figure 2-40)

c. An oxygen-collecting device (reservoir) is attached to the BVM to deliver high concentration oxygen

(1) The reservoir collects a volume of 100% oxygen equal to the capacity of the bag. After squeezing the bag, the bag reexpands, drawing in 100% oxygen from the reservoir into the bag

(2) BVM used with supplemental oxygen (set at a flow rate of 15 L/min) and an attached reservoir will deliver approximately 90% to 100% oxygen to the patient (Figure 2-41)

3. Tidal volumes and inspiratory times (adult patient)

a. If oxygen is available, lower tidal volumes are recommended—a tidal volume of approximately 6 to 7 mL/kg (400 to 600 mL) given over 1 to 2 seconds until the chest rises (Class IIb)[12]

b. If oxygen *is not* available, tidal volumes and inspiratory times for bag-valve-mask ventilation should be approximately 10 mL/kg (700 to 1000 mL) delivered **over 2 seconds** and sufficient to make the chest rise (Class IIa)

In a recent study, researchers concluded that "smaller tidal volumes of approximately 6 mL/kg (−1) (approximately 500 mL) given with a pediatric self-inflatable bag and room air maintain adequate carbon dioxide elimination but do not result in sufficient oxygenation during bag-valve-mask ventilation. Thus, if small (6 mL/kg [−1]) tidal volumes are being used during bag-valve-mask ventilation, additional oxygen is necessary. Accordingly, when additional oxygen during bag-valve-mask ventilation is not available, only large tidal volumes of approximately 11 mL/kg (−1) were able to maintain both sufficient oxygenation and carbon dioxide elimination."[14] The delivery of lower tidal volumes should reduce the risk of gastric inflation and its consequences.

---

4. Advantages

a. Provides a means for delivery of an oxygen-enriched mixture to the patient

b. Conveys a sense of compliance of patient's lungs to the BVM operator

c. Provides a means for immediate ventilatory support

d. Can be used with the spontaneously breathing patient as well as an apneic patient

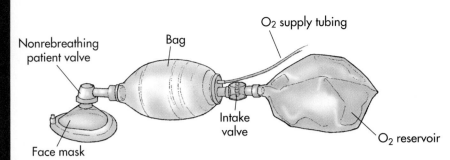

Figure 2-38 Components of a bag-valve-mask device.

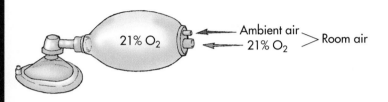

Figure 2-39 A BVM used without supplemental oxygen will deliver 21% oxygen (room air).

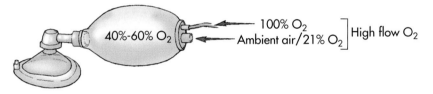

Figure 2-40 A BVM used with supplemental oxygen set at a flow rate of 15 L/min will deliver approximately 40% to 60% oxygen to the patient.

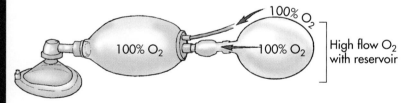

Figure 2-41 A BVM used wih supplemental oxygen (set at a flow rate of 15 L/min) and an attached reservoir will deliver approximately 90% to 100% oxygen to the patient.

5. Disadvantages
   a. The most frequent problem with the BVM is the inability to provide adequate ventilatory volumes. This is caused by difficulty in providing a leak-proof seal to the face while simultaneously maintaining an open airway
   b. Should only be used by trained operators (ideally a two-rescuer operation—one to hold the mask to the face and maintain an open airway, the other to compress the bag with two hands)
      (1) Difficult to use by inexperienced operators
   c. Gastric distention

> *Gastric distention is a complication of positive-pressure ventilation that can lead to regurgitation and subsequent aspiration. Gastric distention also restricts movement of the diaphragm, impeding ventilation.*

6. Technique
   a. Using personal protective equipment, position yourself at the top of the supine patient's head
      (1) Open the patient's airway using a head-tilt/chin-lift or, if trauma is suspected, perform the jaw thrust without head-tilt maneuver
      (2) If needed, clear the patient's airway of secretions or vomitus
      (3) If the patient is unresponsive, insert an OPA
   b. Select a mask of appropriate size and place it on the patient's face
      (1) Apply the narrow portion (apex) of the mask over the bridge of the patient's nose and the wide end (base) of the mask over the groove between the lower lip and chin
      (2) If the mask has a large, round cuff surrounding a ventilation port, center the port over the mouth
      (3) Stabilize the mask in place with your thumb and forefinger, creating a "C." Use the remaining fingers of the same hand to maintain proper head position by lifting the jaw along the bony portion of the mandible. The remaining fingers create an "E"
   c. Connect the bag to the mask, if not already done. Connect the bag to oxygen at 15 L/min and attach a reservoir
   d. If you are alone, squeeze the bag with one hand, or with one hand and your arm or chest (Figure 2-42). If an assistant is available, ask the assistant to squeeze the bag with two hands until the patient's chest rises while you press the mask firmly against the patient's face with both hands and simultaneously maintain proper head position (Figure 2-43)

BVM ventilation is optimally a two-rescuer operation—one to hold the mask to the face (ensuring a good mask-to-face seal) and maintain an open airway, the other to compress the bag with two hands.

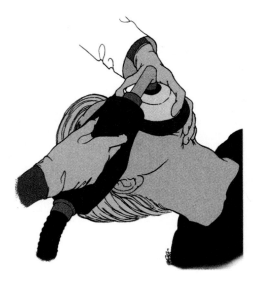

Figure 2-42 Bag-valve-mask ventilation—one-person technique.

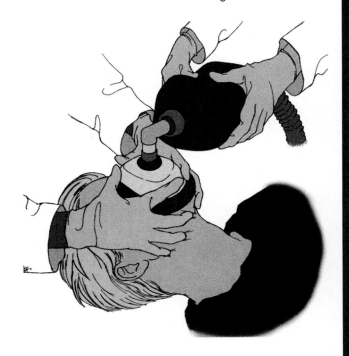

Figure 2-43 Bag-valve-mask ventilation—two-person technique.

Slow, gentle ventilation helps minimize the risk of gastric inflation.

e. Observe the rise and fall of the patient's chest with each ventilation. Stop ventilation when adequate chest rise is observed. Allow for adequate exhalation after each ventilation
  (1) Ventilate the adult patient once every 5 seconds (12 ventilations/min). Ventilations should be delivered slowly, allowing the bag to refill completely between ventilations

7. Troubleshooting bag-valve-mask ventilation
  a. If the chest does not rise and fall with bag-valve-mask ventilation, reevaluate:
    (1) Reassess head position; reposition the airway, and reattempt to ventilate
    (2) Inadequate tidal volume delivery may be the result of an improper mask seal or incomplete bag compression
      (a) If air is escaping from under the mask, reposition fingers and mask
    (3) Reevaluate effectiveness of bag compression
      (a) Check for obstruction
      (b) Lift the jaw
      (c) Suction the airway as needed
  b. If the chest still does not rise, select an alternative method of positive-pressure ventilation (e.g., pocket mask, automatic transport ventilator)

French researchers assessed 1502 patients for 10 potential markers of difficult mask ventilation (DMV) and correlated the findings with actual mask ventilation difficulty during elective anesthesia.[15] DMV was defined as the inability of an unassisted anesthesiologist to maintain oxygen saturation above 92% or to prevent or reverse signs of inadequate ventilation during positive-pressure mask ventilation under general anesthesia.

These researchers identified five factors that can be used to predict difficult mask ventilation: age older than 55 years, body mass index greater than 26 kg/m^2, presence of a beard, lack of teeth, and a history of regular snoring. The presence of any two of these attributes was 72% sensitive and 73% specific for DMV. DMV was reported in 75 patients (5% of patients), with one case of impossible ventilation. The anesthesiologist anticipated DMV in only 13 patients (17% of the DMV cases).

The fact that there was only one case of impossible mask ventilation in this study emphasizes the importance of bag-valve-mask ventilation as a rescue technique when intubation is unsuccessful.

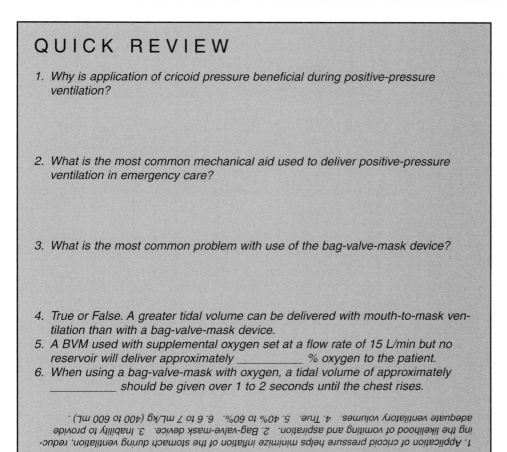

QUICK REVIEW

1. *Why is application of cricoid pressure beneficial during positive-pressure ventilation?*

2. *What is the most common mechanical aid used to deliver positive-pressure ventilation in emergency care?*

3. *What is the most common problem with use of the bag-valve-mask device?*

4. *True or False. A greater tidal volume can be delivered with mouth-to-mask ventilation than with a bag-valve-mask device.*
5. *A BVM used with supplemental oxygen set at a flow rate of 15 L/min but no reservoir will deliver approximately _____ % oxygen to the patient.*
6. *When using a bag-valve-mask with oxygen, a tidal volume of approximately _____ should be given over 1 to 2 seconds until the chest rises.*

1. Application of cricoid pressure helps minimize inflation of the stomach during ventilation, reducing the likelihood of vomiting and aspiration. 2. Bag-valve-mask device. 3. Inability to provide adequate ventilatory volumes. 4. True. 5. 40% to 60%. 6. 6 to 7 mL/kg (400 to 600 mL).

Automatic Transport Ventilators (ATVs)

1. Description and function
   a. The automatic transport ventilator is a device used to provide positive pressure ventilation
      (1) Time-cycled, gas-powered ATVs are used in the prehospital setting or for intrahospital transport when caring for patients who require ventilatory support (Figure 2-44)
      (2) Studies have demonstrated that ATVs and self-inflating bag-valve devices can maintain a satisfactory minute ventilation and adequate arterial blood oxygenation
   b. ATV should have the following minimum features[2]:
      (1) Standard 15- to 22-mm adapter for a face mask, tracheal tube, or other airway adjunct
      (2) Lightweight (4 kg), compact, rugged design
      (3) Capability of operating under temperature extremes
      (4) Default peak inspiratory pressure limit of 60 cm H_2O, adjustable from 20 to 80 cm H_2O
      (5) An audible alarm that sounds when the peak inspiratory limiting pressure is generated. This alerts the rescuer that poor lung compliance or high airway resistance is resulting in a diminished tidal volume delivery
      (6) Minimal gas compression volume in the breathing circuit
      (7) Ability to deliver 50% to 100% oxygen with each ventilation
      (8) Ability to provide a default inspiratory time of 2 seconds in adults and 1 second in children and default inspiratory flow of approximately 30 L/min in adults and 15 L/min in children, with

the ability to adjust inspiratory time and flow once the patient is intubated with a tracheal tube or alternative airway

(9) Ability to provide a default rate of 10 breaths/min for adults and 20 breaths/min for children, with the ability to adjust the rate once the patient is intubated with a tracheal tube or alternative airway

(10) At least two controls (one for rate and one for tidal volume)

(11) Alarms to indicate low pressure in the oxygen cylinder, disconnection from the ventilator, or a low battery

2. Indications

a. Patients requiring ventilatory assistance due to a decreased level of responsiveness or apnea

3. Advantages

a. Frees the rescuer for other tasks when used in intubated patients

b. In patients who are not intubated, the rescuer has both hands free for mask application and airway maintenance

c. Cricoid pressure can be applied with one hand while the other seals the mask on the face

d. Once set, provides a specific tidal volume, respiratory rate, and minute ventilation

4. Disadvantages

a. Need for an oxygen source (or, sometimes, electric power)

b. Some ATVs should not be used in children <5 years of age

5. Technique

a. Test the ATV to ensure it is working properly before using it on any patient

b. If not already set, set the tidal volume and ventilation rate

c. Occlude the outlet adapter. An audible pressure limit alarm should sound with the next cycle (breath) to ensure that the pressure limit is intact and the lungs will not be over-inflated

d. Assess lung compliance and chest rise with a bag-valve device

e. Attach the patient valve assembly to the airway device (ETT, mask, or airway adjunct)

f. Assess ventilations, listen for bilateral lung sounds, and observe for proper chest rise

g. Count the number of ventilator cycles for 1 full minute to ensure proper correlation with the breaths/minute setting on the ATV

h. Monitor the device to ensure delivery of adequate tidal volume and ventilation rate

> ATVs should only be used by persons properly trained in the use of the device.

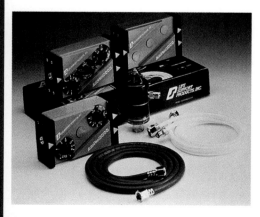

Figure 2-44 Automatic transport ventilators: the Autovent 1000, 2000, and 3000.

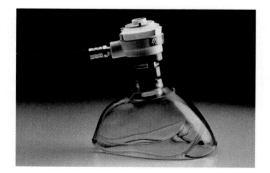

Figure 2-45 Flow-restricted oxygen-powered ventilation device.

Flow-Restricted Oxygen-Powered Ventilation Devices

Class Indeterminate

1. Description and function
   a. Flow-restricted, oxygen-powered ventilation devices were formerly called *demand valves* (Figure 2-45)
   b. Allows positive-pressure ventilation with 100% oxygen
   c. Can be attached to a face mask, ETT, tracheostomy tube
   d. Consists of a high-pressure tubing connecting the oxygen supply and a valve that is activated by a lever or push button; when the valve is open, oxygen flows into the patient
2. Advantages
   a. Easy to use
   b. Provides high oxygen concentrations and good volume delivery
3. Disadvantages
   a. Gastric distention in patients who are not intubated
   b. Inability to feel compliance of patient's lungs
   c. Barotrauma to the lungs (e.g., pneumothorax, subcutaneous emphysema)
4. Contraindications
   a. Not for use in pediatric patients
5. Technique
   a. Using personal protective equipment, open the airway
   b. If no trauma is suspected, use a head-tilt/chin-lift
   c. If trauma is suspected, immobilize the head and neck and ask an assistant to hold the patient's head manually to prevent movement. Open the airway using a jaw thrust without head-tilt maneuver
   d. If the patient is unresponsive, size and insert an OPA
   e. Attach an adult mask and obtain a mask seal. Connect the device to the mask, if not already done
   f. Trigger the device until the patient's chest rises. Repeat once every 5 seconds

CRICOID PRESSURE

1. Purpose
   a. Cricoid pressure (Sellick maneuver) compresses and occludes the esophagus between the cricoid cartilage and the fifth and sixth cervical vertebrae
      (1) Minimizes gastric distention and aspiration during positive-pressure ventilation
      (2) Cricoid pressure is *not* intended to facilitate visualization of the vocal cords during intubation
2. Technique
   a. Locate the cricoid cartilage (Figure 2-46)
   b. Apply firm pressure on the cricoid cartilage with the thumb and index or middle finger, just lateral to the midline (Figure 2-47)
      (1) If active regurgitation occurs while performing the Sellick maneuver, release cricoid pressure to avoid rupture of the stomach or esophagus
   c. During ET intubation, cricoid pressure should be maintained until the ET tube cuff is inflated and proper tube position is verified

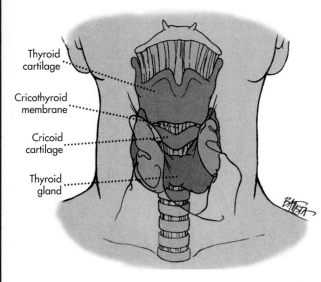

Figure 2-46 Landmarks of the cricoid cartilage.

Thyroid cartilage
Cricothyroid membrane
Cricoid cartilage
Thyroid gland

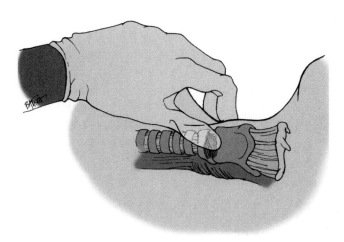

Figure 2-47 Applying cricoid pressure.

3. Complications
   a. Laryngeal trauma with excessive force
   b. Esophageal rupture from unrelieved high gastric pressures
   c. Excessive pressure may obstruct the trachea in small children

> *If active regurgitation occurs while performing the Sellick maneuver, release cricoid pressure to avoid rupture of the stomach or esophagus.*

OXYGEN ADMINISTRATION DEVICES

Low-Flow Oxygen Delivery Systems

Nasal Cannula (Nasal Prongs)

1. Description and function
   a. Piece of plastic tubing with two soft prongs that project from the tubing. The prongs are inserted into the patient's nares, and the tubing secured to the patient's face (Figure 2-48). Oxygen flows from the cannula into the patient's nasopharynx, which acts as an anatomical reservoir
   b. Although the actual inspired oxygen concentration depends on the patient's respiratory rate and depth, the nasal cannula can deliver oxygen concentrations of approximately 25% to 45% at 1 to 6 L/min flow
      (1) In the adult patient, oxygen delivery by means of a nasal cannula does not need to be humidified if the flow rate is ≤4 L/min.
2. Advantages
   a. Comfortable, well tolerated by most patients

Formula = 4 × the oxygen flow rate in L/min + 21% (ambient air)

- 1 L/min = 25%
- 2 L/min = 29%
- 3 L/min = 33%
- 4 L/min = 37%
- 5 L/min = 41%
- 6 L/min = 45%

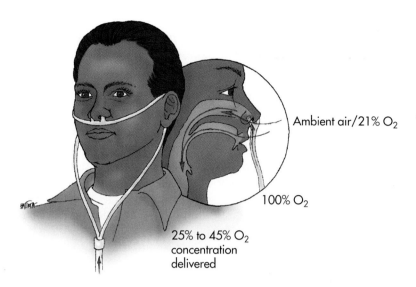

Ambient air/21% O$_2$

100% O$_2$

25% to 45% O$_2$
concentration
delivered

Figure 2-48 At flow rates of 1-6 L/min, a nasal cannula can deliver an oxygen concentration of 25% to 45%.

   b. Does not interfere with patient assessment or impede patient communication with health care personnel
   c. Allows for talking and eating
   d. No rebreathing of expired air
   e. Can be used with mouth breathers
   f. Useful in patients predisposed to carbon dioxide retention (COPD)
  3. Disadvantages
   a. Can only be used in the spontaneously breathing patient
   b. Easily displaced
   c. Nasal passages must be patent
   d. Drying of mucosa
   e. May cause sinus pain

Reservoir Systems

Simple Face Mask (Standard Mask)

  1. Description and function
   a. A plastic reservoir designed to fit over the patient's nose and mouth
   b. The mask is secured around the patient's head by means of an elastic strap
   c. Internal capacity of the mask produces a reservoir effect
   d. Small holes on each side of the mask allow for the passage of inspired and expired air. Supplemental oxygen is delivered through a small diameter tube connected to the base of the mask (Figure 2-49)
   e. At 6 to 10 L/min, the simple face mask can provide an inspired oxygen concentration of approximately 40% to 60%
      (1) Recommended flow rate is 8 to 10 L/min
      (2) Patient's actual inspired oxygen concentration will vary because the amount of air that mixes with supplemental oxygen depends on the patient's inspiratory flow rate

> When using a simple face mask, the oxygen flow rate must be higher than 5 L/min to flush the accumulation of the patient's exhaled carbon dioxide from the mask.

2. Advantages
   a. Delivery of higher oxygen concentration than by nasal cannula
3. Disadvantages
   a. Can only be used with spontaneously breathing patients
   b. Not tolerated well by severely dyspneic patients
   c. Can be uncomfortable
   d. Difficult to hear the patient speaking when the device is in place
   e. Must be removed at meals
   f. Requires a tight face seal to prevent leakage of oxygen
   g. Oxygen flow rates of more than 10 L/min do not enhance delivered oxygen concentration

Partial Rebreather (Rebreathing) Mask

1. Description and function
   a. Provides moderate oxygen concentrations through a low-flow oxygen delivery system
   b. Similar to a simple oxygen mask but has an attached oxygen-collecting device (reservoir) at the base of the mask that is filled before patient use

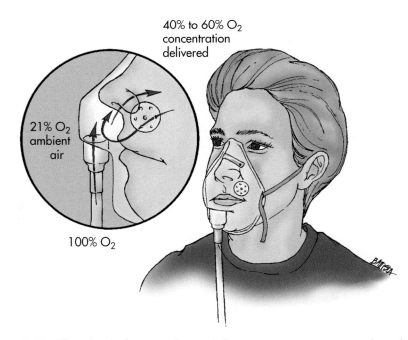

40% to 60% O_2 concentration delivered

21% O_2 ambient air

100% O_2

Figure 2-49 The simple face mask can deliver an oxygen concentration of 40% to 60% with an oxygen flow rate of 6 to 10 L/min. (Recommended flow rate is 8 to 10 L/min).

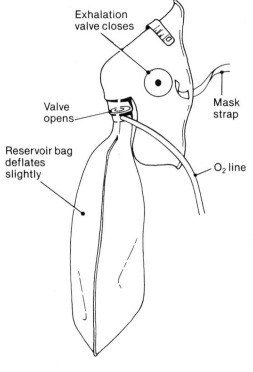

INHALATION

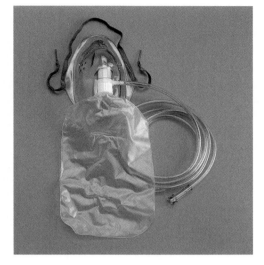

Figure 2-50 The partial rebreather mask has an attached oxygen-collecting device (reservoir) at the base of the mask. The reservoir collects oxygen and allows some of the patient's exhaled air to enter the reservoir bag and be reused.

Figure 2-51 In the nonrebreather mask, oxygen collects in the reservoir (bag) below the mask before inhalation. A one-way valve separates the reservoir from the mask and directs exhaled air out through the side ports of the mask.

    (1) 100% oxygen is delivered through oxygen tubing to the reservoir bag. The reservoir collects the oxygen and allows some of the patient's exhaled air (approximately equal to the volume of the patient's anatomical dead space) to enter the reservoir bag and be reused (Figure 2-50)

    (2) Oxygen concentration of the patient's exhaled air, combined with the supply of 100% oxygen, allows the use of oxygen flow rates lower than those necessary for a nonrebreather mask

    (3) Depending on the patient's respiratory pattern, oxygen concentrations of 35% to 60% can be delivered when a high enough oxygen flow rate (typically 6 to 10 L/min) is used to prevent the reservoir bag from collapsing completely on inspiration

2. Advantages
   a. Delivery of higher oxygen concentration than by nasal cannula
   b. Inspired oxygen is not mixed with ambient air
3. Disadvantages
   a. Can only be used with spontaneously breathing patients
   b. Not tolerated well by severely dyspneic patients
   c. Can be uncomfortable
   d. Difficult to hear the patient speaking when the device is in place
   e. Must be removed at meals
   f. Requires a tight face seal to prevent leakage of oxygen
   g. Oxygen flow rates of more than 10 L/min do not enhance delivered oxygen concentration

Nonrebreather (nonrebreathing) mask

1. Description and function
   a. Provides high oxygen concentrations through a low-flow oxygen delivery system
   b. Similar to partial rebreather masks but do not permit mixing of the patient's exhaled air with 100% oxygen
   c. Has a one-way valve that separates the reservoir (bag) from the mask and directs exhaled air out through the side ports on the mask. This valve prevents the patient's exhaled air from returning to the reservoir bag (thus the term *nonrebreather*), ensuring a supply of 100% oxygen to the patient with minimal dilution from the entrainment of ambient air (Figure 2-51)
   d. Provides a higher inspired oxygen concentration than the nasal cannula, simple face mask, and partial rebreather mask
   e. Delivery device of choice when high concentrations of oxygen are needed in the spontaneously breathing patient because it can consistently deliver an inspired oxygen concentration of up to 100% at 10 to 15 L/min flow
      (1) Fill the reservoir bag with oxygen before placing the mask on the patient
      (2) After placing the mask on the patient, adjust the flow rate so the bag does not completely deflate when the patient inhales.

Despite its ability to deliver high oxygen concentrations, the nonrebreather mask is considered a low-flow device if neither or only one of the side ports on the mask are covered.

> *When using a partial rebreather or nonrebreather mask, ensure that the bag does not collapse when the patient inhales. Should the bag collapse, increase the delivered oxygen by 2-liter increments until the bag remains inflated. The reservoir bag must remain at least two-thirds full so that sufficient supplemental oxygen is available for each breath.*

2. Advantages
   a. Higher oxygen concentration delivered than by nasal cannula, simple face mask, and partial rebreather mask
3. Disadvantages
   a. Can only be used with spontaneously breathing patients
   b. Mask must fit snugly on the patient's face to prevent room air from mixing with oxygen inhaled from the reservoir bag

High-Flow Oxygen Delivery Systems

Venturi Mask

1. Description and function
   a. High-flow oxygen delivery system that delivers low- to medium-concentration oxygen
   b. Mask fits over the patient's nose and mouth and contains a short corrugated hose with a jet orifice that is connected to oxygen supply tubing (Figure 2-52)
      (1) Oxygen under pressure is forced through a small jet orifice entering the mask. As the oxygen passes through the orifice, it draws ambient air into the mask
      (2) Resulting mixture is delivered to the patient through the face mask

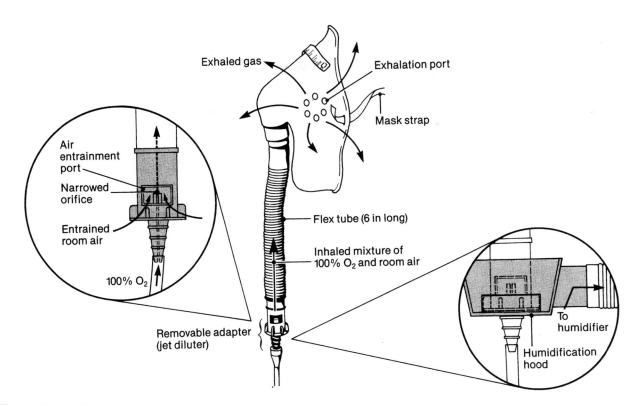

Figure 2-52 The Venturi mask fits over the patient's nose and mouth and contains a short corrugated hose with a jet orifice that is connected to oxygen supply tubing. Oxygen under pressure is forced through a small jet orifice entering the mask. As the oxygen passes through the orifice, it draws ambient air into the mask. The resulting mixture is delivered to the patient through the face mask.

    c. May be supplied with several color-coded adapters that alter the rate of oxygen flow past the air entrainment port
       (1) The mix of air and oxygen delivered to the patient is adjusted by changing adapters that attach to the base of the mask or by having an adjustable, rotating opening that changes the amount of air mixing with oxygen (Figure 2-53)
       (2) Typically delivers oxygen concentrations of 24%, 28%, 35%, 40%, or 50% oxygen
       (3) To obtain a precise inspired oxygen concentration (within 1%), the color-coded adapters indicate the specific flow rate at which the oxygen should be delivered
  2. Advantages
    a. Provides precise inspired oxygen concentration in a selected range
    b. Recommended for patients who rely on a hypoxic respiratory drive (e.g., COPD)
  3. Disadvantages
    a. Can only be used with spontaneously breathing patients
    b. Uncomfortable for prolonged use
    c. Must fit snugly

Table 2-2 provides a summary of oxygen percentage delivery by device.

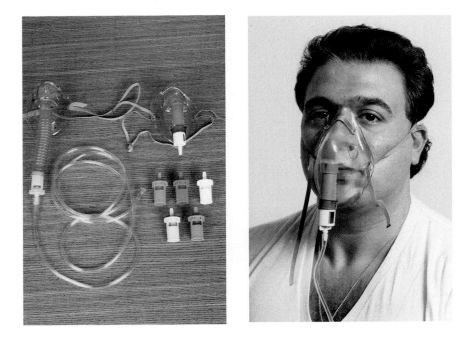

Figure 2-53 The Venturi mask may be supplied with several color-coded adapters that alter the rate of oxygen flow past the air entrainment port. The mix of air and oxygen delivered to the patient is adjusted by changing either the flow of oxygen or the size of the air entrainment port.

Table 2-2   Oxygen Percentage Delivery by Device

Device	Approximate Inspired Oxygen Concentration	Liter Flow (Liters/Minute)
Low-Flow Oxygen Delivery Systems		
Nasal cannula	25% to 45%	1 to 6
Simple face mask	40% to 60%	6 to 10 (8 to 10 recommended)
Partial rebreather mask	35% to 60%	6 to 10
Nonrebreather mask	60% to 100%	10 to 15
High-Flow Oxygen Delivery Systems		
Venturi mask	24% to 50%	4 to 8

ADVANCED AIRWAY MANAGEMENT

Endotracheal (ET) Intubation

1. Description and function
   a. **Endotracheal intubation** is an advanced airway procedure in which a tube is placed directly into the trachea
   b. May be performed for a variety of reasons, including the delivery of anesthesia, assisting a patient's breathing with positive-pressure ventilation, and protection of the patient's airway from aspiration
   c. Requires special equipment and supplies—laryngoscope handle, laryngoscope blades, extra batteries, ET tubes of various sizes, a 10-mL syringe for inflation of the ET tube cuff (if present), a stylet, a bag-valve-mask device with supplemental oxygen and a reservoir, suction equipment, a commercial tube-holder or tape, water-soluble lubricant, a bite-block or OPA, and an end-tidal CO_2 detector and/or esophageal detector
2. Laryngoscope
   a. An instrument that consists of a handle and blade used for examining the interior of the larynx

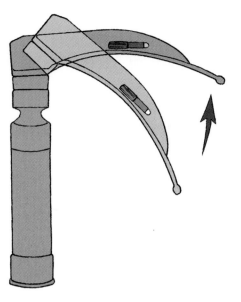

Figure 2-54 The bulb on the laryngoscope blade lights when the blade is attached to the laryngoscope handle and elevated to a right angle.

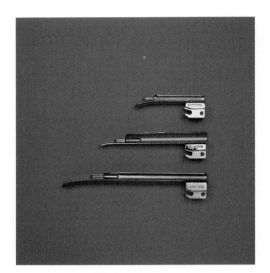

Figure 2-55 Straight laryngoscope blades.

    (1) Used to visualize the glottic opening (the space between the vocal cords)

    (2) A standard laryngoscope is made of plastic or stainless steel

  b. Laryngoscope handle contains the batteries for the light source

    (1) Attaches to a plastic or stainless steel blade that has a bulb located in the blade's distal tip. The point where the handle and the blade attach to make electrical contact is called the *fitting*

    (2) The bulb on the laryngoscope blade lights when the blade is attached to the laryngoscope handle and elevated to a right angle (Figure 2-54)

  c. Laryngoscope blades

    (1) Available in a variety of sizes ranging from 0 to 4.

      (a) Size #0 used for infants; size #4 blade is used for large adults

    (2) Select the appropriate blade size with the larygnoscope blade held next to the patient's face

      (a) Blade of proper size should reach between the patient's lips and larynx

      (b) If unsure of the correct size, it is usually best to select a blade that is too long, rather than too short

    (3) Two types of laryngoscope blades—straight and curved

      (a) Straight blade is also referred to as the *Miller, Wisconsin,* or *Flagg blade* (Figure 2-55)

        (i) During endotracheal intubation, the tip of the straight blade is positioned under the epiglottis. When the laryngoscope handle is lifted anteriorly, the blade directly lifts the epiglottis out of the way to expose the glottic opening (Figure 2-56)

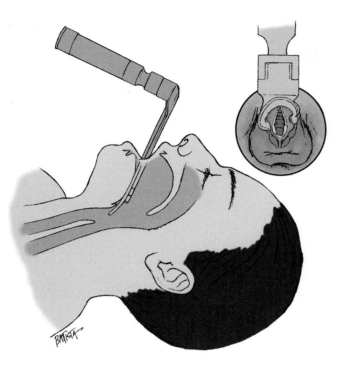

Figure 2-56 The tip of the straight blade is positioned under the epiglottis to expose the glottic opening.

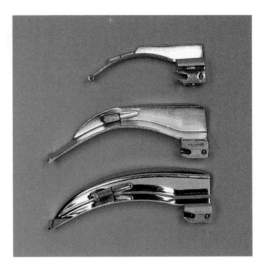

Figure 2-57 Curved laryngoscope blades.

    (b) Curved blade is also called the *MacIntosh blade* (Figure 2-57)
       (i) Inserted into the vallecula, the space, or "pocket" between the base of the tongue and the epiglottis
       (ii) When the laryngoscope handle is lifted anteriorly, the blade elevates the tongue and indirectly lifts the epiglottis, allowing visualization of the glottic opening (Figure 2-58)

3. Endotracheal tube
  a. Curved tube that is open at both ends
    (1) Standard 15-mm connector is located at the proximal end for attachment of various devices for delivery of positive-pressure ventilation
    (2) Distal end of the tube is beveled to facilitate placement between the vocal cords
  b. Cuff
    (1) Some ET tubes have an inflatable balloon cuff that surrounds the distal tip of the tube
      (a) When the distal cuff is inflated, it contacts the wall of the trachea as it expands, sealing off the trachea from the remainder of the pharynx, reducing the risk of aspiration
      (b) Cuff is attached to a one-way valve through a side tube with a pilot balloon that is used to indicate if the cuff is inflated (Figure 2-59)
      (c) Cuffed ET tubes are generally unnecessary in children less than 8 years of age because the narrowing of the cricoid cartilage serves as a natural cuff

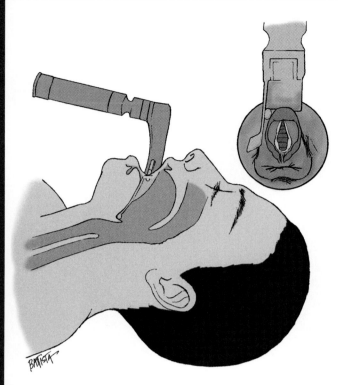

Figure 2-58 The curved blade is inserted into the vallecula, the space or "pocket" between the base of the tongue and the epiglottis.

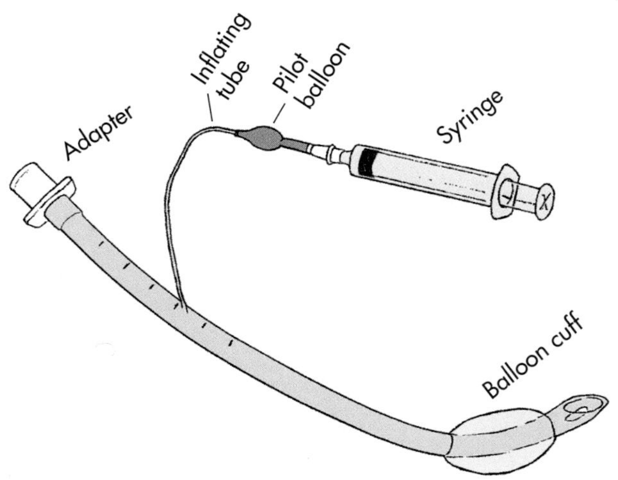

Figure 2-59 Components of the endotracheal tube.

c. Sizing
   (1) ET tubes are measured in millimeters (mm) by their internal diameter (ID) and external diameter (OD). Centimeter markings on the tube indicate the distance from the tip
   (2) ET tubes are available in lengths ranging from 12 cm to 32 cm. Internal tube diameters range from 2.5 mm to 4.5 mm (uncuffed) and 5.0 mm to 10.0 mm (cuffed)
   (3) Selection of an ET tube of the correct size is important
       (a) Select the largest tube size appropriate for the patient because larger tubes facilitate suctioning of secretions and decrease the work of breathing
       (b) An ET tube that is too small may provide too little airflow and may lead to the delivery of inadequate tidal volumes
       (c) A tube that is too large may cause tracheal edema and/or vocal cord damage
       (d) Common internal diameters of ET tubes for adults are typically from 7.0 mm to 8.5 mm. Most common sizes used for adults are:
           (i) Adult female: 7.0 to 8.0 mm ID
           (ii) Adult male: 8.0 to 8.5 mm ID
   (4) Because of the size variation in adults, it is important to have several sizes of tubes on hand
       (a) At a minimum, have the size tube most commonly used (see previously), plus a tube a half size smaller and another half size larger
       (b) When immediate ET tube placement is necessary, most adults can accept an ET tube with an internal diameter of at least 7.5 mm

Emergency Rule:
A 7.5 mm ETT may be used in most adults.

d. Distance or depth of insertion
   (1) When the ET tube has been properly placed, the centimeter markings on the side of the tube should be observed and recorded. This value is typically between the 19- and 23-cm mark at the front teeth
   (b) Average tube depth in males is 23 cm at the lips, 22 cm at the teeth
   (c) Average tube depth in women is 22 cm at the lips, 21 cm at the teeth
e. Stylet
   (1) A **stylet** is a flexible plastic-coated wire inserted into an ET tube and is used for molding and maintaining the shape of the tube (Figure 2-60)
   (2) When a stylet is used, the tip of the stylet must be recessed half an inch from the end of the ET tube to avoid trauma to the airway structures

> Endotracheal medications include:
> **A**tropine
> **L**idocaine
> **O**xygen
> **N**aloxone
> **E**pinephrine

4. Indications
   a. Inability of the patient to protect his or her own airway because of the absence of protective reflexes (e.g., coma, respiratory and/or cardiac arrest)
   b. Inability of the rescuer to ventilate the unresponsive patient with less invasive methods
   c. Present or impending airway obstruction/respiratory failure (e.g., inhalation injury, severe asthma, exacerbation of chronic obstructive pulmonary disease, severe pulmonary edema, severe flail chest, or pulmonary contusion)
   d. When prolonged ventilatory support is required
5. Advantages
   a. Isolates the airway
   b. Keeps the airway patent
   c. Reduces the risk of aspiration
   d. Ensures delivery of a high concentration of oxygen
   e. Permits suctioning of the trachea
   f. Provides a route for administration of some medications (ALONE—atropine, lidocaine, oxygen, naloxone [Narcan], epinephrine)
   g. Ensures delivery of a selected tidal volume to maintain lung inflation

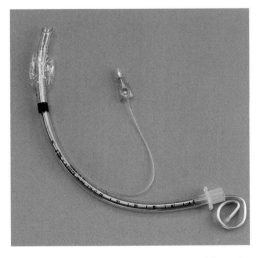

Figure 2-60 Endotracheal tube with stylet.

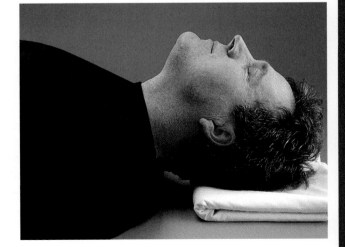

Figure 2-61 The sniffing position aligns the axes of the mouth, pharynx, and trachea.

6. Disadvantages
   a. Considerable training and experience required
   b. Special equipment needed
   c. Bypasses physiologic function of upper airway (e.g., warming, filtering, humidifying of inhaled air)
   d. Requires direct visualization of vocal cords
7. Technique
   a. Using personal protective equipment (at a minimum, use gloves, protective eyewear, and a mask), open the patient's airway with a head-tilt/chin-lift (or jaw thrust without head tilt if trauma is suspected). Ask an assistant to preoxygenate the patient while you auscultate bilateral lung sounds to establish a baseline
   b. While your assistant continues to preoxygenate the patient, assemble and prepare the equipment needed for intubation, including suction equipment
      (1) Select the proper size blade and then assemble the laryngoscope. Attach the blade to the handle and check the blade for a "white, bright light." After verifying the light is in working order, move the blade to its unlocked position to conserve battery life until the light is needed
      (2) Select the proper size ET tube and test the cuff for leaks. If there are no leaks, completely deflate the cuff. Leave the syringe filled with air attached to the inflation valve. If a stylet will be used, insert it into the ET tube, making sure that the end of the stylet is recessed at least half an inch from the tip of the ET tube. Bend the proximal end of the stylet over the ET tube to prevent it from sliding down into the tube. Lubricate the distal end of the ET tube with water-soluble lubricant
   c. Place the patient's head in the "sniffing" position to align the axes of the mouth, pharynx, and trachea (Figure 2-61). Open the patient's mouth and inspect the oral cavity. Remove dentures and/or debris, if present
      (1) Stop ventilations and remove the ventilation face mask and OPA (if present)
      (2) Do not exceed 30 seconds from ventilation to ventilation for each intubation attempt
   d. Direct an assistant to apply cricoid pressure and maintain pressure until the airway is secured
      (1) If the patient begins to actively vomit, discontinue cricoid pressure until the vomiting stops and the airway has been cleared
   e. Holding the laryngoscope in the left hand, and with the tip of the blade pointing away from you, insert the blade into the right side of the patient's mouth between the teeth, sweeping the tongue to the left (Figure 2-62)
   f. Advance the laryngoscope blade until the distal end reaches the base of the tongue (Figure 2-63)
   g. Lift the laryngoscope to elevate the mandible without putting pressure on the front teeth (Figure 2-64) and visualize the epiglottis (Figure 2-65). Suction the laryngopharynx as necessary

---

Margin notes:

A petroleum-based lubricant should *never* be used because it may damage the ET tube and cause tracheal inflammation.

Do **not** place the patient's head in this position if trauma is suspected. If trauma is suspected, a second assistant should apply in-line cervical spine stabilization

The laryngoscope is held in the left hand because most laryngoscopes are designed for right-handed individuals. This allows the dominant (right) hand to be used for manipulation of the ET tube

Do NOT use the patient's teeth or gums as a fulcrum. Do NOT allow the blade to touch the patient's teeth.

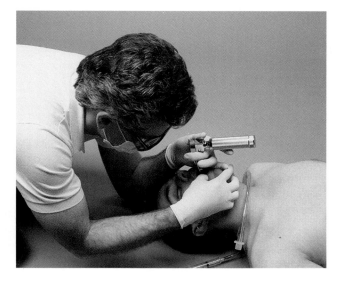

Figure 2-62   Holding the laryngoscope in the left hand and with the tip of the blade pointing away from you, insert the blade into the right side of the patient's mouth between the teeth, sweeping the tongue to the left.

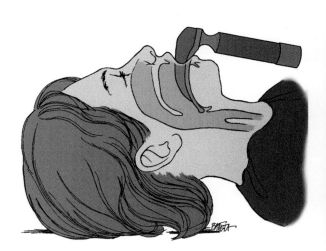

Figure 2-63   Advance the laryngoscope blade until the distal end reaches the base of the tongue.

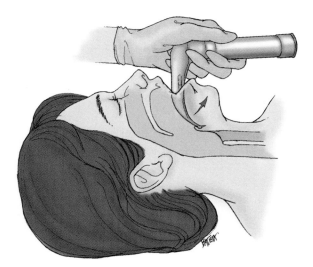

Figure 2-64   Lift the laryngoscope to elevate the mandible without putting pressure on the front teeth.

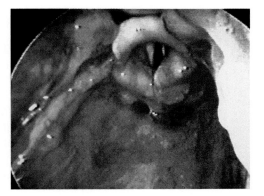

Figure 2-65   View of the epiglottis and vocal cords.

h. After visualizing the epiglottis, identify the vocal cords and place the blade in the proper position
   (1) If using a curved blade, advance the tip of the blade into the vallecula (Figures 2-66 and 2-67)
   (2) If using a straight blade, advance the tip under the epiglottis (Figure 2-68)

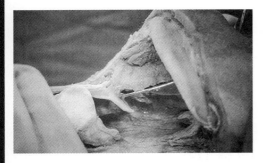

Figure 2-66 The tip of the curved blade is inserted into the vallecula.

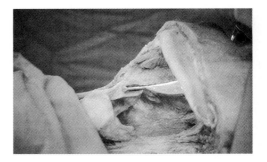

Figure 2-67 The curved blade is lifted anteriorly to expose the vocal cords.

Viewing the vocal cords may be facilitated with the use of the BURP (Backward, Upward, Rightward Pressure) technique. With this maneuver, the larynx is displaced in the three specific directions: (1) posteriorly against the cervical vertebrae, (2) superiorly as possible, and (3) slightly laterally to the right. This maneuver has been shown to improve visualization of the larynx more easily than simple back pressure on the larynx (cricoid pressure)[16,17] because the back-up-right pressure moves the larynx back to the position from which it is displaced by a right-handed (held in operator's left hand) laryngoscope.

The black marker on the ET tube should be at the level of the vocal cords. Advance the ET tube until the proximal end of the cuff lies ½ to 1 inch beyond the cords.

i. Grasp the ET tube with your right hand and introduce it into the right corner of the patient's mouth. Advance the tube through the glottic opening until the distal cuff disappears past the vocal cords (Figure 2-69)
j. While firmly holding the ET tube, remove the stylet (if used) and inflate the distal cuff with approximately 6 to 10 mL of air (volume varies depending on cuff size). Disconnect the syringe from the inflation valve
k. Attach a ventilation device to the ET tube and ventilate the patient. Confirm proper placement of the tube by first auscultating over the epigastrium (should be silent) and then in the midaxillary and anterior chest line on the right and left sides of the patient's chest (Figure 2-70). Observe the patient's chest for full movement with ventilation

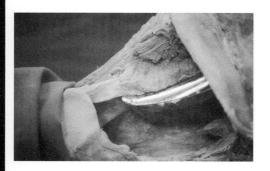

Figure 2-68 The straight blade is advanced under the epiglottis. The blade is then lifted anteriorly, directly exposing the vocal cords.

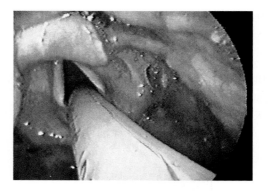

Figure 2-69 An ET tube passing through the glottic opening.

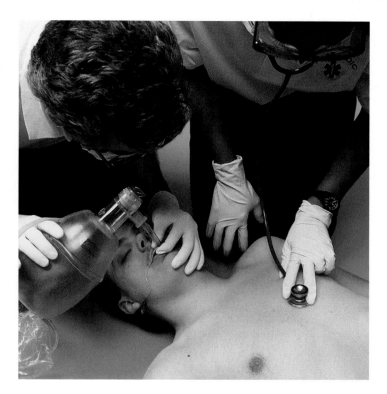

Figure 2-70   Confirm proper placement of the tube by first auscultating over the epigastrium and then in the lateral aspects of the patient's chest at the right and left midaxillary lines.

    (1) Verify placement by at least one additional method (e.g., end-tidal CO_2 [$ETCO_2$] detector or esophageal detector device)

    (2) Once placement is confirmed, note and record the depth (cm marking) of the tube at the patient's teeth

  l. If breath sounds are absent bilaterally after intubation and gurgling is heard over the epigastrium, assume esophageal intubation. Deflate the ET cuff, remove the tube, and preoxygenate the patient before reattempting intubation

  m. If breath sounds are diminished on the left after intubation but present on the right, assume right mainstem bronchus intubation. Deflate the ET cuff, pull back the ETT slightly, reinflate the cuff, and reevaluate breath sounds

  n. Secure the ET tube with a commercial tube-holder or tape and provide ventilatory support with supplemental oxygen (Figure 2-71). After securing the tube, again observe and record the tube depth at the patient's teeth

8. Confirming ET tube placement

  a. Methods used to verify proper placement of an ETT include:

    (1) Visualizing the passage of the ET tube between the vocal cords

    (2) Auscultating the presence of bilateral breath sounds

    (3) Confirming the absence of sounds over the epigastrium during ventilation

    (4) Adequate chest rise with each ventilation

    (5) Absence of vocal sounds after placement of the ET tube

    (6) Monitoring for changes in the color (colorimetric device) or number (digital device) on an $ETCO_2$ detector

    (7) Verification of tube placement by an esophageal detector device

If using an esophageal detector device to confirm placement of the ET tube, do NOT inflate the ET tube cuff before using the esophageal detector. Inflating the cuff moves the distal end of the ET tube away from the walls of the esophagus. If the tube was inadvertently inserted into the esophagus, this movement will cause the detector bulb to reexpand, falsely suggesting that the tube was in the trachea.

$ETCO_2$ monitoring has been suggested as the "sixth vital sign" that should be monitored in patients in addition to heart rate, blood pressure, respiratory rate, body temperature, and blood oxygen saturation.[18]

Confirming Tracheal Tube Placement

It is important to note that auscultation for breath sounds over the lungs and abdomen and observing the chest rise are not always indicative of correct ET tube placement. After visualizing the ETT passing through the vocal cords and confirming placement of the tube by auscultation, verify tube placement by at least one additional method. Consider the following research findings:

- In a 1998 study, researchers sought to evaluate whether condensation on the inner surface of an ET tube (vapor trail) is a reliable indicator of ETT placement.[19] Using mongrel dogs, the researchers noted that vapor trail was observed in 27 (100%) of 27 ETT correctly placed in the trachea and in 23 (83%) of 27 tubes placed in the esophagus. The authors concluded that if these results are confirmed in human studies, the presence of a vapor trail should **not** be used as a clinical indicator of correct ETT placement.

- In Denmark, researchers evaluated various methods used to confirm ETT placement.[20] Forty patients underwent both tracheal and esophageal intubation. Researchers found that auscultation of the upper abdomen and lungs was 100% reliable, independent of which tube was ventilated. Auscultation of the lungs resulted in a wrong conclusion in 15% of the cases when the esophagus was ventilated—the sounds were misinterpreted as normal breath sounds. Suction on the tubes with a 60-mL syringe was also determined a reliable test. Condensation of water vapor in the tube and abnormal upper abdominal movements were determined unreliable.

- Canadian researchers evaluated the reliability of various methods for detecting esophageal intubation in rats.[21] In this study, the esophagus and trachea were simultaneously intubated, and the presence or absence of various clinical signs were noted during tracheal or esophageal ventilation. Arterial blood gases and end-tidal CO_2 were measured. These researchers found that oxygen saturation was the least reliable method for detecting esophageal intubation, chest movement was the most reliable clinical sign for detecting esophageal intubation, and "esophageal rattle" was the second most reliable clinical sign. Moisture condensation in the tracheal tube and abdominal distention were determined to be unreliable. The most reliable method for early detection of esophageal intubation in rats was $ETCO_2$.

- In Austria, researchers compared $ETCO_2$ determination, an esophageal detection device (self-inflating bulb), auscultation, and transillumination using the Trachlight (TL) lighted stylet to verify tracheal tube placement.[22] In this study, a second ETT was placed in the esophagus of each of 38 consecutive tracheally intubated patients. Inexperienced senior medical students and experienced critical care physicians were then asked to assess tube placement. Both examiners correctly diagnosed the position of the tube in 130 of 152 examinations. The wrong result was obtained by *both* examiners 4 times; only the experienced examiner was wrong 4 times; the inexperienced examiner was wrong 14 times. Using $ETCO_2$, both examiners were correct in all cases. Auscultation showed an obvious relation to the examiner's experience: the experienced examiner was correct in all cases, the inexperienced examiner was correct in only 68% of cases. The transillumination technique was associated with a high error rate by both examiners (16% and 13%, respectively). These investigators concluded that capnography was the most reliable method for rapid evaluation of tube position, followed by the esophageal detection method.

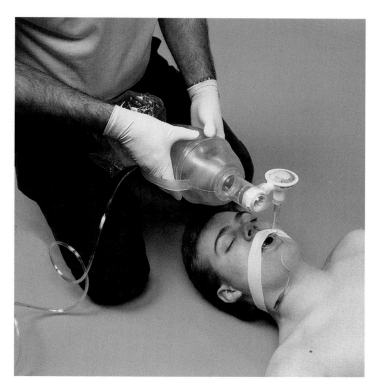

Figure 2-71   Secure the ET tube with a commercial tube-holder and provide ventilatory support with supplemental oxygen.

   b. End-tidal carbon dioxide detection
     (1) **Capnography:** Continuous analysis and recording of CO_2 concentrations in respiratory gases
     (2) **Capnometry:** Measurement of CO_2 concentrations without a continuous written record or waveform
     (3) **Capnometer:** Device used to measure the concentration of CO_2 at the end of exhalation
        (a) End-tidal CO_2 ($ETCO_2$) detector: Capnometer that provides a noninvasive estimate of alveolar ventilation, the concentration of exhaled CO_2 from the lungs, and arterial carbon dioxide content
     (4) $ETCO_2$ monitoring
        (a) Currently used for assessment of conscious sedation safety, evaluation of mechanical ventilation, and verification of ET tube placement
        (b) Because the air in the esophagus normally has very low levels of CO_2, capnometry is considered a rapid method of preventing unrecognized esophageal intubation.
     (5) $ETCO_2$ detectors are available as disposable colorimetric devices (Figure 2-72) or electronic monitors (Figure 2-73)
        (a) Disposable colorimetric devices provide CO_2 readings by chemical reaction on pH-sensitive litmus paper housed in the detector
        (b) The $ETCO_2$ device is placed between an ETT (or Combitube, PTL, etc.) and a ventilation device
     (6) The presence of CO_2 (evidenced by a color change on the colorimetric device or number/light on the electronic monitor) suggests tracheal tube placement

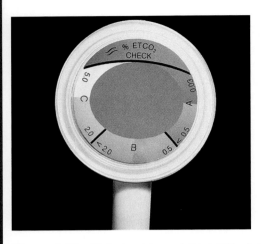

Figure 2-72   Colorimetric end-tidal CO_2 detector.

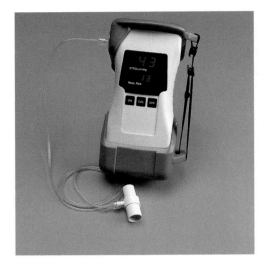

Figure 2-73   Electronic end-tidal CO_2 detector.

Colorimetric capnography is susceptible to inaccurate results because of exposure of the paper to the environment, age, and patient secretions (e.g., vomitus).

(7) A lack of CO_2 (no color change on colorimetric detector or indicator on the electronic monitor) suggests tube placement in the esophagus, particularly in patients with spontaneous circulation

(8) Because CO_2 may inadvertently enter the stomach, it is suggested that the patient be ventilated at least six times before evaluating ETT placement, using an end-tidal CO_2 detector to quickly wash out any retained CO_2.

(9) False-positive results (tube is in the trachea yet the detector indicates the device is in the esophagus) may occur in cardiopulmonary arrest or in a patient with a significant pulmonary embolus.

(10) False-negative results (tube is in the esophagus yet the detector indicates the device is in the trachea) have been reported in patients who ingested carbonated beverages before experiencing a cardiac arrest.

ETCO$_2$ May Predict Death in CPR

End-tidal CO_2 levels are an indirect measure of cardiac output during CPR and may be a predictor of death in cardiac arrest. Researchers prospectively determined whether death could be predicted by monitoring end-tidal CO_2 during resuscitation after cardiac arrest.[23] The study included 150 consecutive victims of cardiac arrest outside the hospital who had electrical activity but no pulse. The patients were intubated and evaluated by mainstream ETCO$_2$ monitoring. When a 20-minute end-tidal CO_2 value of 10 mm Hg or less was used as a screening test to predict death, the sensitivity, specificity, positive predictive value, and negative predictive value were all 100%.

ETCO$_2$ ranged from 18 to 58 mm Hg in survivors and from 0 to 10 mm Hg in nonsurvivors. Of the 150 patients in this study, 35 survived to hospital admission and 115 did not survive. Of the 35 patients who regained circulation, 19 died after hospital arrival and 16 were discharged. Of the 16 discharged, 14 were alive 6 weeks later.

These researchers concluded that an ETCO$_2$ level of 10 mm Hg or less measured 20 minutes after the initiation of ACLS accurately predicted death in patients with cardiac arrest associated with electrical activity but no pulse.

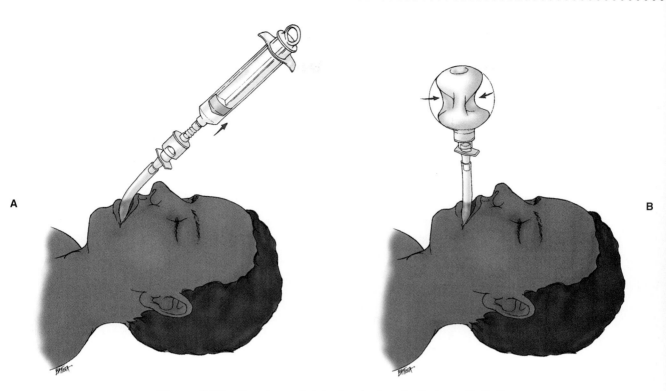

Figure 2-74   Esophageal detector device. **A,** Syringe. **B,** Bulb.

c. Esophageal detector devices (EDD) (Class IIa)
  (1) Simple, inexpensive, and easy-to-use
  (2) Used as an aid in determining if an ET tube is in the trachea or esophagus
    (a) Can also be used to verify correct placement of the esophageal-tracheal Combitube and PTL airway
  (3) There are currently two types of esophageal detectors— a syringe and a bulb (Figure 2-74). These devices operate under the principle that the esophagus is a collapsible tube and the trachea a rigid one
    (a) Syringe device
      (i) Syringe device is connected to an ETT with the plunger fully inserted into the barrel of the syringe
      (ii) If the ETT is in the trachea, the plunger can be easily withdrawn from the syringe barrel
      (iii) If the ETT is in the esophagus, the walls of the esophagus will collapse when negative pressure is applied to the syringe, preventing air from being drawn out of the device
    (b) Bulb device
      (i) Bulb device is compressed before it is connected to an ET tube. A vacuum is created as the pressure on the bulb is released
      (ii) If the ETT is in the trachea, the bulb will refill easily when pressure is released, indicating proper tube placement

            (iii) If the ETT is in the esophagus, the bulb will remain collapsed, indicating improper tube placement

       (3) Special considerations

          (a) Results may be misleading in patients with:

             (i) Morbid obesity

             (ii) Late pregnancy

             (iii) Status asthmaticus

             (iv) Copious tracheal secretions

9. Complications of ET intubation

    a. Bleeding

    b. Laryngospasm

    c. Vocal cord damage

    d. Mucosal necrosis

    e. Barotrauma

    f. Aspiration

    g. Cuff leak

    h. Esophageal intubation

    i. Right mainstem intubation

    j. Occlusion caused by patient secretions or patient biting the tube

    k. Laryngeal or tracheal edema

    l. Tube occlusion

    m. Inability to talk

    n. Hypoxia because of prolonged or unsuccessful intubation

    o. Dysrhythmias

    p. Trauma to the lips, teeth, tongue or soft tissues of the oropharynx

    q. Increased intracranial pressure

QUICK REVIEW

1. When a stylet is used during orotracheal intubation, the tip of the stylet must be recessed _____ from the end of the ET tube to avoid trauma to the airway structures.

2. An endotracheal intubation attempt should not take more than 30 seconds. At what point does this 30-second time interval begin and end?

3. What is the average endotracheal tube size for an adult male? An adult female?

4. An advantage of ventilation with a bag-valve device is a sense of compliance of the lungs is conveyed to the operator. What is meant by compliance?

5. A nasal cannula (prongs) with a liter flow of 1 to 6 L/min will deliver what percentage of oxygen?

6. A bag-valve-mask device used during cardiac arrest should not possess a pop-off (pressure-release) valve. What is the reason for this?

7. Name the three axes of the upper airway that must be aligned during orotracheal intubation.

8. Endotracheal intubation should be accomplished within _____.

1. 1½ inch. 2. The 30-second time interval begins when ventilation ceases to allow insertion of the laryngoscope blade into the patient's mouth and ends when the patient is ventilated on placement of the endotracheal tube. 3. The average endotracheal tube size for an adult male is 8 to 8.5 internal diameter (ID) and 7.0 to 8.0 for an adult female. 4. Compliance refers to the resistance of the patient's lung tissue to ventilation. 5. A nasal cannula can deliver an oxygen concentration of 25% to 45% at a flow rate of 1 to 6 L/min. 6. To properly ventilate patients in cardiac arrest, much higher than usual airway pressures are often needed, the pressure needed to overcome the increase in airway resistance may exceed the limits of the pop-off valve; thus, a pop-off valve may prevent delivery of sufficient tidal volume to properly ventilate the patient in cardiac arrest. 7. Mouth, pharynx, and trachea. 8. 30 seconds.

STOP AND REVIEW

1. Endotracheal intubation:
   a. Is contraindicated in unresponsive patients
   b. Eliminates the risk of aspiration of gastric contents
   c. Should be preceded by efforts to ventilate by another method
   d. When attempted, should be performed in less than 60 seconds

2. Which of the following is NOT a desirable feature of a bag-valve device used during resuscitation attempts?
   a. Nonrebreathing valve
   b. Compressible, self-refilling bag
   c. Functional pop-off (pressure release) valve
   d. Availability in adult and pediatric sizes

3. If oxygen is not available, tidal volumes and inspiratory times for mouth-to-mask ventilation should be approximately _____ delivered over _____ seconds and sufficient to make the chest rise.
   a. 6 to 7 mL/kg; 3
   b. 10 mL/kg; 2
   c. 10 to 15 mL/kg; 1½ to 2
   d. 12 to 15 mL/kg; 2

4. With an oxygen flow rate of 1 to 6 L/minute, a nasal cannula can deliver an estimated oxygen concentration of:
   a. 17% to 21%
   b. 25% to 45%
   c. 40% to 60%
   d. 60% to 100%

5. *True* or *False.* The oropharyngeal airway (OPA) can only be used in the spontaneously breathing patient.

6. When using an $ETCO_2$ detector to confirm placement of an endotracheal tube in a patient with spontaneous circulation, a lack of CO_2 on the detector generally means:
   a. The tube is correctly placed in the trachea
   b. The tube is improperly positioned in the esophagus

The wife of a 72-year-old male reports that her husband "just stopped breathing" moments ago. You find the patient supine in his bed. He does not respond to your voice or to application of a painful stimulus.

7. After determining that the patient is unresponsive, your next course of action should be to:
   a. Open the patient's airway using a jaw thrust without head-tilt maneuver
   b. Open the patient's airway using a head-tilt/chin-lift maneuver
   c. Apply an automated external defibrillator (AED)
   d. Call for help/activate EMS, call for a defibrillator, and continue the Primary ABCD Survey

8. Assessment of your patient reveals gurgling respirations at a rate of 6/min. You prepare to suction the patient. Each suction attempt should last no more than _____ seconds.
   a. 5 to 10
   b. 10 to 15
   c. 15 to 20
   d. 20 to 30

9. Suctioning has cleared the patient's airway. Respirations are 6/min and shallow. Which of the following oxygen delivery devices would be most appropriate to use in this situation?
   a. Nonrebreather mask at 15 L/min
   b. Nasal cannula at 4 L/min
   c. Simple face mask at 4 L/min
   d. Bag-valve-mask device with supplemental oxygen at 15 L/min and a reservoir

10. Which of the following are signs of a complete airway obstruction?
    a. Absence of cough, speech, or breathing
    b. Low-pitched sounds on exhalation
    c. Difficult/labored breathing
    d. High-pitched sounds on inhalation

11. Which of the following statements is INCORRECT regarding the nasopharyngeal airway?
    a. After insertion, the balloon is inflated with 5 mL of air
    b. The nasopharyngeal airway may cause epistaxis if forcefully inserted
    c. Most responsive and semiresponsive patients can tolerate the nasopharyngeal airway
    d. The nasopharyngeal airway should be lubricated with a water-soluble lubricant before insertion

12. Which of the following are examples of multi-lumen (also called *dual lumen*) airways?
    a. Oropharyngeal airway (OPA) and nasopharyngeal airway (NPA)
    b. Esophageal-tracheal Combitube (ETC) and pharyngotracheal lumen airway (PTL)
    c. Laryngeal mask airway (LMA) and esophageal-tracheal Combitube (ETC)
    d. Pharyngotracheal lumen airway (PTL) and nasopharyngeal airway (NPA)

13. *True or False.* A 70-year-old female has suffered a cardiopulmonary arrest. Endotracheal intubation should be performed as the initial step in the management of this patient's airway.

14. Mouth-to-mask breathing combined with supplemental oxygen at a minimum flow rate of 10 L/min can deliver an oxygen concentration of approximately _____ %.
    a. 10
    b. 15
    c. 50
    d. 65

15. Select the CORRECT statement regarding the simple face mask.
    a. The simple face mask provides definitive control of the airway
    b. When using a simple face mask, the O_2 flow rate must be greater than 5 to 6 L/min to avoid accumulation of exhaled air in the mask reservoir
    c. The simple face mask is the preferred device for use in COPD patients because it provides precise O_2 concentrations
    d. The simple face mask can be used effectively to deliver high oxygen concentrations in the patient with apnea

STOP AND REVIEW ANSWERS

1. c. Endotracheal (ET) intubation should be preceded by attempts to ventilate by another method. ET intubation is indicated in situations where the patient is unable to protect his/her own airway. ET intubation reduces but does not eliminate the risk of aspiration of gastric contents and, when attempted, should be performed in less than 30 seconds.

2. c. Pop-off valves are not recommended during resuscitation attempts because higher than usual airway pressures are often needed to ventilate patients in cardiac arrest. Pop-off valves may prevent the creation of airway pressures sufficient to overcome the increase in airway resistance.

3. b. If oxygen *is not* available, tidal volumes and inspiratory times for mouth-to-mask ventilation should be approximately 10 mL/kg (700 to 1000 mL) delivered over 2 seconds (Class IIa) and sufficient to make the chest rise.

4. b. 1 L/min = 25% 4 L/min = 37%
   2 L/min = 29% 5 L/min = 41%
   3 L/min = 33% 6 L/min = 45%

5. False. The oropharyngeal airway should only be used in the unresponsive patient without a gag reflex. Use in a responsive or semi-responsive patient may stimulate vomiting or laryngospasm.

6. b. Because the air in the esophagus normally has very low levels of CO_2, a lack of CO_2 on an $ETCO_2$ detector generally means the ET tube (Combitube or PTL) is improperly positioned in the esophagus.

7. d. After determining that the patient is unresponsive, activate EMS (call 9-1-1 or other emergency number), call for a defibrillator, and continue the Primary ABCD Survey.

8. b. Assessment of your patient reveals gurgling respirations at a rate of 6/min. You prepare to suction the patient. Each suction attempt should last no more than *10 to 15* seconds.

9. d. Remember that an open airway does not assure adequate ventilation. This patient's breathing is inadequate as evidenced by his rate and depth of respirations. The patient with inadequate breathing requires positive-pressure ventilation with 100% oxygen. Of the choices listed, the only device that can provide positive-pressure ventilation is the bag-valve-mask. If readily available, an oropharyngeal airway should be inserted before beginning bag-valve-mask ventilation (if the patient does not have a gag reflex).

10. a. Signs of a complete airway obstruction include the inability to speak, cry, cough, or make any other sound.

11. a. The nasopharyngeal airway is a soft, *uncuffed* rubber or plastic tube. Because the device has no cuff, there is no balloon that should be inflated with air.

12. b. The esophageal-tracheal Combitube (ETC) and pharyngotracheal lumen airway (PTL) are multi-lumen or dual lumen airways.

13. False. Endotracheal intubation should always be preceded by some other form of ventilation (mouth-to-mask, bag-valve-mask).

14. c. Mouth-to-mask breathing combined with supplemental oxygen at a minimum flow rate of 10 L/min can deliver an oxygen concentration of approximately 50%.

15. b. When using the simple face mask, the O_2 flow rate must be greater than 5 to 6 L/min to avoid accumulation of exhaled air in the mask reservoir.

REFERENCES

1. Weil MH, Tang W, editors: *CPR: resuscitation of the arrested heart*, Philadelphia, 1999, WB Saunders.
2. The American Heart Association in Collaboration with the International Liaison Committee on Resuscitation (ILCOR): Advanced cardiovascular life support, Part 6, Section 3: Adjuncts for oxygenation, ventilation, and airway control, *Circulation* 102 (suppl I):1-102, 2000.
3. Perry AG, Potter PA: *Clinical nursing skills & techniques*, ed 3, St Louis, 1994, Mosby.
4. AARC Clinical Practice Guideline: Oxygen therapy in the acute care hospital, *Respir Care* 36:1410-1413, 1991.
5. Staudinger T, Brugger S, Watschinger B, Roggla M, Dielacher C, Lobl T, Fink D, Klauser R, Frass M: Emergency intubation with the Combitube: comparison with the endotracheal airway, *Ann Emerg Med* (10):1573-1575, 1993.
6. Rumball CJ, MacDonald D. The PTL, Combitube, laryngeal mask, and oral airway: a randomized prehospital comparative study of ventilatory device effectiveness and cost-effectiveness in 470 cases of cardiorespiratory arrest, *Prehosp Emerg Care* 1(1):1-10, 1997.
7. Brain AI: The laryngeal mask: a new concept in airway management, *Br J Anaesth* 55:801-805, 1983.
8. Wakeling HG, Butler PJ, Baxter PJ: The laryngeal mask airway: a comparison between two insertion techniques, *Anesth Analg* 85(3):687-690, 1997.
9. Martin PD, Cyna AM, Hunter WAH. Training nursing staff in airway management for resuscitation: a clinical comparison of the face mask and laryngeal mask, *Anaesthesia* 48:33-37, 1993.
10. Alexander R, Hodgson P, Lomax D: A comparison of laryngeal mask airway and Guedel airway, bag and face mask for manual ventilation, *Anaesthesia* 48:231-234, 1993.
11. Yardy N, Hancox D, Strang T: A comparison of two airway aids for emergency use by unskilled personnel. The Combitube and laryngeal mask, *Anaesthesia* 54(2):181-183, 1999.
12. The American Heart Association in Collaboration with the International Liaison Committee on Resuscitation (ILCOR): Adult basic life support, Part 3, *Circulation* 102 (suppl I):1-22, 2000.
13. Klain M, Bircher NG In Weil MH, Tang W, editors: *CPR: resuscitation of the arrested heart*, Philadelphia, 1999, WB Saunders.
14. Dörges V, Ocker H, Hagelberg S, Wenzel V, Idris AH: Smaller tidal volumes with room air are not sufficient to ensure adequate oxygenation during basic life support, *Resuscitation* 44:37-41, 2000.

15. Langeron O, Masso E, Huraux C, Guggiari M, Bianchi A, Coriat P, Riou B: Prediction of difficult mask ventilation, *Anesthesiology* 92(5):1229-1236, 2000.
16. Takahata O, Kubota M, Mamiya K, Akama Y, Nozaka T, Matsumoto H, Ogawa H: The efficacy of the "BURP" maneuver during a difficult laryngoscopy, *Anesth Analg* 419-421, 1997.
17. Cicarelli DD, Stábile Jr SL, Momi T, Pavnocca ML, Miranda SBP, Khouri Filho RA: Tracheal intubation: evaluation of BURP maneuver efficacy, *Rev Bras Anestesiol* 49(1):24-26, 1999.
18. Vardi A, Levin I, Paret G, Barzilay Z: The sixth vital sign: end-tidal CO_2 in pediatric trauma patients during transport, *Harefuah* 139(3-4):85-87, 168, 2000.
19. Kelly JJ, Eynon CA, Kaplan JL, de Garavilla L, Dalsey WC: Use of tube condensation as an indicator of endotracheal tube placement, *Ann Emerg Med* 31(5):575-578, 1998.
20. Andersen KH, Hald A: Assessing the position of the tracheal tube: the reliability of different methods, *Anaesthesia* 44:984-985, 1989.
21. Vaghadia H, Jenkins LC, Ford RW: Comparison of end-tidal carbon dioxide, oxygen saturation and clinical signs for the detection of esophageal intubation, *Can J Anaesth* 36:560-564, 1989.
22. Knapp S, Kofler J, Stoiser B, Thalhammer F, Burgmann H, Posch M, Hofbauer R, Stanzel M, Frass M: The assessment of four different methods to verify tracheal tube placement in the critical care setting, *Anesth Analg* 88(4):766-770, 1999.
23. Levine RL, Wayne MA, Miller CC: End-tidal carbon dioxide and outcome of out-of-hospital cardiac arrest, *N Engl J Med* 31;337(5):301-306, 1997.

BIBLIOGRAPHY

Butman AM, Martin SW, Vomacka RW, McSwain NE: *Comprehensive guide to pre-hospital skills*, Akron, Ohio, 1995, Emergency Training.

Crawford MV, Spence MI: *Common sense approach to coronary care*, ed 6, St Louis, 1995, Mosby.

Gibler WB, Aufderheide TP: *Emergency cardiac care*, St Louis, 1994, Mosby.

Henry MC, Stapleton ER: *EMT prehospital care*, ed 2, Philadelphia, 1997, WB Saunders.

Paradis NA, Halperin HR, Nowak RM, editors: *Cardiac arrest: the science and practice of resuscitation medicine*, Baltimore, 1996, Williams & Wilkins.

Sanders MJ. *Mosby's paramedic textbook*, ed 2, St Louis, 2000, Mosby.

Shade B, Rothenberg MA, Wertz E, Jones S: *Mosby's EMT—Intermediate textbook*, St Louis, 1997, Mosby.

The American Heart Association in Collaboration with the International Liaison Committee on Resuscitation (ILCOR): Adult basic life support, Part 3, *Circulation* 102 (suppl I):1-22, 2000.

The American Heart Association in Collaboration with the International Liaison Committee on Resuscitation (ILCOR): *Advanced cardiovascular life support*, Part 6, Section 3: Adjuncts for oxygenation, ventilation, and airway control, *Circulation* 102 (suppl I):1-95, 2000.

Weil MH, Tang W, editors: *CPR: resuscitation of the arrested heart*, Philadelphia, 1999, WB Saunders Company.

Whitten CE: *Anyone can intubate*, ed 2, San Diego, 1990, Medical Arts Publications.

Woods SL, Sivarajan Froelicher ES, Motzer SA: *Cardiac nursing*, ed 4, Philadelphia, Lippincott Williams & Wilkins, 2000.

Vascular Access

3

OBJECTIVES

On completion of this chapter, you will be able to:

1. Describe the indications for intravenous (IV) therapy.
2. Describe the sites of first choice for cannulation if no IV is in place at the time of cardiac arrest.
3. Describe the advantages of peripheral venipuncture over central venous access.
4. Describe the advantages of central venous access over peripheral venipuncture.
5. Describe the indications for central venous access.
6. Identify anatomical landmarks for cannulation of the femoral, internal jugular, and subclavian veins.
7. List four local complications common to all IV techniques.
8. List four systemic complications common to all IV techniques.
9. Describe the indications for an intraosseous infusion.

VASCULAR ACCESS

1. Various routes may be used for parenteral administration of fluid and/or medications, including the intravenous (IV) route, intraosseous (IO) route, and cutdown
2. **Intravenous cannulation** is the placement of a catheter into a vein to gain access to the body's venous circulation. IV access may be achieved by cannulating a peripheral or central vein
3. When direct IV cannulation is unsuccessful or is taking too long, an intraosseous infusion or venous cutdown are alternative methods of gaining access to the vascular system
   a. An **intraosseous infusion** is the infusion of fluids, medications, or blood directly into the bone marrow cavity
   b. A venous **cutdown** is a surgical procedure that is usually performed by a physician at the patient's bedside. In adults, the median cubital vein in the antecubital fossa or the long saphenous vein are most commonly used for this procedure

INTRAVENOUS THERAPY

1. Indications
   a. Maintain hydration
   b. Restore fluid and electrolyte balance
   c. Provide fluids for resuscitation

 d. Administer medications, blood and blood components, nutrient solutions
 e. Obtain venous blood specimens for laboratory analysis

Peripheral Venous Access

1. Generally considered for short-term use
2. Advantages
 a. Effective route for medications during CPR
 b. Does not require interruption of CPR
 c. Easier to learn than central venous access
 d. If IV attempt unsuccessful, site easily compressible to reduce bleeding
 e. Results in fewer complications than central venous access

---

Routes of Medication Administration

In a 1987 study, 12 patients were randomized to receive intravenous epinephrine administered either in an antecubital vein or via an endotracheal tube. The injection of 1 mg of epinephrine IV increased serum epinephrine levels up to three times the level before administration. By comparison, the maximal increase in epinephrine level after ET administration was less than half the minimal increase in epinephrine levels after IV administration.[2]

Recognizing that animal and clinical CPR studies have not addressed the use of ET epinephrine in doses recommended in the 1992 ACLS guidelines for adults (twice the IV dose), researchers from the UCLA School of Medicine compared the effects of ET and IV drugs on cardiac rhythm in the prehospital setting.[3] In this study, a 3-year (1995-1997) retrospective review of all cardiac arrests transported to a single, municipal teaching institution was performed. Patients >18 years of age in atraumatic cardiac arrest whose first documented field rhythm was asystole with time-to-definitive care of ≤10 minutes (primary asystole) and patients found in VF who developed postcountershock asystole (secondary asystole) were included. Patients were grouped according to route of drug administration (IV, ET, or no drug therapy) as well as rhythm (primary or secondary asystole). A positive response to drug therapy was defined as any subsequent rhythm other than asystole during continued prehospital resuscitation.

One hundred thirty-six patients met inclusion criteria. The following groups were defined:
- Group 1: Primary asystole/IV drugs (39 patients)
- Group 2: Postcountershock asystole/IV drugs (39 patients)
- Group 3: Primary asystole/ET drugs (25 patients)
- Group 4: Postcountershock asystole/ET drugs (18 patients)
- Group 5: Primary or secondary asystole/no drug therapy (15 patients)

Significant differences were not observed between groups with respect to age, gender, witnessed arrest, frequency of bystander CPR, or time-to-definitive care. The positive rhythm response rate was significantly greater in group 1 (64%) and group 2 (69%) than in group 3 (12%) or group 4 (11%). The response rate in the control group was 20% and not significantly different from either ET group. The IV groups also had a significantly greater rate of return of spontaneous circulation (17%) when compared with the ET groups (0%). The researchers concluded that currently recommended doses of epinephrine and atropine administered endotracheally are rarely effective in the setting of cardiac arrest and CPR.

3. Disadvantages
    a. In circulatory collapse, vein may be absent or difficult to access
    b. Phlebitis common with saphenous vein use
    c. Should be used only for administration of isotonic solutions; hypertonic or irritating solutions may cause pain and phlebitis
    d. In cardiac arrest, medications administered from a peripheral vein require 1 to 2 minutes to reach the central circulation
4. Needle size
    a. Gauge—outside diameter of the venipuncture device
        (1) Provides a "rough" indication of flow rate
        (2) Thickness of the wall of the IV catheter varies vary from manufacturer to manufacturer, affecting actual flow rate
        (3) Although IV catheters are color-coded to aid in the visual recognition of the catheter's gauge, the color-coding system is not standard or universal in the medical device industry[4]

Table 3-1   IV Cannula Selection

Gauge	Use	Approximate Flow Rate
14 (large-bore)	• Trauma, surgery, blood administration, administration of viscous medications • Adolescents and adults	315 mL/min
16 (large-bore)	• Trauma, surgery, blood administration, administration of viscous medications • Adolescents and adults	210 mL/min
18	• Trauma, surgery, blood administration • Older children, adolescents, adults	110 mL/min
20	• Suitable for most IV infusions • Older children, adolescents, adults	65 mL/min
22	• Children and elderly patients	38 mL/min
24	• Neonates, infants, children, and adults with fragile veins	24 mL/min

5. Needle types
    a. Over-the-needle catheter (Figure 3-1)
        (1) Widely used
        (2) Soft catheter commonly made of plastic or plastic-like material
        (3) Rigid, plastic hub is color-coded
        (4) Hollow metal needle is preinserted into the catheter; the needle is used to perform the venipuncture. After venipuncture, the catheter is introduced and the needle removed, leaving the catheter in place through which fluid is administered
        (5) Length of catheter limited by length of needle
        (6) Puncture site in vein exactly size of catheter, which reduces possibility of bleeding around venipuncture site
    b. Through-the-needle catheter (Figure 3-2)
        (1) Steel needle used to perform venipuncture; plastic catheter then slides through the needle and into the vein. After the venipuncture is performed, the needle is pulled out of the skin and left attached to the apparatus. A protective device is used to cover the needle to reduce the incidence of catheter shear or trauma to the patient

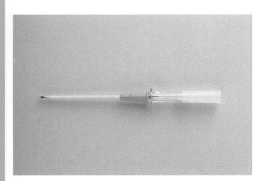

Figure 3-1 An over-the-needle catheter.

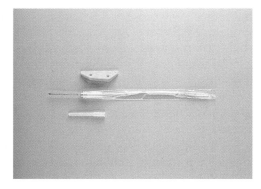

Figure 3-2 Through-the-needle catheter.

(2) Risk of sharp tip of needle shearing off the end of the catheter and producing a catheter-fragment embolus

c. Hollow needle (Figure 3-3)

(1) "Butterfly" or "scalp vein" needle (also called a *winged infusion set*)—common type of hollow needle (steel needle with flexible plastic wings)

(2) May be easier to insert than other types of IV devices because there are no parts to manipulate

(3) Risk of infiltration higher than with other devices because steel needle tip may puncture vasculature after placement

6. Sites

a. Factors to consider when selecting an IV site:

(1) Purpose of the infusion

(2) Amount and type of IV fluid or medications to be infused

(3) Expected duration of IV therapy

(4) Accessibility of the vein

(5) Size and condition of the vein

(6) Patient's age, size, general condition, and preference

(7) Your experience and skill at venipuncture

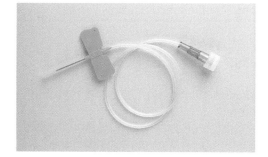

Figure 3-3 Hollow needle – Butterfly type.

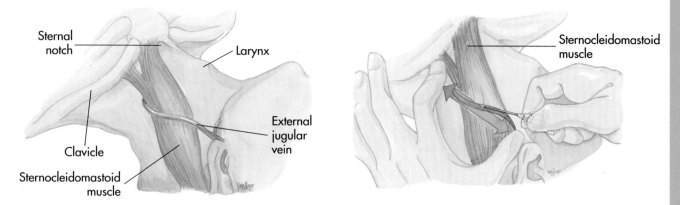

Figure 3-4   A, Anatomy of the external jugular vein. **B,** Cannulation of the external jugular vein.

    b. External jugular (EJ) vein
       (1) Lies superficially along the lateral portion of the neck (Figure 3-4, *A*)
          (a) Extends from behind the angle of the jaw and passes downward across the sternocleidomastoid muscle until it enters the thorax at a point just above the middle third of the clavicle. It joins the subclavian vein just behind the clavicle
       (2) Is considered a peripheral vein
       (3) Is usually easy to cannulate (Figure 3-4, *B*)
          (a) Pressure and tension applied to the external jugular vein just above the clavicle causes the vessel to distend, making cannulation easier
       (4) Provides rapid access to the central circulation
       (5) May not be readily accessible during an arrest situation because of rescuers working to manage the airway
       (6) IV may be easily dislodged
       (7) May be positional with head movement
    c. Upper extremity
       (1) Cephalic vein is located on the lateral (thumb) side (Figure 3-5) and the axillary vein on the medial (little finger) side of the forearm
          (a) Cephalic vein is a large vein, easy to stabilize, and easily accessible. However, motion of the wrist may increase patient discomfort, and irritation to the inner lining of the vessel may result from cannula movement
       (2) Median veins (cephalic, cubital, and basilic) lie in the antecubital fossa
       (3) Antecubital vein
          (a) Usually easily accessible
          (b) Does not interfere with ventilations and chest compressions
          (c) Provides an effective route for administration of IV fluids and medications during cardiac arrest

> *During circulatory collapse or cardiac arrest, the preferred vascular access site is the largest, most accessible vein that does not require the interruption of resuscitation efforts. If no IV is in place before the arrest, establish IV access using a peripheral vein—preferably the antecubital or external jugular vein. In a stable patient, use the more distal veins of the upper extremity first, if accessible. During cardiac arrest, administer IV medications rapidly by bolus injection and follow each medication with a 10- to 20-mL bolus of IV fluid to aid delivery of the medication(s) to the central circulation.*

    d. Lower extremity
      (1) Veins of the lower extremity are not generally used during resuscitation
        (a) Distance from the central circulation
        (b) Cannulation of the veins of the legs, feet, and ankles may compromise lower extremity circulation and cause thrombophlebitis or embolism
      (2) If the lower extremity must be cannulated, the long saphenous vein is the preferred site for IV therapy (Figure 3-6)

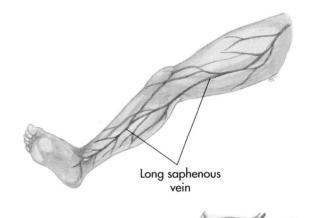

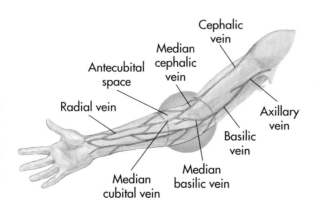

Figure 3-5 Veins of the upper extremity.

Figure 3-6 The saphenous vein.

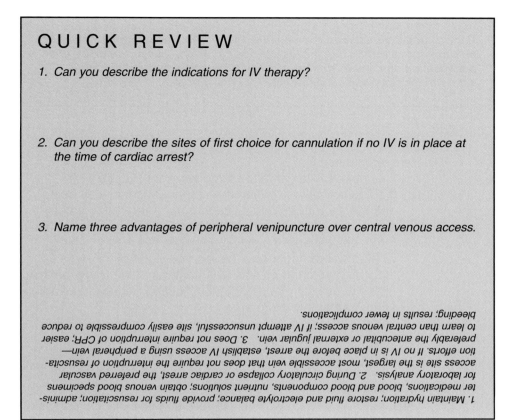

Central Venous Access

1. A central venous catheter (also called a *central line*) is inserted into the vena cava from the subclavian, jugular, or femoral vein
2. Indications
   a. Emergency access to venous circulation when peripheral sites are not readily available
   b. Need for long-term IV therapy
   c. Administration of large volume of fluid
   d. Administration of hypertonic solutions, caustic medications, or parenteral feeding solutions
   e. Placement of transvenous pacemaker electrodes
   f. Placement of central venous pressure or right heart catheters
3. Advantages
   a. Peak medication concentrations are higher and circulation times shorter when medications are administered via a central route compared with peripheral sites
4. Disadvantages
   a. Special equipment (syringe, catheter, needle) required
   b. Excessive time (5 to 10 minutes) for placement
   c. High complication rate
   d. Skill deterioration (frequent practice required to maintain proficiency)
   e. Inability to initiate procedure while other patient care activities in progress

> *During cardiac arrest (and if experienced personnel are available), consider placement of a central line if spontaneous circulation has not returned after defibrillation and administration of medications via a peripheral venous site—unless contraindications exist.*

5. Sites
   a. Femoral vein
      (1) Relevant anatomy
         (a) Lies directly medial to the femoral artery (Figure 3-7)
         (b) If a line is drawn between the anterior superior iliac spine and the symphysis pubis, the femoral artery runs directly across the midpoint—medial to that point is the femoral vein

An acronym used to recall relevant anatomy is NAVEL: *n*erve, *a*rtery, *v*ein, *e*mpty space, *l*igament.

         (c) If the femoral artery pulse is palpable, the artery can be located with a finger and the femoral vein will lie immediately medial to the pulsation. A finger should remain on the artery to assist in landmark identification and avoid insertion of the catheter into the artery
      (2) Advantages
         (a) Does not interrupt CPR
         (b) Vein does not collapse like peripheral veins
         (c) Once cannulated, easy access to the central circulation
      (3) Disadvantages
         (a) If pulse absent, vein may be hard to locate
         (b) Long delivery time of medications into the central circulation unless a long line that extends above the diaphragm is used (because of decreased flow to the extremities)
         (c) Complication rate may be higher, especially involving thrombosis and infection, than for peripheral veins
      (4) Complications

Local complications of IV therapy are most often seen at or near the IV insertion site and are more common than systemic complications. Some local complications can lead to more serious systemic complications.

         (a) Local complications
            (i) Hematoma (from the vein itself or adjacent femoral artery)
            (ii) Thrombosis may extend to deep veins and lead to edema of leg
            (iii) Phlebitis may extend to deep veins
            (iv) Use of femoral vein frequently precludes subsequent use of saphenous vein

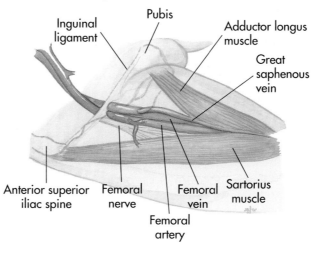

Figure 3-7 Femoral vein anatomy.

Femoral Venous Access

In two studies, the success rate for correct placement of femoral vein catheters during human cardiac arrest was low. "Jastremski et al[5] studied physicians of various backgrounds and found that femoral catheters were correctly placed in the femoral vein in only 31% of cases: 5 of 16 catheters were placed in the femoral artery while 1 was in the soft tissue. Significantly, the physicians did not recognize the malplacement of the catheters in 3 of 6 cases. In a larger study[6] with radiopaque dye injection to verify catheter placement, femoral vein catheters were correctly placed 77% of the time as compared to 94% of subclavian vein catheters. The success rate did not improve during the course of the study, although all of the catheters were placed by either attending physicians or by critical care fellows."[2]

    (b) Systemic complications
       (i) Systemic complications of IV therapy occur within the vascular system, usually distant from the IV insertion site
       (ii) Thrombosis or phlebitis may extend proximally to the iliac vein or inferior vena cava
       (iii) Cannulation of femoral artery may result in loss of limb
  b. Internal jugular vein
    (1) Relevant anatomy
      (a) Runs from the base of the skull downward along the carotid artery until it enters the chest to meet the subclavian vein behind the clavicle (Figure 3-8)
      (b) Cannulation of the right side of the neck is preferred
       (i) Dome of the right lung and pleura are lower than the left
       (ii) More or less a straight line to the right atrium
       (iii) Thoracic duct not in the way (empties on the LEFT side)

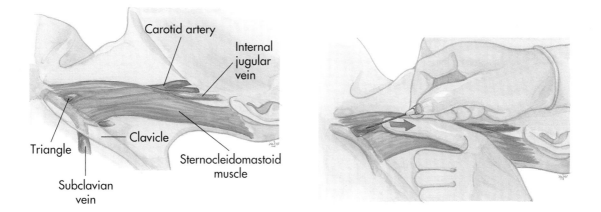
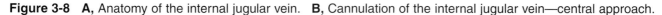

Figure 3-8 **A,** Anatomy of the internal jugular vein. **B,** Cannulation of the internal jugular vein—central approach.

(2) Advantages
    (a) Less risk of pneumothorax with this technique vs. subclavian
    (b) Hematomas in the neck are visible and more easily compressible
    (c) Easier access during CPR than subclavian
    (d) Usually remains patent even when peripheral veins are collapsed
(3) Disadvantages
    (a) Adjacent structures easily damaged
    (b) More training required than peripheral venipuncture
    (c) May interrupt CPR
    (d) Higher complication rate than with peripheral venipuncture
    (e) Higher complications with fibrinolytic therapy
    (f) Limits patient neck movement

c. Subclavian vein
  (1) Relevant anatomy
    (a) Subclavian vein is a continuation of the axillary vein at the outer border of the first rib
    (b) Joins the internal jugular vein behind the medial end of the clavicle to form the brachiocephalic (innominate) vein (Figure 3-9)
    (c) Approximately 3 to 4 cm long and 2 cm in diameter
    (d) Immobilized by small attachments to the first rib and clavicle
    (e) Lies anterior to the subclavian artery and is separated from it by the anterior scalene muscle
  (2) Advantages
    (a) Usually remains patent even when peripheral veins are collapsed
    (b) More subsequent patient neck movement with prolonged cannulation

A recent study demonstrated that approximately a fourth of patients undergoing cannulation of the internal jugular vein develop internal jugular vein valve incompetence, regardless of the insertion site, and the condition usually persists, presumably permanently.[7]

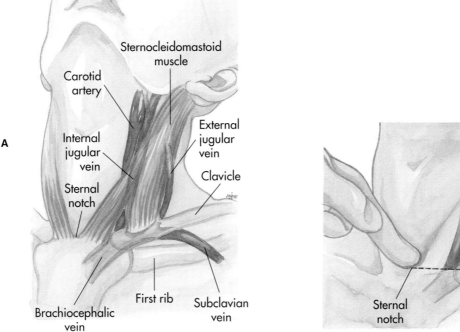

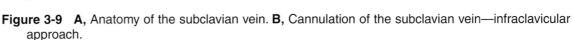

Figure 3-9 **A,** Anatomy of the subclavian vein. **B,** Cannulation of the subclavian vein—infraclavicular approach.

(3) Disadvantages
   (a) Significant risk of pneumothorax, hemothorax, subclavian artery puncture
   (b) More training required than peripheral venipuncture
   (c) May interrupt CPR
   (d) Higher complication rate than with peripheral venipuncture
   (e) Higher complications with fibrinolytic therapy
(4) Internal jugular and subclavian venipuncture complications
   (a) Local complications
      (i) Hematoma (from the vein itself or from an adjacent artery) may compromise airway
      (ii) Damage to adjacent artery, nerve, or lymphatic duct
      (iii) Perforation of endotracheal tube cuff

When cannulating the internal jugular vein, inadvertent puncture of the carotid artery may occur. If a hematoma occurs on one side of the neck, attempting a venipuncture on the opposite side may be hazardous because of the possibility of airway compromise caused by the presence of bilateral hematomas.

   (b) Systemic complications
      (i) Pneumothorax
      (ii) Hemothorax
      (iii) Air embolism
      (iv) Infiltration into mediastinum or pleural space
      (v) Dysrhythmias from catheter tip

QUICK REVIEW

1. Name three indications for central venous access.

2. Name an advantage of central venous access over peripheral venipuncture.

3. Name three possible systemic complications of internal jugular or subclavian venipuncture.

4. Where is the external jugular vein located?

1. *Emergency access to venous circulation when peripheral sites are not readily available and there is a need for long-term IV therapy and administration of large volume of fluid; administration of hypertonic solutions, caustic medications, or parenteral feeding solutions; placement of transvenous pacemaker electrodes and placement of central venous pressure or right heart catheters.* 2. *Peak medication concentrations are higher and circulation times shorter when medications are administered via a central route compared with peripheral sites.* 3. *Hemothorax, air embolism, pneumothorax, dysrhythmias from the catheter tip, infiltration into the mediastinum or pleural space* 4. *The external jugular vein lies superficially along the lateral portion of the neck. It extends from the angle of the mandible and passes downward until it enters the thorax at a point just above the middle of the clavicle and ends in the subclavian vein.*

Complications Common to All IV Techniques

Local Complications

1. Pain and irritation
2. Hematoma formation (Figure 3-10)
   a. *Possible causes:* Advancing the needle completely through the vein or inadequate application of pressure to prevent leakage of blood from the vein when the catheter is removed
   b. *Signs and symptoms:* Ecchymosis over and around the insertion site, pain at the site, swelling and hardness at the insertion site, inability to flush the IV line, inability to advance the cannula all the way into the vein during insertion
3. Infiltration and extravasation
   a. **Infiltration** is the intentional or unintentional process by which a substance enters or infuses into another substance or a surrounding area (Figure 3-11)
   b. **Extravasation** is the actual (unintentional) escape or leakage of an agent that is irritating and causes blistering (a vesicant) from a vessel into the surrounding tissue (Figure 3-12)
   c. *Possible causes:* Venipuncture device dislodged from vein, puncture of distal vein wall during venipuncture, leakage of solution into the surrounding tissue from the cannula's insertion site, poorly secured IV, poor vein or site selection, irritating solution or medication that inflames the intima of the vein and causes it to weaken, improper cannula size, high delivery rate or pressure of the solution or medication
   d. *Signs and symptoms:* Coolness of skin around IV site; swelling at the IV site, with or without pain; sluggish or absent flow rate; infusion continues to infuse when pressure is applied to the vein above the tip of the cannula; no backflow of blood into IV tubing when clamp fully opened and solution container lowered below IV site
4. Thrombosis and thrombophlebitis (Figure 3-13)
   a. *Possible causes:* Clotting at catheter tip and inflammation, injury to endothelial cells of vein wall allowing platelet aggregation and thrombus formation

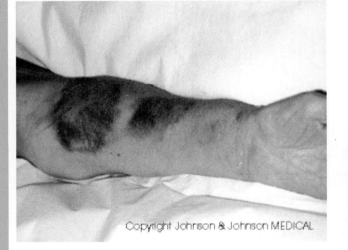

Copyright Johnson & Johnson MEDICAL

Figure 3-10   Bruising/hematoma formation.

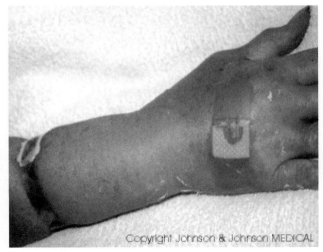

Copyright Johnson & Johnson MEDICAL

Figure 3-11   Infiltration.

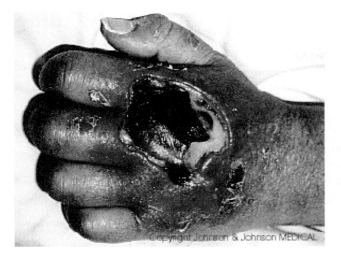

Figure 3-12 Extravasation.

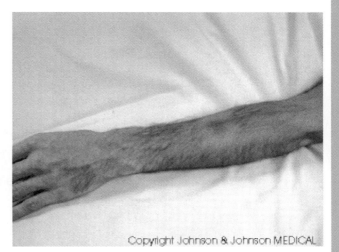

Figure 3-13 Infusion phlebitis.

    b. *Signs and symptoms:* Slowed or stopped infusion rate, aching or burning sensation at infusion site, skin warm and red around IV site, swelling of the extremity, and/or throbbing pain in the limb

5. Venous spasm
    a. *Possible causes:* Severe irritation from irritating medications or fluids, administration of cold fluids or blood
        (1) Examples: Substances with a high or low pH, diazepam (Valium), phenytoin (Dilantin), and dextrose solutions with concentrations higher than 12.5%
    b. *Signs and symptoms:* Sluggish or stopped infusion rate when the clamp is completely open, severe pain from the IV site radiating up the extremity, blanching of the skin over the IV site, or redness over and around the IV site

6. Vessel collapse
    a. *Signs and symptoms:* Inability to see and/or feel a vein, loss of vessel elasticity, vessel feels flat or flaccid, or reduced or stopped infusion flow

7. Inadvertent arterial puncture
    a. If administered arterially, some medications crystallize and may completely occlude the arterial blood supply distal to the point of injection, resulting in permanent interruption of the blood supply to the affected area

8. Cellulitis
    a. **Cellulitis** is a diffuse inflammation and infection of cellular and subcutaneous connective tissue that can lead to abscess formation and ulceration of deeper tissues
    b. *Signs and symptoms:* Pain, tenderness, warmth, edema, red streaking on skin (if spread to lymphatics), roughened appearance of the skin (like that of an orange peel), fever, and chills

9. Nerve, tendon, ligament, and/or limb damage
    a. *Possible causes:* Improper venipuncture technique, improper securing and stabilization of the cannula and IV line after insertion, extravasated IV solution, cellulitis
    b. *Signs and symptoms:* Tingling, numbness, and loss of sensation, loss of movement, cyanosis, pallor, deformity, or paralysis

Systemic Complications

1. Sepsis
2. Contamination and infection (Figure 3-14)
3. Hypersensitivity reactions
   a. *Possible causes:* Can occur as a response to the IV solution, its preservatives, or IV medications; patient may have an allergy to the cannula, antiseptic preparation, or tape
   b. *Signs and symptoms:* Range from mild to severe, affect several body systems, and may develop rapidly, gradually, or be delayed hours after the allergen has been administered
4. Speed shock
   a. *Speed shock* is a systemic reaction to the rapid or excessive infusion of medication or solution into the circulation
   b. *Signs and symptoms:* Flushing of head and neck, apprehension, hypertension, pounding headache, dyspnea, chest pain, chills, loss of responsiveness, and cardiac arrest
5. Emboli (blood clot, catheter, air)
   a. Pulmonary embolism
      (1) *Possible causes:* May result from a thrombus that forms from trauma to the intima of a vein; blood flow past the thrombus can cause a portion of the clot to break off and become an embolus
      (2) *Signs and symptoms:* Dyspnea, tachypnea, dysrhythmias, hypotension, diaphoresis, anxiety, and/or a cough
   b. Catheter embolism
      (1) *Possible causes:* May occur because of catheter shear in which a portion of the catheter is sheared off, usually because of a back-and-forth movement through the needle
      (2) *Signs and symptoms:* Sudden, severe pain at the IV site and/or a reduced or absent blood return when checking placement of the IV catheter
         (a) If catheter does not travel, patient may be asymptomatic
         (b) If catheter lodges in a heart chamber or the pulmonary circulation, patient may experience hypotension, tachycardia, chest pain, cyanosis, and/or a loss of responsiveness

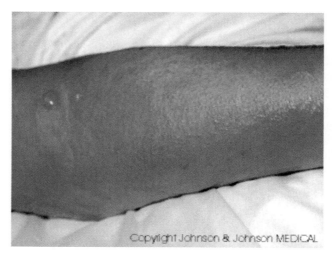

Figure 3-14   Infection.

   c. Air embolism

     (1) *Possible causes:* IV solution container empty; air enters bloodstream by means of the IV catheter tubing

       (a) It is possible for air to enter the circulation during catheter insertion or when the tubing is disconnected to replace IV solutions or IV tubing

       (b) Risk of an air embolus is greatest when central venous cannulation is performed because negative pressure during cannulation may actually pull air into the vein

     (2) *Signs and symptoms:* Hypotension, extreme anxiety, light headedness and confusion, tachypnea, cyanosis, a weak and rapid pulse, and/or a loss of responsiveness

---

- **The Centers for Disease Control and Prevention has reported 159 cases of occupational HIV transmission.[8]**
- **As many as 40% of health care workers who sustain needle sticks become infected with hepatitis B virus (HBV).[9]**
- **Health care workers are at highest risk of exposure to hepatitis C virus (HCV).[10]**

INTRAOSSEOUS INFUSION

1. **Intraosseous infusion** is the process of infusing medications, fluids, and blood products into the bone marrow cavity for subsequent delivery to the venous circulation

2. Site

   a. Traditionally, IO infusion has been accepted as a rapid, reliable method of achieving vascular access under emergency conditions in children

   b. In recent years, studies have been performed to evaluate the use of IO infusions in adult medical emergencies

     (1) Various sites have been studied to evaluate the effectiveness of IO infusion in adults including the clavicle, ilium, and tibia,[11] an area proximal to the medial malleolus,[12,13] and the manubrium (the top bone of the sternum)[14]

     (2) In adults, the cortex of the tibia is thick and bony making it difficult to penetrate, and its marrow is less vascular than that of the sternum

     (3) The sternum may be a better site for IO infusion in adults because it is large, thin, and flat; contains a high proportion of vascular red marrow; is easy to penetrate and less likely to be fractured; and is closer to the central circulation (the manubrium is the site used for placement of the FAST 1 device) (Figure 3-15)

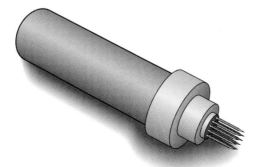

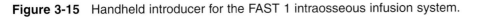

Figure 3-15 Handheld introducer for the FAST 1 intraosseous infusion system.

In some areas, IO infusion is indicated in the management of an adult medical arrest patient in whom peripheral IV access is unsuccessful after 90 seconds.

3. Indications
   a. Emergency administration of fluids and/or medications, especially in the setting of circulatory collapse where rapid vascular access is essential
   b. Difficult, delayed, or impossible IV access
   c. Burns or other injuries preventing venous access at other sites
4. Contraindications
   a. Anatomical anomaly of the sternum
   b. Previous midline sternotomy
   c. Chest trauma with a suspected fractured sternum
   d. Burns over the sternum
   e. Severe osteoporosis or bone-softening conditions
   f. Extremely small adult
5. Possible complications of IO infusion
   a. Extravasation of fluids into subcutaneous tissue
   b. Local abscess or cellulitis
   c. Osteomyelitis (related to long-term IO infusion administration)

A Canadian study[14] reported the results of a new system of IO infusion into the adult sternum called the *First Access for Shock and Trauma (FAST) 1* (See Figure 3-15). The device was evaluated in 50 consecutive patients aged 14 to 84 years at six emergency departments and five EMS sites in Canada and the United States. Indications for use of the device included an adult patient, an urgent need for fluids or medications, and an unacceptable delay or inability to achieve standard vascular access.

With this device, a handheld introducer is used to insert a flexible infusion tube with a stainless-steel tip to a predetermined depth in the manubrium. Fluids and medications are administered through the tube into the marrow space. Generally, the device can be inserted in the sternum in less than 2 minutes and remain in place for a maximum of 24 hours (or until conventional IV access is established). CPR can be performed while fluids are being infused. The FAST 1 (sternal infusion) device *cannot* be used if the patient has:

- Tissue damage directly over the manubrium
- Fracture of the manubrium
- Flail chest involving the sternum
- Previous sternotomy for cardiovascular surgery
- Severe osteoporosis

The overall success rate for achieving vascular access with the system was 84%. Success rates were 74% for first-time users and 95% for experienced users. Failure to achieve vascular access occurred most frequently in patients (5 of 9) described subjectively by the user as "very obese," in whom there was a thick layer of tissue overlying the sternum. Mean time to achieve vascular access was 77 seconds (range 30 to 300). Flow rates of up to 80 mL/min were reported for gravity drip and more than 150 mL/min by syringe bolus.

Early complications included localized bleeding, bruising, swelling, redness, and tenderness. In 12 cases, the operators had difficulty using the removal tool. No complications or complaints were reported at 2-month follow-up. The manufacturer (Pyng Medical Corporation of Vancouver, British Columbia) provided equipment and training support for the study.

Medication dosages administered via the IO route are the same as those administered IV. Any medication or fluid that can be administered IV can be administered IO. Substances infused into the sternum reach the central circulation via the internal mammary and azygos venous systems within seconds. The main contraindication to IO infusion using sites other than the sternum is the presence of a fracture in the pelvis or extremity proximal to or in the bone chosen for IO needle insertion.

STOP AND REVIEW

1. An advantage of central venous access over the peripheral route is:
   a. Easier to learn
   b. Results in fewer complications
   c. Does not require interruption of CPR
   d. More rapid arrival of medications at their sites of action

2. Which of the following is NOT an advantage of internal jugular vein cannulation over subclavian vein cannulation?
   a. Less risk of pleural puncture
   b. Easier to cannulate during CPR
   c. Allows more free movement for the patient
   d. Hematomas are visible and easily compressible

3. Where is the femoral vein relative to the femoral artery?
   a. Medial
   b. Lateral
   c. Anterior
   d. Posterior

4. Which of the following statements regarding central venous access is INCORRECT?
   a. If a femoral pulse is absent, the vein may be difficult to locate
   b. Central venous lines may be successfully placed, even when peripheral perfusion is poor
   c. Central venous access technique requires more training than peripheral venipuncture technique
   d. The central circulation should be accessed through an internal jugular site or infraclavicular subclavian site

5. Local complications common to all intravenous techniques include:
   a. Sepsis
   b. Phlebitis
   c. Air embolism
   d. Catheter-fragment embolism

6. Leg veins are generally avoided for IV therapy because of:
   a. Discomfort
   b. Inadequate flow rates
   c. Increased likelihood and severity of venous thrombosis
   d. Increased likelihood of extravasation caused by motion and downward position

7. Which of the following is considered a peripheral vein?
   a. Femoral
   b. Subclavian
   c. Internal jugular
   d. External jugular

8. _____ is the unintentional escape or leakage of an agent that is irritating and causes blistering (a vesicant) from a vessel into the surrounding tissue.

9. During cardiac arrest, IV medications should be administered rapidly by bolus injection and followed with a _____ bolus of IV fluid.
   a. 3 to 5 mL
   b. 5 to 10 mL
   c. 10 to 20 mL
   d. 20 to 30 mL

10. You have established an IV in a 43-year-old patient complaining of chest pain. Which of the following would indicate speed shock?
    a. Dizziness, acute drop in systolic blood pressure
    b. Flushing of the head and neck, apprehension, pounding headache, dyspnea
    c. Pain, tenderness, warmth, edema, and red streaking on the skin at the IV site
    d. Absence of a backflow of blood when the IV bag is lowered

STOP AND REVIEW ANSWERS

1. d. Advantages of the central venous route over the peripheral route include more rapid arrival of medications at their sites of action and successful placement, even when perfusion is poor.

2. c. Cannulation of the internal jugular vein does not allow free movement for the patient.

3. a. The femoral vein is medial to the femoral artery.

4. d. Access the central circulation through an internal jugular site or *supra*clavicular subclavian site. These sites/approaches should require less interruption of chest compressions than the *infra*clavicular approach.

5. b. Local complications common to all IV techniques include pain and irritation, hematoma formation, infiltration and extravasation, thrombosis and thrombophlebitis, venous spasm, vessel collapse, inadvertent arterial puncture, cellulitis, and nerve, tendon, ligament, and/or limb damage.

6. c. Leg veins are generally avoided because of their distance from the central circulation and because blood flow from the distal extremities is markedly diminished, increasing the likelihood and severity of venous thrombosis.

7. d. The external jugular is considered a peripheral vein. The femoral, subclavian, and internal jugular veins are central veins.

8. *Extravasation* is the actual (unintentional) escape or leakage of an agent that is irritating and causes blistering (a vesicant) from a vessel into the surrounding tissue.

9. c. During cardiac arrest, IV medications should be administered rapidly by bolus injection and followed with a *10- to 20-mL* bolus of IV fluid.

10. b. Speed shock is a systemic reaction to the rapid or excessive infusion of medication or solution into the circulation. Signs and symptoms may include flushing of the head and neck, apprehension, hypertension, pounding headache, dyspnea, chest pain, chills, loss of responsiveness, and cardiac arrest.

REFERENCES

1. Quinton DN, O'Byrne G, Aitkenhead AR: Comparison of endotracheal and peripheral intravenous adrenaline in cardiac arrest. Is the endotracheal route reliable? *Lancet* 11;1(8537):828-829, 1987.
2. Emerman CL, Kerz T, Dick W: In Paradis NA, Halperin HR, Nowak RM, editors: *Cardiac arrest: the science and practice of resuscitation medicine*, Baltimore, 1996, Williams & Wilkins.
3. Niemann JT, Stratton SJ: Endotracheal versus intravenous epinephrine and atropine in out-of-hospital "primary" and postcountershock asystole, *Crit Care Med* 28(6):1815-1819, 2000.
4. Terry J, Baranowski L, Lonsway RA, Hedrick C: *Intravenous therapy: clinical principles and practice*, Philadelphia, 1995, WB Saunders.

5. Jastremski MS, Matthias HD, Randell PA: Femoral venous catheterization during cardiopulmonary resuscitation: a critical appraisal, *J Emerg Med* 1(5):387-391, 1984.
6. Emerman CL, Bellon EM, Lukens TW, May TE, Effron D: A prospective study of femoral versus subclavian vein catheterization during cardiac arrest, *Ann Emerg Med* 19(1):26-30, 1990.
7. Wu X, Studer W, Erb T, Skarvan K, Seeberger MD: Competence of the internal jugular vein valve is damaged by cannulation and catheterization of the internal jugular vein, *Anesthesiology* 93(2):319-324, 2000.
8. *HIV/AIDS surveillance report*, Atlanta, Ga: Centers for Disease Control 8(1):15, 1996.
9. Gerberding JL: Management of occupational exposures to blood-borne viruses, *N Engl J Med* 332:444-451, 1995.
10. Ippolito G, Puro V, Petrosillo N, et al: *Prevention, management and chemoprophylaxis of occupational exposure to HIV*, Charlottesville, Va, 1997, International Health Care Worker Safety Center, University of Virginia.
11. Iwama H, Katsumi A, Shinohara K, Kawamae K, Ohtomo Y, Akama Y, Tase C, Okuaki A: Clavicular approach to intraosseous infusion in adults, *Fukushima J Med Sci* 40(1):1-8, 1994.
12. Iserson KV, Criss E: Intraosseous infusions: a usable technique, *Am J Emerg Med* 4(6):540-542, 1986.
13. Glaeser PW, Hellmich TR, Szewczuga D, Losek JD, Smith DS: Five-year experience in prehospital intraosseous infusions in children and adults, *Ann Emerg Med* 22(7):1119-1124, 1993.
14. Macnab A, Christenson J, Findlay J, Horwood B, Johnson D, Jones L, Phillips K, Pollack C Jr, Robinson DJ, Rumball C, Stair T, Tiffany B, Whelan M: A new system for sternal intraosseous infusion in adults, *Prehosp Emerg Care* 4(2):173-177, 2000.

BIBLIOGRAPHY

Driscoll P, Gwinnutt C, Mackway-Jones K, Wardle T, editors: *Advanced cardiac life support: the practical approach*, ed 2, London, 1997, Chapman & Hall Medical.

Paradis NA, Halperin HR, Nowak RM, editors: *Cardiac arrest: the science and practice of resuscitation medicine*, Baltimore, 1996, Williams & Wilkins.

Sanders MJ: *Mosby's paramedic textbook*, ed 2, St Louis, 2000, Mosby.

Shade B, Rothenberg MA, Wertz E, Jones S: *Mosby's EMT—intermediate textbook*, St Louis, 1997, Mosby.

Snell RS, Smith MS: *Clinical anatomy for emergency medicine*, St Louis, 1993, Mosby.

Terry J, Baranowski L, Lonsway RA, Hedrick C, editors. *Intravenous therapy: clinical principles and practice*, Philadelphia, 1995, WB Saunders.

Weil MH, Tang W, editors: *CPR: resuscitation of the arrested heart*, Philadelphia, 1999, WB Saunders.

Woods SL, Sivarajan Froelicher ES, Motzer SA: *Cardiac nursing*, ed 4, Philadelphia, 2000, Lippincott Williams & Wilkins.

Dysrhythmia Recognition

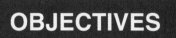

4

On completion of this chapter, you will be able to:

1. Name the primary branches of the right and left coronary arteries.
2. Describe the two types of myocardial cells and the function of each.
3. Describe the significance of each waveform in the cardiac cycle.
4. Describe the normal duration of the PR interval, QRS complex, and QT interval.
5. Describe at least two methods of determining heart rate.
6. Name the primary and escape pacemakers of the heart and the inherent rates of each.
7. Define the absolute and relative refractory periods and their location in the cardiac cycle.
8. Describe correct electrode positioning for leads I, II, III and MCL_1.
9. Describe the primary characteristics of sinus, atrial, junctional, and ventricular dysrhythmias.
10. Name four dysrhythmias that may be observed during an adult cardiac arrest.
11. Describe the primary characteristics of first-, second-, and third-degree atrioventricular (AV) blocks.
12. Describe differentiation of right and left bundle branch block, using lead V_1 or MCL_1.

ANATOMY REVIEW

Coronary Arteries

1. Right coronary artery (RCA)
   a. Originates from the right side of the aorta and passes along the atrioventricular sulcus between the right atrium and right ventricle (Figure 4-1)
      (1) Supplies the inferior wall of the left ventricle
      (2) Marginal branch supplies right atrium and right ventricle
      (3) In 50% to 60% of individuals, a branch of the RCA supplies the SA node
      (4) In 85% to 90% of hearts, the RCA also branches into the AV node artery
      (5) Posterior descending branch supplies blood to the walls of both ventricles
      (6) Has several branches, including the septal branch, that supplies the posterior one-third of the interventricular septum

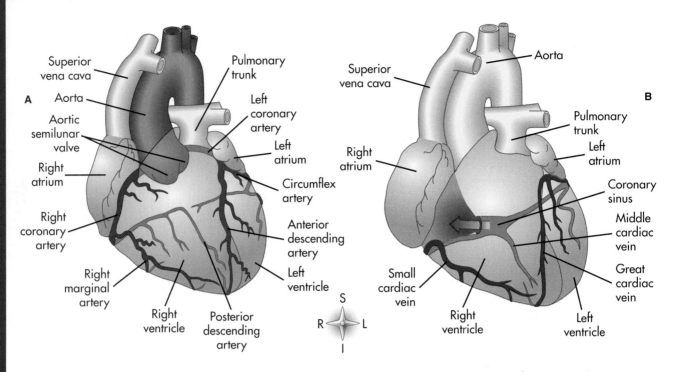

Figure 4-1   Anterior views of the coronary circulation. **A,** Coronary arteries. **B,** Coronary veins.

Occlusion of the left main coronary artery has been referred to as the "widow maker" because of its association with sudden death.

If the posterior wall of the left ventricle is damaged, a cardiac catheterization is usually necessary to determine which coronary artery is involved because both the RCA and LC supply blood to this area.

     b. Occlusion of the RCA can result in:
       (1) Inferior wall MI
       (2) Disturbances in AV nodal conduction
  2. Left coronary artery (LCA)
     a. Originates from the left side of the aorta and consists of the left main coronary artery that divides into two main branches: the left anterior descending (also called the *anterior interventricular*) artery and the left circumflex artery
     b. The left anterior descending (LAD) branch travels to the anterior interventricular sulcus and its branches supply blood to the anterior surfaces of both ventricles. Branches of the LAD include the diagonal and septal arteries
       (1) Occlusion of the septal branch of the LAD can result in a septal MI
       (2) Occlusion of the diagonal branch of the LAD can result in an anterior wall MI
       (3) Occlusion of the LAD can result in pump failure and/or intraventricular conduction delays
     c. The left circumflex (LC) branch follows the coronary sulcus between the right and left ventricle and supplies blood to the left atrium and left ventricle
       (1) Supplies the lateral wall of the left ventricle. Thus, occlusion can result in a lateral wall MI
       (2) In some patients, the circumflex artery may also supply the inferior portion of the left ventricle
         (a) A posterior wall MI may occur because of occlusion of the right coronary artery or the left circumflex artery
       (3) Supplies the SA node in 40% to 60% of individuals and the AV node in 10% to 15% of individuals

Location of MI	Affected Coronary Artery
Lateral	Left coronary artery, circumflex branch
Inferior	Right coronary artery, posterior descending branch
Septum	Left coronary artery, left anterior descending artery, septal branch
Anterior	Left coronary artery, left anterior descending artery, diagonal branch
Posterior	Right coronary artery or left circumflex artery
Right ventricle	Right coronary artery, proximal branches

QUICK REVIEW

1. An inferior wall MI is usually the result of occlusion of the _____ coronary artery.
2. An anterior wall MI is usually the result of occlusion of the _____ _____ coronary artery.
3. Occlusion of the left circumflex coronary artery usually results in a(n) _____ wall MI.
4. True or False. A septal MI is usually the result of occlusion of the right coronary artery.

1. Right. 2. Left anterior descending. 3. Lateral. 4. False.

BASIC ELECTROPHYSIOLOGY

Cardiac Cell Types (Table 4-1)

1. Myocardial cells
   a. Also called *working* or *mechanical cells*
   b. Contain contractile filaments
   c. When electrically stimulated, these filaments slide together and the myocardial cell contracts
   d. Do not normally spontaneously generate electrical impulses, depending on pacemaker cells for this function
2. Pacemaker cells
   a. Specialized cells of the electrical conduction system
   b. Responsible for the spontaneous generation and conduction of electrical impulses
   c. Found in nodes, bundles, bundle branches, and branching networks (fascicles) in the heart

Table 4-1	Cardiac Cell Types		
Kinds of Cardiac Cells	**Where Found**	**Primary Function**	**Primary Property**
Myocardial cells	Myocardium	Contraction and relaxation	Contractility
Pacemaker cells	Electrical conduction system	Generation and conduction of electrical impulses	Automaticity and conductivity

Modified from Huszar RJ: *Basic dysrhythmia: interpretation and management*, ed 2, St Louis, 1994, Mosby.

Cardiac Action Potential

1. Cell membranes contain membrane channels
   a. These channels are pores through which specific ions or other small, water-soluble molecules can cross the cell membrane from outside to inside (Figure 4-2)
   b. Electrical impulses are the result of brief but rapid flow of charged ions back and forth across the cell membrane
   c. Cardiac action potential is an illustration of these events in a single cardiac cell during polarization, depolarization, and repolarization. The stimulus that alters the gradient across the cell membrane may be electrical, mechanical, or chemical
2. Polarization
   a. Also called the *resting membrane potential*
   b. Polarization is the resting state during which no electrical activity occurs in the heart
   c. When a cardiac muscle cell is polarized, the inside of the cell is more negative than the outside because of the numbers and types of ions found inside the cell (Figure 4-3)
3. Depolarization
   a. Before the heart can mechanically contract and pump blood, cardiac muscle cell depolarization must take place

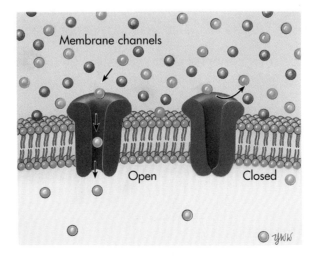

Figure 4-2   Cell membranes contain membrane channels. These channels are pores through which specific ions or other small, water-soluble molecules can cross the cell membrane from outside to inside.

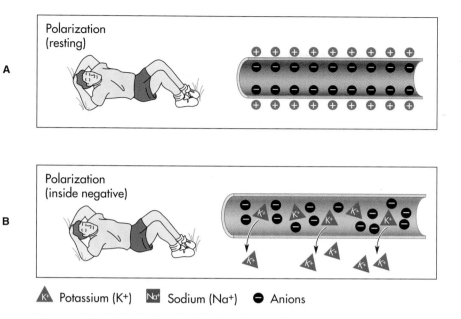

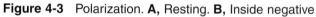

Potassium (K+)   Sodium (Na+)   ● Anions

Figure 4-3   Polarization. **A,** Resting. **B,** Inside negative

b. When the cardiac muscle cell is stimulated, the cell is said to **depolarize** (Figure 4-4)

c. The inside of the cell becomes more positive because of the entry of sodium (Na+) ions into the cell through Na+ membrane channels

d. Depolarization proceeds from the innermost layer of the heart (endocardium) to the outermost layer (epicardium)

e. On the ECG, the P wave represents atrial depolarization, and the QRS complex represents ventricular depolarization.

Depolarization = stimulation.

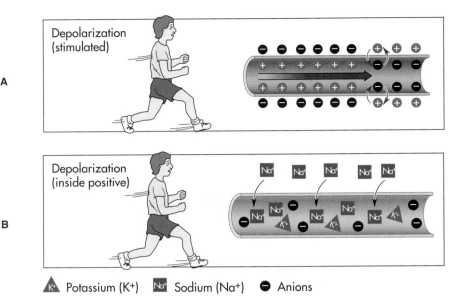

Figure 4-4   Depolarization. **A,** Stimulated. **B,** Inside positive.

      f. Depolarization is **not** the same as contraction.
         (1) Depolarization is an electrical event *expected* to result in contraction (a mechanical event)
         (2) It is possible to view organized electrical activity on the cardiac monitor, yet evaluation of the patient reveals no palpable pulse. This clinical situation is termed **pulseless electrical activity (PEA)**
  4. Repolarization
      a. After the cell depolarizes, the diffusion of Na^+ into the cell stops
      b. Potassium (K^+) is allowed to diffuse out of the cell, leaving negatively charged ions inside the cell. Thus **repolarization** occurs because of the outward diffusion of K^+
      c. The membrane potential of the cell returns to its negative resting level (Figure 4-5)
      d. This causes the contractile proteins to separate (relax). The cell can then be stimulated again if another electrical impulse arrives at the cell membrane
      e. Repolarization proceeds from the epicardium to the endocardium
      f. On the ECG, the ST-segment represents early ventricular repolarization, and the T wave represents ventricular repolarization

Repolarization = recovery.

Refractory Periods

  1. **Refractoriness:** The extent to which a cell is able to respond to a stimulus
  2. *Absolute* **refractory period** (also known as the *effective refractory period*)
      a. Corresponds with the onset of the QRS complex to the peak of the T wave
      b. During this period, the myocardial cell will not respond to further stimulation, no matter how strong the stimulus

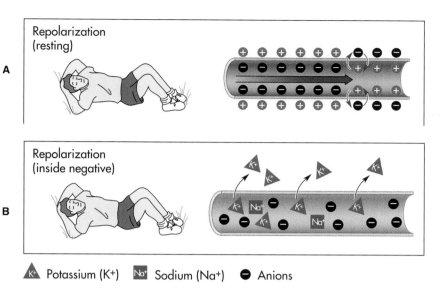

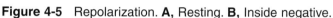

Figure 4-5   Repolarization. **A,** Resting. **B,** Inside negative.

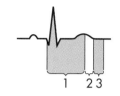

Figure 4-6   **1,** The absolute refractory period; **2,** relative refractory period; and **3,** the supernormal period.

3. *Relative* **refractory period** (also known as the *vulnerable period*)
   a. Corresponds with the downslope of the T wave
   b. During this period, some cardiac cells have repolarized to their threshold potential and can be stimulated to respond (depolarize) if subjected to a stronger than normal stimulus
4. Supernormal period
   a. After the relative refractory period is a **supernormal period** during which a weaker than normal stimulus can cause depolarization of cardiac cells
   b. Corresponds with the end of the T wave. It is possible for cardiac dysrhythmias to develop during this period (Figure 4-6)

Properties of Cardiac Cells

1. **Automaticity**
   a. Ability of cardiac pacemaker cells to spontaneously initiate an electrical impulse without being stimulated from another source (such as a nerve)
   b. SA node, AV junction, and Purkinje fibers normally possess this characteristic
2. **Excitability** (or **irritability**)
   a. Characteristic shared by all cardiac cells
   b. Refers to the ability of cardiac muscle cells to respond to an external stimulus, such as that from a chemical, mechanical, or electrical source
3. **Conductivity**
   a. Refers to the ability of a cardiac cell to receive an electrical stimulus and conduct that impulse to an adjacent cardiac cell
   b. All cardiac cells possess this characteristic
4. **Contractility**
   a. Refers to the ability of cardiac cells to shorten, causing cardiac muscle contraction in response to an electrical stimulus
   b. Contractility can be enhanced with certain medications, such as digitalis, dopamine, and epinephrine

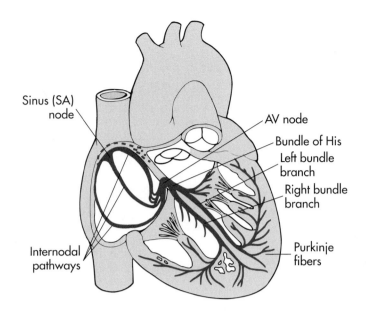

Figure 4-7   The conduction system.

QUICK REVIEW

1. *Name the two types of cardiac cells; and describe their function.*

2. *What is the significance of the "absolute" refractory period?*

3. *Define automaticity.*

4. *Is depolarization the same as contraction?*

1. Myocardial (working) cells (also known as **mechanical cells**) are found in the myocardium. These cells contain contractile filaments that contract when the cells are electrically stimulated. Electrical (pacemaker) cells are found in the electrical conduction system. Their primary function is generation and conduction of electrical impulses.   2. During this period, cardiac cells have not yet repolarized and, no matter how strong a stimulus, cannot be stimulated to depolarize.   3. The ability of cardiac cells to spontaneously initiate an electrical impulse without being stimulated by an external source (such as a nerve).   4. No. Depolarization is an electrical event; contraction is a mechanical event.

The Conduction System (Figure 4-7)

Table 4-2 Summary of the Conduction System		
Structure	**Location**	**Function**
Sinoatrial node	Right atrial wall just inferior to opening of superior vena cava	Primary pacemaker; initiates impulse that is normally conducted throughout the left and right atria. Intrinsic rate 60 to 100 beats/min
Atrioventricular node	Posterior septal wall of the right atrium, immediately behind the tricuspid valve and near the opening of the coronary sinus	Receives impulse from SA node and delays relay of the impulse to the bundle of His, allowing time for the atria to empty their contents into the ventricles before the onset of ventricular contraction
Bundle of His	Superior portion of interventricular septum	Receives impulse from AV node and relays it to right and left bundle branches. Intrinsic pacemaker ability of 40 to 60 beats/min
Right and left bundle branches	Interventricular septum	Receives impulse from bundle of His and relays it to Purkinje fibers in ventricular myocardium
Purkinje fibers	Ventricular myocardium	Receives impulse from bundle branches and relays it to ventricular myocardium. Intrinsic pacemaker ability of 20 to 40 beats/min

ELECTROCARDIOGRAM (ECG)

1. The ECG records the electrical activity of a large mass of atrial and ventricular cells as specific waveforms and complexes
2. The ECG monitoring may be used to monitor a patient's heart rate, evaluate the effects of disease or injury on heart function, evaluate pacemaker function, evaluate the response to medications (e.g., antiarrhythmics), and/or obtain a baseline recording before, during, and after a medical procedure
3. The ECG *can* provide information about:
   a. Orientation of the heart in the chest
   b. Conduction disturbances
   c. Electrical effects of medications and electrolytes
   d. Mass of cardiac muscle
   e. Presence of ischemic damage
4. The ECG does *not* provide information about the mechanical (contractile) condition of the myocardium. The effectiveness of the heart's mechanical activity is evaluated by assessment of the patient's pulse and blood pressure

Electrodes

1. Electrodes are applied at specific locations on the patient's chest wall and extremities in combinations of two, three, four, or five to view the heart's electrical activity from different angles and planes
2. One end of a monitoring cable is attached to the electrode and the other end to an ECG machine

Leads

1. A **lead** is a record of electrical activity between two electrodes
2. A lead has a negative (−) and positive (+) electrode (pole)
   a. Moving the lead selector on the ECG machine allows us to make any of the electrodes positive or negative
   b. Position of the positive electrode on the body determines the portion of the heart "seen" by each lead
   c. Each lead senses the magnitude and direction of the electrical forces caused by the spread of waves of depolarization and repolarization throughout the heart (Figure 4-8)
3. Three types of leads—standard limb leads, augmented leads (Figure 4-9), and precordial (chest) leads:
   a. Allow viewing of the heart's electrical activity in two different planes: frontal or horizontal (transverse)
      (1) Frontal plane leads view the heart from the front of the body
      (2) Horizontal plane leads view the heart as if the body were sliced in half horizontally
   b. A 12-lead ECG provides views of the heart in both the frontal and horizontal planes and views the surfaces of the left ventricle from 12 different angles
      (1) Six leads view the heart in the frontal plane as if the body were flat: three bipolar leads and three unipolar leads
         (a) **Bipolar lead** consists of a positive and negative electrode. Each lead records the difference in electrical potential between two selected electrodes
         (b) Leads I, II, and III are called *standard limb leads* (Table 4-3) or *bipolar leads*

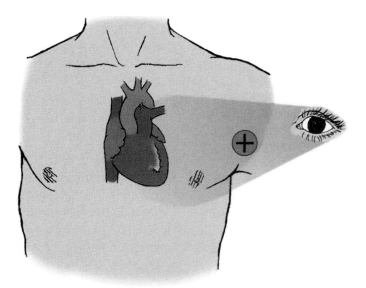

Figure 4-8 Each lead has a negative (−) and positive (+) electrode. The position of the positive electrode on the body determines the portion of the heart "seen" by each lead.

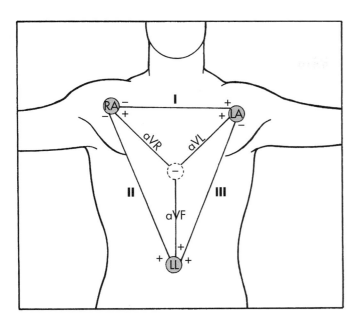

Figure 4-9   View of the standard limb leads and augmented leads.

Table 4-3   Summary of Standard Limb Leads

Lead	Positive Electrode	Negative Electrode	Heart Surface Viewed
Lead I	Left arm	Right arm	Lateral
Lead II	Left leg	Right arm	Inferior
Lead III	Left leg	Left arm	Inferior

(2) **Unipolar lead** consists of a single positive electrode and a reference point
   (a) These leads are also called *unipolar limb leads* or *augmented limb leads* (Table 4-4). The reference point for these leads lies in the center of the heart's electrical field (left of the interventricular septum and below the AV junction)
   (b) Leads aVR, aVL, and aVF are augmented limb leads

Table 4-4   Summary of Augmented Leads

Lead	Positive Electrode	Heart Surface Viewed
Lead aVR	Right arm	None
Lead aVL	Left arm	Lateral
Lead aVF	Left leg	Inferior

     (c) The augmented leads record the difference in electrical potential at one location relative to zero potential rather than relative to the electrical potential of another extremity, as in the bipolar leads

(3) Six precordial (chest or V) leads view the heart in the horizontal plane, allowing a view of the front and left side of the heart (Table 4-5)

(4) Precordial leads are identified as V_1, V_2, V_3, V_4, V_5, and V_6. (Figure 4-10)

(5) Precordial leads are unipolar leads

Table 4-5   Summary of Precordial Leads

Lead	Positive Electrode Position	Heart Surface Viewed
Lead V_1	Right side of sternum, fourth intercostal space	Septum
Lead V_2	Left side of sternum, fourth intercostal space	Septum
Lead V_3	Midway between V_2 and V_4	Anterior
Lead V_4	Left midclavicular line, fifth intercostal space	Anterior
Lead V_5	Left anterior axillary line at same level as V_4	Lateral
Lead V_6	Left midaxillary line at same level as V_4	Lateral

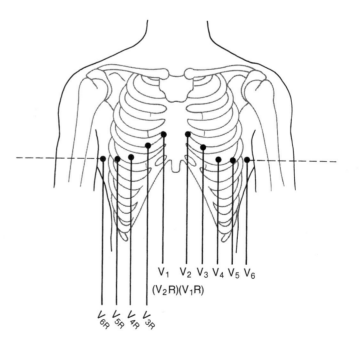

V_1 V_2 V_3 V_4 V_5 V_6
$(V_2R)(V_1R)$

V_{6R} V_{5R} V_{4R} V_{3R}

Figure 4-10 Anatomic placement of the left and right precordial leads.

QUICK REVIEW

1. A _____ is a record of electrical activity between two electrodes
2. The position of the _____ electrode on the body determines the portion of the heart "seen" by each lead.
3. Name three leads that look at the inferior wall of the left ventricle.

4. Name two leads that look at the anterior wall of the left ventricle.

5. Name four leads that look at the lateral wall of the left ventricle.

6. _____ plane leads view the heart as if the body were sliced in half.

1. Lead. 2. Positive. 3. Leads II, III, and aVF. 4. V₃ and V₄. 5. Lead I, aVL, V₅, V₆. 6. Horizontal/transverse.

ECG PAPER

1. ECG paper is graph paper made up of small and large boxes
2. Smallest boxes are 1 millimeter wide and 1 millimeter high
3. Horizontal axis of the paper corresponds with *time*. Time is stated in seconds (Figure 4-11)
   a. ECG paper normally records at a constant speed of 25 mm/sec; thus, each horizontal unit (1-mm box) represents 0.04 sec (25 mm/sec × 0.04 sec = 1 mm)
   b. There are five small boxes in each large box on the paper
   c. A large box represents 0.20 second; five large boxes, each consisting of five small boxes, represent 1 second; 15 large boxes equal an interval of 3 seconds; 30 large boxes represent 6 seconds

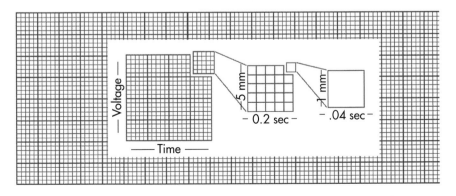

Figure 4-11 The horizontal axis represents time. The vertical axis represents amplitude or voltage.

4. Vertical axis of the paper represents *voltage* or *amplitude* of the ECG waveforms or deflections
    a. Voltage may appear as a positive or negative value
    b. Size or amplitude of a waveform is measured in millivolts (mv) or millimeters (mm)

QUICK REVIEW

1. In Lead II, where is the positive electrode located?

2. True or False. A unipolar lead consists of a single positive electrode and a reference point.
3. True or False. On ECG graph paper, time is measured on the vertical axis.
4. On the horizontal axis, each small square on ECG graph paper represents
   _____.
5. There are _____ small boxes in each large box on ECG graph paper.
6. Each square on ECG paper is _____ mm in height and width.

1. Left leg. 2. True. 3. False. 4. 0.04 sec. 5. Five. 6. 1 mm.

WAVEFORMS

P Wave

1. First wave in the cardiac cycle (Figure 4-12)
    a. First half of the P wave is recorded when the electrical impulse that originated in the SA node stimulates the right atrium and reaches the AV node
    b. Downslope of P wave reflects stimulation of left atrium
2. Represents atrial depolarization and the spread of the electrical impulse throughout the right and left atria
3. Normal characteristics
    a. Smooth and rounded
    b. No more than 2.5 mm in height
    c. No more than 0.11 sec in duration (width)
    d. Positive in leads I, II, aVF, and V_2 through V_6
    e. May be positive, negative, or biphasic in leads III, aVL, and V_1

PR Segment and PR Interval

1. Segment: Line between waveforms; named by the waveform that precedes or follows it
2. PR segment
    a. Part of the PR interval—the horizontal line between the end of the P wave and the beginning of the QRS complex
    b. Normally isoelectric (flat)
    c. His-Purkinje system is activated during the PR segment
3. Interval: Waveform and a segment
    a. P wave plus the PR segment equals the PR interval (PRI) (Figure 4-13)

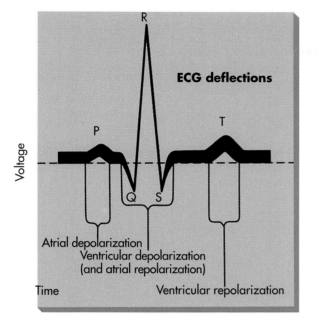

Figure 4-12 The ECG waveforms—P, QRS, and T.

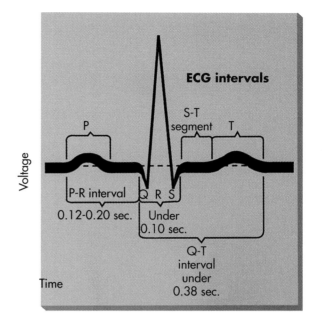

Figure 4-13 The ECG segments and intervals—PR interval, QRS duration, ST segment, QT interval.

    b. PR interval reflects depolarization of the right and left atria (P wave) and the spread of the impulse through the AV node, bundle of His, right and left bundle branches, and the Purkinje fibers (PR segment)

    c. Measured from the point where the P wave leaves the baseline to the beginning of the QRS complex

  4. Normal characteristics

    a. A normal PR interval indicates the electrical impulse was conducted normally through the atria, AV node, bundle of His, bundle branches, and Purkinje fibers

    b. Normally measures 0.12 to 0.20 sec in adults; may be shorter in children and longer in older persons

    c. Normally shortens as heart rate increases

QUICK REVIEW

1. A _____ is a line between waveforms.
2. The _____ reflects atrial depolarization.
3. A waveform and a segment is called a(n) _____.
4. True or False. The PR interval represents atrial depolarization and the spread of the impulse through the AV node, bundle of His, right and left bundle branches, and the Purkinje fibers.
5. What is the normal duration of the PR interval?

6. PR interval is measured from _____ to _____.

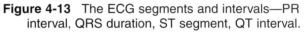

1. Segment. 2. P wave. 3. Interval. 4. True. 5. 0.12 to 0.20 sec. 6. Beginning of P wave to beginning of QRS complex.

QRS Complex

1. QRS complex consists of the Q wave, R wave, and S wave
    a. Q wave is the first deflection of the QRS complex—always negative (below the baseline)
    b. R wave is the first positive deflection (above the baseline) in the QRS complex
    c. S wave is a negative deflection following the R wave
    d. One or even two of the three waveforms that make up the QRS complex may not always be present
2. Represents the spread of the electrical impulse through the ventricles (ventricular depolarization)
3. Normal characteristics
    a. In adults, normally measures between 0.06 and 0.10 sec
    b. With the exception of leads III and aVR, a normal Q wave is less than 0.04 sec in duration and less than 25% of the amplitude of the R wave in that lead

ST-segment

1. Portion of the ECG tracing between the end of the QRS complex and the T wave
2. Represents early part of repolarization of the right and left ventricles
3. Normal ST-segment begins at the isoelectric line, extends from the end of the S wave, and curves gradually upward to the beginning of the T wave
4. Point where QRS complex and ST-segment meet is called the *junction* or *J* point (Figure 4-14)
5. Determining ST-segment elevation or depression
    a. PR segment is used as the baseline from which to evaluate the degree of displacement of the ST-segment from the isoelectric line (Figure 4-15)
    b. Measure at a point 0.04 sec (one small box) after the end of the QRS complex (the J point)
    c. ST-segment is considered *elevated* if the segment deviates above the baseline of the PR segment and *depressed* if the segment deviates below it
    d. ST-segment elevation or depression is considered "significant" if the displacement is more than 1 mm (one box) and is seen in two or more leads facing the same anatomical area of the heart

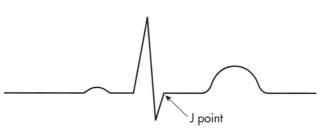
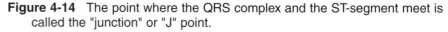

Figure 4-14   The point where the QRS complex and the ST-segment meet is called the "junction" or "J" point.

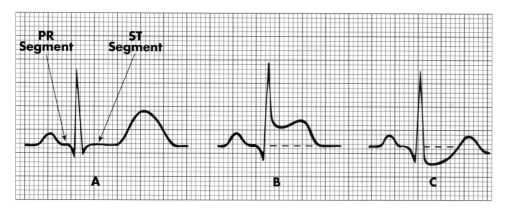

Figure 4-15   The ST segment. **A,** The PR segment is used as the baseline from which to determine the presence of ST segment elevation or depression. **B,** ST segment elevation. **C,** ST segment depression.

- *ST-segment depression of more than 1 mm is suggestive of myocardial ischemia.*
- *ST-segment elevation of more than 1 mm is suggestive of myocardial injury.*
- *Horizontal ST-segment (forms a sharp angle with the T wave) is suggestive of ischemia.*
- *Digitalis causes a depression (scoop) of the ST-segment sometimes referred to as a "dig dip."*

T Wave

1. T wave represents ventricular repolarization
2. Absolute refractory period is still present during the beginning of the T wave
3. At the peak of the T wave, the relative refractory period has begun
4. Normal characteristics:
   a. Slightly asymmetrical
   b. Not normally more than 5 mm in height in any limb leads or 10 mm in any precordial lead. T waves are not normally less than 0.5 mm in height in leads I and II
   c. Generally upright in all leads except lead aVR; may be positive or negative in leads III and V_1
5. Negative (inverted) T waves suggest myocardial ischemia
6. Tall, pointed (peaked) T waves are commonly seen in hyperkalemia

QT Interval

1. QT interval represents total ventricular activity: The time from ventricular depolarization (activation) to repolarization (recovery)
2. Measured from the beginning of the QRS complex to the end of the T wave
   a. In the absence of a Q wave, the QT interval is measured from the beginning of the R wave to the end of the T wave
3. Duration varies according to age, gender, and particularly heart rate
   a. As heart rate increases, QT interval decreases; as heart rate decreases, QT interval increases

4. To determine if the QT interval is short or long:
   a. Measure the QT interval in the leads that show the largest amplitude T waves.
   b. Measure from the beginning of the QRS complex to the end of the T wave. In the absence of a Q wave, the QT interval is measured from the beginning of the R wave to the end of the T wave.
   c. If the measured QT interval is less than half the R-R interval, it is probably normal (Figure 4-16). This method of QT interval measurement works well as a general guideline until the ventricular rate exceeds 100 beats/minute.

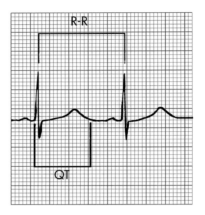

Figure 4-16 Measuring the QT interval. Abnormal QT interval prolongation in a patient taking quinidine.

QUICK REVIEW

1. What does the QRS complex represent?

2. The _____ is the portion of the ECG tracing between the end of the QRS complex and the T wave.
3. Where is the absolute refractory period on the ECG?
4. What is the normal duration of the QRS complex in an adult?

5. True or False. Tall, pointed (peaked) T waves are commonly seen in hyperkalemia.
6. The _____ is used as the baseline from which to evaluate the degree of displacement of the ST-segment from the isoelectric line.
7. What does the QT interval represent?

1. *Ventricular depolarization.* 2. *ST-segment.* 3. *Absolute refractory period (also known as the effective refractory period) extends from the onset of the QRS complex to approximately the peak of the T wave.* 4. *Between 0.06 and 0.10 sec.* 5. *True.* 6. *PR segment.* 7. *Total ventricular activity—the time from ventricular depolarization (activation) to repolarization (recovery).*

RATE MEASUREMENT

1. Six-second method
   a. Most ECG paper in use today is printed with 1-sec or 3-sec markers on the top or bottom of the paper
   b. To determine the ventricular rate, count the number of R-R intervals within a period of 6 seconds and multiply that number by 10 to find the number of complexes in 1 minute (Figure 4-17)

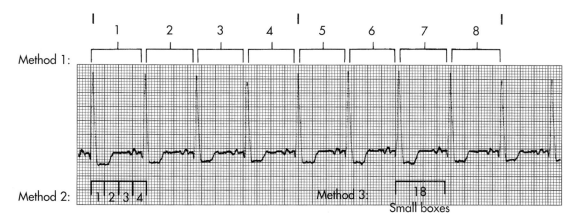

Figure 4-17 Calculating heart rate. Method 1: Number of R-R intervals in 6 seconds × 10 (e.g., 8 × 10 = 80/min). Method 2: Number of large boxes between QRS complexes divided into 300 (e.g., 300 divided by 4 = 75/min). Method 3: Number of small boxes between QRS complexes divided into 1500 (e.g., 1500 divided by 18 = 84/min).

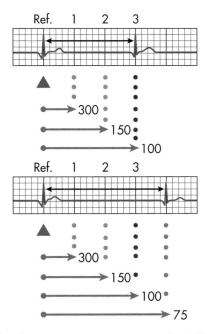

Figure 4-18 Determining heart rate—sequence method. To measure the ventricular rate, find a QRS complex that falls on a heavy dark line. Count 300, 150, 100, 75, 60, and 50 until a second QRS complex occurs. This will be the heart rate. **A,** Heart rate = 100. **B,** Heart rate = 75.

2. Large boxes
   a. To determine the ventricular rate, count the number of large boxes between two R-R intervals and divide into 300
   b. To determine the atrial rate, count the number of large boxes between two consecutive P waves (P-P interval) and divide into 300
3. Small boxes
   a. Each 1-mm box on the graph paper represents 0.04 sec. There are 1500 boxes in 1 minute. 60 seconds/minute divided by 0.04 sec/box = 1500 boxes/min
   b. To calculate the ventricular rate, count the number of small boxes between two consecutive R waves and divide into 1500
   c. To determine the atrial rate, count the number of small boxes between two consecutive P waves and divide into 1500
4. Sequence method
   a. To determine ventricular rate, select an R wave that falls on a dark vertical line
   b. Number the next 6 consecutive dark vertical lines as follows: 300, 150, 100, 75, 60, and 50
   c. Note where the next R wave falls in relation to the 6 dark vertical lines already marked. This is the heart rate (Figure 4-18)

QUICK REVIEW

1. You are viewing a rhythm strip and observe that an R wave falls on a dark vertical line. The next R wave falls on a dark vertical line three boxes to the right of the first. What is the ventricular rate?

2. What is the ventricular rate if there are 12 QRS complexes in a 6-sec strip?

1. 100. 2. 120.

RHYTHM/REGULARITY

1. Waveforms on an ECG strip are evaluated for regularity by measuring the distance between the P waves and QRS complexes
2. If the rhythm is regular, the R-R intervals (or P-P intervals if assessing atrial rhythm) are the same. Generally, a variation of plus or minus 10% is acceptable

ANALYZING A RHYTHM STRIP

1. Assess the rate
   a. A **tachycardia** exists if the rate is more than 100 beats/min
   b. A **bradycardia** exists if the rate is less than 60 beats/min
2. Assess rhythm/regularity
   a. To determine if the ventricular rhythm is regular or irregular, measure the distance between two consecutive R-R intervals and compare that distance with the other R-R intervals
   b. To determine if the atrial rhythm is regular or irregular, measure the distance between two consecutive P-P intervals and compare that distance with the other P-P intervals
3. Identify and examine P waves
   a. To locate P waves, look to the left of each QRS complex
   b. Normally, one P wave precedes each QRS complex; they occur regularly and appear similar in size, shape, and position
   c. If no P wave is present, the rhythm originated in the AV junction or the ventricles
4. Assess intervals (evaluate conduction)
   a. PR interval
      (1) Measure the PR interval from the point where the P wave leaves the baseline to the beginning of the QRS complex
      (2) Normal is 0.12 to 0.20 sec
      (3) If the PR intervals are the same, they are said to be *constant*.
      (4) If the PR intervals are different, is there a pattern?
          (a) In some dysrhythmias, the duration of the PR interval will increase until a P wave appears with no QRS after it. This is referred to as *lengthening* of the PR interval
          (b) PR intervals that vary in duration and have no pattern are said to be *variable*
   b. Identify the QRS complexes and measure their duration
      (1) QRS is narrow (normal) if it measures 0.10 sec or less and is considered wide if it measures more than 0.10 sec
   c. Measure the QT interval in the leads that show the largest amplitude T waves
      (1) If the measured QT interval is less than half the R-R interval, it is probably normal
      (2) This method of QT interval measurement works well as a general guideline until the ventricular rate exceeds 100 beats/min
5. Evaluate the overall appearance of the rhythm
   a. Is the ST-segment elevated or depressed?
   b. Are the T waves upright and of normal height?
      (1) T wave following an abnormal QRS complex is usually opposite in direction of the QRS
6. Interpret the rhythm and evaluate its clinical significance
   a. Interpret the rhythm specifying the site of origin (pacemaker site) of the rhythm (sinus), the mechanism (bradycardia), and the ventricular rate (e.g., "sinus bradycardia at 38 beats/min")
   b. Evaluate the patient's clinical presentation to determine how he or she is tolerating the rate and rhythm

Cardiac output is the amount of blood pumped into the aorta each minute by the heart. It is defined as the stroke volume (amount of blood ejected from a ventricle with each heart beat) times the heart rate. Thus a change in either the heart rate or stroke volume may affect cardiac output. Signs and symptoms of decreased cardiac output include cold, clammy skin; color changes in the skin and mucous membranes; dyspnea, orthopnea, and crackles (rales); changes in mental status; changes in blood pressure; dysrhythmias; jugular venous distention; fatigue; and restlessness.

QUICK REVIEW

1. List the six steps valued in analyzing a rhythm strip.

1. Assess the rate, assess rhythm/regularity, identify and examine P waves, assess intervals (evaluate conduction—PR interval, QRS duration, QT interval), evaluate overall appearance of the rhythm (ST-segment elevation/depression, T wave inversion), interpret rhythm and evaluate clinical significance.

DYSRHYTHMIA RECOGNITION

Sinus Rhythm

Figure 4-19 demonstrates a **sinus rhythm**. Characteristics of sinus rhythm are outlined in Table 4-6.

Table 4-6   Characteristics of Sinus Rhythm

Rate	60 to 100 beats/min
Rhythm	Regular
P waves	Uniform in appearance, positive (upright) in lead II, one precedes each QRS complex
PR interval	0.12 to 0.20 sec and constant from beat to beat
QRS duration	0.10 sec or less

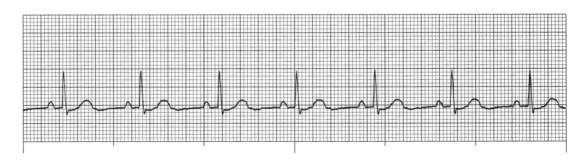

Figure 4-19   Sinus rhythm at 70 beats/min.

Sinus Bradycardia

Causes and Clinical Significance

Sinus bradycardia (Figure 4-20) (Table 4-7) may be normal in physically conditioned adults and during sleep. Sinus bradycardia is a common dysrhythmia associated with inferior and posterior acute myocardial infarction.[1] Other causes of sinus bradycardia include disease of the SA node, increased vagal (parasympathetic) tone (vomiting, increased intracranial pressure, vagal maneuvers, carotid sinus pressure), hypoxia, hypothermia, hypothyroidism, hyperkalemia, uremia, glaucoma, sleep apnea syndrome, and administration of medications such as calcium channel blockers (verapamil, diltiazem), digitalis, and beta-blockers (propranolol).

Clinical signs and symptoms of hemodynamic compromise include hypotension, chest pain, shortness of breath, changes in mental status, left ventricular failure, a fall in urine output, and cold, clammy skin.

Table 4-7	Characteristics of Sinus Bradycardia
Rate	Less than 60 beats/min
Rhythm	Regular
P waves	Uniform in appearance, positive (upright) in lead II, one precedes each QRS complex
PR interval	0.12-0.20 sec and constant from beat to beat
QRS duration	0.10 sec or less unless an intraventricular conduction delay exists

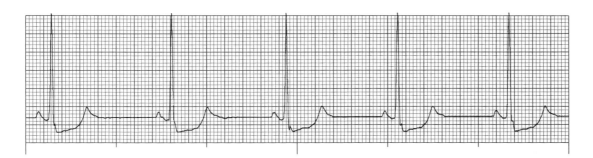

Figure 4-20   Sinus bradycardia at 48 beats/min.

Sinus Tachycardia

Causes and Clinical Significance

Sinus tachycardia (Figure 4-21)(Table 4-8) occurs as a normal response to the body's demand for increased oxygen because of fever, pain and anxiety, hypoxia, congestive heart failure, acute myocardial infarction, infection, sympathetic stimulation, shock, hypovolemia, dehydration, exercise, and fright. Sinus tachycardia may also occur as the result of administration of medications such as epinephrine, atropine, dopamine, and dobutamine, or substances such as caffeine-containing beverages, nicotine, and cocaine.

Sinus tachycardia is seen in about one third of patients with acute myocardial infarction,[2] especially those with an anterior infarction.[3] In the setting of acute MI, sinus tachycardia is a warning signal for heart failure, hypovolemia, and increased risk for serious dysrhythmias.

Table 4-8	Characteristics of Sinus Tachycardia
Rate	101 to 180 beats/min
Rhythm	Regular
P waves	Uniform in appearance, positive (upright) in lead II, one precedes each QRS complex; at very fast rates, it may be difficult to distinguish a P wave from a T wave
PR interval	0.12-0.20 second and constant from beat to beat
QRS duration	0.10 second or less unless an intraventricular conduction delay exists

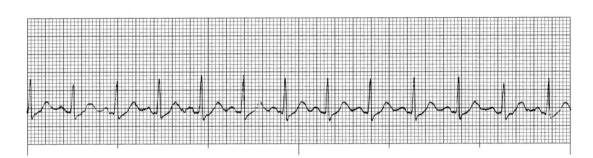

Figure 4-21   Sinus tachycardia at 129 beats/min.

Sinus Arrhythmia

Causes and Clinical Significance

Respiratory sinus arrhythmia is a normal phenomenon that occurs with respiration and changes in intrathoracic pressure. The heart rate increases with inspiration (R-R intervals shorten) and decreases with expiration (R-R intervals lengthen). **Sinus arrhythmia** is most commonly observed in infants and children, but may be seen in any age group (Figure 4-22) (Table 4-9).

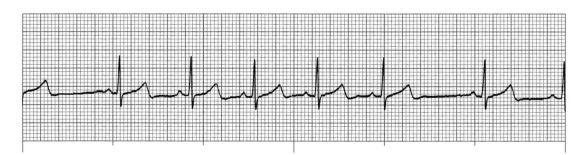

Figure 4-22   Sinus arrhythmia at 54-88 beats/min.

Table 4-9   Characteristics of Sinus Arrhythmia

Rate	Usually 60 to 100 beats/min but may be slower or faster
Rhythm	Irregular, phasic with respiration; heart rate increases gradually during inspiration (R-R intervals shorten) and decreases with expiration (R-R intervals lengthen)
P waves	Uniform in appearance, positive (upright) in lead II, one precedes each QRS complex
PR interval	0.12 to 0.20 sec and constant from beat to beat
QRS duration	0.10 second or less unless an intraventricular conduction delay exists

Nonrespiratory sinus arrhythmia is more likely seen in older individuals and in those with heart disease. It is common after acute inferior wall MI and may be seen with increased intracranial pressure. Nonrespiratory sinus arrhythmia may be the effect of medications such as digitalis and morphine, and carotid sinus pressure.[2]

Sinoatrial (SA) Block

Causes and Clinical Significance

SA block (Figure 4-23) (Table 4-10) is relatively uncommon but may occur because of acute MI; digitalis, quinidine, procainamide, or salicylate administration; coronary artery disease; myocarditis; congestive heart failure; carotid sinus sensitivity; or increased vagal tone. If the episodes of SA block are frequent and/or accompanied by a slow rate, the patient may show signs and symptoms of hemodynamic compromise.

Table 4-10   Characteristics of Sinoatrial (SA) Block

Rate	Usually normal but varies because of the pause
Rhythm	Irregular because of the pause(s) caused by the SA block; the pause is the same as (or an exact multiple of) the distance between two other P-P intervals
P waves	Uniform in appearance, positive (upright) in lead II; when present, one precedes each QRS complex
PR interval	0.12 to 0.20 sec and constant from beat to beat
QRS duration	0.10 second or less unless an intraventricular conduction delay exists

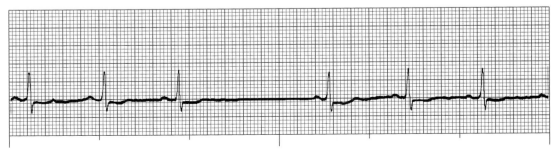

Figure 4-23   Sinoatrial (SA) block.

Sinus Arrest

Causes and Clinical Significance

Causes of **sinus arrest** (Figure 4-24) (Table 4-11) include hypoxia, myocardial ischemia or infarction, hyperkalemia, digitalis toxicity, reactions to medications such as beta-blockers and calcium channel blockers, carotid sinus sensitivity, or increased vagal tone. Signs of hemodynamic compromise such as weakness, lightheadedness, dizziness, or syncope may be associated with this dysrhythmia.

Table 4-11	Characteristics of Sinus Arrest
Rate	Usually normal but varies because of the pause
Rhythm	Irregular—the pause is of undetermined length (more than one PQRST complex is omitted) and is not the same distance as other P-P intervals
P waves	Uniform in appearance, positive (upright) in lead II; when present, one precedes each QRS complex
PR interval	0.12 to 0.20 sec and constant from beat to beat
QRS duration	0.10 second or less unless an intraventricular conduction delay exists

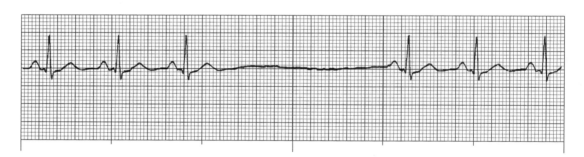

Figure 4-24   Sinus arrest.

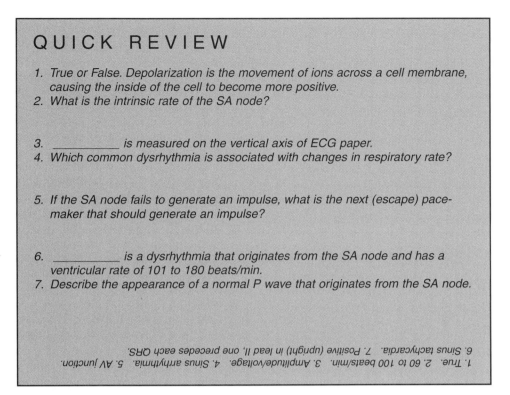

QUICK REVIEW

1. True or False. Depolarization is the movement of ions across a cell membrane, causing the inside of the cell to become more positive.
2. What is the intrinsic rate of the SA node?

3. _____ is measured on the vertical axis of ECG paper.
4. Which common dysrhythmia is associated with changes in respiratory rate?

5. If the SA node fails to generate an impulse, what is the next (escape) pacemaker that should generate an impulse?

6. _____ is a dysrhythmia that originates from the SA node and has a ventricular rate of 101 to 180 beats/min.
7. Describe the appearance of a normal P wave that originates from the SA node.

1. *True.* 2. *60 to 100 beats/min.* 3. *Amplitude/voltage.* 4. *Sinus arrhythmia.* 5. *AV junction.* 6. *Sinus tachycardia.* 7. *Positive (upright) in lead II, one precedes each QRS.*

Premature Atrial Complexes (PACs)

Causes and Clinical Significance

Premature Atrial Complexes (PACs) (Figure 4-25) (Table 4-12) are very common and may occur because of emotional stress, congestive heart failure, myocardial ischemia or injury, mental and physical fatigue, atrial enlargement, digitalis toxicity, hypokalemia, hypomagnesemia, hyperthyroidism, and excessive intake of caffeine, tobacco, or alcohol.

Table 4-12   Characteristics of Premature Atrial Complexes (PACs)

Rate	Usually within normal range but depends on underlying rhythm
Rhythm	Regular with premature beats
P waves	Premature (occurring earlier than the next expected sinus P wave), positive (upright) in lead II, one precedes each QRS complex, often differ in shape from sinus P waves—may be flattened, notched, pointed, biphasic, or lost in the preceding T wave
PR interval	May be normal or prolonged, depending on the prematurity of the beat
QRS duration	Usually less than 0.10 sec but may be wide (aberrant) or absent, depending on the prematurity of the beat; the QRS of the PAC is similar in shape to those of the underlying rhythm unless the PAC is abnormally conducted

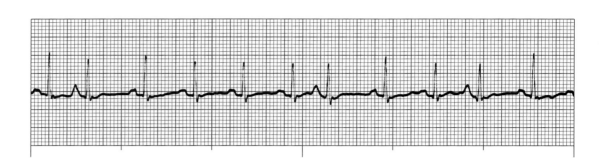

Figure 4-25 Sinus tachycardia with three PACs. From the *left*, beats 2, 7, and 10 are PACs.

Wandering Atrial Pacemaker

Causes and Clinical Significance

Wandering atrial pacemaker (Figure 4-26) (Table 4-13) may be observed in normal, healthy hearts (particularly in athletes) and during sleep. It may also occur with some types of organic heart disease and with digitalis toxicity. This dysrhythmia usually produces no signs and symptoms unless it is associated with a bradycardic rate.

Table 4-13	Characteristics of Wandering Atrial Pacemaker (Multiformed Atrial Rhythm)
Rate	Usually 60 to 100 beats/min but may be slow; if the rate is greater than 100 beats/min, the rhythm is termed *multifocal* (or *chaotic*) *atrial tachycardia*
Rhythm	May be irregular as the pacemaker site shifts from the SA node to ectopic atrial locations and the AV junction
P waves	Size, shape, and direction may change from beat to beat. At least three different P wave configurations are required for a diagnosis of wandering atrial pacemaker or multifocal atrial tachycardia
PR interval	Variable
QRS duration	Usually less than 0.10 second unless an intraventricular conduction delay exists

Lead II (continuous)

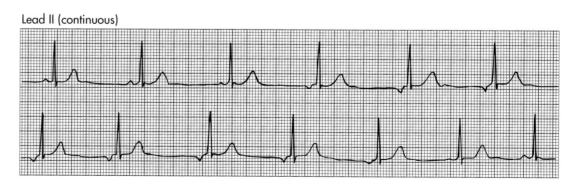

Figure 4-26 Wandering atrial pacemaker. Continuous strip (lead II).

Multifocal Atrial Tachycardia (MAT)

When wandering atrial pacemaker is associated with a ventricular response of 100 beats/min or greater, the rhythm is termed **multifocal atrial tachycardia (MAT)** (Figure 4-27). MAT is also called *chaotic atrial tachycardia*. In MAT, multiple ectopic sites stimulate the atria. Multifocal atrial tachycardia may be confused with atrial fibrillation because both rhythms are irregular; however, P waves (although varying in size, shape, and direction) are clearly visible in MAT.

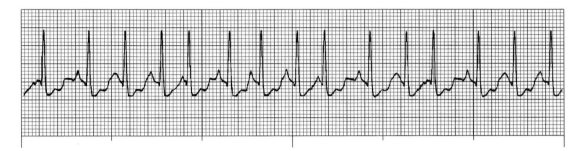

Figure 4-27   Multifocal atrial tachycardia (MAT).

Causes and Clinical Significance

Multifocal atrial tachycardia is most commonly observed in elderly individuals and those with severe chronic obstructive pulmonary disease (COPD), acute myocardial infarction, hypoxia, and theophylline toxicity. Electrolyte imbalances, such as hypokalemia and hypomagnesemia, have also been reported as causes of this dysrhythmia.[2]

Supraventricular Tachycardia (SVT)

The term **supraventricular tachycardia (SVT)** (Table 4-14) may be used in two ways. First, it describes all tachydysrhythmias that originate above the bifurcation of the bundle of His. Second, the term refers to a dysrhythmia with a rapid ventricular rate (tachycardia) and a narrow QRS complex, but whose specific origin (atrial or junctional) is uncertain. The term **paroxysmal** is used to describe the sudden onset or cessation of a dysrhythmia. Correct use of the term *paroxysmal* requires observing the onset or cessation of the dysrhythmia and identification of the underlying rhythm that preceded it. SVT that starts or ends suddenly is called **paroxysmal supraventricular tachycardia (PSVT)** (Figure 4-28). In PSVT, the QRS is narrow unless there is an intraventricular conduction delay (bundle branch block).

Table 4-14	Characteristics of Supraventricular Tachycardia (SVT)
Rate	150 to 250 beats/min
Rhythm	Regular
P waves	Atrial P waves may be observed that differ from sinus P waves
PR interval	If P waves are seen, the PRI will usually measure 0.12 to 0.20 sec
QRS duration	Less than 0.10 sec unless an intraventricular conduction delay exists

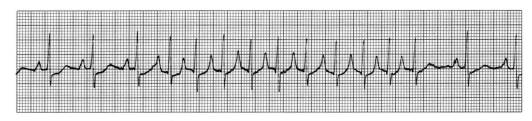

Figure 4-28 Paroxysmal supraventricular tachycardia (PSVT).

Types of PSVT

Three primary types of PSVT are *atrial tachycardia, atrioventricular nodal reentrant tachycardia (AVNRT),* and *AV reentrant tachycardia (AVRT).*

"Supraventricular tachycardias can be classified into those that are AV nodal passive and those that are AV nodal active. AV nodal **passive** SVTs are those in which the AV node does not play a part in the maintenance of the tachycardia but serves only to conduct passively the supraventricular rhythm into the ventricles. AV nodal passive SVTs include atrial tachycardia, atrial flutter, and atrial fibrillation, all of which arise from within the atria and do not need the AV node's participation to sustain the atrial arrhythmia. AV nodal **active** tachycardias require participation of the AV node in the maintenance of the tachycardia."[4] Regular, narrow QRS supraventricular tachycardias are most commonly caused by AVNRT and AVRT, both of which require the AV node as part of the reentry circuit that sustains the tachycardia.

Atrial Tachycardia

Atrial tachycardia (AT) is three or more sequential premature atrial complexes (PACs) occurring at a rate of more than 100beats/min. Atrial tachycardia that starts or ends suddenly is called *paroxysmal atrial tachycardia* (PAT). Paroxysmal atrial tachycardia may last for minutes, hours, or days.

Atrial tachycardia (Figure 4-29) (Table 4-15) is a series of rapid beats from an atrial ectopic focus, often precipitated by a PAC. This very rapid atrial rate overrides the SA node and becomes the pacemaker. Conduction of the atrial impulse to the ventricles is frequently 1:1 (i.e., every atrial impulse is conducted to the ventricles). When used in an attempt to slow this type of paroxysmal atrial tachycardia, carotid sinus pressure will either abruptly convert the dysrhythmia to a sinus rhythm or have no effect.

Ectopic atrial tachycardia (also called *automatic atrial tachycardia* or *benign slow paroxysmal atrial tachycardia*) is a type of AT characterized by abnormal P waves that appear different from sinus P waves. The atrial rate is usually between 100 to 180 beats/min and the ventricular rhythm is regular. Most patients with this dysrhythmia have evidence of organic heart disease.

A rhythm that lasts from 3 beats up to 30 seconds is called *nonsustained.* A *sustained* rhythm is one that lasts more than 30 seconds.

As the heart rate increases, ventricular filling time decreases, resulting in decreased stroke volume.

Table 4-15	Characteristics of Atrial Tachycardia
Rate	150 to 250 beats/min
Rhythm	Regular
P waves	One positive P wave precedes each QRS complex in lead II but the P waves differ in shape from sinus P waves. With rapid rates, it is difficult to distinguish P waves from T waves
PR interval	May be shorter or longer than normal and may be difficult to measure because P waves may be hidden in T waves
QRS duration	0.10 second or less unless an intraventricular conduction delay exists

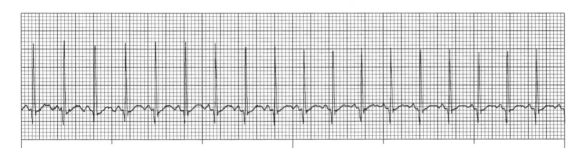

Figure 4-29   Atrial tachycardia.

Causes and Clinical Significance

Atrial tachycardia most often occurs because of rapid firing of an ectopic pacemaker in either the left or the right atrium. The patient may complain of lightheadedness and/or may experience a syncopal episode. Angina or CHF may be induced in susceptible individuals.

AV Nodal Reentrant Tachycardia (AVNRT)

AV nodal reentrant tachycardia (AVNRT) (Table 4-16) is the most common type of PSVT. As its name implies, AV nodal reentrant tachycardia is caused by a reentrant focus in the area of the AV node.

Two conduction pathways exist within the AV node that conduct impulses at different speeds and recover at different rates. The fast pathway conducts impulses rapidly but has a long refractory period (slow recovery time). The slow pathway conducts impulses slowly but has a short refractory period (fast recovery time)[5] (Figure 4-30).

Under the right conditions, the fast and slow pathways can form an electrical circuit or loop. As one side of the loop is repolarizing, the other is depolarizing. Normally, conduction occurs down the fast pathway to activate the bundle of His and ventricles.

Table 4-16   Characteristics of AV Nodal Reentrant Tachycardia (AVNRT)

Rate	150 to 250 beats/min; typically 170 to 250 beats/min
Rhythm	Ventricular rhythm is usually very regular
P waves	P waves are often hidden in the QRS complex. If the ventricles are stimulated first and then the atria, a negative (inverted) P wave will appear after the QRS in leads II, III, and aVF. When the atria are depolarized after the ventricles, the P wave typically distorts the end of the QRS complex
PR interval	P waves are not seen before the QRS complex; therefore the PR interval is not measurable
QRS duration	Less than 0.10 second unless an intraventricular conduction delay exists

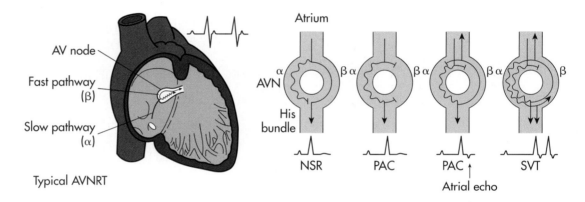

Figure 4-30   Schematic for typical AV nodal reentrant tachycardia (AVNRT). AV = AV node, NSR = normal sinus rhythm, PAC = premature atrial complex, SVT = supraventricular tachycardia. (From Braunwald E, Schneiman M, editors: *Arrhythmias: electrophysiologic principles*, vol IX, Singapore, 1996, Current Medicine/Mosby.)

Causes and Clinical Significance

Cardiac output = stroke volume × heart rate. In a patient with a very rapid ventricular rate, diastolic filling time is shortened, thereby reducing stroke volume and, ultimately, cardiac output.

AVNRT is common in young, healthy individuals with no structural heart disease as well as in individuals with atherosclerotic or hypertensive heart disease. AVNRT is often precipitated by a premature complex. The primary symptom during AVNRT is palpitations. Rapid ventricular rates may be associated with lightheadedness, dyspnea, weakness, nervousness, chest pain or pressure, nausea, diaphoresis, dizziness, syncope, and possible signs of shock depending on the duration and rate of the tachycardia and the presence of structural heart disease. Recurrent episodes vary in frequency, duration, and severity from several times a day to every 2 to 3 years.

Vagal Maneuvers

Vagal maneuvers (Table 4-17) are methods used to stimulate baroreceptors located in the internal carotid arteries and the aortic arch. Stimulation of these receptors results in reflex stimulation of the vagus nerve and release of acetylcholine. Acetylcholine slows conduction through the AV node, resulting in slowing of the heart rate.

Examples of vagal maneuvers include:
- Coughing
- Squatting
- Carotid sinus pressure
- Pulling of the tongue
- Digital rectal massage
- Bearing down (Valsalva maneuver)
- Breath-holding
- Immersion of the face in ice water
- Stimulation of the gag reflex

When using vagal maneuvers, keep the following points in mind:
- Before attempting a vagal maneuver, an IV should be established and emergency medications readily available
- Continuous monitoring of the patient's ECG is essential; note the onset and end of the vagal maneuver on the ECG rhythm strip
- In general, a vagal maneuver should not be continued for more than 10 seconds and should not be used in patients with known myocardial ischemia or recent infarction

Carotid Sinus Pressure

Procedure   The patient's neck should be auscultated for bruits before applying carotid pressure. If there are no contraindications to the procedure, the patient is placed in a supine position with the head turned to the left. Firm pressure is applied to the carotid sinus (just below the angle of the jaw) for 3 to 5 seconds. Simultaneous, bilateral carotid pressure should ***never*** be performed.

Although there is some overlap of the right and left vagus nerves, it is thought that the right vagus nerve has more fibers to the SA node and atrial muscle and the left vagus more fibers to the AV node and some ventricular muscle.

Complications

- Syncope
- Transient ischemic attack/stroke
- Bradydysrhythmias (e.g., sinus arrest, AV block, asystole)

Contraindications

- Avoid in the elderly
- Carotid bruits
- History of cerebrovascular disease

Table 4-17   Effects of Vagal Maneuvers on Different Types of Tachycardias

Dysrhythmia	Effects of Vagal Maneuvers
Sinus tachycardia	Gradual slowing and return to previous rate on cessation of maneuver
AV nodal reentrant tachycardia	Abrupt cessation of the tachycardia or no effect
AV reentrant tachycardia	Abrupt cessation of the tachycardia or no effect
Atrial flutter	Ventricular rate unchanged or temporarily slowed; flutter waves may be revealed during maneuver
Atrial fibrillation	Ventricular rate unchanged or temporarily slowed
Ventricular tachycardia	No effect

AV Reentrant Tachycardia (AVRT)

The next most common type of PSVT is called **atrioventricular reentrant tachycardia (AVRT)**. **Preexcitation** is a term used to describe rhythms that originate from above the ventricles but in which the impulse travels via a pathway other than the AV node and bundle of His. Thus the supraventricular impulse excites the ventricles earlier than would be expected if the impulse traveled by way of the normal conduction system. Patients with preexcitation syndromes are prone to AVRT.

During fetal development, strands of myocardial tissue form connections between the atria and ventricles, outside the normal conduction system. These strands normally become nonfunctional shortly after birth; however, in patients with preexcitation syndrome, these connections persist as congenital malformations of working myocardial tissue. Because these connections bypass part or all of the normal conduction system, they are called **accessory pathways**. The term **bypass tract** is used when one end of an accessory pathway is attached to normal conductive tissue. This pathway may connect the right atrial and ventricular walls, the left atrial and ventricular walls, or connect the atrial and ventricular septa on either the right or the left side.

There are three major forms of preexcitation syndrome, each differentiated by their accessory pathways or bypass tracts[6] (Figure 4-31).

1. In **Wolff-Parkinson-White (WPW) syndrome** (Table 4-18), the accessory pathway is called the *Kent bundle*. This bundle connects the atria directly to the ventricles, completely bypassing the normal conduction system.

2. In **Lown-Ganong-Levine (LGL) syndrome**, the accessory pathway is called the *James bundle*. This bundle connects the atria directly to the lower portion of the AV node, thus partially bypassing the AV node. In LGL syndrome, one end of the James bundle is attached to normal conductive tissue. This congenital pathway may be called a *bypass tract*.

3. Another unnamed preexcitation syndrome involves the **Mahaim fibers**. These fibers do not bypass the AV node but originate below the AV node and insert into the ventricular wall, bypassing part or all of the ventricular conduction system.

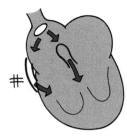
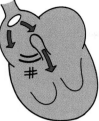
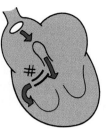

| Kent (W-P-W) short P-R with Δ wave | James (L-G-L) short P-R without Δ wave | Mahaim normal P-R with Δ wave |

Figure 4-31 The three major forms of preexcitation. Location of the accessory pathways and corresponding ECG characteristics.

Table 4-18   Characteristics of Wolff-Parkinson-White (WPW) Syndrome

Rate	Usually 60 to 100 beats/min, if the underlying rhythm is sinus in origin
Rhythm	Regular, unless associated with atrial fibrillation
P waves	Normal and positive in lead II unless WPW is associated with atrial fibrillation
PR interval	If P waves are observed, less than 0.12 sec
QRS duration	Usually greater than 0.12 sec, slurred upstroke of the QRS complex (delta wave) may be seen in one or more leads

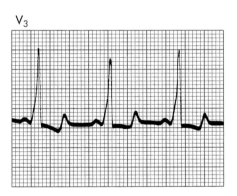

V_3

Figure 4-32 Lead V_3. Typical WPW pattern showing the short PR interval, delta wave, wide QRS complex and secondary ST, and T-wave changes.

Delta waves are produced by accessory pathways that insert directly into ventricular muscle. A delta wave is the initial slurred deflection at the beginning of the QRS complex that results from initial activation of the QRS by conduction over the accessory pathway[7] (Figure 4-32).

Causes and Clinical Significance

Individuals with preexcitation syndrome are predisposed to tachydysrhythmias because there is a loss of the protective blocking mechanism provided by the AV node and because the accessory pathway provides a mechanism for reentry. Signs and symptoms associated with rapid ventricular rates may include palpitations, anxiety, weakness, dizziness, chest pain, shortness of breath, and shock.

PSVT and atrial fibrillation are the two most common tachydysrhythmias seen in WPW. Atrial fibrillation and atrial flutter that occur in the presence of an accessory pathway are particularly dangerous because of the extremely rapid ventricular rate than can result from conduction of the atrial impulses directly into the ventricles. The ventricular rate can be 250 to 300 beats/min and can deteriorate into ventricular fibrillation, resulting in sudden death.[4]

Atrial Flutter

Atrial flutter (Figure 4-33) (Table 4-19) is an ectopic atrial rhythm in which an irritable site depolarizes regularly at an extremely rapid rate. Atrial flutter has been classified into two types. Type I atrial flutter is caused by a reentrant circuit that is localized in the right atrium. Type I atrial flutter is also called *typical* or *classical atrial flutter*. Type II atrial flutter is called *atypical* or *very rapid atrial flutter*. Patients with Type II atrial flutter often develop atrial fibrillation. The precise mechanism of Type II atrial flutter has not been defined.

Table 4-19 Characteristics of Atrial Flutter	
Rate	Atrial rate 250 to 450 beats/min, typically 300 beats/min; ventricular rate variable—determined by AV blockade; the ventricular rate will usually not exceed 180 beats/min because of the intrinsic conduction rate of the AV junction
Rhythm	Atrial regular, ventricular regular or irregular depending on AV conduction/blockade
P waves	No identifiable P waves; saw-toothed "flutter" waves are present
PR interval	Not measurable
QRS duration	Usually less than 0.10 sec but may be widened if flutter waves are buried in the QRS complex or an intraventricular conduction delay exists

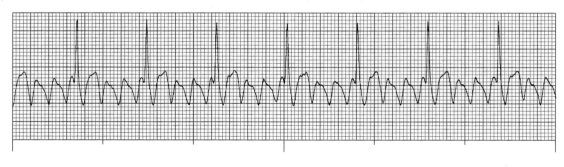

Figure 4-33 Atrial flutter.

Causes and Clinical Significance

Atrial flutter is usually a paroxysmal rhythm precipitated by a PAC that may last for seconds to hours, and occasionally 24 hours or more. Chronic atrial flutter is unusual because the rhythm usually reverts to sinus rhythm or atrial fibrillation, either spontaneously or with treatment.[5]

Severity of signs and symptoms associated with atrial flutter vary, depending on the ventricular rate, the duration of the dysrhythmia, and the patient's cardiovascular status. The more rapid the ventricular rate, the more likely the patient is to be symptomatic with this dysrhythmia. The patient may be asymptomatic and not require treatment or may experience serious signs and symptoms or the patient may complain of palpitations or skipped beats, weakness, dizziness, or chest pressure/pain.

Atrial Fibrillation (Afib)

Causes and Clinical Significance

Atrial fibrillation (Figure 4-34) (Table 4-20) occurs because of multiple reentry circuits in the atria. This dysrhythmia may occur acutely (lasting less than 48 hours), paroxysmally (intermittent), or chronically (lasting at least one month). In atrial fibrillation, the atria are depolarized at a rate of 400 to 600 beats/min. These rapid impulses cause the muscles of the atria to quiver (fibrillate), resulting in ineffectual atrial contraction, a subsequent decrease in cardiac output, and loss of atrial kick.

Conditions commonly associated with atrial fibrillation include rheumatic heart disease, coronary artery disease, hypertension, mitral or tricuspid valve disease, congestive heart failure, pericarditis, pulmonary embolism, cardiomyopathy, and hypoxia. Other precipitants of atrial fibrillation include drugs or intoxicants (e.g., alcohol, carbon monoxide), acute or chronic pulmonary disease, enhanced vagal tone, enhanced sympathetic tone, hypokalemia, and hyperthyroidism. Paroxysmal atrial fibrillation has been associated with excessive alcohol consumption in otherwise healthy individuals ("holiday heart syndrome").[8]

Table 4-20	Characteristics of Atrial Fibrillation
Rate	Atrial rate usually greater than 400-600 beats/min; ventricular rate variable
Rhythm	Ventricular rhythm usually irregularly irregular
P waves	No identifiable P waves; fibrillatory waves present. Erratic, wavy baseline
PR interval	Not measurable
QRS duration	Usually less than 0.10 second but may be widened if an intraventricular conduction delay exists

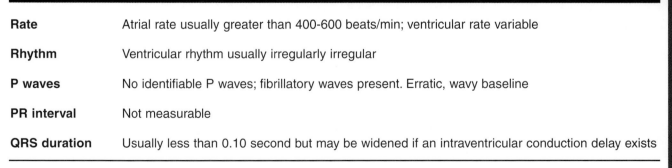

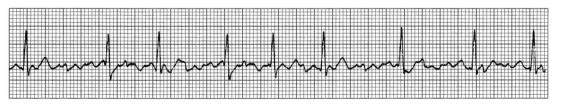

Figure 4-34   Atrial fibrillation.

Patients experiencing Afib may develop intra-atrial emboli because the atria are not contracting and blood stagnates in the atrial chambers. This predisposes the patient to systemic emboli, particularly stroke, if the clots dislodge spontaneously or because of conversion to a sinus rhythm. It is estimated that 15% to 20% of strokes in patients without rheumatic heart disease are caused by atrial fibrillation, and the incidence is even higher for those with rheumatic heart disease.[7]

The severity of signs and symptoms associated with atrial fibrillation vary, depending on the ventricular rate, the duration of the dysrhythmia, and the patient's cardiovascular status. The more rapid the ventricular rate, the more likely the patient is to be symptomatic with this dysrhythmia.

The patient may be asymptomatic or may experience serious signs and symptoms. Atrial fibrillation with a rapid ventricular response may produce signs and symptoms including lightheadedness, palpitations, dyspnea, chest pressure/pain, and hypotension.

QUICK REVIEW

1. A _____ is an early beat initiated by an irritable atrial site.

2. What dysrhythmia is characterized by a ventricular rhythm that may be regular or irregular and waveforms resembling teeth of a saw or picket fence before each QRS?

3. What is the significance of the relative refractory period?

4. How would you determine if the ventricular rhythm on a rhythm strip was regular or irregular?

5. Describe the appearance of atrial activity in atrial fibrillation on the ECG.

6. Name three possible causes of premature atrial complexes (PACs).

7. Name a consequence of decreased ventricular filling time.

8. _____ is a term that refers to the sudden onset or cessation of a dysrhythmia.

9. What is the most common preexcitation syndrome?

10. True or False. Multifocal atrial tachycardia is another name for atrial fibrillation.

1. Premature atrial complex (PAC). 2. Atrial flutter. 3. During this period, most (but not all) cardiac cells have repolarized and can be stimulated to depolarize if a stimulus is strong enough. Should a stimulus precipitate depolarization during this period, chaos may result. 4. Measure the distance between two consecutive R-R intervals and compare that distance with another R-R interval. If the ventricular rhythm is regular, the R-R intervals will measure the same. 5. In atrial fibrillation, the atria are not contracting; they are quivering; this produces an erratic, wavy baseline (fibrillatory waves, f waves) on the ECG. P waves are not visible. 6. Often unknown, hypoxia, digitalis toxicity, sympathomimetic drugs, CHF, myocardial ischemia or injury, use of stimulants (excess coffee, tobacco, alcohol). 7. Decreased stroke volume, decreased cardiac output. 8. Paroxysmal. 9. Wolff-Parkinson-White syndrome. 10. False.

Premature Junctional Complexes (PJCs)

Causes and Clinical Significance

Premature Junctional Complexes (PJCs) (Figure 4-35) (Table 4-21) are less common than either PACs or PVCs. PJCs may occur because of excessive caffeine, tobacco, or alcohol intake; valvular disease; ischemia; congestive heart failure; digitalis toxicity; increased vagal tone; acute myocardial infarction; hypoxia; electrolyte imbalance (particularly magnesium and potassium); exercise; and rheumatic heart disease.

Most individuals with PJCs are asymptomatic. However, PJCs may lead to symptoms of palpitations or the feeling of skipped beats. The sensation of skipped beats may be caused by ineffective contraction resulting from poor filling of the left ventricle during the premature beat.[5] Lightheadedness, dizziness, and other signs of decreased cardiac output may be evident if PJCs are frequent.

Table 4-21	Characteristics of Premature Junctional Complexes (PJCs)
Rate	Usually within normal range but depends on underlying rhythm
Rhythm	Regular with premature beats
P waves	May occur before, during, or after the QRS; if visible, the P wave is inverted in leads II, III, and aVF
PR interval	If a P wave occurs before the QRS, the PR interval will usually be less than or equal to 0.12 sec; if no P wave occurs before the QRS, there will be no PR interval
QRS duration	Usually 0.10 sec or less unless an intraventricular conduction delay exists

Lead II

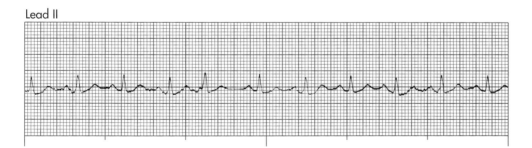

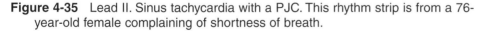

Figure 4-35 Lead II. Sinus tachycardia with a PJC. This rhythm strip is from a 76-year-old female complaining of shortness of breath.

Junctional Escape Beats/Rhythm

A **junctional escape beat** (Figure 4-36) (Table 4-22) originates in the AV junction and appears LATE (after the next expected sinus beat). A junctional escape rhythm is several sequential junctional escape beats. Junctional escape beats and rhythms occur when the SA node fails to pace the heart or AV conduction fails. **Junctional escape rhythms** occur at a very regular rate of 40 to 60 beats/min (Figure 4-37) (Table 4-23).

Table 4-22 Characteristics of Junctional Escape Beats

Rate	Usually within normal range but depends on underlying rhythm
Rhythm	Regular with *LATE* beats
P waves	May occur before, during, or after the QRS; if visible, the P wave is inverted in leads II, III, and aVF
PR interval	If a P wave occurs before the QRS, the PR interval will usually be less than or equal to 0.12 sec; if no P wave occurs before the QRS, there will be no PR interval
QRS duration	Usually 0.10 sec or less unless an intraventricular conduction delay exists

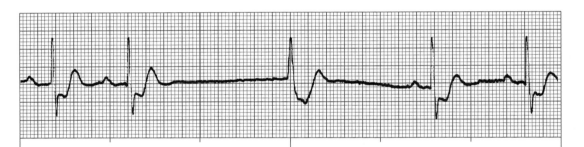

Figure 4-36 Sinus rhythm at 71 beats/min with a prolonged PR interval (0.24 sec), 3.36 sec period of sinus arrest and a junctional escape beat.

Table 4-23 Characteristics of Junctional Escape Rhythm

Rate	40 to 60 beats/min
Rhythm	Very regular
P waves	May occur before, during, or after the QRS; if visible, the P wave is inverted in leads II, III, and aVF
PR interval	If a P wave occurs before the QRS, the PR interval will usually be less than or equal to 0.12 sec; if no P wave occurs before the QRS, there will be no PR interval
QRS duration	Usually 0.10 sec or less unless an intraventricular conduction delay exists

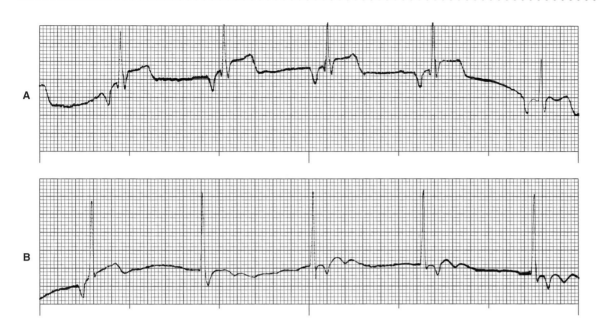

Figure 4-37   Junctional escape rhythm. Lead II—continuous strips. **A,** Note the retrograde P waves before the QRS complexes. **B,** Note the change in the location of the P waves. In the first beat, the retrograde P wave is observed before the QRS. In the second beat, no P wave is observed. In the remaining beats, the P wave is observed after the QRS complexes.

Causes and Clinical Significance

Junctional escape beats frequently occur during episodes of sinus arrest or follow pauses of nonconducted PACs. Junctional escape beats may also be observed in healthy individuals during a sinus bradycardia. A junctional escape rhythm may be seen in acute myocardial infarction (particularly inferior wall MI), rheumatic heart disease, valvular disease, disease of the SA node, hypoxia, increased parasympathetic tone, immediately post-cardiac surgery, and in patients taking digitalis, quinidine, beta-blockers, or calcium channel blockers.

The patient may be asymptomatic with a junctional escape rhythm or may experience signs and symptoms that may be associated with the slow heart rate and decreased cardiac output. Signs and symptoms may include weakness, chest pain or pressure, syncope, an altered level of consciousness, and hypotension.

Accelerated Junctional Rhythm

Causes and Clinical Significance

Causes of **accelerated junctional rhythm** (Figure 4-38) (Table 4-24) include digitalis toxicity, acute myocardial infarction, cardiac surgery, rheumatic fever, COPD, and hypokalemia. The patient may be asymptomatic with this dysrhythmia because the ventricular rate is 60 to 100 beats/min; however, the patient should be monitored closely.

Table 4-24	**Characteristics of Accelerated Junctional Rhythm**
Rate	60 to 100 beats/min
Rhythm	Very regular
P waves	May occur before, during, or after the QRS; if visible, the P wave is inverted in leads II, III, and aVF
PR interval	If a P wave occurs before the QRS, the PR interval will usually be less than or equal to 0.12 sec; if no P wave occurs before the QRS, there will be no PR interval
QRS duration	Usually 0.10 sec or less unless an intraventricular conduction delay exists

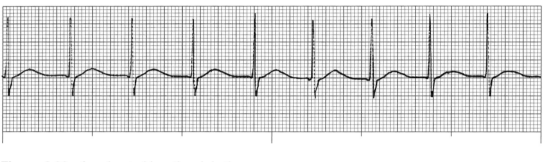

Figure 4-38   Accelerated junctional rhythm.

Junctional Tachycardia

Causes and Clinical Significance

Junctional tachycardia (Figure 4-39) (Table 4-25) is an ectopic rhythm that originates in the pacemaker cells found in the bundle of His. This dysrhythmia may occur because of myocardial ischemia or infarction, congestive heart failure, or digitalis toxicity (common cause).

With sustained ventricular rates of 150 beats/min or more, the patient may complain of a sudden feeling of a "racing heart" and severe anxiety. Because of the fast ventricular rate, the ventricles may be unable to fill completely, resulting in decreased cardiac output. Junctional tachycardia associated with acute myocardial infarction may increase myocardial ischemia and the frequency and severity of chest pain, extend the size of the infarction, cause congestive heart failure, hypotension, cardiogenic shock, and/or predispose the patient to ventricular dysrhythmias.

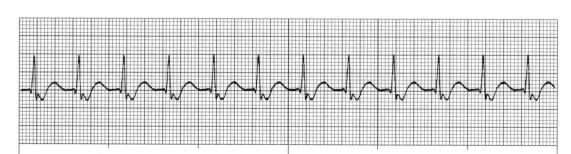

Figure 4-39   Junctional tachycardia.

Table 4-25 Characteristics of Junctional Tachycardia

Rate	101 to 180 beats/min
Rhythm	Very regular
P waves	May occur before, during, or after the QRS; if visible, the P wave is inverted in leads II, III, and aVF
PR interval	If a P wave occurs before the QRS, the PR interval will usually be less than or equal to 0.12 sec; if no P wave occurs before the QRS, there will be no PR interval
QRS duration	Usually 0.10 sec or less unless an intraventricular conduction delay exists

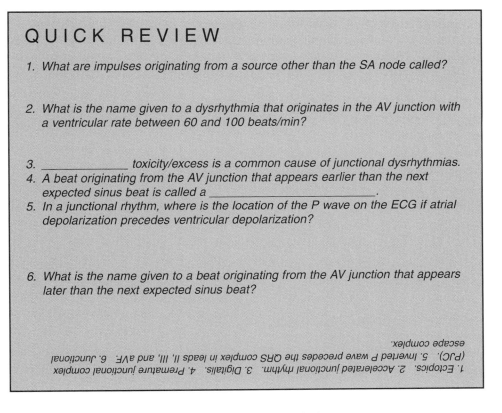

QUICK REVIEW

1. What are impulses originating from a source other than the SA node called?

2. What is the name given to a dysrhythmia that originates in the AV junction with a ventricular rate between 60 and 100 beats/min?

3. _____ toxicity/excess is a common cause of junctional dysrhythmias.
4. A beat originating from the AV junction that appears earlier than the next expected sinus beat is called a _____.
5. In a junctional rhythm, where is the location of the P wave on the ECG if atrial depolarization precedes ventricular depolarization?

6. What is the name given to a beat originating from the AV junction that appears later than the next expected sinus beat?

1. Ectopics. 2. Accelerated junctional rhythm. 3. Digitalis. 4. Premature junctional complex (PJC). 5. Inverted P wave precedes the QRS complex in leads II, III, and aVF. 6. Junctional escape complex.

Premature Ventricular Complexes (PVCs)

Premature ventricular complexes (PVCs) (Table 4-26) may occur in patterns:

- Pairs (couplets): Two sequential PVCs
- Runs or bursts: Three or more sequential PVCs is called *ventricular tachycardia (VT)*
- Bigeminal PVCs (ventricular bigeminy): Every other beat is a PVC
- Trigeminal PVCs (ventricular trigeminy): Every third beat is a PVC
- Quadrigeminal PVCs (ventricular quadrigeminy): Every fourth beat is a PVC

Table 4-26 Characteristics of Premature Ventricular Complexes (PVCs)

Rate	Usually within normal range but depends on underlying rhythm
Rhythm	Essentially regular with premature beats; if the PVC is an interpolated PVC, the rhythm will be regular
P waves	Usually absent or, with retrograde conduction to the atria, may appear after the QRS (usually upright in the ST-segment or T wave)
PR interval	None with the PVC because the ectopic originates in the ventricles
QRS duration	Greater than 0.12 sec, wide and bizarre, T wave frequently in opposite direction of the QRS complex

Premature ventricular beats that look the same in the same lead and originate from the same anatomic site (focus) are called **uniform** PVCs (Figure 4-40). PVCs that appear different from one another in the same lead are called **multiform** PVCs (Figure 4-41). Multiform PVCs often, but do not always, arise from different anatomic sites. The terms *unifocal* and *multifocal* are sometimes used to describe PVCs that are similar or different in appearance. Uniform PVCs are unifocal, but multiform PVCs are not necessarily multifocal.[8]

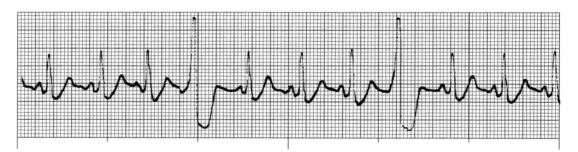

Figure 4-40 Sinus tachycardia with frequent uniform PVCs.

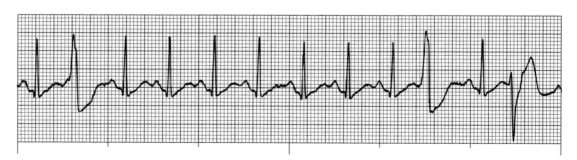

Figure 4-41 Sinus tachycardia with multiform PVCs.

R-on-T PVCs occur when the R wave of a PVC falls on the T wave of the preceding beat (Figure 4-42). Because the T wave is vulnerable (relative refractory period) to any electrical stimulation, it is possible that a PVC occurring during this period of the cardiac cycle will precipitate VT or VF; however, VT and VF most commonly occur without a preceding R-on-T PVC, and most R-on-T PVCs do not precipitate a sustained ventricular tachydysrhythmia.[8]

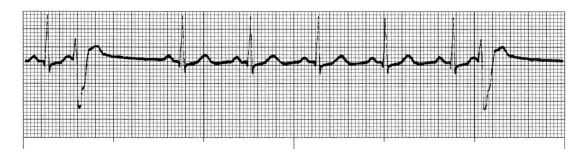

Figure 4-42   Sinus rhythm with two R-on-T PVCs.

A pair of PVCs occurring in immediate succession is called a *couplet* or *paired* PVCs (Figure 4-43). The appearance of couplets indicates the ventricular ectopic site is extremely irritable. Three or more PVCs occurring in immediate succession at a rate of more than 100 beats/min is considered a "salvo," "run," or "burst" of ventricular tachycardia.

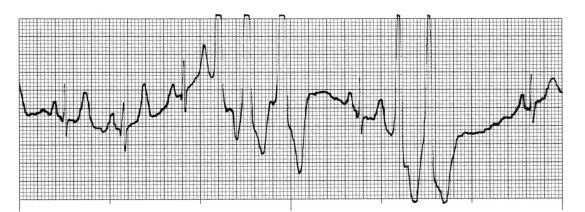

Figure 4-43   Sinus rhythm with a run of VT and one episode of couplets.

Causes and Clinical Significance

PVCs can occur in healthy persons with apparently normal hearts and for no apparent cause. PVCs may occur because of hypoxia, stress, an increase in catecholamines, stimulants (alcohol, caffeine, tobacco), acid-base imbalance, electrolyte imbalance, digitalis toxicity, medications (epinephrine, dopamine, phenothiazines, isoproterenol), ischemia, myocardial infarction, or congestive heart failure.

Patients experiencing PVCs may be asymptomatic or complain of palpitations, a "racing heart," skipped beats, or chest or neck discomfort.

Ventricular Escape Beats/Rhythm

Causes and Clinical Significance

Ventricular escape (idioventricular) beats/rhythm (Figure 4-44 and 4-45) (Tables 4-27 and 4-28) may occur when the SA node and the AV junction fail to initiate an electrical impulse, when the rate of discharge of the SA node or AV junction becomes less than the inherent ventricular rate, or when impulses generated by a supraventricular site are blocked. An idioventricular rhythm may also occur because of myocardial infarction, digitalis toxicity, or metabolic imbalances.

Because the ventricular rate associated with this rhythm is slow (20 to 40 beats/min) and there is loss of atrial kick, the patient may experience severe hypotension, weakness, disorientation, lightheadedness, or loss of responsiveness because of decreased cardiac output.

Table 4-27   Characteristics of Ventricular Escape Beats

Rate	Usually within normal range but depends on underlying rhythm
Rhythm	Essentially regular with late beats; the ventricular escape beat occurs after the next expected sinus beat
P waves	Usually absent or, with retrograde conduction to the atria, may appear after the QRS (usually upright in the ST-segment or T wave)
PR interval	None with the ventricular escape beat because the ectopic beat originates in the ventricles
QRS duration	Greater than 0.12 sec, wide and bizarre, T wave frequently in opposite direction of the QRS complex

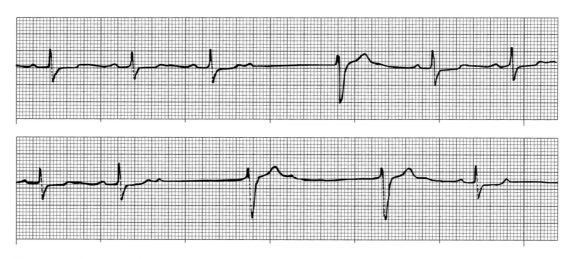

Figure 4-44   Ventricular escape beats following nonconducted premature atrial complexes.

Table 4-28   Characteristics of Ventricular Escape (Idioventricular) Rhythm

Rate	20 to 40 beats/min
Rhythm	Essentially regular
P waves	Usually absent or, with retrograde conduction to the atria, may appear after the QRS (usually upright in the ST-segment or T wave)
PR interval	None
QRS duration	Greater than 0.12 sec, T wave frequently in opposite direction of the QRS complex

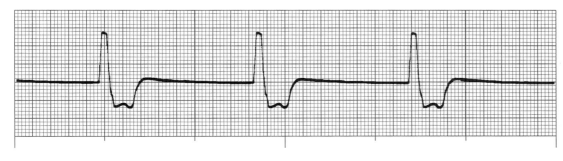

Figure 4-45   Idioventricular rhythm (IVR).

Accelerated Idioventricular Rhythm (AIVR)

Causes and Clinical Significance

Accelerated Idioventricular Rhythm (AIVR) (Figure 4-46) (Table 4-29) is usually considered a benign escape rhythm that appears when the sinus rate slows and disappears when the sinus rate speeds up. AIVR is often seen during the first 12 hours of a myocardial infarction and is particularly common after successful reperfusion therapy. AIVR is seen in both anterior and inferior MI and in 90% of patients during the first 24 hours after reperfusion. AIVR has been reported in 10% to 40% of patients with acute MI.[3] AIVR has been reported in patients with digitalis toxicity, subarachnoid hemorrhage, and in patients with rheumatic and hypertensive heart disease.

Table 4-29   Characteristics of Accelerated Idioventricular Rhythm (AIVR)

Rate	41 to 100 beats/min
Rhythm	Essentially regular
P waves	Usually absent or, with retrograde conduction to the atria, may appear after the QRS (usually upright in the ST-segment or T wave)
PR interval	None
QRS duration	Greater than 0.12 sec, T wave frequently in opposite direction of the QRS complex

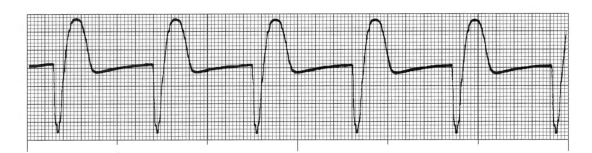

Figure 4-46 Accelerated idioventricular rhythm (AIVR).

Ventricular Tachycardia (VT)

Ventricular tachycardia (VT) exists when three or more PVCs occur in immediate succession at a rate greater than 100 beats/min. VT may occur as a short run lasting less than 30 seconds (non-sustained), but more commonly persists for more than 30 seconds (sustained) VT may occur with or without pulses, and the patient may be stable or unstable with this rhythm.

Ventricular tachycardia, like PVCs, may originate from an ectopic focus in either ventricle. In VT, the QRS complex is wide and bizarre. P waves, if visible, bear no relationship to the QRS complex. The ventricular rhythm is usually regular but may be slightly irregular. When the QRS complexes of VT are of the same shape and amplitude, the rhythm is termed **monomorphic VT**. When the QRS complexes of VT vary in shape and amplitude, the rhythm is termed **polymorphic VT**.

Monomorphic Ventricular Tachycardia

Causes and Clinical Significance

Sustained **monomorphic VT** (Figure 4-47) (Table 4-30) is often associated with underlying heart disease, particularly myocardial ischemia, and rarely occurs in patients without underlying structural heart disease. The most common cause of sustained monomorphic VT in American adults is coronary artery disease with prior myocardial infarction.[8] Other causes of VT include cardiomyopathy, cyclic antidepressant overdose, digitalis toxicity, valvular heart disease, mitral valve prolapse, trauma (e.g., myocardial contusion, invasive cardiac procedures), acid-base imbalance, electrolyte imbalance (e.g., hypokalemia, hyperkalemia, hypomagnesemia), and increased production of catecholamines (e.g., cocaine abuse).[2]

Table 4-30 Characteristics of Monomorphic Ventricular Tachycardia

Rate	101 to 250 beats/min
Rhythm	Essentially regular
P waves	May be present or absent; if present, they have no set relationship to the QRS complexes appearing between the QRSs at a rate different from that of the VT
PR interval	None
QRS duration	Greater than 0.12 sec, often difficult to differentiate between the QRS and T wave

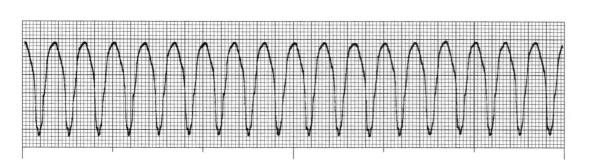

Figure 4-47   Monomorphic ventricular tachycardia (VT).

Signs and symptoms of hemodynamic compromise related to the tachycardia may include shock, chest pain, hypotension, shortness of breath, pulmonary congestion, congestive heart failure, acute myocardial infarction, and/or a decreased level of responsiveness.

Polymorphic Ventricular Tachycardia

Polymorphic VT refers to a rapid ventricular dysrhythmia with beat-to-beat changes in the shape and amplitude of the QRS complexes. Polymorphic VT is further divided into two classifications based on its association with a normal or prolonged QT interval:

> A typical cycle consists of 5 to 20 QRS complexes.

1. Long QT syndrome (LQTS)
   - Acquired (iatrogenic)
   - Congenital (idiopathic)
2. Normal QT

Polymorphic VT that occurs in the presence of a long QT interval is called **torsade de pointes (TdP)** (Table 4-31). TdP is a dysrhythmia intermediary between ventricular tachycardia and ventricular fibrillation.[2] *Torsade de pointe* is French for "twisting of the points," which describes the QRS that changes in shape, amplitude, and width and appears to "twist" around the isoelectric line, resembling a spindle. The singular form, *torsade de pointes*, refers to one episode (several [5 to 10] "pointes").[9] The plural form, *torsades de pointes*, refers to more than one episode or to a prolonged attack[10] (Figure 4-48).

Table 4-31	Characteristics of Polymorphic Ventricular Tachycardia
Rate	150 to 300 beats/min, typically 200 to 250 beats/min
Rhythm	May be regular or irregular
P waves	None
PR interval	None
QRS duration	Greater than 0.12 sec, gradual alteration in amplitude and direction of the QRS complexes

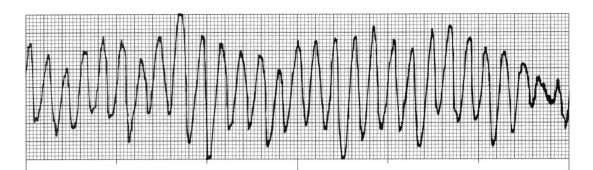

Figure 4-48 Torsade de Pointes (TdP). This rhythm strip is from a 77-year-old male three days post myocardial infarction (MI). His chief complaint at the onset of this episode was chest pain. He had a past medical history of a previous MI and an abdominal aortic aneurysm repair. The patient was given lidocaine and defibrillated several times without success. Lab work revealed a serum potassium (K^+) level of 2.0. IV K^+ was administered and the patient converted to a sinus rhythm with the next defibrillation.

> Polymorphic VT that occurs in the presence of a normal QT interval is simply referred to as **polymorphic VT**.

"The normal QT type of polymorphic VT has a pattern similar to that of TdP. However, unlike TdP it is not related to sinus bradycardia, preceding pauses, or electrolyte abnormalities. It is important to distinguish between long QT syndrome and normal QT because they have different mechanisms and treatments."[10] Standard antiarrhythmic medications are administered in the management of normal QT polymorphic VT.

Causes and Clinical Significance

TdP may be precipitated by slow heart rates and is associated with medication or electrolyte disturbances that prolong the QT interval. A prolonged QT interval indicates a lengthened relative refractory period (vulnerable period), which puts the ventricles at risk for TdP. A prolonged QT interval may be congenital or acquired. Lengthening of the QT interval may be the only warning sign suggesting impending TdP.

Symptoms associated with TdP are usually related to the decreased cardiac output that occurs because of the fast ventricular rate. Patients may complain of palpitations, lightheadedness, or experience a syncopal episode or seizures. TdP may be initiated by a PVC and may occasionally terminate spontaneously and recur after several seconds or minutes or may deteriorate to VF.

Ventricular Fibrillation (VF)

Ventricular fibrillation (VF) (Table 4-32) is a chaotic rhythm that originates in the ventricles. In VF, there is no organized depolarization of the ventricles. The ventricular myocardium quivers, and, as a result, there is no effective myocardial contraction and no pulse. The resulting rhythm is irregularly irregular with chaotic deflections that vary in shape and amplitude. No normal-looking waveforms are visible.

VF with low amplitude waves (less than 3 mm) is frequently called *"fine" ventricular fibrillation* (Figure 4-49). Waves that are more easily visible are described as "coarse" (greater than 3 mm) (Figure 4-50).

Table 4-32   Characteristics of Ventricular Fibrillation (VF)

Rate	Cannot be determined because there are no discernible waves or complexes to measure
Rhythm	Rapid and chaotic with no pattern or regularity
P waves	Not discernible
PR interval	Not discernible
QRS duration	Not discernible

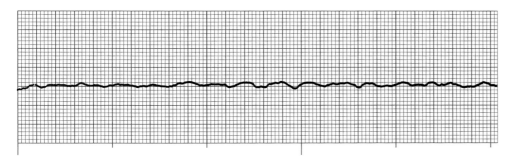

Figure 4-49   Fine VF.

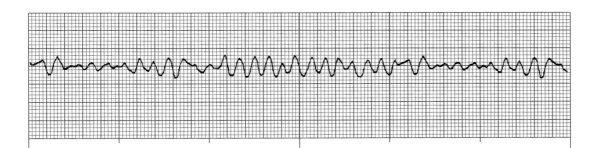

Figure 4-50   Coarse VF.

Causes and Clinical Significance

The patient in VF is unresponsive, apneic, and pulseless. Extrinsic factors that enhance the vulnerability of the myocardium to fibrillate include increased sympathetic nervous system activity, vagal stimulation, metabolic abnormalities (e.g., hypokalemia, hypomagnesemia), antiarrhythmics and other medications (e.g., psychotropics, digitalis, sympathomimetics), and environmental factors (e.g., electrocution). Intrinsic factors include hypertrophy, ischemia, myocardial failure, enhanced AV conduction (e.g., bypass tracts, "fast" AV node), abnormal repolarization, and bradycardia.[11]

It has been demonstrated that patients whose initial fibrillation amplitudes were greater than 0.2 mV (2 mm) had a significantly greater likelihood of resuscitation and that this amplitude declined over time.[12] Factors influencing fibrillation amplitude include electrode size, location, resistance of the chest wall to current, the shape of the chest, and skin condition.[1]

A return of spontaneous circulation is more frequently associated with *early* defibrillation of VF.[1] Defibrillation later in the course of VF is more likely to result in asystole or pulseless electrical activity.[12]

Asystole (Cardiac Standstill)

Causes and Clinical Significance

The term *bradyasystolic rhythm* is a cardiac rhythm in which the ventricular rate is less than 60 beats/min and/or there are periods of asystole.[13]

Asystole (Figure 4-51) (Table 4-33) may occur because of extensive myocardial damage (possibly from ischemia or infarction), hypoxia, hypokalemia, hyperkalemia, hypothermia, acidosis, drug overdose, ventricular aneurysm, acute respiratory failure, or traumatic cardiac arrest (among other causes). Ventricular asystole may occur temporarily following termination of a tachydysrhythmia because of medication administration, defibrillation, or synchronized cardioversion.

Table 4-33   Characteristics of Asystole

Rate	Ventricular usually not discernible but atrial activity may be observed ("P-wave" asystole)
Rhythm	Ventricular not discernible, atrial may be discernible
P waves	Usually not discernible
PR interval	Not measurable
QRS duration	Absent

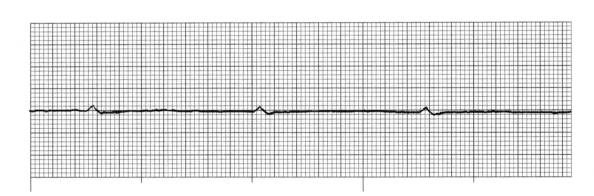

Figure 4-51   "P-wave" asystole.

Whenever a flat line is observed on an ECG, it has been recommended that the rhythm be confirmed in two leads because ventricular fibrillation may be "masquerading" as asystole. In a 1988 study,[14] emergency medical technicians (EMTs) trained in defibrillation were instructed to inspect the lead connections to the patient and defibrillator, check the calibration and battery status of the ECG monitor, and record the ECG rhythm in three different leads whenever an initial flat line was noted on the monitor. VF was documented in 3 of 118 patients (2.5%) when the monitor lead was switched. The authors concluded that VF masquerading as asystole is rare.

Pulseless Electrical Activity (PEA)

Pulseless electrical activity (PEA) is a clinical situation, not a specific dysrhythmia. PEA exists when organized electrical activity (other than VT) is observed on the cardiac monitor, but the patient is pulseless (Figure 4-52).

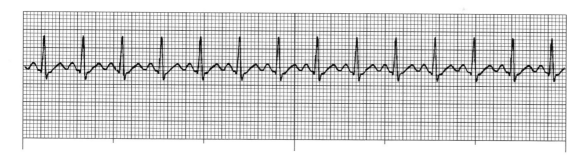

Figure 4-52   The rhythm shown is a sinus tachycardia however, if no pulse is associated with the rhythm, the clinical situation is termed *pulseless electrical activity (PEA)*.

Causes and Clinical Significance

Many conditions may cause PEA. The acronym PATCH-4-MD (see box) can be used as an aid in memorizing many of the possible causes of PEA. The most common cause of PEA is hypovolemia. The second most common cause is myocardial contractile failure, usually because of extensive ischemic or metabolic injury.[1] PEA has a poor prognosis unless the underlying cause can be rapidly identified and appropriately managed. "Irrespective of PEA etiology, the more normal the ECG complex and the shorter the time from cardiac arrest, the higher is the likelihood of successful resuscitation or survival. Conversely, the more abnormal the ECG complex, the longer time from cardiac arrest and the lower the likelihood of successful resuscitation or survival."[15]

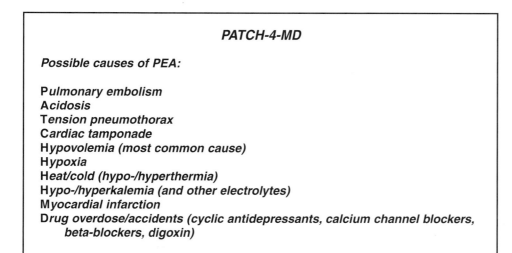

PATCH-4-MD

Possible causes of PEA:

Pulmonary embolism
Acidosis
Tension pneumothorax
Cardiac tamponade
Hypovolemia (most common cause)
Hypoxia
Heat/cold (hypo-/hyperthermia)
Hypo-/hyperkalemia (and other electrolytes)
Myocardial infarction
Drug overdose/accidents (cyclic antidepressants, calcium channel blockers, beta-blockers, digoxin)

QUICK REVIEW

1. Two sequential PVCs are called a _____.
2. What is the name given to the clinical situation in which organized electrical activity (other than VT) is observed on the cardiac monitor, but the patient has no pulse?

3. What is the name given a PVC falling on the T wave of the preceding beat?

4. PVCs of similar configuration in the same lead are called _____.
5. _____ is a pattern in which every third beat is an ectopic beat.
6. True or False. Ventricular tachycardia is an essentially regular ventricular rhythm with a ventricular rate of more than 100 beats/min.
7. A(n) _____ PVC is a type of PVC that occurs between two normal beats and does not interrupt the underlying rhythm.
8. _____ is a type of polymorphic VT associated with a prolonged QT interval.

1. Couplet. 2. Pulseless electrical activity (PEA). 3. R-on-T PVC. 4. Uniform PVCs. 5. Trigeminy. 6. True. 7. Interpolated PVC. 8. Torsades de pointes.

First-Degree AV Block

The **AV junction** is an area of specialized conduction tissue that provides the electrical links between the atrium and ventricle. If a delay or interruption in impulse conduction occurs within the AV node, bundle of His, or His-Purkinje system, the resulting dysrhythmia is called an **atrioventricular (AV) block**. AV blocks have been traditionally classified in two ways: according to the degree of block and/or according to the site of block.

Causes and Clinical Significance

First-degree AV block (Figure 4-53) (Table 4-34) may be a normal finding in individuals with no history of cardiac disease, especially in athletes. First-degree AV block may also occur because of ischemia or injury to the AV node or junction, medication therapy (e.g., quinidine, procainamide, beta-blockers, calcium channel blockers, digitalis, and amiodarone), rheumatic heart disease, hyperkalemia, acute myocardial infarction (often inferior wall MI), or increased vagal tone.

Table 4-34   Characteristics of First-Degree AV Block

Rate	Usually within normal range but depends on underlying rhythm
Rhythm	Regular
P waves	Normal in size and shape; one positive (upright) P wave before each QRS in leads II, III, and aVF
PR interval	Prolonged (greater than 0.20 sec) but constant
QRS duration	Usually 0.10 sec or less unless an intraventricular conduction delay exists

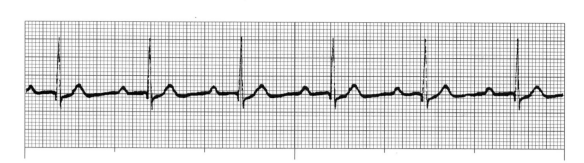

Figure 4-53   Sinus rhythm at 60 beats/min with a first-degree AV block.

Second-Degree AV Block, Type I (Wenckebach, Mobitz Type I)

Second-degree AV block occurs when some, but not all, atrial impulses are blocked from reaching the ventricles. Because the SA node is generating impulses in a normal manner, each P wave will occur at a regular interval across the rhythm strip (all P waves will plot through on time) although not every P wave will be followed by a QRS complex. This suggests that the atria are being depolarized normally, but not every impulse is being conducted to the ventricles. As a result, more P waves than QRS complexes are visible on the ECG rhythm strip.

Causes and Clinical Significance

Second-degree AV block type I (Figure 4-54) (Table 4-35) is caused by conduction delay within the AV node and is most commonly associated with AV nodal ischemia secondary to occlusion of the right coronary artery.[5] Second-degree AV block type I may also occur because of increased parasympathetic tone or the effects of medication (e.g., digitalis, beta-blockers, verapamil). When associated with an acute inferior wall myocardial infarction, this rhythm occurs because of increased parasympathetic stimulation rather than injury to the conduction system and develops within the first 24 to 48 hours of infarction. This dysrhythmia is usually transient, resolving within 48 to 72 hours as the effects of parasympathetic stimulation disappear.

Table 4-35	Characteristics of Second-Degree AV Block, Type I
Rate	Atrial rate is greater than the ventricular rate
Rhythm	Atrial regular (Ps plot through); ventricular irregular
P waves	Normal in size and shape; some P waves are not followed by a QRS complex (more Ps than QRSs)
PR interval	**Lengthens with each cycle** (although lengthening may be very slight), until a P wave appears without a QRS complex; the PRI *after* the nonconducted beat is shorter than the interval preceding the nonconducted beat
QRS duration	Usually 0.10 second or less but is periodically dropped

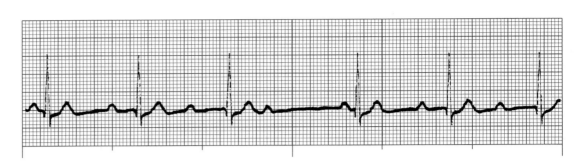

Figure 4-54 Second-degree AV block type I.

Second-Degree AV Block, Type II (Mobitz Type II)

Causes and Clinical Significance

The bundle branches receive their primary blood supply from the left coronary artery. Thus, disease of the left coronary artery or an anterior myocardial infarction is usually associated with blocks that occur within the bundle branches. **Second-degree AV block type II** (Figure 4-55) (Table 4-36) may also occur because of acute myocarditis or other types of organic heart disease. The patient's response to this dysrhythmia is usually related to the ventricular rate. If the ventricular rate is within normal limits, the patient may be asymptomatic. More commonly, the ventricular rate is significantly slowed, and serious signs and symptoms result (low blood pressure, shortness of breath, congestive heart failure, pulmonary congestion, decreased level of consciousness) because of the slow rate and decreased cardiac output.

Table 4-36 Characteristics of Second-Degree AV Block, Type II	
Rate	Atrial rate is greater than the ventricular rate, ventricular rate is often slow
Rhythm	Atrial regular (Ps plot through); ventricular irregular
P waves	Normal in size and shape; some P waves are not followed by a QRS complex (more Ps than QRSs)
PR interval	Within normal limits or slightly prolonged but **constant** for the conducted beats; there may be some shortening of the PR interval that follows a nonconducted P wave
QRS duration	Usually 0.10 sec or greater, periodically absent after P waves

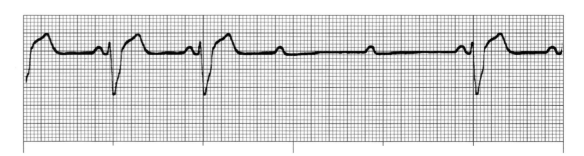

Figure 4-55 Second-degree AV block type II.

Second-Degree AV Block, 2:1 Conduction (2:1 AV Block)

Two conducted P waves must occur ***consecutively*** and the PR intervals of the consecutive beats compared to identify either type I or type II second-degree AV block. When two P waves occur for every one QRS complex (2:1 conduction), the decision as to what to term the rhythm is based on the width of the QRS complex.

A 2:1 AV conduction pattern associated with a narrow QRS complex (0.10 sec or less) usually represents a form of second-degree AV block type I. A 2:1 AV conduction pattern associated with wide QRS complexes (greater than 0.10 sec) is usually associated with a delay in conduction below the bundle of His—thus it is usually a type II block.

Causes and Clinical Significance

In **second-degree AV block with 2:1 conduction** (Table 4-37) the causes and clinical significance are those of type I or type II block previously described. Clinically, conduction usually improves in response to exercise or administration of atropine or catecholamines in type I AV block (Figure 4-56). In type II AV block, conduction typically worsens with exercise or administration of atropine or catecholamines (Figure 4-57).

Table 4-37	Characteristics of Second-Degree AV Block, 2:1 Conduction
Rate	Atrial rate is twice the ventricular rate
Rhythm	Atrial regular (Ps plot through); ventricular regular
P waves	Normal in size and shape; every other P wave is followed by a QRS complex (more Ps than QRSs)
PR interval	Constant
QRS duration	Within normal limits if the block occurs above the bundle of His (probably type I); wide if the block occurs below the bundle of His (probably type II); absent after every other P wave

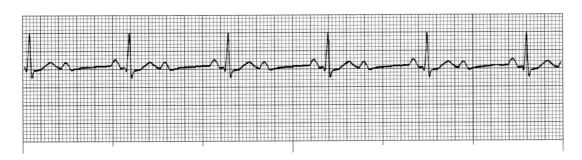

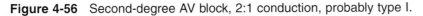

Figure 4-56   Second-degree AV block, 2:1 conduction, probably type I.

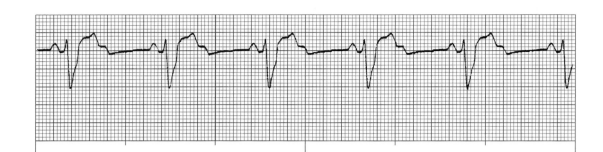

Figure 4-57 Second-degree AV block, 2:1 conduction, probably type II.

Complete AV Block

First- and second-degree AV blocks are types of *incomplete* blocks because the AV junction conducts at least some impulses to the ventricles.[8] With complete AV block, the atria and ventricles beat independently of each other. Impulses generated by the sinoatrial node are blocked before reaching the ventricles. The block may occur at the AV node, bundle of His, or bundle branches. A secondary pacemaker (either junctional or ventricular) stimulates the ventricles; therefore, the QRS may be narrow or wide, depending on the location of the escape pacemaker and the condition of the intraventricular conduction system.

Causes and Clinical Significance

Complete AV block has an incidence of 5.8% in the early period of acute MI and is nearly twice as common with inferior/posterior infarctions compared with anterior infarction.[5] When associated with an inferior MI, complete AV block often resolves on its own within 1 week. Complete AV block associated with an anterior MI may develop suddenly and without warning, usually 12 to 24 hours after the onset of acute ischemia.

Generally, complete AV block (Figure 4-58) (Table 4-38) with narrow QRS complexes (junctional escape pacemaker with a ventricular rate of more than 40 beats/min) is a more stable rhythm than a complete AV block (Figure 4-59) with wide QRS complexes (ventricular pacemaker with a ventricular rate that is usually less than 40 beats/min) because the ventricular escape pacemaker is usually slower and less consistent. The patient's signs and symptoms will depend on the origin of the escape pacemaker (junctional vs. ventricular), and the patient's response to a slower ventricular rate.

Table 4-38 Characteristics of Complete AV Block

Rate	Atrial rate is greater than ventricular rate; the ventricular rate is determined by the origin of the escape rhythm
Rhythm	Atrial regular (Ps plot through); ventricular regular; there is no relationship between the atrial and ventricular rhythms
P waves	Normal in size and shape
PR interval	**None**—atria and ventricles beat independently of each other; thus there is no true PR interval
QRS duration	Narrow or wide, depending on the location of the escape pacemaker and the condition of the intraventricular conduction system; narrow indicates junctional pacemaker, wide indicates ventricular pacemaker

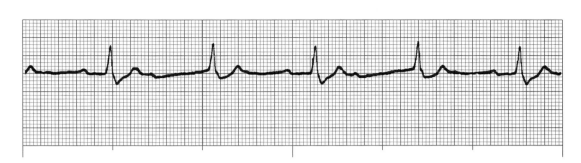

Figure 4-58 Complete AV block with a junctional escape pacemaker (QRS 0.08 to 0.10 sec.).

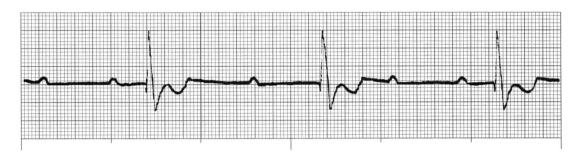

Figure 4-59 Complete AV block with a ventricular escape pacemaker (QRS 0.12 to 0.14 sec.).

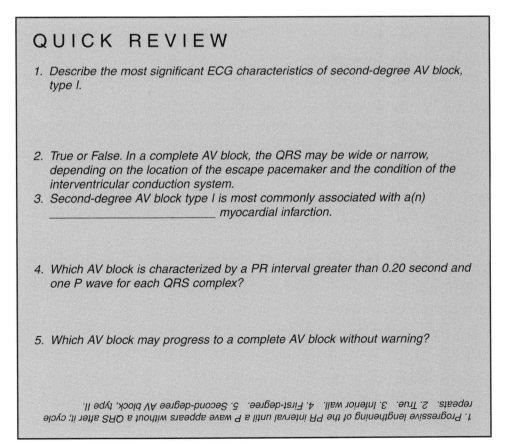

QUICK REVIEW

1. Describe the most significant ECG characteristics of second-degree AV block, type I.

2. True or False. In a complete AV block, the QRS may be wide or narrow, depending on the location of the escape pacemaker and the condition of the interventricular conduction system.
3. Second-degree AV block type I is most commonly associated with a(n) _____ myocardial infarction.

4. Which AV block is characterized by a PR interval greater than 0.20 second and one P wave for each QRS complex?

5. Which AV block may progress to a complete AV block without warning?

1. Progressive lengthening of the PR interval until a P wave appears without a QRS after it; cycle repeats. 2. True. 3. Inferior wall. 4. First-degree. 5. Second-degree AV block, type II.

Intraventricular Conduction Defects

A delay or block can occur in any part of the intraventricular conduction system. A block in only one of the fascicles of the bundle branches is called a **monofascicular block**. A block in any two divisions of the bundle branches is a **bifascicular block**.

A delay in conduction in the right bundle branch causes right ventricular activation to occur after left ventricular activation is completed, producing a R' deflection. A delay in the left bundle branch markedly postpones left ventricular activation, resulting in an abnormally prominent S wave.[16]

If a delay or block occurs in one of the bundle branches, the ventricles will be depolarized asynchronously. The impulse travels first down the unblocked branch and stimulates that ventricle. Because of the block, the impulse must then travel from cell to cell through the myocardium (rather than through the normal conduction pathway) to stimulate the other ventricle. This means of conduction is slower than normal, and the QRS complex appears widened on the ECG. The ventricle with the bundle branch block (BBB) is the last to be depolarized.

QRS measuring 0.10 to 0.12 sec is called an **incomplete** right or left bundle branch block. A QRS measuring more than 0.12 sec is called a **complete** right or left bundle branch block. If the QRS is wide but there is no BBB pattern, the term *wide QRS* or *intraventricular conduction delay* is used to describe the QRS.

ECG characteristics

Width of a QRS complex is most accurately determined when it is viewed and measured in more than one lead. The measurement should be taken from the QRS complex with the longest duration and clearest onset and end.

ECG criteria for identification of a right or left BBB are:
- QRS duration of more than 0.12 sec (if a complete BBB)
- QRS complexes produced by supraventricular activity (i.e., the QRS complex is not a paced beat nor did it originate in the ventricles)

In LBBB, septal activation is altered, and the right ventricle depolarizes before the left. Thus abnormal Q waves originating from the left ventricle may be obscured. Further, ST-segment and T wave changes are often present with LBBB, making the diagnosis of an acute MI even more difficult.

Determining right vs. left BBB
1. View lead V_1 or MCL_1
2. Move from the J-point back into the QRS complex and determine if the terminal portion (last 0.04 sec) of the QRS complex is a positive (upright) or negative (downward) deflection (Figures 4-60 and 4-61)
   a. If the two criteria for bundle branch block are met and the terminal portion of the QRS is positive, a RBBB is most likely present (Figure 4-62) If the terminal portion of the QRS is negative, a LBBB is most likely present (Figure 4-63)

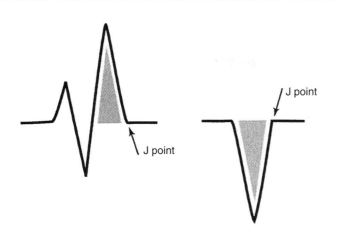

Figure 4-60 Move from the J-point back into the QRS complex and determine if the terminal portion (last 0.04 second) of the QRS complex is a positive (upright) or negative (downward) deflection. If the two criteria for bundle branch block are met and the terminal portion of the QRS is positive, a RBBB is most likely present. If the terminal portion of the QRS is negative, a LBBB is most likely present.

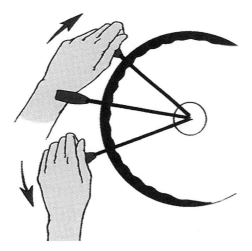

Figure 4-61 Differentiating right versus left BBB. The "turn signal theory"—right is up, left is down.

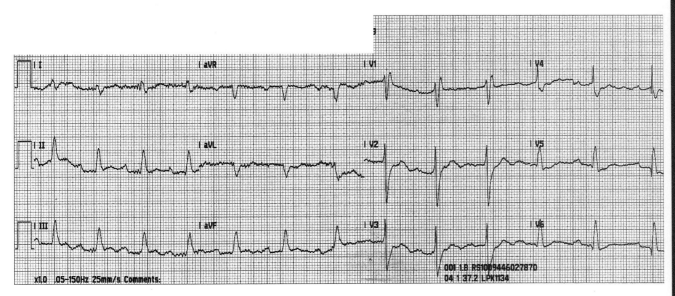

Figure 4-62 Right bundle branch block.

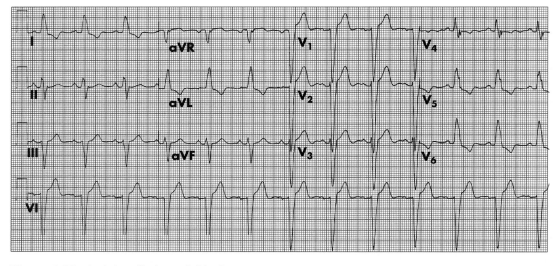

Figure 4-63   Left bundle branch block.

See Tables 4-39 tp 4-43 for a summary of the characteristics of sinus mechanisms, atrial rhythms, junctional rhythms, ventricular rhythms, and AV blocks.

Table 4-39 Sinus Mechanisms: Summary of Characteristics

	Sinus Rhythm	Sinus Bradycardia	Sinus Tachycardia	Sinus Arrhythmia	SA Block	Sinus Arrest
Rate	60 to 100 beats/min	<60 beats/min	101 to 180 beats/min	Usually 60 to 100 beats/min	Varies	Varies
Rhythm	Regular	Regular	Regular	Irregular, typically phasic with respiration	Regular except for the event; pause is the same (or an exact multiple of) the distance between two P-P intervals of underlying rhythm	Regular except for the event; pause of undetermined length, not a multiple of other P-P intervals.
P waves (lead II)	Positive, one precedes each QRS	Positive, one precedes each QRS	Positive, one precedes each QRS	Positive, one precedes each QRS	When present, positive, one precedes each QRS	When present, positive, one precedes each QRS
PR interval	0.12 to 0.20 sec	0.12 to 0.20 sec	0.12 to 0.20 sec	0.12 to 0.20 sec	When present, 0.12 to 0.20 sec	When present, 0.12 to 0.20 sec
QRS	0.10 sec or less	0.10 sec or less	0.10 sec or less	0.10 sec or less	0.10 sec or less	0.10 sec or less
Clinical significance		May be asymptomatic; if decreased cardiac output occurs because of the slow rate, may result in fatigue, syncope, lightheadedness, and/or hypotension	Normal response to demand for increased oxygen caused by fever, pain, anxiety, hypoxia, CHF, fright, stress, etc.; may be asymptomatic	Does not usually require intervention unless accompanied by a bradycardia that causes hemodynamic compromise	Usually asymptomatic; May be associated with signs/symptoms of decreased cardiac output, including altered mental status, dizziness, near-syncope, syncope, and/or hypotension	May be associated with signs/ symptoms of decreased cardiac output, including altered mental status, dizziness, near-syncope, syncope, and/or hypotension

Table 4-40 Atrial Rhythms: Summary of Characteristics

	PACs	Wandering Atrial Pacemaker	SVT	WPW	Atrial Flutter	Atrial Fibrillation
Rate	Usually within normal range, but depends on underlying rhythm	Usually 60 to 100 beats/min; if rate greater than 100 beats/min, the rhythm is termed *multifocal atrial tachycardia*	150 to 250 beats/min	Usually 60 to 100 beats/min if the underlying rhythm is sinus in origin	Atrial rate 250 to 450 beats/min, typically 300 beats/min; ventricular rate variable—determined by AV blockade	Atrial rate 400 to 600 beats/min; ventricular rate variable
Rhythm	Regular with premature beats	May be irregular as pacemaker site shifts from SA node to ectopic atrial locations and AV junction	Regular	Regular, unless associated with atrial fibrillation	Atrial regular, ventricular regular or irregular	Ventricular rhythm, usually irregularly irregular
P waves (lead II)	Premature, positive in lead II, one precedes each QRS, differ from sinus P waves, may be lost in preceding T wave	Size, shape, and direction may change, from beat to beat	Atrial P waves may be observed that differ from sinus P waves	Normal and positive in lead II unless WPW is associated with atrial fibrillation	No identifiable P waves; saw-toothed "flutter" waves present; "saw-tooth" "picket fence"	No identifiable P waves; fibrillatory waves present; erratic, wavy baseline
PR interval	May be normal or prolonged	Variable	If P waves are seen, the PRI will usually measure 0.12 to 0.20 sec	If P waves are seen, <0.12 sec	Not measureable	Not measureable
QRS	0.10 sec or less unless abnormally conducted	Usually <0.10 sec	Usually <0.10 sec	Usually >0.12 sec; delta wave may be seen in one or more leads	Usually <0.10 sec	Usually <0.10 sec
Clinical significance	Very common; presence does not imply underlying cardiac disease	Usually produces no signs and symptoms unless associated with bradycardic rate	Rapid ventricular rate may decrease cardiac output	Extremely rapid ventricular rates possible, producing serious signs and symptoms	If accompanied by a rapid ventricular rate, decreased cardiac output; may deteriorate to Afib	If accompanied by a rapid ventricular rate, decreased cardiac output; increased stroke risk

Table 4-41   Junctional Rhythms: Summary of Characteristics

	PJCs	Junctional Escape Beat	Junctional Escape Rhythm	Accelerated Junctional Rhythm	Junctional Tachycardia
Rate	Usually within normal range, but depends on underlying rhythm	Usually within normal range, but depends on underlying rhythm	40 to 60 beats/min	60 to 100 beats/min	101 to 180 beats/min
Rhythm	Regular with premature beats	Regular with late beats	Regular	Regular	Regular
P waves (lead II)	May occur before, during, or after the QRS; if visible, the P wave is inverted in leads II, III, and aVF	May occur before, during, or after the QRS; if visible, the P wave is inverted in leads II, III, and aVF	May occur before, during, or after the QRS; if visible, the P wave is inverted in leads II, III, and aVF	May occur before, during, or after the QRS; if visible, the P wave is inverted in leads II, III, and aVF	May occur before, during, or after the QRS; if visible, the P wave is inverted in leads II, III, and aVF
PR interval	If P wave is present before the QRS, usually less than or equal to 0.12 sec; if no P wave occurs before the QRS, there will be no PR interval	If P wave is present before the QRS, usually less than or equal to 0.12 sec; if no P wave occurs before the QRS, there will be no PR interval	If P wave is present before the QRS, usually less than or equal to 0.12 sec; if no P wave occurs before the QRS, there will be no PR interval	If P wave is present before the QRS, usually less than or equal to 0.12 sec; if no P wave occurs before the QRS, there will be no PR interval	If P wave is present before the QRS, usually less than or equal to 0.12 sec; if no P wave occurs before the QRS, there will be no PR interval
QRS	Usually 0.10 sec or less unless an intraventricular conduction delay exists	Usually less than 0.10 sec	Usually 0.10 sec or less unless an intraventricular conduction delay exists	Usually 0.10 sec or less unless an intraventricular conduction delay exists	Usually 0.10 sec or less unless an intraventricular conduction delay exists
Clinical significance	Most individuals with PJCs are asymptomatic; lightheadedness, dizziness, and other signs of decreased cardiac output may be evident if PJCs are frequent; if the patient is taking digitalis, check digoxin level	Signs and symptoms of decreased cardiac output may be present due to underlying bradycardic rate and/or SA node dysfunction. If the patient is taking digitalis, check digoxin level.	Signs and symptoms of decreased cardiac output may be present because of bradycardic rate and/or SA node dysfunction; if the patient is taking digitalis, check digoxin level	Most individuals are asymptomatic as the ventricular rate is within normal limits; if the patient is taking digitalis, check digoxin level	The more rapid the rate, the greater the incidence of symptoms caused by increased myocardial oxygen demand; signs of decreased cardiac output may be evident because of the increased rate; if the patient is taking digitalis, check digoxin level

Table 4-42 Ventricular Rhythms: Summary of Characteristics

	PVCs	Ventricular Escape Beat	Ventricular Escape (Idioventricular Rhythm (IVR)	Accelerated Idioventricular Rhythm (AIVR)	Monomorphic Ventricular Tachycardia	Torsades de Pointes	Ventricular Fibrillation	Asystole
Rate	Usually within normal range but depends on underlying rhythm	Usually within normal range but depends on underlying rhythm	20 to 40 beats/min	41 to 100 beats/min	101 to 250 beats/min	150 to 300 beats/min	Not discernible	None
Rhythm	Regular with premature beats	Regular with *late* beats	Essentially regular	Essentially regular	Usually regular	Irregular	Chaotic	None
P waves (lead II)	Usually absent or, with retrograde conduction to the atria, may appear after the QRS (usually upright in the ST-segment or T wave)	Usually absent or, with retrograde conduction to the atria, may appear after the QRS (usually upright in the ST-segment or T wave)	Usually absent or, with retrograde conduction to the atria, may appear after the QRS (usually upright in the ST-segment or T wave)	Usually absent or, with retrograde conduction to the atria, may appear after the QRS (usually upright in the ST-segment or T wave)	May be present or absent; if present, they have no set relationship to the QRS complexes, appearing between the QRSs at a rate different from that of the VT	Independent or none	Absent	Atrial activity may be observed ("P-wave" asystole)
PR interval	None	None	None	None	None	None	None	None
QRS	>0.12 sec	>0.12 sec	>0.12 sec	>0.12 sec	>0.12 sec	>0.12 sec	Not discernible	Absent
Clinical significance	PVCs may or may not produce palpable pulses; patient may be asymptomatic or complain of palpitations, a "racing heart," skipped beats, or chest or neck discomfort	A *protective* mechanism, protecting the heart from more extreme slowing or even asystole	Possible severe hypotension, weakness, disorientation, lightheadedness, or loss of consciousness because of decreased cardiac output as a result of slow rate	Usually asymptomatic; however, possible dizziness, lightheadedness, or other signs of hemodynamic compromise may result from loss of atrial kick	Possible palpitations, shortness of breath, chest pain, or discomfort; loss of consciousness, especially if VT is prolonged or sustained	Possible palpitations, syncope, and/or dizziness	Unresponsive, apneic, and pulseless	Unresponsive, apneic, and pulseless

Table 4-43 AV Blocks: Summary of Characteristics

	First-Degree	Second-Degree, Type I	Second-Degree, Type II	Second-Degree, 2:1 Conduction	Complete (Third-Degree)
Rate	Usually within normal range, but depends on underlying rhythm	Atrial rate greater than ventricular rate; both often within normal limits	Atrial rate is greater than the ventricular rate; ventricular rate often slow	Atrial rate greater than ventricular rate	Atrial rate greater than ventricular rate; ventricular rate determined by origin of escape rhythm
Rhythm	Atrial regular, ventricular regular	Atrial regular, ventricular irregular	Atrial regular, ventricular irregular	Atrial regular, ventricular regular	Atrial regular, ventricular regular
P waves (lead II)	Normal, one P wave precedes each QRS	Normal in size and shape; some P waves are not followed by a QRS complex (more Ps than QRSs)	Normal in size and shape; some P waves are not followed by a QRS complex (more Ps than QRSs)	Normal in size and shape; every other P wave is not followed by a QRS complex (more Ps than QRSs)	Normal in size and shape; some P waves are not followed by a QRS complex (more Ps than QRSs)
PR interval	>0.20 sec and constant	Lengthens with each cycle until a P wave appears without a QRS	Normal or slightly prolonged but constant for conducted beats	Constant	None; the atria and ventricles beat independently of each other, thus there is no true PR interval
QRS	Usually <0.10 sec unless an intraventricular conduction delay exists	Usually <0.10 sec unless an intraventricular conduction delay exists	Usually >0.10 sec, periodically absent after P waves	Within normal limits if block above bundle of His (probably type I); wide if block below bundle of His (probably type II); absent after every other P wave	Narrow or wide, depending on location of escape pacemaker and condition of intraventricular conduction system
Clinical significance	Patient often asymptomatic, but first-degree AV block that occurs with acute MI should be monitored closely for increasing heart block	Usually asymptomatic	May rapidly progress to complete AV block without warning	Signs and symptoms depend on the origin of the escape pacemaker and patient's response to ventricular rate	Signs and symptoms will depend on the origin of escape pacemaker and patient's response to ventricular rate

STOP AND REVIEW

1. The R wave:
   a. Is the first negative deflection after the P wave on the ECG
   b. Is the second negative deflection after the P wave on the ECG
   c. May be a positive or negative waveform that follows the P wave on the ECG
   d. Is the first positive deflection after the P wave on the ECG

2. On the ECG, the P wave represents _____ depolarization and the QRS complex represents _____ depolarization.

3. In most adults, the normal QRS complex measures no more than _____ in duration.
   a. 0.04 sec
   b. 0.06 sec
   c. 0.10 sec
   d. 0.14 sec

4. When viewing a rhythm strip, where is the ST-segment found?

   _____

   _____

   _____

5. Which of the following statements regarding vagal maneuvers is INCORRECT?
   a. Carotid sinus pressure should be avoided in older patients
   b. Carotid sinus pressure should be avoided if carotid bruits are present
   c. Continuous ECG monitoring should be used when carotid sinus pressure is performed
   d. Simultaneous bilateral carotid pressure is applied to ensure slowing of conduction through the AV node

6. The duration of the normal PR interval is:
   a. 0.04 to 0.06 sec
   b. 0.06 to 0.10 sec
   c. 0.12 to 0.20 sec
   d. 0.20 to 0.24 sec

7. What is meant by the term *pulseless electrical activity (PEA)*?

   _____

   _____

8. Identify the following rhythm (lead II):

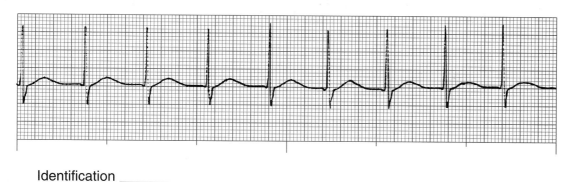

Identification _____

9. In sinus arrhythmia, a gradual increasing of the heart rate is usually associated with:
   a. Expiration
   b. Inspiration
   c. Excessive caffeine intake
   d. Early signs of congestive heart failure

10. Identify the following rhythm (lead II).

Lead II (continuous)

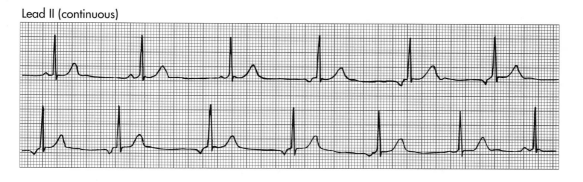

Identification _____

11. Identify the following rhythm (lead II).

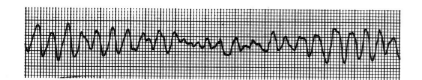

Identification _____

12. Identify the following rhythm (lead II).

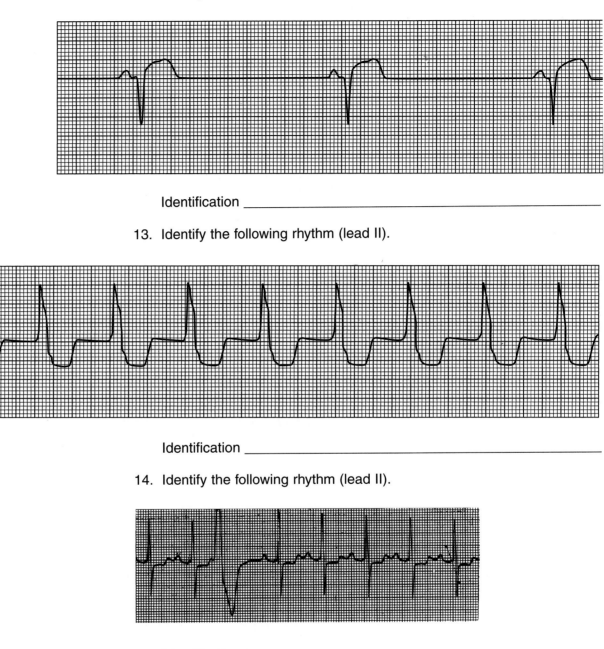

Identification _____

13. Identify the following rhythm (lead II).

Identification _____

14. Identify the following rhythm (lead II).

Identification _____

15. Identify the following rhythm (lead II).

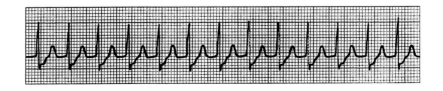

Identification _____

16. Identify the following rhythm (lead II).

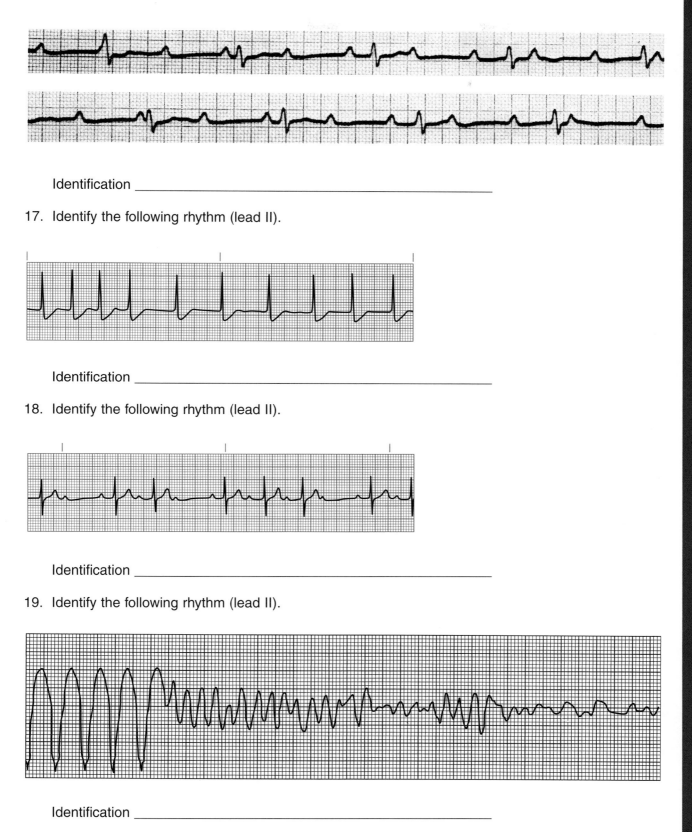

Identification _____

17. Identify the following rhythm (lead II).

Identification _____

18. Identify the following rhythm (lead II).

Identification _____

19. Identify the following rhythm (lead II).

Identification _____

20. Identify the following rhythm (lead II).

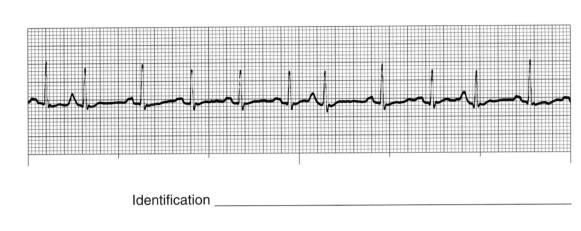

Identification _____

21. Match the following dysrhythmias with their respective ECG characteristics.

Rhythm	**ECG Characteristics**

_____ Sinus bradycardia

_____ Premature ventricular complex (PVC)

_____ Second-degree AV block, type I

_____ Polymorphic ventricular tachycardia

_____ Premature junctional complex (PJC)

_____ Complete (third-degree) AV block

_____ Atrial fibrillation

_____ Sinus tachycardia

_____ Idioventricular (ventricular escape) rhythm

_____ Ventricular fibrillation

_____ Atrial flutter

_____ Monomorphic ventricular tachycardia

_____ Premature atrial complex (PAC)

_____ Second-degree AV block, type II

a. One upright P wave before each QRS, ventricular rate 101 to 180 beats/min

b. Early complex characterized by an upright P wave before the QRS; QRS usually narrow

c. Ventricular rhythm may be regular or irregular, waveforms resembling teeth of a saw or picket fence before QRS

d. More P waves than QRSs, P waves occur regularly, regular ventricular rhythm, no pattern to PR intervals, QRS narrow or wide

e. Early complex characterized by no P wave before the QRS; QRS usually wide

f. Absent P waves, wide QRS, ventricular rate 40 beats/min or less

g. More P waves than QRSs, P waves occur regularly, irregular ventricular rhythm, constant PR intervals, QRS usually wide

h. More P waves than QRSs, P waves occur regularly, irregular ventricular rhythm, lengthening PR intervals, QRS usually narrow

i. Early complex characterized by no P wave or an inverted P wave before or after the QRS; QRS usually narrow

j. Rapid rhythm in which the QRS complex is wide and usually regular; QRS complexes are of same shape and amplitude

k. One upright P wave before each QRS, ventricular rate <60 beats/min, QRS narrow

l. Rapid rhythm in which the QRS complexes are wide and twist from upright to negative or negative to upright and back

m. Irregularly irregular ventricular rhythm, no identifiable P waves

n. Irregularly irregular rhythm with no normal-looking waveforms; chaotic deflections vary in shape and amplitude

STOP AND REVIEW ANSWERS

1. d. The QRS complex consists of the Q wave, R wave, and S wave and represents the spread of the electrical impulse through the ventricles (ventricular depolarization). The QRS complex begins as a downward deflection, the Q wave. A Q wave is **always** a negative waveform. The QRS complex continues as a large, upright, triangular waveform called the *R wave*. The S wave is the negative waveform following the R wave. An R wave is **always** positive and an S wave is **always** negative. Thus the R wave is the first positive deflection after the P wave on the ECG.

2. On the ECG, the P wave represents **atrial** depolarization and the QRS complex represents **ventricular** depolarization.

3. c. The normal duration of the QRS complex in an adult varies between 0.06 and 0.10 sec. About half of all adults have a QRS duration of 0.08 sec. A 0.11 sec duration may sometimes be observed in healthy individuals. Men tend to have slightly longer QRS durations than women.[39]

4. On the ECG, a segment is a line between waveforms. The segment is named by the waveform that precedes or follows it. The ST-segment begins with the end of the QRS complex and ends with the onset of the T wave.

5. d. When carotid sinus pressure is performed, simultaneous, bilateral carotid pressure should **NEVER** be applied.

6. c. PR interval normally measures 0.12 to 0.20 sec and reflects depolarization of the right and left atria (P wave) and the spread of the impulse through the AV node, bundle of His, right and left bundle branches, and the Purkinje fibers (PR segment). The PR interval is measured from the point where the P wave leaves the baseline to the beginning of the QRS complex.

7. Pulseless electrical activity is a clinical situation not a specific dysrhythmia. PEA exists when organized electrical activity (other than VT) is observed on the cardiac monitor, but the patient is pulseless.

8. Accelerated junctional rhythm. The ECG criteria for an accelerated junctional rhythm are the same as for a junctional escape rhythm. The only difference between the two rhythms is the increase in the ventricular rate. The ventricular rate of a junctional rhythm is between 40 to 60 beats/min. An accelerated junctional rhythm has a regular ventricular rate of 61 to 100 beats/min.

9. b. Respiratory sinus arrhythmia is a normal phenomenon that occurs with respiration and changes in intrathoracic pressure. The heart rate increases with inspiration (R-R intervals shorten) and decreases with expiration (R-R intervals lengthen). Sinus arrhythmia is most commonly observed in infants and children but may be seen in any age group.

10. Wandering atrial pacemaker (multiformed atrial rhythm). With this rhythm, the size, shape, and direction of the P waves vary, sometimes from beat to beat. The differences in P wave configuration reflect gradual shifting of the dominant pacemaker between the SA node, the atria, and/or the AV junction.

11. Coarse ventricular fibrillation (VF). In VF, there is no organized depolarization of the ventricles. The ventricular myocardium quivers and, as a result, there is no effective myocardial contraction and no pulse. The resulting rhythm is irregularly irregular with chaotic deflections that vary in shape and amplitude. No normal-looking waveforms are visible. VF with low amplitude waves (less than 3 mm) is frequently called *fine* ventricular fibrillation. Waves that are more easily visible are described as *coarse* (greater than 3 mm).

12. Sinus bradycardia with ST-segment elevation.

13. Accelerated idioventricular rhythm (AIVR). AIVR exists when three or more sequential ventricular escape beats occur at a rate of 41 to 100 beats/min. P waves are usually absent but, with retrograde conduction to the atria, may appear after the QRS (usually upright in the ST-segment or T wave). The ventricular rhythm is essentially regular with a QRS that is greater than 0.12 sec in duration. The T wave is frequently in a direction opposite the QRS complex.

14. Sinus rhythm with an R-on-T PVC. R-on-T PVCs occur when the R wave of a PVC falls on the T wave of the preceding beat.

15. Supraventricular tachycardia (SVT) with ST-segment depression.

16. Complete (third-degree) AV block. The QRS measures 0.12 sec in duration, suggesting the escape rhythm is ventricular in origin.

17. Atrial fibrillation with a ventricular response of 110 beats/min.

18. Second-degree AV block type 1 with a ventricular response of approximately 60 beats/min.

19. Ventricular tachycardia deteriorating to ventricular fibrillation.

20. Sinus tachycardia with three PACs. From the left, beats 2, 7, and 10 are PACs.

21. Answers to the matching exercise.

Rhythm	**ECG Characteristics**

k   Sinus bradycardia

e   Premature ventricular complex (PVC)

h   Second-degree AV block, type I

l   Polymorphic ventricular tachycardia

i   Premature junctional complex (PJC)

d   Complete (third-degree) AV block

m   Atrial fibrillation

a   Sinus tachycardia

f   Idioventricular (ventricular escape) rhythm

n   Ventricular fibrillation

c   Atrial flutter

j   Monomorphic ventricular tachycardia

b   Premature atrial complex (PAC)

g   Second-degree AV block, type II

a. One upright P wave before each QRS, ventricular rate 101 to 180 beats/min

b. Early complex characterized by an upright P wave before the QRS; QRS usually narrow

c. Ventricular rhythm may be regular or irregular, waveforms resembling teeth of a saw or picket fence before QRS

d. More P waves than QRSs, P waves occur regularly, regular ventricular rhythm, no pattern to PR intervals, QRS narrow or wide

e. Early complex characterized by no P wave before the QRS; QRS usually wide

f. Absent P waves, wide QRS, ventricular rate 40 beats/min or less

g. More P waves than QRSs, P waves occur regularly, irregular ventricular rhythm, constant PR intervals, QRS usually wide

h. More P waves than QRSs, P waves occur regularly, irregular ventricular rhythm, lengthening PR intervals, QRS usually narrow

i. Early complex characterized by no P wave or an inverted P wave before or after the QRS; QRS usually narrow

j. Rapid rhythm in which the QRS complex is wide and usually regular; QRS complexes are of same shape and amplitude

k. One upright P wave before each QRS, ventricular rate <60 beats/min, QRS narrow

l. Rapid rhythm in which the QRS complexes are wide and twist from upright to negative or negative to upright and back

m. Irregularly irregular ventricular rhythm, no identifiable P waves

n. Irregularly irregular rhythm with no normal-looking waveforms; chaotic deflections vary in shape and amplitude

REFERENCES

1. Weil MH, Tang W, editors: *CPR: resuscitation of the arrested heart*, Philadelphia, 1999, WB Saunders.
2. Chou T, Knilans TK: *Electrocardiography in clinical practice: adult and pediatric*, Philadelphia, 1996, WB Saunders.
3. Murphy JG: *Mayo clinical cardiology review*, ed 2, Philadelphia, 2000, Lippincott, Williams & Wilkins.
4. Woods SL, Sivarajan Froelicher ES, Motzer SA: *Cardiac nursing*, ed 4, Philadelphia, 2000, Lippincott, Williams & Wilkins.
5. Padrid PJ, Kowey PR, editors: *Cardiac arrhythmia: mechanisms, diagnosis, and management*, Baltimore, 1995, Williams & Wilkins.
6. Crawford MV, Spence MI: *Common sense approach to coronary care*, ed 6, St Louis, 1995, Mosby.
7. Goldman L, Braunwald E: *Primary cardiology*, Philadelphia, 1998, WB Saunders.
8. Goldberger AL: *Clinical electrocardiography: a simplified approach*, ed 6, St Louis, 1999, Mosby.
9. Conover MB: *Understanding electrocardiography*, ed 7, St Louis, 1996, Mosby.
10. Marriott HJL, Conover MB: *Advanced concepts in arrhythmias*, ed 3, St Louis, 1998, Mosby.
11. Paradis NA, Halperin HR, Nowak RM, editors: *Cardiac arrest: the science and practice of resuscitation medicine*, Baltimore, 1996, Williams & Wilkins.
12. Weaver WD, Cobb LA, Dennis D, et al: Amplitude of ventricular fibrillation waveform and outcome after cardiac arrest, *Ann Intern Med* 102:53-55, 1985.
13. Ornato JP, Peberdy MA: in Paradis NA, Halperin HR, Nowak RM, editors: *Cardiac arrest: the science and practice of resuscitation medicine*, Baltimore, 1996, Williams & Wilkins.
14. Cummins RO, Austin D Jr: The frequency of "occult" ventricular fibrillation masquerading as a flat line in prehospital cardiac arrest, *Ann Emerg Med* 17(8):813-817, 1988.
15. Aufderheide TP: in Paradis NA, Halperin HR, Nowak RM, editors: *Cardiac arrest: the science and practice of resuscitation medicine*, Baltimore, 1996, Williams & Wilkins.
16. Wagner GS: *Marriott's practical electrocardiography*, ed 9, Baltimore, 1994, Williams & Wilkins.

BIBLIOGRAPHY

Berne RM, Levy MN: *Cardiovascular physiology*, ed 7, St Louis, 1997, Mosby.

Braunwauld E, Scheinman M, editors: *Arrhythmias: electrophysiologic principles*, vol IX, Singapore, 1996, Current Medicine/Mosby.

Chou T, Knilans TK: *Electrocardiography in clinical practice: adult and pediatric*, Philadelphia, 1996, WB Saunders.

Driscoll P, Gwinnutt C, Mackway-Jones K, Wardle T, editors: *Advanced cardiac life support: the practical approach*, ed 2, London, 1997, Chapman & Hall Medical.

Goldberger AL: *Clinical electrocardiography: a simplified approach*, ed 6, St Louis, 1999, Mosby.

Goldman L, Braunwald E: *Primary cardiology*, Philadelphia, 1998, WB Saunders.

Marriott HJL, Conover MB: *Advanced concepts in arrhythmias*, ed 3, St Louis, 1998, Mosby.

Murphy JG: *Mayo clinical cardiology review*, ed 2, Philadelphia, 2000, Lippincott, Williams & Wilkins.

Paradis NA, Halperin HR, Nowak RM, editors: *Cardiac arrest: the science and practice of resuscitation medicine*, Baltimore, 1996, Williams & Wilkins.

Sanders MJ: *Mosby's paramedic textbook*, ed 2, St Louis, 2000, Mosby.

Snell RS, Smith MS: *Clinical anatomy for emergency medicine*, St Louis, 1993, Mosby.

Weil MH, Tang W, editors: *CPR: resuscitation of the arrested heart*, Philadelphia, 1999, WB Saunders.

Willerson JT, Cohn JN, editors: *Cardiovascular medicine*, New York, 1995, Churchill Livingstone.

Woods SL, Sivarajan Froelicher ES, Motzer SA: *Cardiac nursing*, ed 4, Philadelphia, 2000, Lippincott, Williams & Wilkins.

Electrical Therapy

OBJECTIVES

On completion of this chapter, you will be able to:

1. Define the terms *countershock*, *defibrillation*, and *synchronized cardioversion*.
2. Discuss the primary differences between monophasic and biphasic defibrillation.
3. Describe four factors affecting transthoracic resistance.
4. Describe proper placement of hand-held defibrillator paddles or self-adhesive monitoring/defibrillation pads.
5. Define and describe the procedure for performing a "quick-look."
6. Identify indications for defibrillation.
7. Describe the procedure for defibrillation.
8. Describe the differences in the delivery of energy relative to the cardiac cycle with synchronized cardioversion and defibrillation.
9. Identify indications for delivery of synchronized cardioversion.
10. Describe the procedure for synchronized cardioversion.
11. Explain the precautions that should be taken when defibrillating a patient with a permanent pacemaker.
12. Explain the rationale for early defibrillation.
13. Differentiate between a fully automated external defibrillator and a semi-automated external defibrillator.
14. List the steps in the operation of an automated external defibrillator.
15. Explain the considerations for interruption of CPR when using an automated external defibrillator.
16. For each of the following dysrhythmias, identify the energy levels currently recommended and indicate if the shock delivered should be a synchronized or unsynchronized countershock.
    a. Pulseless VT/VF
    b. Monomorphic VT
    c. Polymorphic VT
    d. Paroxysmal supraventricular tachycardia
    e. Atrial fibrillation
    f. Atrial flutter
17. Briefly describe an implantable cardioverter-defibrillator.
18. Explain the precautions that should be taken when defibrillating a patient with an implantable cardioverter-defibrillator.
19. Discuss indications for transcutaneous pacing.
20. List possible complications of transcutaneous pacing.
21. Describe the indications, technique, and precautions for administering a precordial thump.

COUNTERSHOCK

Countershock is the delivery of an electrical current through the myocardium over a very brief period to terminate a cardiac dysrhythmia. There are two types of countershock: defibrillation (also called unsynchronized countershock or asynchronous countershock) and cardioversion.

DEFIBRILLATION

Definition and Purpose

1. **Defibrillation:** Therapeutic delivery of unsynchronized (the delivery of energy has no relationship to the cardiac cycle) electrical current through the myocardium over a very brief period to terminate a cardiac dysrhythmia
   a. Does not "jump start" the heart
   b. The shock attempts to deliver a uniform electrical current of sufficient intensity to simultaneously depolarize ventricular cells, including fibrillating cells, causing momentary asystole
   c. Provides an opportunity for the heart's natural pacemakers to resume normal activity
   d. Pacemaker with the highest degree of automaticity then assumes responsibility for pacing the heart
2. **Defibrillator:** Device used to administer an electrical shock at a preset voltage to terminate a cardiac dysrhythmia (Figure 5-1)
   a. Consists of:
      (1) **Capacitor** that stores energy
      (2) An adjustable high-voltage power supply that allows the operator to select an energy level
      (3) Charge switch/button that allows the capacitor to charge
      (4) Discharge switches/buttons that allow the capacitor to discharge
      (5) Hand-held paddles or self-adhesive monitoring/defibrillator pads
         (a) Energy is delivered from the defibrillator to the patient through paddles of various types, including hand-held paddles, internal paddles or "spoons," or self-adhesive disposable monitoring/defibrillation pads
         (b) Self-adhesive pads (Figure 5-2)
            (i) Have a dual function: to record/monitor the cardiac rhythm and to deliver the shock
            (ii) These pads are used during "hands-free" or "hands-off" defibrillation and consist of a flexible metal "paddle," a layer of conductive gel, and an adhesive ring that holds them in place on the patient's chest
         (c) "Hands-free" defibrillation
            (i) Enhances operator safety by physically separating the operator from the patient
            (ii) Instead of leaning over the patient with hand-held paddles, the operator delivers a shock to the patient by means of discharge buttons located on a remote cable, an adapter, or on the defibrillator itself

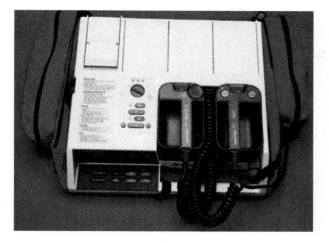

Figure 5-1 A defibrillator is used to administer an electrical shock at a preset voltage to terminate a cardiac dysrhythmia.

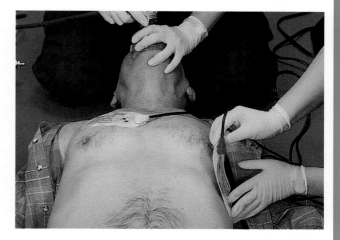

Figure 5-2 Self-adhesive monitoring/defibrillation pads record the cardiac rhythm and deliver the shock.

Energy, Current, and Voltage

1. When defibrillation is performed, the electrical shock passes a large flow of electrons (current) through the heart over a brief period
   a. Defibrillation threshold is the least amount of energy in joules or volts delivered to the heart that reproducibly reverts VF to normal rhythm. This differs from the cardioversion energy requirement, which is defined as the least amount of energy necessary to revert VT to sinus rhythm[1]
2. Monophasic vs. biphasic defibrillation
   a. Defibrillators deliver energy or current in "waveforms" that flow between two electrode patches (or paddles)
   b. There are three general types or classes of waveforms: *monophasic*, *biphasic*, and *triphasic*[2]
      (1) Waveforms are classified by whether the current flow delivered is in one direction, two directions, or multiple directions
      (2) Monophasic waveforms use energy delivered in one *(mono)* direction through the patient's heart
      (3) With biphasic waveforms, energy is delivered in two *(bi)* phases: the current moves in one direction for a specified period, stops, and then passes through the heart a second time in the opposite direction
         (a) When delivered at appropriate energy levels, biphasic success rates can equal those of conventional devices[3,4]
      (4) Triphasic waveforms were introduced in 1997 and deliver multi-directional shocks

Transthoracic Resistance (Impedance)

1. Strength of the electrical shock delivered is expressed in joules (J)
2. Impedance refers to the resistance to the flow of current
3. Transthoracic impedance (resistance) refers to the natural resistance of the chest wall to the flow of current. Impedance is measured in ohms

Energy (joules) = Power (watts) × Duration (seconds)

Historically, transthoracic defibrillation protocols used in the management of pulseless VT and VF have called for an initial shock with 200 joules and the use of increasing energy levels in an attempt to terminate the dysrhythmia. Monophasic waveforms have been predominantly used for both manually operated and automated external defibrillation. In animal experiments conducted in 1983, researchers replaced the monophasic waveform with a biphasic waveform and found the biphasic waveform significantly reduced the energy and the number of shocks needed to successfully defibrillate. Biphasic waveforms have replaced monophasic waveforms for implantable defibrillators because of proven advantages in energy requirements, size, and weight. Biphasic waveforms are now being used clinically, and their safety and efficacy have been demonstrated in both experimental and clinical settings.

Researchers have demonstrated that for both monophasic and biphasic shocks, increasing shock strength does not always improve the probability of successful defibrillation and may in fact increase the incidence of post-shock dysrhythmias.[5] In dogs, researchers have demonstrated that the time until the heart recovered hemodynamically after a defibrillation episode was shorter for biphasic than for monophasic shocks. These researchers also demonstrated that hemodynamic recovery took longer after high energy shocks than after low energy shocks.[6] Further, evidence exists that transthoracic defibrillation with biphasic shocks resulted in less post-shock ECG evidence of myocardial dysfunction (injury or ischemia) than standard monophasic shocks.[7]

4. The amount of current penetrating the chest wall to shock the heart depends on the energy chosen (joules) and the resistance of the chest wall to the passage of that current
   a. If the resistance of the chest wall is increased, less energy will be delivered through the chest wall to the heart
   b. Transthoracic resistance varies considerably among individuals
      (1) Only about 4% to 20% of the total current flow delivered to the thorax actually reaches the heart during defibrillation[6]
      (2) The remainder is dissipated by parallel pathways in the thoracic cage (82%) and lungs (14%)[8]
      (3) The average transthoracic resistance of adult humans is 70 to 80 ohms, with a range from 15 to 150 ohms
5. Factors known to affect transthoracic resistance

Factors Known To Affect Transthoracic Resistance[9]

- Paddle (electrode) size
- Presence of conductive media between the paddles (electrodes) and the patient's skin
- Selected energy
- Number and time interval of previous shocks
- Phase of the patient's respiration
- Chest size (distance between paddles)
- Paddle pressure

   a. Paddle size
      (1) To a point, transthoracic resistance decreases with increased paddle size
      (2) For adults, the optimal paddle size ranges from 8.5 to 12 cm in diameter[9-11]

b. Use of conductive media
   (1) Aids the passage of current at the interface between the defibrillator paddles/electrodes and the body surface (Figure 5-3)
   (2) Types of conductive material available include gels, pastes, and prepackaged defibrillator pads
   (3) Do not use alcohol-soaked pads for defibrillation—they may ignite!
   (4) Failure to use conductive material results in:
       (a) Very high transthoracic impedance and a lack of penetration of current
       (b) Burns to the skin surface
   (5) Use of improper pastes, creams, gels, or pads can cause burns or sparks and pose a risk of fire in an oxygen-enriched environment[12]
   (6) Use of excessive gel may result in spreading of the material across the chest wall during resuscitation, leading to arcing of the current from one paddle to the other
       (a) May produce a potentially dangerous spark or burns
   (7) Damp skin and air pockets beneath hand-held paddles or self-adhesive defibrillation pads increase transthoracic resistance and may cause an uneven delivery of current[13]
c. Selected energy, number, and time interval of previous shocks
   (1) Defibrillation is the definitive treatment and single most important factor in surviving cardiac arrest caused by pulseless VT or VF
   (2) Initial management of pulseless VT or VF includes CPR and delivery of three serial shocks in rapid succession without pausing to check for the presence of a pulse between each shock (assuming the rhythm is unchanged)
   (3) When treating cardiac dysrhythmias using electrical therapy, selecting the appropriate energy (joules) is important
       (a) If the energy and current selected is too low, the shock delivered will not terminate the dysrhythmia
       (b) The use of excessive energy and current may induce cardiac damage[14]

> Appropriate use of conductive gel reduces transthoracic resistance by more than 60%[8]

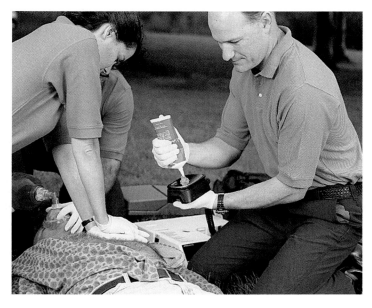

Figure 5-3 Use conductive material to aid the passage of current at the interface between the defibrillator paddles/electrodes and the body surface.

Studies have demonstrated that the use of shocks of 200 J or less is as effective as shocks of 300 J or more.[15,16] A 1982 study compared the effects of initial electrical shocks using 175 J and 320 J in 249 patients with VF and found that initial shocks using 175 J were as effective as shocks of nearly twice that energy level.[17] These researchers noted that repeated shocks at the higher energy level resulted in a higher incidence of AV block after defibrillation than in those patients receiving shocks with 175 J.

Research has shown that a biphasic waveform defibrillator delivering lower energy (150 J) nonescalating (150 J, 150 J, 150 J) biphasic shocks achieved clinical outcomes equivalent to those of monophasic shocks with increasing energy levels. Today, both escalating (increasing energy levels) and nonescalating (no increase in energy level) biphasic waveform defibrillators are available; however, there is insufficient data to recommend one type of device over another.

    (4) In the management of pulseless VT/VF:
        (a) Recommended energy level for the first monophasic shock is 200 J
        (b) Repeated countershocks result in a progressive decrease in transthoracic resistance that depends on the time interval between countershocks[18]
        (c) Regardless of the energy level used, if pulseless VT/VF is not terminated with the first two monophasic shocks, the third monophasic shock is delivered using 360 J
        (d) In pulseless VT/VF, pause only to confirm the rhythm on the monitor between serial shocks

If one of the shocks delivered successfully terminates pulseless VT/VF but the dysrhythmia recurs, begin defibrillation at the last energy level used that resulted in successful defibrillation.

  d. Phase of respiration
    (1) Phase of the patient's respiration is another determinant of transthoracic resistance[19]
    (2) Inspiration increases transthoracic resistance, and resistance is lowered during exhalation
        (a) Because air is a poor conductor of electricity, the greater the volume of air in the lungs when a shock is delivered, the greater the resistance to the flow of current[20]
        (b) Resistance may be lowest when a shock is delivered during the expiratory phase of respiration because the distance between the paddles and the heart is decreased
  e. Distance between paddles
    (1) An individual's chest size or the distance between paddles (electrodes) determines how effectively current is transmitted through tissue to the heart
    (2) A larger chest results in higher transthoracic resistance
  f. Paddle position
    (1) Location of defibrillation paddles (electrodes) affects the magnitude of the shock necessary to defibrillate the heart[6]
    (2) Hand-held paddles or self-adhesive defibrillator pads may be placed in one of three positions for transthoracic defibrillation:

(a) *Apex-anterior position*
  (i)   Anterior (sternum) paddle is placed to the right of the upper sternum below the clavicle
  (ii) Other (apex) paddle is placed to the left of the patient's left nipple with the center of the paddle in the left mid-axillary line (Figure 5-4)
  (iii) If the paddles are placed too close together on the anterior surface of the chest, a substantial amount of current shunts between them and an insufficient amount reaches the left ventricle (Figure 5-5)
  (iv) Placement of the paddles further apart allows a sufficient amount of current to reach the left ventricle (Figure 5-6)
(b) *Apex-posterior position*
  (i)   Anterior paddle is placed over the cardiac apex and the other paddle is placed posteriorly below the right scapula (Figure 5-7)
(c) *Anterior-posterior position*
  (i)   One paddle is placed over the left precordium and the other posteriorly below the right or left scapula

Apex-anterior position is most commonly used during resuscitation because the anterior chest is usually readily accessible. The apex-anterior position is also referred to as the *anterolateral* or *sternum-apex position.*

Paddles may be labeled according to their position on the chest (e.g., sternum, apex) or according to their polarity (e.g., positive, negative). Reversal of the position of the paddles is not important during defibrillation, provided the heart is located between the paddles [21]

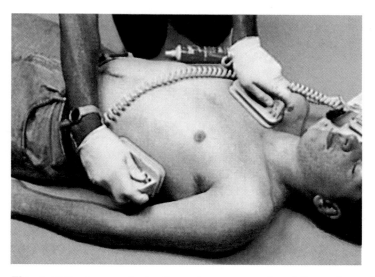

Figure 5-4 Apex-anterior (i.e., sternum-apex) paddle position. The anterior (sternum) paddle is placed to the right of the upper sternum below the clavicle and the other (apex) paddle is placed to the left of the nipple in the left midaxillary line.

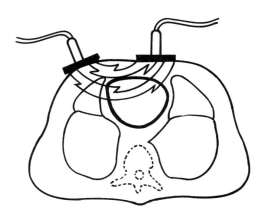

Figure 5-5 If the paddles are placed too close together on the anterior surface of the chest, a substantial amount of current shunts between them and an insufficient amount reaches the left ventricle.

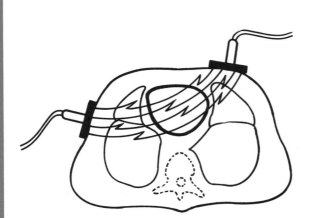

Figure 5-6 Placement of the paddles further apart allows a sufficient amount of current to reach the left ventricle.

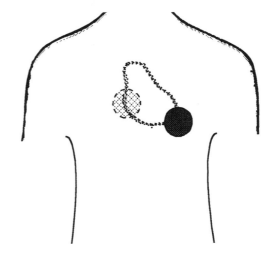

Figure 5-7 Apex-posterior paddle position.

      (ii) In a 1998 study, researchers found that transthoracic resistance and current flow should be similar using any of these electrode positions. Further, the posterior electrode may be placed in either the right or the left infrascapular position without affecting transthoracic resistance. They also determined that patients with a high body surface area and transthoracic resistance might require higher energy selection to achieve defibrillation[22]

  (d) Defibrillation in women

      (i) Elevate the left breast and place the apex defibrillator paddle or self-adhesive defibrillator pad lateral to or underneath the breast

      (ii) Placement of the defibrillation paddles or pads directly on the tissues of the breast results in higher transthoracic resistance, reducing current flow[23]

 g. Paddle pressure

  (1) When using hand-held defibrillator paddles in cardiac arrest caused by pulseless VT or VF, firm paddle-to-chest contact pressure lowers transthoracic resistance

    (a) Improves contact between the skin surface and the paddles

    (b) Decreases the amount of air in the lungs (Figure 5-8)

  (2) No pressure is applied when using self-adhesive monitoring/defibrillation pads

    (a) Despite the absence of pressure, these pads appear to be as effective as hand-held paddles[24]

Firm pressure on hand-held paddles reduces transthoracic resistance by as much as 25%[8]

Defibrillation: Indications

1. Pulseless ventricular tachycardia
2. Ventricular fibrillation
3. Sustained polymorphic VT
4. Unstable or refractory ventricular tachycardia with a pulse
5. Undue delay in delivery of synchronized cardioversion

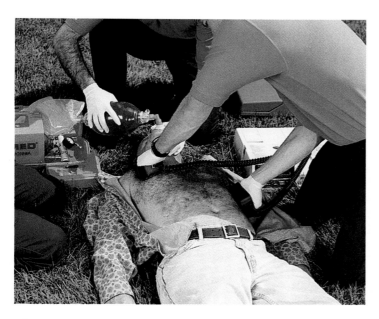

Figure 5-8 When using hand-held defibrillator paddles, use firm paddle-to-chest contact pressure to lower transthoracic resistance.

"Quick-Look"

1. Used to determine a patient's cardiac rhythm without taking the time to apply monitoring leads to the patient's chest
2. The paddles (instead of monitoring leads) will function as electrodes, monitoring the patient's cardiac rhythm
3. To perform a "quick-look":
   a. Turn the power on to the ECG monitor
   b. Turn the lead selector on the monitor to "paddles"
   c. Apply conductive gel to the defibrillator paddles or apply disposable pre-gelled defibrillator pads to the patient's chest
   d. Place the paddles firmly on the patient's chest in the sternum-apex position
   e. Adjust the ECG size (gain) to the desired height
   f. Ensure that all movement around the patient ceases while assessing the patient's rhythm
   g. Observe the patient's rhythm and check for the presence of a pulse
   h. If the rhythm observed is VF or pulseless VT, proceed with defibrillation

Note: When performing a "quick-look," removal of the paddles from the patient's chest while in "paddle" mode will result in artifact display on the cardiac monitor. The paddles must remain in contact with the patient's chest to monitor the patient's cardiac rhythm.

When a *flat line* is observed on an ECG:
   • Ensure power to monitor is on
   • Check the lead/cable connections
   • Ensure the correct lead is selected
   • Turn up the gain (ECG size) on the monitor
   If the rhythm appears to be asystole, confirm the rhythm in second lead. This is done because it is possible (although rare) that coarse VF may be present in some leads (called *occult VF*).[25] A 1988 study noted that a flat line produced by technical errors such as no power, leads unconnected, gain set to low, or incorrect lead selection *(false asystole)*, was far more frequent than occult VF.[26]
   When performing a "quick-look," if the rhythm appears to be asystole, confirm the rhythm in another lead by positioning the paddles in a lead I or lead III position. If electrodes and lead wires are already connected to the patient, confirming the rhythm in another lead simply requires changing the lead selector switch on the monitor to at least one other lead.

QUICK REVIEW

1. What is the purpose of defibrillation?

2. Name four possibilities to consider if the cardiac monitor displays a flat line.

3. Name four factors that affect transthoracic resistance.

4. A 75-year-old female has suffered a cardiac arrest. You have applied conventional defibrillator paddles to the chest for a "quick-look." The cardiac monitor displays asystole. You recall that you should confirm this rhythm in another lead. Using the quick-look paddles, how will you do this?

1. The purpose of defibrillation (unsynchronized countershock) is to produce momentary asystole; the shock attempts to completely depolarize the myocardium at once and provide an opportunity for the natural pacemaker centers of the heart to resume normal activity. 2. Possibilities include no power, loose leads, true asystole, no connection to the patient, no connection to the defibrillator/monitor. 3. Paddle (electrode) size, presence of conductive medium between the paddles (electrodes) and the patient's skin, selected energy, number and time interval of previous shocks, phase of the patient's respiration, chest size (distance between paddles), paddle pressure. 4. Assuming the initial quick-look was performed with the paddles simulating electrode positioning for lead II, rotate the paddles to simulate electrode placement for lead I or lead III.

Defibrillation: Procedure

1. Operating the defibrillator
   a. Before using a defibrillator, become familiar with standard defibrillator components
   b. Locate:
      (1) On/off switch
      (2) Energy selector
      (3) Charge button (on paddles and/or on machine)
      (4) Discharge buttons
      (5) Lead-select switch
      (6) Synchronization button
      (7) ECG size (gain) control
2. Defibrillation with hand-held paddles: procedure
   a. Turn the power on to the monitor/defibrillator
   b. Apply conductive material to the defibrillator paddles (gel) or patient's chest wall (disposable pre-gelled defibrillator pads)
      (1) Remove nitroglycerin paste/patches from the patient's chest if present

   c. Verify the presence of a shockable rhythm on the monitor
(Figure 5-9)

   d. Verify the patient's hemodynamic status

   e. Select the appropriate energy level for the clinical situation/
dysrhythmia

   f. Place the defibrillator paddles on the patient's chest and apply firm
pressure

   g. Charge the defibrillator and recheck the ECG rhythm

   h. If the rhythm is unchanged, call "clear!" and look (360 degrees) to
be sure everyone is clear of the patient, bed, and any equipment
connected to the patient (Figure 5-10)

   i. Depress both discharge buttons simultaneously to deliver the shock.
After the shock has been delivered, release the buttons

     (1) In pulseless VT/VF, leave the paddles in place on the chest
between the first three shocks

     (2) Visually reconfirm the rhythm between defibrillations

     (3) If the rhythm on the monitor changes (is not VF) or if there is any
question about the rhythm displayed, assess the patient's pulse

     (4) If defibrillation terminates pulseless VT/VF and then recurs,
defibrillate at the last successful energy setting

4. "Hands-free" defibrillation: procedure

   a. Remove nitroglycerin paste/patches from the patient's chest if
present

   b. Remove the self-adhesive monitoring/defibrillation pads from their
sealed package

     (1) Check the pads for the presence of adequate gel

   c. Attach the pads to the hands-free defibrillation cable

   d. Attach the self-adhesive monitoring/defibrillation pads to the
patient's chest in a sternum-apex or anterior-posterior position
(per manufacturer's instructions)

Do not lean on the paddles—they may slip!

Never hand charged paddles to a coworker.

If the patient's rhythm changes, run a rhythm strip for placement in the patient's medical record.

Disposable self-adhesive monitoring/defibrillation pads are pre-gelled and do not require the application of additional gel to the patient's chest.

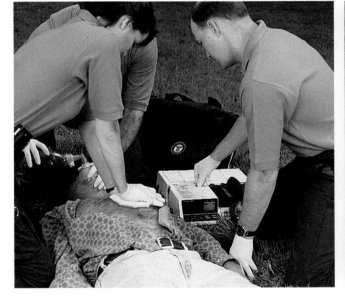

Figure 5-9 Verify the presence of a shockable rhythm on the monitor and then select the appropriate energy level for the clinical situation/dysrhythmia.

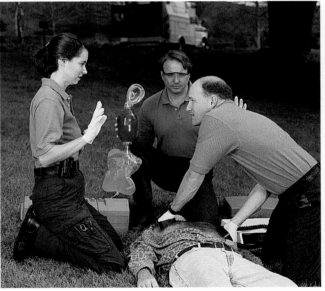

Figure 5-10 Charge the paddles and recheck the ECG rhythm. Call "clear!" and look to be sure everyone is clear of the patient.

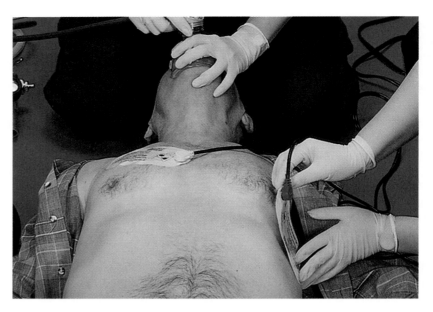

Figure 5-11 Attach the self-adhesive monitoring/defibrillation pads to the patient's chest in a sternum-apex or anterior-posterior position (per manufacturer's instructions).

    (1) When applying the adhesive pads, press from one edge of the pad across the entire surface to remove all air and avoid the development of air pockets (Figure 5-11)

e. Attach the hands-free defibrillation cable to the monitor/defibrillator
f. Turn the power of the monitor/defibrillator on
g. Turn the lead selector to "paddles" or "lead II" as needed (per manufacturer's instructions)
h. Verify the presence of a shockable rhythm on the monitor
i. Verify the patient's hemodynamic status
j. Select the appropriate energy level for the clinical situation/dysrhythmia
k. Charge defibrillator and recheck the ECG rhythm
l. If the rhythm is unchanged, call "clear!" and look (360 degrees) to be sure everyone is clear of the patient, bed, and any equipment connected to the patient
m. Depress both discharge buttons on the defibrillator simultaneously to deliver the shock; after the shock has been delivered, release the buttons
n. Reassess the ECG rhythm

SYNCHRONIZED CARDIOVERSION

1. Description and purpose
   a. Reduces the potential for delivery of energy during the vulnerable period of the T wave (relative refractory period)
      (1) Synchronizing circuit allows the delivery of a shock to be "programmed"
      (2) Machine searches for the highest (R wave deflection) or deepest (QS deflection) part of the QRS complex and delivers the shock a few milliseconds after this portion of the complex

2. Indications
   a. Unstable supraventricular tachycardia
   b. Unstable atrial fibrillation
   c. Unstable atrial flutter
   d. Unstable wide-complex tachycardia
   e. Unstable ventricular tachycardia with a pulse

A patient in VT with a pulse who is unresponsive, hypotensive, or in severe pulmonary edema should receive unsynchronized shocks to avoid the delay associated with attempts to synchronize.

---

3. Procedure
   a. If awake and time permits, administer sedation
   b. Turn the power of the monitor/defibrillator on
   c. Attach monitoring leads to the patient or self-adhesive monitoring/defibrillation pads
   d. Remove nitroglycerin paste/patches from the patient's chest if present
   e. Apply conductive gel to the defibrillator paddles or place pre-gelled defibrillator pads on the patient's chest wall
   f. Select a lead with an optimum QRS complex amplitude (positive or negative) and no artifact
   g. Identify the dysrhythmia and verify the patient's hemodynamic status
      (1) Run an ECG strip to document the patient's rhythm
   h. Press the "sync" button on the defibrillator
      (1) Verify the machine is "marking" or "flagging" each QRS complex
      (2) If sync markers do not appear, or appear elsewhere on the ECG display, adjust the gain until the markers occur within each QRS complex
      (3) If adjusting the gain does not result in sync markers within each QRS complex, select another lead or reposition the ECG electrodes
   i. Select the appropriate energy level for the clinical situation/ dysrhythmia
   j. If using hand-held paddles, place defibrillator paddles on the patient's chest and apply firm arm pressure
      (1) Do not lean on the paddles—they may slip!
   k. Charge the defibrillator and recheck the ECG rhythm
   l. If the rhythm is unchanged, call "clear!" and look (360 degrees) to be sure everyone is clear of the patient, bed, and any equipment connected to the patient
   m. Press and hold both discharge buttons simultaneously until the shock is delivered
      (1) There may be a slight delay while the machine detects the next QRS complex
      (2) After the shock has been delivered, release the buttons
   n. Reassess the ECG rhythm
      (1) If the tachycardia persists, increase the energy level according to the appropriate algorithm and ensure the machine is in sync mode before delivering another shock
      (2) If VF occurs during the course of synchronization, check the patient's pulse and rhythm (verify all electrodes and cable connections are secure), turn off the sync control, and defibrillate

When VT is rapid and the R wave is wide and bizarre in appearance, the monitor may not be able to differentiate the T wave from the QRS complex. In such cases, there is a greater likelihood that a synchronized shock may occur on the T wave (because of misidentification by the monitor) than a random unsynchronized shock. Thus defibrillation may be safer in this situation than synchronized cardioversion.[13]

If the patient's rhythm changes, run a rhythm strip for placement in the patient's medical record.

> *Some defibrillators revert to the defibrillation mode after the delivery of a synchronized shock to allow immediate defibrillation in case cardioversion produces VF. Other defibrillators remain in the synchronized mode after a synchronized shock. If VF occurs when using this type of defibrillator, ensure the sync button is off before attempting to defibrillate.*

4. Defibrillation and synchronized cardioversion: special considerations

Contact may cause electrical arcing and patient skin burns during defibrillation

a. Keep monitoring electrodes and wires away from the area where defibrillator pads or self-adhesive monitoring/defibrillation pads will be placed

Removing excessive chest hair has been shown to reduce transthoracic resistance when using self-adhesive defibrillation electrodes

b. If the patient has excessive chest hair, it may be necessary to quickly shave the areas of the chest where the hand-held paddles or self-adhesive monitoring/defibrillation pads will be placed to ensure proper contact and penetration of current

Wipe the area clean—do not use alcohol or alcohol-based cleansers

c. Remove transdermal patches, bandages, necklaces, or other materials from the sites used for paddle placement—do not attempt to defibrillate through them
d. Do not discharge the defibrillator with the paddles pressed together or into the open air
   (1) Discharging the defibrillator with the paddles together may pit or damage the surface of the paddle plates, possibly resulting in patient skin burns during defibrillation
e. When defibrillating a patient with a permanent (implanted) pacemaker, defibrillator paddles or self-adhesive monitoring/defibrillation pads should be placed at least 5 inches from the pacemaker's pulse generator (bulge under the patient's skin)
   (1) If the permanent pacemaker is located in the patient's left pectoral area, standard sternum-apex paddle placement for defibrillation is acceptable.
   (2) If the patient's pacemaker is located in the right pectoral area, anterior-posterior paddle placement can be used for defibrillation

After defibrillation, the patient with a permanent pacemaker should have the pacemaker checked to ensure proper function

f. When defibrillating a patient with an implantable cardioverter-defibrillator (ICD), defibrillator paddles or self-adhesive monitoring/defibrillation pads should be placed at least one inch from the ICD
g. Electrical interventions (defibrillation and synchronized cardioversion) of a patient receiving digoxin therapy should be avoided unless the situation is life threatening. If it is not prudent to delay cardioversion, the lowest possible energy level (10 to 20 joules) should be selected to avoid provoking ventricular dysrhythmias
5. Defibrillation and synchronized cardioversion: possible complications
   a. Skin burns because of lack of conductive medium, gel "bridging" (i.e., the gel forms a "bridge" on the skin); risk of fire from combination of electrical and oxygen sources
   b. Myocardial damage/dysfunction
   c. Embolic episodes
   d. Dysrhythmias including asystole, AV block, bradycardia, or VF following cardioversion
   e. Injury to the operator and/or team members if improper technique used
6. Defibrillation and synchronized cardioversion: possible errors
   a. Operator unfamiliar with equipment
   b. Failure to properly maintain equipment (e.g., battery maintenance, paddle cleaning)

c. Failure to remove transdermal patches, bandages, or other materials from the site used for paddle placement
d. Failure to confirm patient's hemodynamic status before performing electrical therapy (i.e., treating the monitor, not the patient)
e. Other procedures performed (e.g., establishing an IV, endotracheal intubation) before defibrillation in the patient with pulseless VT/VF
f. Improper paddle/electrode position (insufficient current reaches the left ventricle)
g. Excessive use of conductive gel on the patient's chest or on the paddles
h. Inappropriate energy level or type of countershock (i.e., defibrillation, synchronized cardioversion) selected for dysrhythmia/clinical situation
i. Failure to "clear" self and team members before delivery of each shock
j. Failure to assess for the presence of a pulse with each rhythm change observed on the cardiac monitor
k. Failure to assess the patient's vital signs on return of a pulse

---

Defibrillation should not be performed around a magnetic resonance imaging (MRI) unit. "The high magnetic field created by an MRI device will attract the equipment with a force sufficient to cause death or serious personal injury to persons between the equipment and the MRI device."[13] Store emergency equipment outside the scan room door and move the patient away from the scanner if resuscitation is needed.

Table 5-1   Electrical Therapy: Summary

Type of Countershock	Dysrhythmia	Recommended Energy Levels
Defibrillation	Pulseless VT/VF	200 J, 200-300 J, 360 J or equivalent biphasic energy
	Sustained polymorphic VT	200 J, 200-300 J, 360 J or equivalent biphasic energy
	Unstable VT with a pulse	100 J, 200 J, 300 J, 360 J or equivalent biphasic energy
	Undue delay in delivery of synchronized countershock	Depends on rhythm
Synchronized cardioversion	Paroxysmal supraventricular tachycardia (PSVT)	50 J, 100 J, 200 J, 300 J, 360 J or equivalent biphasic energy
	Atrial flutter	50J, 100 J, 200 J, 300 J, 360 J or equivalent biphasic energy
	Atrial fibrillation	100 J, 200 J, 300 J, 360 J or equivalent biphasic energy
	Stable VT with a pulse	100 J, 200 J, 300 J, 360 J or equivalent biphasic energy

QUICK REVIEW

A 53-year-old female is complaining of chest pain and begins losing conscious-ness. Her BP is now 50/P, respirations 12. The cardiac monitor displays a narrow QRS tachycardia at 220 beats/min. Oxygen therapy was initiated and an IV was established before the patient's collapse. You promptly deliver a synchronized countershock at 50 joules; however, reassessment reveals the patient to be pulse-less and apneic. The cardiac monitor reveals VF. What course of action should you take at this time?

Ensure the leads are securely in place, verify the patient is pulseless and apneic, ensure the syn-chronizer switch is off, and defibrillate with 200 joules (or equivalent biphasic energy). Reassess.

AUTOMATED EXTERNAL DEFIBRILLATORS (AEDs)

The European Resuscitation Council, the American Heart Association, and the International Liaison Committee on Resuscitation have advocated the widespread dissemination of automated external defibrillators (AEDs). **Early defibrillation** is the delivery of a shock within 5 minutes of the time EMS receives the call.[31]

The rationale for early defibrillation is based on four factors:[31]
1. The most frequent initial rhythm seen in witnessed sudden cardiac arrest is VF
2. Defibrillation is the definitive treatment for VF
3. The probability of successful defibrillation decreases rapidly over time
4. VF tends to convert to asystole within a few minutes

What is an AED?

1. An AED is an external defibrillator with a computerized cardiac rhythm analysis system
   a. Patient's cardiac rhythm is analyzed by a microprocessor in the defibrillator that uses an algorithm to distinguish rhythms that should be shocked from those that do not require defibrillation
   b. Standard AEDs should be used for patients that are apneic, pulse-less, and ≥8 years of age (approximately >25 kg body weight)
   c. The Food and Drug Administration has approved AEDs for use in children. These devices are equipped with a specially designed defib pad and cable system that reduces the energy delivered by the AED to an appropriate dose for a child
2. The AED microprocessor analyzes multiple features of the patient's cardiac rhythm, including the frequency, amplitude, and integration of the frequency and amplitude (e.g., such as slope or wave morphology)
   a. Safety "filters" check for false signals (e.g., radio transmissions, poor electrode contact, 60-cycle interference, and loose electrodes)

Public access defibrillation (PAD) programs necessitate the use of AEDs by the lay public. In a Seattle study, researchers endeavored to improve their understanding of AED use in naive users by measuring the mean time to defibrillation and the appropriateness of AED pad placement. They selected sixth-grade students to simulate an extreme circumstance of unfamiliarity with the problem of out-of-hospital cardiac arrest and defibrillation. Using a mock cardiac arrest scenario, use of the AED by 15 children was compared with that of 22 emergency medical technicians (EMTs) or paramedics. Each subject's time from entry onto the cardiac arrest scene to delivery of the shock into simulated VF and the appropriateness of AED pad placement were evaluated. All performances were videotaped to assess safety of use and compliance with AED prompts to remain clear of the mannequin during shock delivery.

The mean time to defibrillation was 90+/−14 seconds for the children and 67+/−10 seconds for the EMTs/paramedics. Electrode pad placement was appropriate for all subjects and all remained clear of the "patient" during shock delivery. The researchers concluded, "During mock cardiac arrest, the speed of AED use by untrained children is only modestly slower than that of professionals. The difference between the groups is surprisingly small, considering the naiveté of the children as untutored first-time users. These findings suggest that widespread use of AEDs will require only modest training."[32]

    b. Some AEDs detect spontaneous movement by the patient or movement of the patient by others

    c. If a shock is indicated, the AED defibrillates or advises the operator to initiate a defibrillation

    d. The shock is delivered by means of two self-adhesive monitoring/defibrillation pads applied to the patient's chest

3. Types of AEDs
    a. AEDs may be fully automated or semi-automated
       (1) Both devices typically have a power control and an "analyze" control
       (2) When the fully automated defibrillator recognizes VF, monomorphic VT, or polymorphic VT above a preset rate, it charges its capacitors and delivers a shock without further input from the operator (Figure 5-12)
    b. Semi-automated (shock-advisory) external defibrillators (SAEDs)
       (1) Require operator intervention at specific points in the treatment sequence, depending on the brand of AED
       (2) Some AEDs require the operator to press an "analyze" control to initiate rhythm analysis while others automatically begin analyzing the patient's cardiac rhythm when the electrode pads are attached to the patient's chest
       (3) If a shockable rhythm is present, the SAED will notify the operator that a shock is indicated by means of visual and/or audible signals (Figure 5-13)
       (4) In most AEDs, the capacitors charge automatically if a shockable rhythm is detected. The operator then presses a "shock" control to deliver the shock

4. AED: operation
    a. Use personal protective equipment
    b. Assess responsiveness. If unresponsive, call for help
    c. Open the airway and check for breathing
    d. If the patient is not breathing, deliver two slow breaths
    e. Assess for the presence of a pulse; if the patient is pulseless, begin chest compressions and attach the AED (Figure 5-14)

Do not delay defibrillation to perform endotracheal intubation, establish an IV, or other interventions.

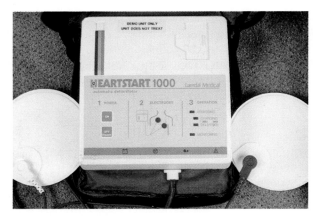

Figure 5-12   Fully automated external defibrillator.

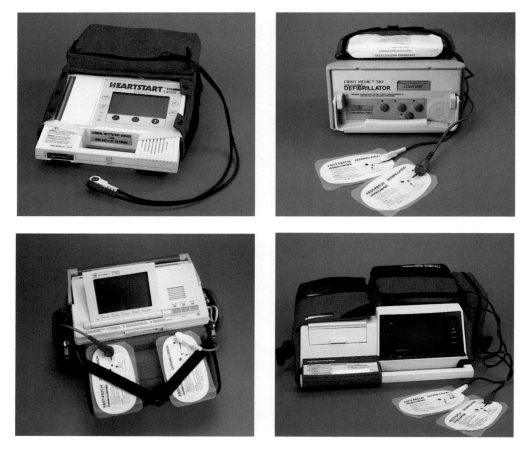

Figure 5-13   Semi-automated external defibrillators.

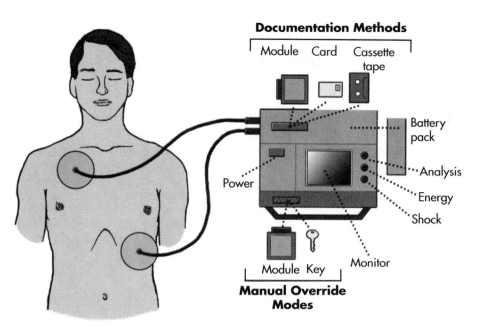

Figure 5-14   Automated external defibrillator.

f. Turn the power on to the AED. Depending on the brand of AED, this is accomplished by either pressing the "on" button or lifting up the monitor screen or lid

g. Open the package containing the self-adhesive monitoring/defibrillation pads

   (1) Connect the pads to the AED cables (if not pre-connected) and then apply the pads to the patient's chest (upper-right sternal border, lower-left ribs over the cardiac apex) (Figure 5-15). Stop CPR to allow placement of the pads on the patient's chest

   (2) Some models require connection of the AED cable to the AED before use

h. Analyze the ECG rhythm: (Figure 5-16)

> Interruption of CPR to analyze the patient's rhythm and deliver shocks is acceptable because the benefits of defibrillation outweigh the possible negative effects of a brief delay in CPR.

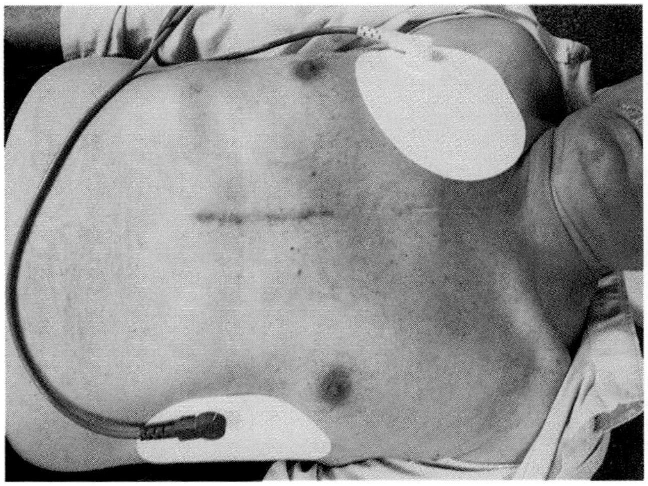

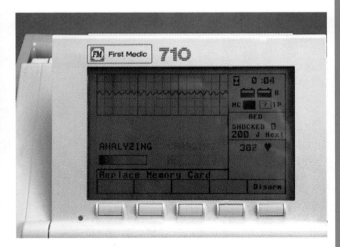

Figure 5-15   Connect the adhesive pads to the AED cables and then apply the pads to the patient's chest at the upper-right sternal border and the lower-left ribs over the cardiac apex.

Figure 5-16   Analyze the rhythm.

(1) Some AEDs require the operator to press an "analyze" control to begin analysis of the patient's rhythm while others automatically begin analysis when the adhesive monitoring/defibrillation pads are attached to the patient's chest

(2) Time required for rhythm analysis ranges from 5 to 15 seconds

---

AEDs take multiple "looks" at the patient's rhythm—each lasting a few seconds. If several "looks" confirm the presence of a shockable rhythm, the AED will signal that a shock is indicated. Artifact caused by motion or 60-cycle interference may simulate VF and interfere with accurate rhythm analysis. While the AED is analyzing the patient's cardiac rhythm, all movement (including chest compressions, artificial ventilations, and movement associated with patient transport) must cease. If analysis of the patient's rhythm is necessary during patient transport, stop the emergency vehicle and reanalyze the rhythm.

---

i. If the AED detects a shockable rhythm, it will advise that a shock is indicated

(1) Clear the area surrounding the patient and, if using a semi-automated external defibrillator, press the shock control to deliver a shock (Figure 5-17)

Depending on the manufacturer and battery condition, the time required for charging of the AEDs capacitors is approximately 10 to 30 seconds.

Both monophasic and biphasic AEDs are currently available. If the AED used is a monophasic waveform defibrillator, the recommended energy for the first shock is 200 J, 200 J to 300 J for the second shock, and 360 J for the third shock. Depending on the manufacturer, biphasic waveform AEDs may deliver nonescalating shocks.

---

j. After delivering the first shock, reanalyze the rhythm

(1) If the AED advises a shock is indicated, deliver a second shock and then reanalyze the rhythm. If the AED advises a third shock, deliver the shock as indicated

k. After delivery of the third shock, reassess the patient's pulse

(1) If there is no pulse, perform CPR for 1 minute and then reanalyze the rhythm

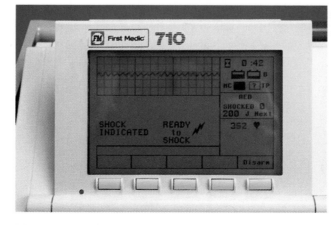

Figure 5-17 Clear the patient and press the shock control to deliver a shock if indicated.

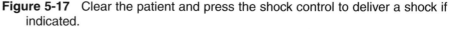

(2) If a pulse is present, assess breathing; if breathing is inadequate, provide assisted ventilation

(3) Reassess the patient's pulse every 30 to 60 seconds

5. AED: advantages
   a. Voice prompts the user
   b. Easy to learn; memorizing treatment protocol is easier than recalling the steps of CPR
   c. Less training required to operate and maintain skills than with conventional defibrillators
   d. Speed of operation (delivery of first shock) faster than that with conventional defibrillators
   e. Promotes rescuer safety by permitting remote, "hands-free" defibrillation

6. AEDs: special considerations
   a. If the patient has a pacemaker or ICD, the AED may be used, but the adhesive AED pads should be placed at least 1 inch from the implanted device
      (1) If an ICD is in the process of delivering shocks to the patient, allow it approximately 30 to 60 seconds to complete its cycle
   b. If a transdermal medication patch is present on the patient's chest, do *not* attempt to defibrillate through it. Remove the patch and wipe the area clean before applying the AED pads

   > Do not use alcohol or alcohol-based cleansers.

   c. If the patient has excessive chest hair, the AED pads may not adhere to the patient's chest resulting in a "check electrodes" message from the AED
      (1) If pressing down firmly on each AED pad does not correct the problem, quickly remove the AED pads (simultaneously removing some of the chest hair) and apply a second set of AED pads
      (2) If the problem persists, remove the AEDs pads and quickly shave the areas of the chest where the AED pads will be placed and then apply a new set of AED pads
   d. If the patient is lying in water or on a wet surface, remove the patient from contact with the water and quickly dry the patient's chest before attaching the AED
   e. If the patient is lying on a metal surface, remove the patient from contact with the metal surface before attaching the AED

Integration of ACLS with an AED

If the patient remains in VF after the delivery of three serial shocks by the AED, ACLS personnel should enter the ACLS VF sequence at that point—i.e., continue CPR, intubate, establish IV access, administer medications, etc.

A recent study retrospectively examined the effect of equipping the aircraft of a major U.S. airline with AEDs and training its flight attendants in their use.[33] Flight attendants applied the AED when passengers had a lack of consciousness, pulse, or respiration. The AED was also used as a monitor for other medical emergencies, generally at the direction of a passenger who was a physician. Two arrhythmia specialists analyzed the ECG obtained during each use of the device for appropriateness of use.

Nearly 71 million passengers were carried by the airline during the 2-year study period. AEDs were used for 200 patients (191 on the aircraft and 9 in the terminal), including 99 with documented loss of consciousness. ECG data were available for 185 patients. The administration of a shock was advised in all 14 patients who had electrocardiographically documented VF, and no shock was advised in the remaining patients (sensitivity and specificity of the defibrillator in identifying VF, 100%). The first shock successfully defibrillated the heart in 13 patients (defibrillation was withheld in one case at the family's request). The rate of survival to discharge from the hospital after shock with the AED was 40%. A total of 36 patients either died or were resuscitated after cardiac arrest, and no complications arose from use of the AED as a monitor in conscious passengers.

In another study,[34] investigators studied a prospective series of cases of sudden cardiac arrest in casinos. Casino security officers were trained to use AEDs that had been placed with the intent of achieving a collapse-to-shock time of 3 minutes or less. The protocol used in the study called for defibrillation first (if feasible), followed by manual CPR. AEDs were used in 105 patients whose initial cardiac rhythm was VF. Fifty-six patients (53%) survived to hospital discharge, and all survivors could function without assistance. The survival rate was 74% for those patients who received their first defibrillation no later than 3 minutes after a witnessed collapse and 49% for those who received their first defibrillation after more than 3 minutes.

IMPLANTABLE CARDIOVERTER-DEFIBRILLATOR (ICD)

ICD treats dysrhythmias—
it does not prevent them.

1. What is an ICD?
   a. An implantable cardioverter-defibrillator (ICD) is an electronically programmed device capable of identifying and terminating dysrhythmias including VT and VF
   b. **ICD:** part of a system that consists of three main parts: the ICD (pulse generator), leads, and a programmer
      (1) Pulse generator contains the circuitry, battery, and capacitors
      (2) Leads
         (a) Insulated wires attached to the ICD
         (b) Used to sense the patient's cardiac rhythm and deliver therapy
         (c) Depending on the type of ICD implanted, one or more leads may be used
      (3) Programmer: Separate device located in a physician's office that is used to alter the function of the ICD during follow-up care
   c. ICD typically weighs about 8 oz and is placed subcutaneously in the left upper quadrant of the patient's abdomen (Figure 5-18) or the left pectoral region (Figure 5-19)
      (1) Patients with an ICD are asked to wear medical identification insignia with information regarding the ICD model and manufacturer and carry an ICD identification card

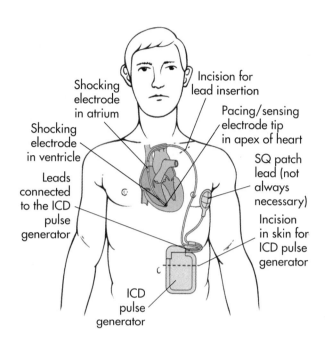

Figure 5-18 ICD implanted in the left upper abdominal quadrant. (Adapted from Medtronic, Inc., Minneapolis, MN.)

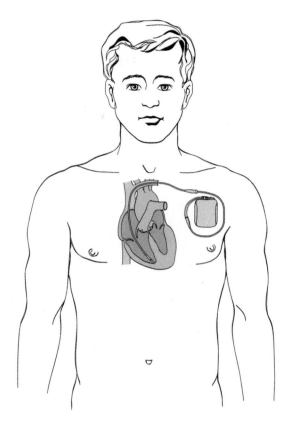

Figure 5-19 ICD implanted in the left pectoral region. (Adapted from Cardiac Pacemakers, Inc., St. Paul, MN.)

   d. ICD can deliver a range of therapies (called *tiered-therapy*), including defibrillation, antitachycardia (overdrive) pacing, synchronized cardioversion, and bradycardia pacing, depending on the dysrhythmia detected and how the device is programmed (Figure 5-20)

     (1) A physician determines the appropriate therapies for each patient

     (2) The energy used for synchronized cardioversion is programmable: 0.1 to 37 J depending on the device

     (3) The energy used for defibrillation is also programmable: up to 37 J

     (4) The number of defibrillation attempts varies by device

   e. ICD has an electronic memory that stores information for retrieval by a physician, including the number and types of treatments received, how successful each therapy was in terminating a tachydysrhythmia, what the heart was doing during the most recent episodes, and the status of the ICD batteries and programmed settings

   f. The patient with an ICD should stay away from sources of magnetic and electromagnetic radiation, including MRI, diathermy, and arc welding equipment to avoid possible underdetection, inappropriate therapy delivery, and/or electrical reset of the device

2. External electrical therapy and the patient with an ICD

   a. Treatment of the patient with an ICD is no different from the treatment of patients without them; however, care should be taken to ensure that hand-held paddles or self-adhesive monitoring/defibrillation pads are not placed directly over the device

> Depending on the manufacturer, the ICD may deliver a maximum of six shocks for VF. After a dysrhythmia is detected, most devices require up to 10 seconds before beginning electrical therapy

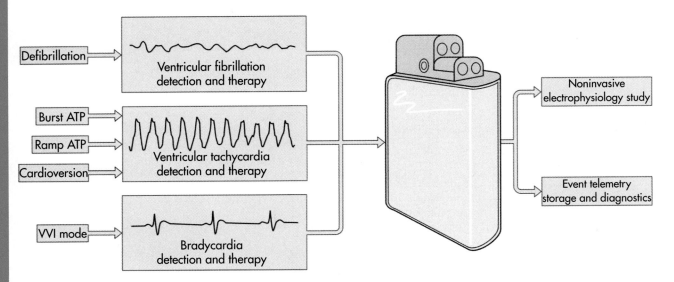

Figure 5-20 ICD can deliver a range of therapies including defibrillation, antitachycardia (overdrive) pacing (ATP), synchronized cardioversion, and bradycardia pacing, depending on the dysrhythmia detected and how the device is programmed. *VVI*, ventricular pacing, sensing, inhibiting.

    b. Approximately 2 J of energy are delivered at the body surface when the ICD discharges internally
        (1) Rescuers in contact with the patient may feel a tingling sensation when the ICD delivers a shock
        (2) Although the energy is enough to be felt by the rescuer, it is not enough to cause physiologic harm
        (3) Rubber gloves worn by rescuers while caring for the patient will insulate them from the tingling sensation,[35] although rescuers may feel the patient's muscles twitch as the device discharges[36]

QUICK REVIEW

1. Where is the pulse generator of an implantable-cardioverter defibrillator typically located?

2. An 80-year-old male has suffered a cardiac arrest. The cardiac monitor displays VF. You have exposed the patient's chest and are preparing to defibrillate when you note the patient has a permanent pacemaker in place. What distance from the pacemaker generator should the defibrillator paddles be placed?

3. What is an AED?

1. *Subcutaneously in the left upper quadrant of the patient's abdomen or the left pectoral region.*
2. *At least 5 inches (12.5 cm) from the pacemaker generator.* 3. *AED is an external defibrillator with a cardiac rhythm analysis system that senses and records the rhythm and, if indicated, delivers an electrical shock. The shock is delivered by means of two adhesive pads applied to the patient.*

PACEMAKER THERAPY

1. Pacemaker systems
   a. **Pacemaker**—Artificial pulse generator that delivers an electrical current to the heart to stimulate depolarization
   b. Pacemaker systems are usually named according to where the electrodes are located and the route the electrical current takes to the heart (Figures 5-21 to 5-23)
   c. Pacemaker system consists of a pulse generator (power source) and pacing lead(s)
      (1) Pulse generator houses a battery and electronic circuitry to sense and analyze the patient's **intrinsic** rhythm and the timing circuitry for pacing stimulus output
      (2) Pacing lead is an insulated wire used to carry an electrical impulse from the pacemaker to the patient's heart and back to the pacemaker
         (a) The exposed portion of the pacing lead is called an *electrode*, which is placed in direct contact with the heart
2. Permanent pacemakers
   a. Implanted into subcutaneous tissue of anterior thorax just below right or left clavicle
   b. Circuitry housed in a hermetically sealed case made of titanium that is airtight and impermeable to fluid
   c. Common indications for insertion of a permanent pacemaker include permanent or intermittent complete AV block, permanent or intermittent second-degree AV block type II, or sinus node dysfunction including sick sinus syndrome that may be manifested as severe sinus bradycardia, bradycardia-tachycardia syndrome, sinus arrest, or sinus block
3. Temporary pacemakers
   a. Temporary pacing can be accomplished through transvenous, epicardial, or transcutaneous means
      (1) Transvenous pacemakers stimulate the endocardium of the right atrium or ventricle (or both) by means of an electrode introduced into a central vein
      (2) Epicardial pacing is the placement of pacing leads directly onto or through the epicardium under direct visualization
      (3) Transcutaneous pacing (TCP) delivers pacing impulses to the heart using electrodes placed on the patient's thorax. TCP is also called *temporary external pacing* or *noninvasive pacing*
   b. Indications for emergent temporary pacing include hemodynamically significant bradycardia (blood pressure <80 mm Hg systolic, change in mental status, pulmonary edema, angina); bradycardia with escape rhythms unresponsive to drug therapy; **overdrive pacing** of tachycardia—supraventricular or ventricular—refractory to pharmacologic therapy or electrical countershock; and bradyasystolic cardiac arrest
   c. Prophylactic pacing, in the setting of acute MI, is indicated in symptomatic sinus node dysfunction, second-degree AV block type II, complete AV block, and new left, right, or alternating bundle branch block
4. Pacemaker modes
   a. **Fixed-rate pacemaker**
      (1) Continuously discharges at a preset rate (usually 70 to 80 per min) regardless of the patient's heart rate

During overdrive pacing, the heart is paced briefly (seconds) at a rate faster than the rate of the tachycardia. The pacemaker is then stopped to allow return of the heart's intrinsic pacemaker.

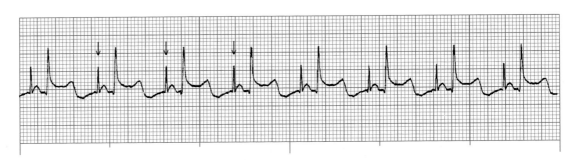

Figure 5-21 Atrial pacing.

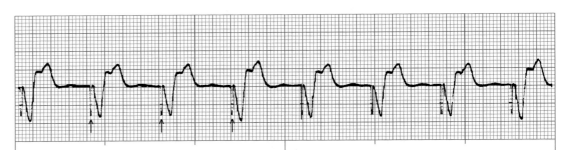

Figure 5-22 Ventricular pacing.

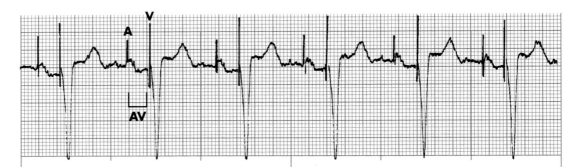

Figure 5-23 AV sequential pacing. *A,* Atrial pacing; *V,* ventricular pacing; *AV,* AV interval.

       (2) Simple circuitry, reducing the risk of pacemaker failure
       (3) Does not sense the patient's own cardiac rhythm
          (a) May result in competition between the patient's cardiac rhythm and that of the pacemaker
          (b) VT or VF may be induced if the pacemaker were to fire during the T wave (vulnerable period) of a preceding patient beat
          (c) Not often used today
   b. **Demand pacemaker**
       (1) Discharges only when the patient's heart rate drops below the pacemaker's preset (base) rate
          (a) For example, if the demand pacemaker's pulse generator were preset at a rate of 70 impulses/min, it would sense the patient's heart rate and allow electrical impulses to flow from the pacemaker through the pacing lead to stimulate the heart only when the rate fell below 70 beats/min
       (2) May be programmable or nonprogrammable
          (a) Voltage level and impulse rate are preset at the time of manufacture in nonprogrammable pacemakers

5. Transcutaneous pacing (TCP)
   a. Indications
      (1) TCP is recommended as the initial pacing method of choice in emergency cardiac care because it is effective, quick, safe, and is the least invasive pacing technique currently available
      (2) Indicated for significant bradycardias unresponsive to atropine therapy or when atropine is not immediately available
      (3) May be used as a "bridge" until transvenous pacing can be accomplished or the cause of the bradydysrhythmia is reversed (as in cases of drug overdose or hyperkalemia)
      (4) May be considered in asystolic cardiac arrest (less than 10 minutes in duration) and witnessed asystolic arrest
   b. Technique
      (1) Electrode placement
         (a) Two large pacing electrodes (approximately 8- to 10-cm in diameter) are attached to the skin surface of the patient's outer chest wall
            (i) Place the anterior (negative) chest electrode to the left of the sternum, halfway between the xiphoid process and left nipple (Figure 5-24)
            (ii) In female patients, the anterior electrode should be positioned under the left breast
            (iii) Place the posterior (positive) electrode on the left posterior thorax directly behind the anterior electrode
            (iv) Electrodes should fit completely on the patient's torso, have a minimum of 1 to 2 inches of space between electrodes, and should not overlap bony prominences of the sternum, spine, or scapula
            (v) If the anterior-posterior electrode position is contraindicated, the anterior-lateral position may be used
            (vi) Anterior (negative) electrode is placed on the left anterior thorax, just lateral to the left nipple in the midaxillary line
            (vii) Posterior (positive) electrode is placed on the right anterior upper thorax in the subclavicular area (Figure 5-25)
         (b) Connect the patient to an ECG monitor, obtain a rhythm strip, and verify the presence of a paceable rhythm

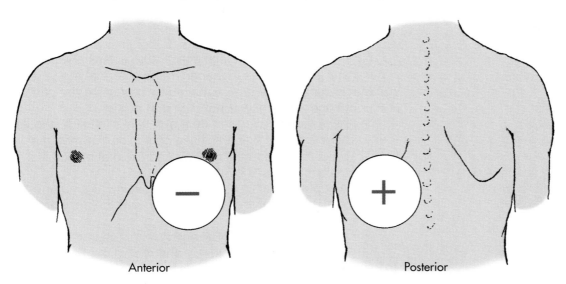

Anterior   Posterior

Figure 5-24 Anterior-posterior positioning of transcutaneous electrodes.

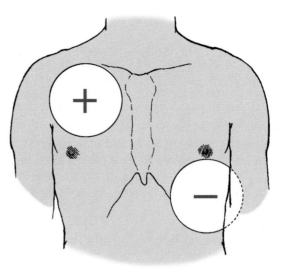

Figure 5-25 Anterior-lateral positioning of transcutaneous electrodes.

(c) Connect the pacing cable to the adhesive electrodes on the patient and the pulse generator
(d) Turn the power on to the pulse generator and set the pacing rate
   (i) In a patient with a pulse, the rate is generally set at a nonbradycardic rate between 60 and 80 beats/min
   (ii) In an asystolic patient, the rate is typically set between 80 and 100 beats/min
(e) After the rate has been regulated, set the stimulating current (output or milliamperes)
   (i) In a patient with a pulse, the current is increased slowly but steadily until capture is achieved
   (ii) Sedation or analgesia may be needed to minimize the discomfort associated with this procedure (common with currents of 50 mA or more)
   (iii) For the asystolic patient, it is reasonable to set the current to maximal output and then decrease the output if capture is achieved
(f) Observe the cardiac monitor for **electrical** capture
   (i) Usually evidenced by a wide QRS and broad T waves (Figure 5-26)
   (ii) In some patients, electrical capture is less obvious—indicated only as a change in the shape of the QRS
(g) **Mechanical** capture is evaluated by assessing the patient's right upper extremity or right femoral pulses
   (i) Assessment of pulses on the patient's left side should be avoided to help minimize confusion between the presence of an actual pulse and skeletal muscle contractions caused by the pacemaker
(h) Once capture is achieved, continue pacing at an output level slightly higher (approximately 2 mA) than the threshold of initial electrical capture
   (i) Assess the patient's BP and level of responsiveness
   (ii) Monitor the patient closely and record the ECG rhythm
(i) If defibrillation is necessary, place the defibrillation paddles 2 to 3 cm (¾ to 1 inch) away from the pacemaker electrodes to prevent arcing

---

Chest compressions can be performed during TCP without risk of injury to the health care provider.

If electrical capture is achieved **without** mechanical capture, the patient should be treated according to the resuscitation guidelines for pulseless electrical activity.

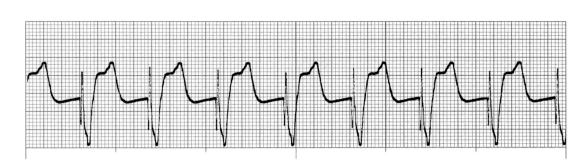

Figure 5-26 100% ventricular-paced rhythm.

      (i) Some pacemaker models should be turned off or disconnected before defibrillating

      (j) Documentation should include the date and time pacing was initiated (including baseline and pacing rhythm strips), the current required to obtain capture, the pacing rate selected, the patient's responses to electrical and mechanical capture, medications administered during the procedure, and the date and time pacing was terminated

c. TCP: Limitations

  (1) Primary limitation is patient discomfort

    (a) Discomfort is proportional to the intensity of skeletal muscle contraction and the direct electrical stimulation of cutaneous nerves

    (b) Degree of discomfort varies with the device used and the stimulating current required to achieve capture

  (2) Capture may be difficult to achieve or increased stimulating current may be required in patients with increased chest wall muscle mass, chronic obstructive pulmonary disease (COPD), pleural effusions, dilated cardiomyopathy, hypoxia, or metabolic acidosis because of the extremely high current thresholds required[37,38]

d. TCP: Complications

  (1) Coughing

  (2) Skin burns

  (3) Interference with sensing because of patient agitation or muscle contractions

  (4) Pain from electrical stimulation of the skin and muscles

  (5) Failure to recognize that the pacemaker is not capturing

  (6) Failure to recognize the presence of underlying treatable VF

  (7) Tissue damage, including third-degree burns, has been reported in pediatric patients with improper or prolonged TCP[39]

  (8) Prolonged pacing has been associated with pacing threshold changes, leading to capture failure

e. TCP: Contraindications

  (1) Children weighing less than 15 kg (33 lb) unless pediatric pacing electrodes are used

  (2) Flail chest

  (3) Bradycardia in the setting of severe hypothermia

  (4) Bradyasystolic cardiac arrest of more than 20 minutes in duration (relative contraindication)

The energy requirements for TCP vary widely. In one study of 35 patients, energy requirements for pacing varied from 30 to 110 mA, and patients requiring more than 50 mA for pacing needed sedation.

Hypothermia-induced bradycardia is the result of decreased spontaneous depolarization of the pacemaker cells and is refractory to atropine and other cardiostimulatory drugs.[41] Hypotension associated with hypothermia is a result of direct cold-induced myocardial depression, bradycardia, and decreased left ventricular stroke volume.[42,43]

In a study published in 1997, researchers evaluated the hemodynamic response of 20 mongrel dogs to transcutaneous pacing during rewarming from hypothermia.[44] Rewarming was accomplished significantly faster in the paced group (171.5 +/– 31.5 minutes) than in the control group (254 +/– 55.9 minutes). After rewarming, the mean cardiac index in the paced dogs returned to 84% of baseline, compared with 63% of baseline in the non-paced group. None of the paced animals demonstrated significant hemodynamic deterioration, potentially lethal dysrhythmias, or other evidence of myocardial injury.

Pacemaker Malfunction

1. Failure to Pace
   a. **Failure to pace:** Pacemaker malfunction that occurs when the pacemaker fails to deliver an electrical stimulus or when it fails to deliver the correct number of electrical stimulations/min
   b. Recognized on the ECG as an absence of pacemaker spikes (even though the patient's intrinsic rate is less than that of the pacemaker) and a return of the underlying rhythm for which the pacemaker was implanted
   c. Patient signs and symptoms may include syncope, chest pain, bradycardia, and hypotension
   d. Causes of failure to pace
      (1) Battery failure, fracture of the pacing lead wire, displacement of the electrode tip, pulse generator failure, a broken or loose connection between the pacing lead and the pulse generator, electromagnetic interference, and/or the sensitivity setting set too high
   e. Treatment may include adjusting the sensitivity setting, replacing the pulse generator battery, replacing the pacing lead, replacing the pulse generator unit, tightening connections between the pacing lead and pulse generator, performing an electrical check, and/or removing the source of electromagnetic interference

Patient Responses to Current with Transcutaneous Pacing

Output (mA)*	Response
20	Prickly sensation on skin
30	Slight thump on chest
40	Definite thump on chest
50	Coughing
60	Diaphragm pacing and coughing
70	Coughing and knock on chest
80	More uncomfortable than 70 mA
90	Strong, painful knock on chest
100	Leaves bed because of pain

*Responses with Zoll-NTP.

From Flynn JB: *Introduction to critical care skills.* St Louis, 1993, Mosby.

2. Failure to capture
   a. **Failure to capture**: Inability of the pacemaker stimulus to depolarize the myocardium
   b. Recognized on the ECG by visible pacemaker spikes not followed by P waves (if the electrode is located in the atrium) or QRS complexes (if the electrode is located in the right ventricle) (Figure 5-27)
   c. Patient signs and symptoms may include fatigue, bradycardia, and hypotension
   d. Causes of failure to capture
      (1) Battery failure, fracture of the pacing lead wire, displacement of pacing lead wire (common cause), perforation of the myocardium by a lead wire, edema or scar tissue formation at the electrode tip, output energy (mA) set too low (common cause), and/or increased stimulation threshold because of medications, electrolyte imbalance, or increased fibrin formation on the catheter tip
   e. Treatment may include repositioning the patient, slowly increasing the output setting (mA) until capture occurs or the maximum setting is reached, replacing the pulse generator battery, replacing or repositioning of the pacing lead, or surgery
3. Failure to sense
   a. **Sensitivity**: Extent to which a pacemaker recognizes intrinsic electrical activity
   b. **Failure to sense**: Occurs when the pacemaker fails to recognize spontaneous myocardial depolarization (Figure 5-28)

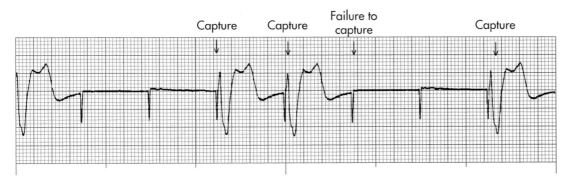

Figure 5-27   Failure to capture.

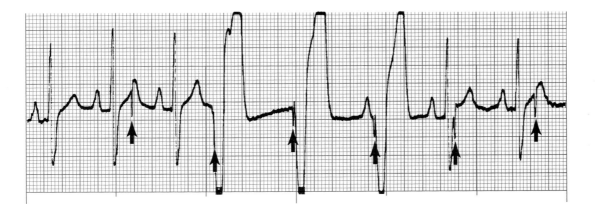

Figure 5-28   Failure to sense.

c. Recognized on the ECG by pacemaker spikes that follow too closely behind the patient's QRS complexes (earlier than the programmed escape interval)

R-on-T phenomenon may precipitate VT or VF

   (1) Because pacemaker spikes occur when they should not, this type of pacemaker malfunction may result in pacemaker spikes that fall on T waves (R-on-T phenomenon) and/or competition between the pacemaker and the patient's own cardiac rhythm

d. Patient may complain of palpitations or skipped beats

e. Causes of failure to sense[45]

   (1) Battery failure, fracture of pacing lead wire, displacement of the electrode tip (most common cause), decreased P wave or QRS voltage, circuitry dysfunction (generator unable to process QRS signal), increased sensing threshold from edema or fibrosis at the electrode tip, antidysrhythmic medications, severe electrolyte disturbances, or myocardial perforation

f. Treatment may include increasing the sensitivity setting, replacing the pulse generator battery, and/or replacing or repositioning of the pacing lead

4. Oversensing

a. Oversensing: Results from inappropriate sensing of extraneous electrical signals

   (1) Atrial sensing pacemakers may inappropriately sense ventricular activity, ventricular sensing pacemakers may misidentify a tall, peaked intrinsic T wave as a QRS complex

b. Recognized on the ECG as pacemaker spikes at a rate slower than the pacemaker's preset rate (paced QRS complexes that come later than the pacemaker's preset escape interval) or no paced beats even though the pacemaker's preset rate is greater than the patient's intrinsic rate

c. The patient with a pacemaker should avoid strong electromagnetic fields such as arc welding equipment and a magnetic resonance imaging (MRI) machine

d. Treatment includes adjustment of the pacemaker's sensitivity setting or possible insertion of a bipolar lead if oversensing is caused by unipolar lead dysfunction

PRECORDIAL THUMP

1. Description

a. **Precordial thump** (also called *thumpversion*[46-48]): Forceful blow delivered to the center of the sternum to terminate VT or VF

b. Use of this technique is controversial

   (1) There is some evidence that VT has been converted to a sinus rhythm with this technique[49,50]; however, there are also reports that VT has been converted to asystole or PEA[50,51] or the technique has no effect[52]

2. Indications

Delivery of a precordial thump should never delay defibrillation.

a. If used, this technique should be limited to **witnessed** cardiac arrest where the patient is pulseless and a defibrillator is not immediately available

3. Technique

a. Precordial thump is delivered to the junction of the lower and middle third of the sternum of an adult using a clenched fist from a height of 8 to 10 inches (Figure 5-29)

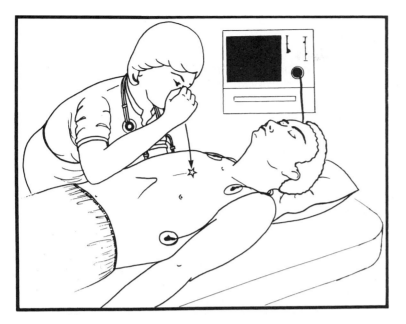

Figure 5-29 Precordial thump.

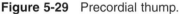

    b. After delivery of a precordial thump, recheck the patient's pulse and rhythm

4. Special considerations
    a. Should not be performed in infants and children
    b. Should not be taught to lay rescuers

STOP AND REVIEW

1. If an unstable patient presented with each of the following dysrhythmias, identify the dysrhythmia for which synchronized cardioversion is indicated:
    a. Paroxysmal supraventricular tachycardia (PSVT)
    b. Sustained torsades de pointes (TdP)
    c. Ventricular fibrillation (VF)
    d. Pulseless ventricular tachycardia (VT)

2. A 73-year-old male is found pulseless and apneic. CPR is initiated. The cardiac monitor shows VF. The proper energy levels for delivery of the initial "serial" shocks to this patient would be:
    a. 50, 100, and 200 J or equivalent biphasic energy
    b. 100, 200, and 360 J or equivalent biphasic energy
    c. 100, 200, and 300 J or equivalent biphasic energy
    d. 200, 200 to 300, and 360 J or equivalent biphasic energy

3. When placing hand-held defibrillator paddles on a patient's chest in the sternum-apex position, the apex paddle should be placed:
    a. To the left of the sternum with the center of the paddle just below the left clavicle
    b. To the left of the nipple with the center of the paddle in the left midaxillary line
    c. With the center of the paddle in the midclavicular line
    d. With the center of the paddle in the anterior axillary line

4. An implantable defibrillator-cardioverter (ICD):
   a. Is an external defibrillator with a computerized cardiac rhythm analysis system
   b. Is part of the "early defibrillation" link of the sequence of survival
   c. Delivers shocks by means of two self-adhesive monitoring/defibrillation pads applied to the patient's chest
   d. Can deliver a range of therapies including defibrillation, antitachycardia pacing, synchronized cardioversion, and bradycardia pacing, depending on the rhythm detected and how the device is programmed

5. Select the INCORRECT statement regarding defibrillation.
   a. Transthoracic resistance is affected by the time interval between successive shocks
   b. In the pulseless patient with VF or VT, three "serial" shocks are delivered with a brief pause for a pulse check between each shock
   c. When using hand-held defibrillator paddles, firm paddle pressure helps decrease transthoracic resistance
   d. To a point, transthoracic resistance decreases with increased paddle size

6. _____ is the therapeutic delivery of unsynchronized electrical current through the myocardium over a very brief period to terminate a cardiac dysrhythmia.
   a. Defibrillation
   b. ECG monitoring
   c. Transcutaneous pacing
   d. Transvenous pacing

7. A 56-year-old male has a permanent pacemaker in place. Should it be necessary to defibrillate this patient, hand-held defibrillator paddles should be placed:
   a. Directly over the pacemaker generator
   b. 5 inches from the pacemaker generator
   c. 6 to 12 inches from the pacemaker generator
   d. It makes no difference where the paddles are placed

8. You have delivered a synchronized countershock. The rhythm on the cardiac monitor now reveals VF. Your best course of action at this time will be to:
   a. Confirm the rhythm in two leads
   b. Immediately deliver another synchronized countershock
   c. Establish an IV, perform CPR for 1 minute, then defibrillate
   d. Quickly confirm the patient is apneic and pulseless, then defibrillate immediately

9. Transcutaneous pacing is indicated in which of the following situations?
   a. Prolonged asystole (>20 minutes)
   b. Accelerated junctional rhythm, BP 108/64
   c. Second-degree AV block, type II, BP 68/42
   d. Ventricular fibrillation (VF)

10. Energy levels recommended in the management of an unstable patient in atrial flutter are:
    a. 50, 100, 200, 300, and 360 J or equivalent biphasic energy
    b. 50, 100, 200, and 360 J or equivalent biphasic energy
    c. 100, 200, and 300 J or equivalent biphasic energy
    d. 200, 200 to 300, and 360 J or equivalent biphasic energy

STOP AND REVIEW ANSWERS

1. a. Synchronized cardioversion is indicated in the management of the patient in PSVT who is exhibiting serious signs and symptoms related to the tachycardia. Defibrillation (unsynchronized counter-shock) is indicated for sustained torsades de pointes, ventricular fibrillation, and pulseless ventricular tachycardia.

2. d. The proper energy levels for delivery of the initial "serial" shocks to a patient in pulseless VT or VF are 200, 200 to 300, and 360 J or equivalent biphasic energy.

3. b. When placing hand-held defibrillator paddles on a patient's chest in the sternum-apex position, the apex paddle should be placed to the left of the nipple with the center of the paddle in the left midaxillary line.

4. d. An **implantable** defibrillator-cardioverter (ICD) can deliver a range of therapies including defibrillation, antitachycardia pacing, synchronized cardioversion, and bradycardia pacing, depending on the rhythm detected and how the device is programmed. An **automated external defibrillator (AED)** is part of the sequence of survival. The AED is an external defibrillator with a computerized cardiac rhythm analysis system. The device delivers shocks by means of two self-adhesive monitoring/defibrillation pads applied to the patient's chest.

5. b. Initial management of pulseless VT or VF includes CPR and delivery of three "serial" shocks in rapid succession **without** pausing to check for the presence of a pulse between each shock (assuming the rhythm is unchanged). The amount of current penetrating the chest wall to shock the heart depends on the energy chosen (joules) and the resistance of the chest wall to the passage of that current, and decreasing the time interval between successive shocks. When using hand-held defibrillator paddles, firm paddle pressure helps decrease transthoracic resistance. To a point, transthoracic resistance decreases with increased paddle size. For adults, the optimal paddle size ranges from 8.5 to 12 cm in diameter.

6. a. **Defibrillation** is the therapeutic delivery of unsynchronized (the delivery of energy has no relationship to the cardiac cycle) electrical current through the myocardium over a very brief period to terminate a cardiac dysrhythmia.

7. b. When defibrillating a patient with a permanent (implanted) pacemaker, defibrillator paddles or self-adhesive monitoring/defibrillation pads should be placed at least 5 inches from the pacemaker's pulse generator.

8. d. If VF occurs after delivery of a synchronized cardioversion, quickly confirm the patient is apneic and pulseless, ensure that the "sync" button is off, and then defibrillate immediately.

9. c. Transcutaneous pacing is not indicated in the management of VF or an accelerated junctional rhythm and is unlikely to be of benefit in prolonged asystole. In second-degree AV block type II, TCP may be used as a "bridge" until transvenous pacing can be accomplished.

10. a. Energy levels recommended in the management of an unstable patient in atrial flutter include synchronized shocks with 50, 100, 200, 300, and 360 J or equivalent biphasic energy.

REFERENCES

1. Willerson JT, Cohn JN, editors: *Cardiovascular medicine*, New York, 1995, Churchill-Livingstone Inc.

2. Huang J, KenKnight BH, Rollins DL, Smith WM, Ideker RE: Ventricular defibrillation with triphasic waveforms, *Circulation* 101(11):1324-1328, 2000.

3. Schneider T, Martens PR, Paschen H, Kuisma M, Wolcke B, Gliner BE, Russell JK, Weaver WD, Bossaert L, Chamberlain D: Multicenter, randomized, controlled trial of 150-J biphasic shocks compared with 200- to 360-J monophasic shocks in the resuscitation of out-of-hospital cardiac arrest victims, *Circulation* 102(15):1780-1787, 2000.

4. Gliner BE, Jorgenson DB, Poole JE, White RD, Kanz KG, Lyster TD, Leyde KW, Powers DJ, Morgan CB, Kronmal RA, Bardy GH: Treatment of out-of-hospital cardiac arrest with a low-energy impedance-compensating biphasic waveform automatic external defibrillator, The LIFE Investigators, *Biomed Instrum Technol* 32(6):631-644, 1998.

5. Cates AW, Wolf PD, Hillsley RE, Souza JJ, Smith WM, Ideker RE: The probability of defibrillation success and the incidence of postshock arrhythmia as a function of shock strength. *Pacing Clin Electrophysiol* 17(7):1208-1217, 1994.

6. Ellenbogen KA, Kay GN, Wilkoff BL: *Clinical cardiac pacing and defibrillation*, ed 2, Philadelphia, 2000, WB Saunders.

7. Reddy RK, Gleva MJ, Gliner BE, Dolack GL, Kudenchuk PJ, Poole JE, Bardy GH: Biphasic transthoracic defibrillation causes fewer ECG ST-segment changes after shock, *Ann Emerg Med* 30(2):127-134, 1997.

8. Weil MH, Tang W, editors: *CPR: resuscitation of the arrested heart*, Philadelphia, 1999, WB Saunders.

9. Kerber RE, Grayzel J, Hoyt R, Marcus M, Kennedy J: Transthoracic resistance in human defibrillation: influence of body weight, chest size, serial shocks, paddle size and paddle contact pressure, *Circulation* 63:676–682, 1981.

10. Thomas ED, Ewy GA, Dahl CF, Ewy MD: Effectiveness of direct current defibrillation: role of paddle electrode size, *Am Heart J* 93:463-467, 1977.

11. Connell PN, Ewy GA, Dahl CF, Ewy MD: Transthoracic impedance to defibrillator discharge: effect of electrode size and electrode-chest wall interface, *J Electrocardiol* 6(4):313-M, 1973.

12. Hummell RS, Ornato JP, Wienberg SM, Clarke AM: Spark-generating properties of electrode gels used during defibrillation: a potential fire hazard, *JAMA* 260(20):3021-3024, 1988.

13. Crockett PJ, Droppert BM, Higgins SE, Richards RK: *Defibrillation: what you should know*. Redmond, WA, 1996, Physio-Control Corporation.

14. Kerber RE: Transthoracic cardioversion of atrial fibrillation and flutter: standard techniques and new advances, *Am J Cardiol* 78(8A):22-26, 1996.

15. Adgey AAJ, Campbell NPS, Webb SW: Transthoracic ventricular fibrillation in the adult, *Med Instrum* 2:7; 12:17-19, 1978.

16. Campbell NPS, Webb SW, Adgey AAJ, et al: Transthoracic ventricular defibrillation in adults, *Br Med J* Nov 26; 2(6099) 1379-1381, 1977.

17. Weaver WD, Cobb LA, Copass MK, Hallstrom AP: Ventricular defibrillation: a comparative trial using 175-J and 320-J shocks, *N Engl J Med* 307:1101-1106, 1982.

18. Dahl CF, Ewy GA, Ewy MD, Thomas ED: Transthoracic impedance to direct current discharge: effect of repeated countershocks, *Med Instrum* 10(3):151-154, 1976.

19. Ewy GA, Hellman DA, McClung S, Tarren D: Influence of ventilation phase on transthoracic impedance and defibrillation effectiveness, *Crit Care Med* 8(3):164-166, 1980.

20. Sirna SJ, Ferguson DW, Charbonnier F, Kerber RE: Factors affecting transthoracic impedance during electrical cardioversion, *Am J Cardiol* 62(16):1048-1052, 1988.

21. Olsovsky MR, Shorofsky SR, Gold MR: The effect of shock configuration and delivered energy on defibrillation impedance, *Pacing Clin Electrophysiol* 22(1 Pt 2):165-168, 1999.

22. Garcia LA, Kerber RE: Transthoracic defibrillation: does electrode adhesive pad position alter transthoracic impedance? *Resuscitation* 37(3): 139-143, 1998.

23. Pagan-Carlo LA, Spencer KT, Robertson CE, Dengler A, Birkett C, Kerber RE: Transthoracic defibrillation: importance of avoiding electrode placement directly on the female breast, *J Am Coll Cardiol* 27(2):449-452, 1996.

24. Stults KR, Brown DD, Cooley F, Kerber RE: Self-adhesive monitor/defibrillation pads improve prehospital defibrillation success, *Ann Emerg Med* 16(8):872-877, 1987.

25. Ewy GA, Dahl CF, Zimmermann M, Otto C: Ventricular fibrillation masquerading as ventricular standstill, *Crit Care Med* 841-844, 1981.

26. Cummins RO, Austin D Jr. The frequency of "occult" ventricular fibrillation masquerading as a flat line in prehospital cardiac arrest. *Ann Emerg Med* 17:813-817, 1988.

27. The American Heart Association in Collaboration with the International Liaison Committee on Resuscitation (ILCOR): Advanced Cardiovascular Life Support Section 2: Defibrillation, *Circulation* 102 (suppl I):1-92-93, 2000.

28. Bissing JW, Kerber RE: Effect of shaving the chest of hirsute subjects on transthoracic impedance to self-adhesive defibrillation electrode pads, *Am J Cardiol* 86(5):587-589, A10, 2000.

29. *Physicians GenRx: The Complete Drug Reference*, ed 10, 2000, Mosby.

30. Kerber RE, Kienzle MG, Olshansky B, Waldo AL, Wilber D, Carlson MD, Aschoff AM, Birger S, Fugatt L, Walsh S, et al: Ventricular tachycardia rate and morphology determine energy and current requirements for transthoracic cardioversion, *Circulation* 85(1):158-163, 1992.

31. The American Heart Association in Collaboration with the International Liaison Committee on Resuscitation (ILCOR): The automated external defibrillator, Part 4, *Circulation* 102 (suppl I):1-60, 2000.

32. Gundry JW, Comess KA, DeRook FA, Jorgenson D, Bardy GH: Comparison of naive sixth-grade children with trained professionals in the use of an automated external defibrillator, *Circulation* 19;100(16):1703-1707, 1999.

33. Page RL, Joglar JA, Kowal RC, Zagrodzky JD, Nelson LL, Ramaswamy K, Barbera SJ, Hamdan MH, McKenas DK: Use of automated external defibrillators by a US airline, *N Engl J Med* 343(17):1210-1216, 2000.

34. Valenzuela TD, Roe DJ, Nichol G, Clark LL, Spaite DW, Hardman RG: Outcomes of rapid defibrillation by security officers after cardiac arrest in casinos, *N Engl J Med* 343(17):1206-1209, 2000.

35. Moser SA, Crawford D, Thomas A: Caring for patients with implantable cardioverter defibrillators, *Crit Care Nurse* 8:52-65, 1988.

36. Wallace M: Treating AICD patients. Are you in for a shock? *JEMS* 20(2):59-61, 64, 1995.

37. Crawford MV, Spence MI: *Common sense approach to coronary care*, ed 6, St Louis, 1995, Mosby.

38. Wilson JG, Macgregor DC, Goldman BS, et al: Factors affecting patient recovery following pacemaker implantation, *Clin Prog Pacing Electrophysiol* 2(6):554, 1984.

39. Beland MJ, Hesslein PS, Finlay CD, Faerron-Angel JE, Williams WG, Rowe RD: Noninvasive transcutaneous cardiac pacing in children, *Pacing Clin Electrophysiol* 10:1262-1270, 1987.

40. Madsen JK, Meibom J, Videbak R, Pedersen F, Grande P: Transcutaneous pacing: experience with the Zoll noninvasive temporary pacemaker, *Am Heart J* 116(1 Pt 1):7-10, 1988.

41. Danzel DF: Accidental hypothermia, In Rosen P, editor: Emergency medicine: concepts and clinical practice, St Louis, 1988, Mosby.

42. Dixon RG, Dougherty JM, White LJ, Lombino D, Rusnak RR: Transcutaneous pacing in a hypothermic-dog model, *Ann Emerg Med* 29(5): 602-606, 1997.

43. Kolodzik PW, Mullin MJ, Krohmer JR, et al: The effects of anti-shock trouser inflation during hypothermic cardiovascular depression in the canine model, *Am J Emerg Med* 6:584-590, 1988.

44. Dixon RG, Dougherty JM, White LJ, Lombino D, Rusnak RR: Transcutaneous pacing in a hypothermic-dog model, *Ann Emerg Med* 29(5): 602-606, 1997.

45. Gibler WB: *Emergency cardiac care*, St Louis, 1994, Mosby.

46. Kerber RE, Robertson CE: In Paradis NA, Halperin HR, Nowak RM, editors: *Cardiac arrest: the science and practice of resuscitation medicine*, Baltimore, 1996, Williams & Wilkins.

47. Barold SS: Atrioventricular block following thumpversion of ventricular tachycardia, *Pacing Clin Electrophysiol* 28(11 Pt 1):1703-1704, 2000.

48. Gupta PR, Sinha PR, Somani PN: Chronic atrial fibrillation reverting to sinus rhythm following thumpversion in a case of rheumatic heart disease, *Indian Heart J* 42(3):199-200, 1990.

49. Caldwell G, Millar G, Quinn E, Vincent R, Chamberlain DA: Simple mechanical methods for cardioversion: defense of the precordial thump and cough version, *Br Med J Clin Res* 291:627-630, 1985.

50. Miller J, Tresch D, Horwitz L, Thompson BM, Aprahamian C, Darin JC: The precordial thump, *Ann Emerg Med* 13:791-794, 1984.

51. Yakaitis RW, Redding JS: Precordial thumping during cardiac resuscitation, *Crit Care Med* 1:22-26, 1973.

52. Miller J, Addas A, Akhtar M: Electrophysiology studies: precordial thumping patients paced into ventricular tachycardia, *J Emerg Med* 3(3):175-179, 1985.

BIBLIOGRAPHY

Ellenbogen KA, Kay GN, Wilkoff BL: *Clinical cardiac pacing and defibrillation*, ed 2, Philadelphia, 2000, WB Saunders.

Gibler WB, Aufderheide TP: *Emergency cardiac care*, St Louis, 1994, Mosby.

Goldman L, Braunwald E: *Primary cardiology*, Philadelphia, 1998, WB Saunders.

Kinney MR, Packa DR, editors: *Andreoli's comprehensive cardiac care*, ed 8, St Louis, 1996, Mosby.

Messerli, Franz H: *Cardiovascular drug therapy*, ed 2, Philadelphia, 1996, WB Saunders.

Murphy JG: *Mayo clinical cardiology review*, ed 2, Philadelphia, 2000, Lippincott, Williams & Wilkins.

Paradis NA, Halperin HR, Nowak RM, editors: *Cardiac arrest: the science and practice of resuscitation medicine*, Baltimore, 1996, Williams & Wilkins.

Schurig L, Gura M, Taibi B, editors: *NASPE Council of Associated Professionals. Educational guidelines:pacing and electrophysiology*, ed 2, Armonk, NY, 1997, Futura Publishing.

Weil MH, Tang W, editors: *CPR: resuscitation of the arrested heart*, Philadelphia, 1999, WB Saunders.

Willerson JT, Cohn JN, editors: *Cardiovascular medicine*, New York, 1995, Churchill-Livingstone.

Woods SL, Sivarajan Froelicher ES, Motzer SA: *Cardiac nursing*, ed 4, Philadelphia, 2000, Lippincott Williams & Wilkins.

Myocardial Ischemia, Injury, and Infarction

6

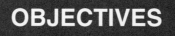

OBJECTIVES

On completion of this chapter, you will be able to:

1. Define *acute coronary syndromes*.
2. Describe the pathophysiology of coronary artery disease and the process of atherosclerosis.
3. Differentiate the characteristics of stable (classic) angina, unstable angina, and acute myocardial infarction.
4. Explain why pain relief is a high priority in the management of acute coronary syndromes.
5. Explain *atypical presentation* and its significance in acute coronary syndromes.
6. Identify the ECG changes associated with myocardial ischemia, injury, and infarction.
7. Explain the ECG criteria for significant ST-segment changes.
8. Describe methods for measuring ST-segment elevation and depression.
9. Describe the initial assessment and immediate general treatment of acute coronary syndromes.
10. List the characteristics of a patient eligible for fibrinolytic therapy.
11. Describe the initial management of a patient experiencing ST-elevation MI, non–ST-elevation MI, and unstable angina.
12. Identify the most common complications of an acute myocardial infarction.
13. Describe the management of a patient experiencing acute pulmonary edema.
14. Describe the management of a patient experiencing hypotension/shock caused by a volume problem or pump problem.
15. Explain the importance of the 12-lead ECG in acute coronary syndromes.
16. Identify the leads that comprise the standard 12-lead ECG.
17. List the leads that view the anterior wall, inferior wall, lateral wall, and septum.
18. Explain the clinical and ECG features of right ventricular infarction.

CARDIOVASCULAR DISEASE

Cardiovascular diseases (CVD) include coronary heart disease (coronary artery disease, ischemic heart disease), stroke (brain attack), hypertension, and rheumatic heart disease. To understand the significance of cardiovascular disease, consider the following facts from the American Heart Association[1]:

- According to 1997 estimates, 59,700,000 Americans have one or more forms of cardiovascular disease
- In 1997, cardiovascular disease claimed 953,110 lives in the United States (41.2% of all deaths)
- About one sixth of the individuals who die of CVD are under age 65
- Coronary heart disease caused 466,101 deaths in 1997 and is the single leading cause of death in America today
- Annually, an estimated 1,100,000 Americans experience a new or recurrent coronary attack (acute MI or fatal coronary heart disease), and more than 40% of them will die from the event
- It is estimated that 225,000 individuals/year die of coronary heart disease without being hospitalized; these are sudden deaths caused by cardiac arrest, usually resulting from ventricular fibrillation (VF)

INTRODUCTION TO ACUTE CORONARY SYNDROMES (ACS)

1. Acute coronary syndromes (ACS) include unstable angina, non–ST-segment elevation MI and ST-segment elevation MI
2. These syndromes represent a physiologic continuum of clinical disease and share the common pathophysiology of atherosclerotic plaque rupture and intracoronary thrombosis
3. Sudden cardiac death may occur with each of these syndromes

Arterial Structure

1. Arteries consist of three layers (Figure 6-1)
   a. *Outer layer:* Tunica adventitia
      (1) Consists of flexible fibrous connective tissue
      (2) Helps hold the vessel open
      (3) Origin of the vasa vasorum, which supplies the layers of the arterial wall with blood
   b. *Middle layer:* Tunica media
      (1) Consists of smooth muscle tissue and elastic connective tissue
      (2) This layer, encircled by smooth muscle and innervated by fibers of the autonomic nervous system, allows constriction and dilation of the vessel
      (3) Medium-sized muscular arteries (e.g., coronary, brachial, radial, femoral) contain substantially more smooth muscle than conductance vessels (large elastic arteries)
      (4) Smooth muscle cells function to maintain vascular tone and regulate local blood flow based on metabolic requirements; however, these cells are capable of producing collagen, elastin, and other substances important in the formation of atherosclerotic plaques
   c. *Innermost layer:* Tunica intima
      (1) Consists of endothelium that lines the vascular system
      (2) Endothelium is a single layer of cells in direct contact with the blood
      (3) Functions of normal endothelium are:
         (a) Presents a barrier between the blood and the arterial wall
         (b) Prevents platelets from sticking and aggregating and forming clots, because of antithrombotic properties

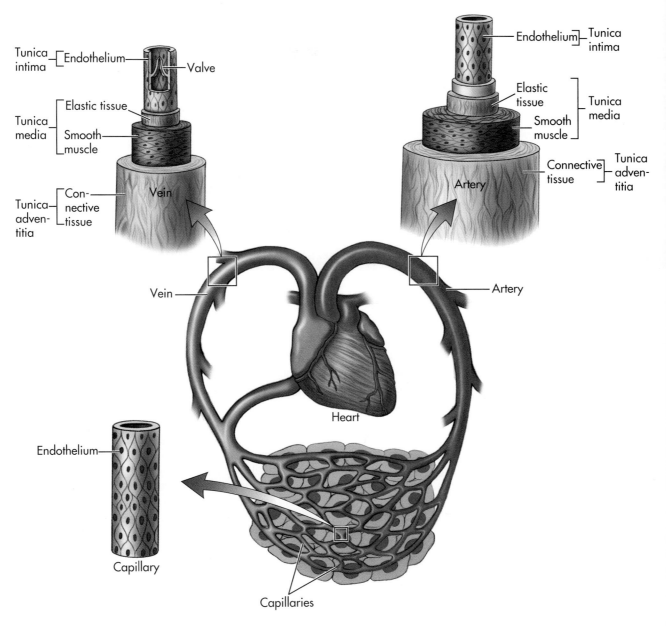

Figure 6-1 Blood vessel wall layers.

   (c) Produces vasodilating factors
     (i) Endothelium-derived relaxing factor (EDRF) is a powerful vasodilator synthesized by endothelial cells. It is thought that EDRF contributes to regulation of blood flow by relaxing of vascular smooth muscle and preventing platelet aggregation and release of platelet factors that promote thrombus formation
     (ii) Reported stimuli for release of EDRF include thrombin, histamine, norepinephrine, acetylcholine, vessel distention, and shear stress (the frictional force from blood flow)
     (iii) Atherosclerosis tends to replace EDRF-producing endothelial cells

(d) Produce vasoconstricting factors
  (i) Thrombin, epinephrine, and vasopressin stimulate the formation of vasoconstricting factors (endothelins) in the endothelium
  (ii) Vasoconstricting factors are also reportedly produced by activated cells (macrophages) in atherosclerotic lesions of individuals with acute ischemic coronary disease and plaque rupture[2]
  (iii) Elevated levels of vasoconstricting factors are found in atherosclerosis, acute MI, CHF, and hypertension
(e) Releases platelet factors that promote thrombus formation
(f) Prevents migration and proliferation of smooth muscle cells
(g) Prevents inflammation

PATHOGENESIS OF ACUTE CORONARY SYNDROMES

Atherosclerosis

Athero = gruel or paste; *sclerosis* = hardness.

1. **Arteriosclerosis:** Chronic disease of the arterial system, characterized by abnormal thickening and hardening of the vessel walls
2. **Atherosclerosis:** Form of arteriosclerosis in which the thickening and hardening of the vessel walls are caused by an accumulation of fibro-fatty deposits in the intimal lining of large and middle-sized muscular arteries
3. As the fatty deposits build up, the artery opening gradually narrows and blood flow to the muscle decreases. A decreased supply of oxygenated blood to a body part or organ is called **ischemia**
4. Any artery in the body can develop atherosclerosis
   a. If the coronary arteries are involved (coronary artery disease or coronary heart disease) and blood flow to the heart is decreased, angina (chest pain) or more serious signs and symptoms may result
   b. If the arteries in the leg are involved (peripheral vascular disease), leg pain (claudication) may result
   c. If the arteries supplying the brain are involved (carotid artery disease), a stroke or transient ischemic attack (TIA) may result

Coronary Artery Pathology

1. The usual cause of an acute coronary syndrome is the rupture of an atherosclerotic plaque. Atherosclerotic lesions occur primarily in the innermost layer of an artery and include the fatty streak, fibrous plaque, and the advanced (complicated) lesion (Figure 6-2)
2. Fatty streaks
   a. Thin, flat yellow lesions composed of lipid-containing (mostly cholesterol) macrophages or smooth muscle cells that protrude slightly into the arterial lumen
   b. Appear in all populations, even those with a low incidence of CAD and have been found in individuals of all ages, from premature infants to the elderly
   c. Do not obstruct the vessel and are not associated with any clinical symptoms. Controversy exists about whether fatty streaks are precursors of atherosclerotic lesions.

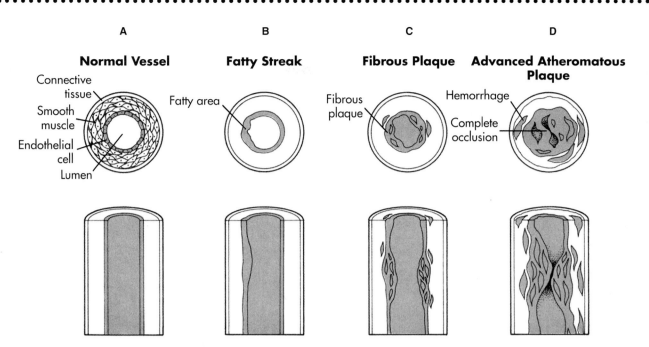

Figure 6-2 Progression of atherosclerosis. **A,** Normal vessel. **B,** Fatty streaks. **C,** Fibrous plaque development. **D,** Advanced (complicated) lesions.

3. Fibrous plaques and advanced lesions
   a. Atherosclerotic plaques differ in composition, consistency, "vulnerability," and their propensity to generate a thrombus
   b. "Stable" plaques are hard, primarily consist of collagen-rich sclerotic tissue, and have a relatively thick fibrous cap over the center of the plaque material that separates the material from contact with the blood, making it less likely to rupture (Figure 6-3)
      (1) Many of these plaques are not hemodynamically significant because they do not impede arterial flow; however, as they increase in size, they can produce severe narrowing of the arterial lumen. Seventy percent diameter stenosis is generally required to produce anginal symptoms
      (2) Research has shown that the walls of an artery remodel, or outwardly expand, as plaque accumulates inside it. This process occurs so that the size of the vessel stays relatively constant, despite the increased plaque volume. When the plaque fills approximately 40% of the vessel lumen, remodeling ceases because the artery can no longer expand to accommodate the increase in plaque size
      (3) Complete occlusion of the vessel may cause infarction; however, because the plaque typically increases in size over months and years, collateral arteries may develop to supply tissue, thus preventing infarction despite complete vessel occlusion
   c. "Vulnerable" (prone to rupture) plaques are soft, primarily consist of lipid-rich atheromatous material (lipid pool or "gruel"), and have a thin cap of fibrous tissue that separates the material from the vessel lumen (Figure 6-4)
      (1) Rupture of a plaque is unpredictable. Determinants of a plaque's vulnerability to rupture are thought to include the size of the atheromatous core and the thickness of the fibrous cap. Contributing factors to plaque rupture may include shear stress (the

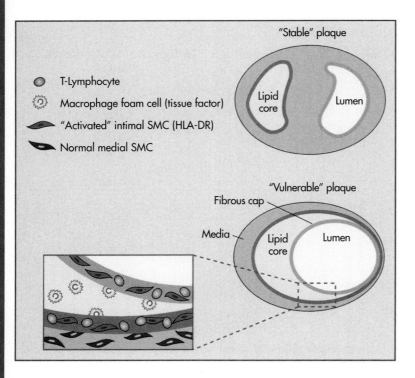

Figure 6-3 Comparison of "stable" and "vulnerable" plaques. A stable plaque has a relatively thick fibrous cap separating the lipid core from contact with the blood. A vulnerable plaque typically has a large lipid core and a thin cap of fibrous tissue that separates it from the vessel lumen. *SMC*, smooth muscle cell.

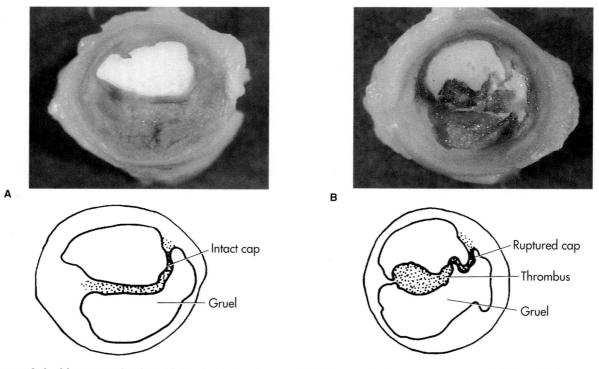

Figure 6-4 Macroscopic view of a vulnerable plaque. **A,** Yellow, soft atheromatous material ("gruel") is separated from the opening of the vessel only by a thin, but intact, fibrous cap. The vessel opening contains white radiographic contrast medium. **B,** This specimen was just a few millimeters distal to the one shown in **A**. Here the thin fibrous cap is ruptured; a big cap fragment and some of the soft atheromatous gruel are missing (because of downstream embolization), and a mural thrombus has evolved where the thrombogenic atheromatous gruel has been exposed. White contrast medium has penetrated the soft gruel through the ruptured cap. (Falk E, Anderson HR: Pathology of atherosclerotic plaque: stable, unstable, and infarctional. In *Interventional cardiovascular medicine: principles and practice.* Edited by Roubin GS, Califf RM, O'Neill NW, et al. New York: Churchill Livinstone 1994.)

frictional force from blood flow), coronary spasm at the site of the plaque, internal plaque changes, and the effects of risk factors (e.g., hypertension, hyperlipidemia)

  (a) Plaques located at vessel bifurcations are more likely to rupture because of the speed of blood flow and turbulence created at these areas (Figure 6-5)

(2) If the fibrous cap ruptures, the contents of the plaque (including collagen and other tissue factors) are exposed to flowing blood, which promotes platelet adhesion and aggregation. The coagulation cascade then begins, resulting in additional platelet aggregation and thrombosis (Figure 6-6)

  (a) When an atherosclerotic plaque ruptures or erodes, platelets adhere to the damaged lining of the vessel and to each other within 1 to 5 seconds, forming a plug

  (b) "Sticky platelets" secrete several chemicals including thromboxane A_2. These substances stimulate vasoconstriction, reducing blood flow at the site

  (i) At this stage, antiplatelet agents are most effective. Aspirin blocks the synthesis of thromboxane A_2, inhibiting platelet aggregation. Fibrinolytic therapy is not effective at this stage and may accelerate occlusion of the vessel by causing the release of thrombin, further activating platelets.

  (ii) Despite the absence of thromboxane A_2, platelets may still be induced to aggregate by triggers such as thrombin, subendothelial collagen, or stainless steel from intracoronary stents.[3]

  (c) Once platelets are activated, glycoprotein IIb/IIIa receptors that are essential for platelet aggregation appear on the surface of the platelet. Fibrinogen molecules bind to these receptors to form bridges ("cross-links") between adjacent platelets, allowing them to aggregate

  (i) Glycoprotein IIb/IIIa receptor inhibitors prevent fibrinogen binding and platelet aggregation, regardless of the trigger responsible for platelet aggregation[4]

  (d) As the process continues, fibrinogen cross-links platelets, thrombin is then generated, fibrin is formed and ultimately a thrombus is produced (Figure 6-7)

  (i) Once an active thrombosis has developed, heparin can inhibit further clotting by inactivating thrombin and preventing the conversion of fibrinogen to fibrin (Figure 6-8)

  (ii) Coumadin interferes with the clotting mechanism but at a different step in the process than heparin. Coumadin decreases the synthesis of prothrombin in the liver, decreasing prothrombin levels in the blood. This ultimately results in formation of less thrombin and diminished blood clotting

  (iii) Aspirin has little effect on thrombin-induced platelet aggregation

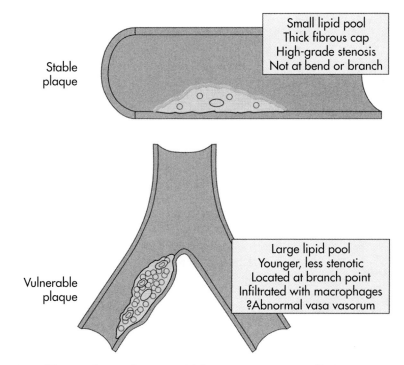

Figure 6-5 Plaques located at vessel bifurcations are more likely to rupture because of the speed of blood flow and the turbulence created at these areas. (From Mandel WJ: Cardiac arrhythmias, Philadelphia, JB Lippincott, 1980: 21, 214.)

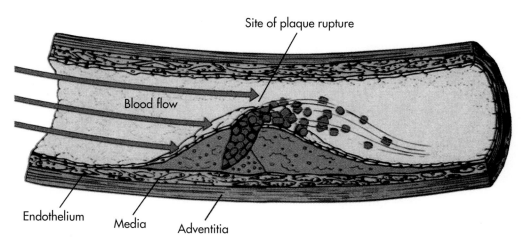

Figure 6-6 Arterial thrombus responsible for acute MI. Rupture of a vulnerable plaque results in adhesion of platelets at the site and activation of additional platelets (aggregation). The coagulation cascade then begins, resulting in additional platelet aggregation and thrombosis.

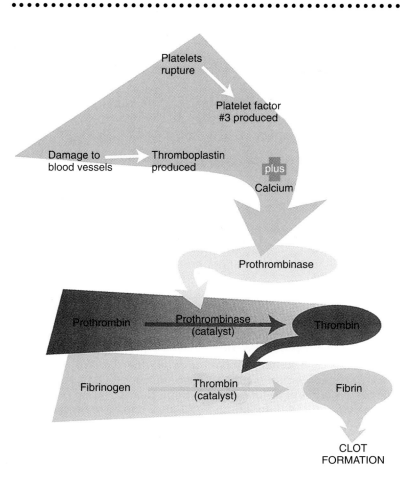

Figure 6-7 Simplified illustration of the process of clot formation.

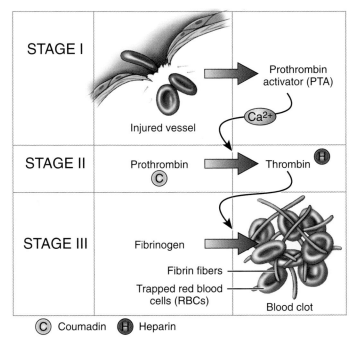

Figure 6-8 Once active thrombosis has developed, heparin can inhibit further clotting by inactivating thrombin and preventing the conversion of fibrinogen to fibrin. Coumadin *(C)* and heparin *(H)* activity are indicated.

(e) Clots are dissolved by a process called **fibrinolysis**. Fibrinolytics (formerly called *thrombolytics*) stimulate the conversion of plasminogen to plasmin, which dissolves the clot (Figure 6-9)

d. "Rupture of the plaque surface occurs frequently during plaque growth and is probably the most significant mechanism underlying rapid progression of coronary lesions. In the great majority of cases, it may be clinically silent. Only if significant *thrombosis* evolves will plaque rupture give rise to an acute ischemic (coronary) syndrome"[5]

(1) Occlusion of a coronary artery by a thrombus may be complete or incomplete

(a) Complete occlusion of the coronary artery may result in a Q-wave MI (ST-elevation MI) or sudden death

(b) Incomplete occlusion of the coronary artery by a thrombus may result in no clinical signs and symptoms (silent), unstable angina, non–Q-wave MI (non–ST-segment elevation MI) or, possibly, sudden death

(2) The patient's clinical presentation and outcome depend on factors including:

(a) Amount of myocardium supplied by the affected artery

(b) Severity and duration of myocardial ischemia

(c) Electrical instability of the ischemic myocardium

(d) Degree and duration of coronary obstruction

(e) Presence (and extent) or absence of collateral coronary circulation

> The extent of arterial narrowing and reduction in blood flow are critical determinants of coronary artery disease.

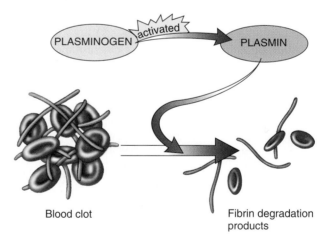

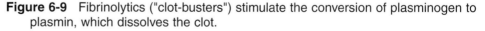

Figure 6-9 Fibrinolytics ("clot-busters") stimulate the conversion of plasminogen to plasmin, which dissolves the clot.

MYOCARDIAL ISCHEMIA

Angina

1. Angina pectoris is chest discomfort or other related symptoms caused by myocardial ischemia. Myocardial ischemia results when the heart's demand for oxygen exceeds its supply from the coronary circulation
2. Angina is typically described as heaviness, pressure, squeezing, constriction, or pain. Some patients have difficulty describing their discomfort or deny their discomfort is truly pain[6]
3. Common sites for anginal pain include upper part of chest, beneath sternum radiating to neck and jaw; beneath sternum radiating down left arm; epigastric; epigastric radiating to neck, jaw, and arms; neck and jaw; left shoulder; and intrascapular (Figure 6-10)
4. Angina can occur because of a decreased myocardial oxygen supply or an increase in myocardial oxygen demand. If the process is not reversed and blood flow restored, severe myocardial ischemia may lead to cellular injury and, eventually, infarction.
5. Ischemia can quickly resolve by:
   a. Reducing the oxygen needs of the heart (by resting or slowing the heart rate with medications such as beta-blockers) or
   b. Increasing blood flow by dilating the coronary arteries with medications such as nitroglycerin (NTG)

Stable (classic) angina

1. Remains relatively constant and predictable in terms of severity, presentation, character, precipitating events, response to therapy
2. Characterized by transient episodes of chest pain or discomfort related to activities that increase myocardial oxygen demand (e.g., emotional upset, exercise/exertion, exposure to cold weather) and may be associated with shortness of breath, palpitations, sweating, nausea, or vomiting
3. Duration of symptoms typically 2 to 5 minutes, occasionally 5 to 15 minutes; prolonged discomfort (>30 min) uncommon in stable angina

Myocardial ischemia, injury, and infarction are referred to as *the 3 I's* of an acute coronary event.

Angina is not a disease but a **symptom** of myocardial ischemia.

Ask the patient to describe the severity of his/her discomfort using a numeric scale from 1 to 10 (1 = least, 10 = worst pain). Use of such a scale allows evaluation of the effectiveness of interventions.

The pain associated with angina pectoris occurs because of the stimulation of nerve endings by lactic acid and carbon dioxide that accumulates in ischemic tissue.

Silent ischemia is a term used to describe objective evidence of myocardial ischemia, without the patient experiencing any symptoms of angina.

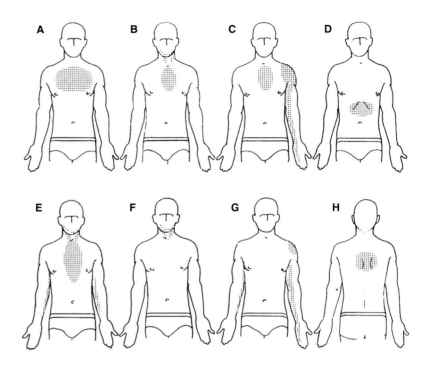

Figure 6-10 Common sites for anginal pain. **A,** Upper part of chest. **B,** Beneath sternum radiating to neck and jaw. **C,** Beneath sternum radiating down left arm. **D,** Epigastric. **E,** Epigastric radiating to neck, jaw, and arms. **F,** Neck and jaw. **G,** Left shoulder. **H,** Intrascapular.

Assessing Chest Pain

The **OPQRST** mnemonic may be used to recall pertinent questions to ask when obtaining a history from a patient experiencing chest pain.

1. **O**nset: "When did your symptoms begin?" "What were you doing when they began?" "Did your symptoms begin suddenly or gradually?"

2. **P**rovocation/Palliative: "Did anything bring on the pain?" "Does anything make the pain better or worse?" (Associated with respiration, movement)

3. **Q**uality: "How would you describe your discomfort?" (Pressure, pain, crushing, dull, burning, tearing, throbbing, squeezing, stabbing, vise-like)

4. **R**egion/Radiation/Referral: "Where is your discomfort?" (Ask the patient to point to it) "Does it go anywhere else?" (Neck, shoulders, arm, back)

5. **S**everity: "On a scale of 1 to 10, with 1 being the least and 10 being the worst, what number would you assign your pain or discomfort?"

6. **T**iming: "Does your discomfort come and go or is it constant?"

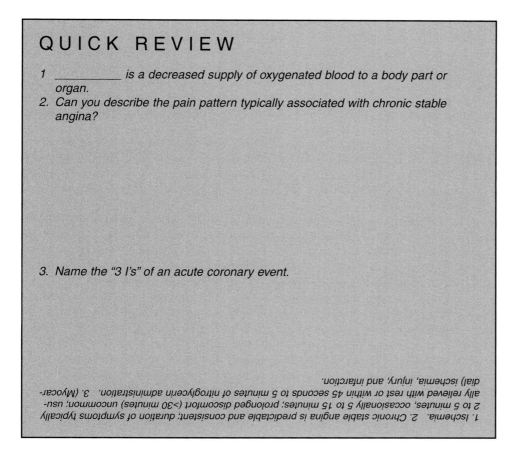

QUICK REVIEW

1 _____ is a decreased supply of oxygenated blood to a body part or organ.

2. Can you describe the pain pattern typically associated with chronic stable angina?

3. Name the "3 I's" of an acute coronary event.

1. Ischemia.   2. Chronic stable angina is predictable and consistent; duration of symptoms typically 2 to 5 minutes, occasionally 5 to 15 minutes; prolonged discomfort (>30 minutes) uncommon; usually relieved with rest or within 45 seconds to 5 minutes of nitroglycerin administration.   3. (Myocardial) ischemia, injury, and infarction.

Unstable angina

1. Syndrome of intermediate severity between stable angina and acute myocardial infarction
2. Usually occurs as a result of plaque rupture and thrombus formation in a coronary artery that causes a sudden decrease in myocardial blood flow
   a. Less common causes of unstable angina include coronary artery spasm, severe hypertension, hyperthyroidism, and hypertrophic cardiomyopathy
3. Occurs most often in men and women 60 to 80 years of age who have one or more of the major risk factors for coronary artery disease (e.g., hypertension, hyperlipidemia, cigarette smoking, diabetes mellitus)
4. Characterized by one or more of the following:
   a. Symptoms of angina at rest (usually >20 minutes)
   b. Progressive worsening of preexisting stable angina
   c. New onset (<2 months) angina that is severe and brought on by minimal exertion
5. Episodes of pain occur with increased frequency
   a. Pain usually lasts longer (up to 30 minutes)
   b. Pain generally radiates more widely
   c. May be accompanied by dyspnea

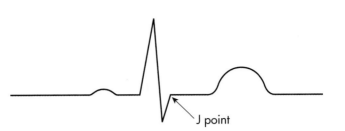

Figure 6-11 Point where the QRS complex and the ST segment meet is called the "junction" or "J" point.

6. ECG changes
   a. Myocardial ischemia delays repolarization; thus ECG changes characteristic of ischemia include temporary changes in the ST segment and T wave
   b. On the ECG, the J point is the point where the QRS ends and the ST segment begins (Figure 6-11). ST-segment **depression** is suggestive of myocardial ischemia and is considered significant when the ST segment is more than 1 mm below the baseline at a point 0.04 sec (one small box) to the right of the J point
   c. If ischemia is present through the full thickness of the myocardium, a negative (inverted) T wave will be present in the leads facing the affected area of the ventricle. In leads opposite the affected area, reciprocal (mirror image) changes may be seen
   d. If ischemia is present only in the subendocardial layer, the T wave is usually positive (upright) because the direction of repolarization is unaffected (repolarization normally occurs from epicardium to endocardium) but may be abnormally tall
7. In the early acute phase, distinguishing patients with unstable angina from those with acute MI is often impossible because their clinical presentations and ECG findings may be identical
8. Features that are *not* characteristic of discomfort caused by myocardial ischemia include[7]:
   a. Sharp or knife-like pain brought on by respiratory movements or cough
   b. Primary or sole location of discomfort in the middle or lower abdominal region
   c. Pain reproduced with movement or palpation of the chest wall or arms
   d. Constant pain that lasts for many hours
   e. Very brief episodes of pain that last a few seconds or less
   f. Pain that radiates into the lower extremities

> *"Although typical characteristics substantially raise the probability of CAD, features not characteristic of chest pain, such as sharp stabbing pain or reproduction of pain on palpation, do not exclude the possibility of acute coronary syndrome."*[7]

Anginal equivalent

1. Patient has no specific chest pain or discomfort
2. Manifestations of cardiac ischemia are characterized by excessive fatigue or weakness, dyspnea, or isolated arm or jaw pain
3. Elderly are likely to present with these above symptoms or palpitations, excessive sweating, dizziness, or syncope

---

QUICK REVIEW

1. Describe the characteristics of unstable angina.

2. A 55-year-old male is complaining of chest discomfort that radiates to his left arm and jaw. Signs suggestive of myocardial ischemia appear on the ECG as _____ in leads facing the affected area.

1. Unstable angina is characterized by one or more of the following: symptoms of angina at rest (usually >20 minutes), progressively worsening of preexisting stable angina, or new onset (<2 months) angina that is severe and brought on by minimal exertion.   2. ST-segment depression and, sometimes, T wave changes.

MYOCARDIAL INJURY

1. Ischemia prolonged more than just a few minutes results in myocardial injury.
   a. Injured myocardial cells can live or die depending on how quickly blood flow is restored to the affected tissue. If blood flow is restored, no tissue death occurs. However, without rapid intervention, the injured area will become necrotic.
   b. Methods to restore blood flow may include administration of fibrinolytic agents, coronary angioplasty, or a coronary artery bypass graft (CABG), among others.
2. ECG changes
   a. Injured myocardium does not function normally, affecting both muscle contraction and the conduction of electrical impulses
   b. Injured myocardium depolarizes incompletely and remains electrically more positive than the uninjured areas surrounding it
      (1) Viewed on the ECG as ST-segment **elevation** in the leads facing the affected area. In leads opposite the affected area, ST-segment depression (reciprocal changes) may be seen.
   c. ST-segment elevation is considered significant when the ST segment is ≥ one millimeter above the baseline at a point 0.04 second (one small box) to the right of the J-point (Figure 6-12)

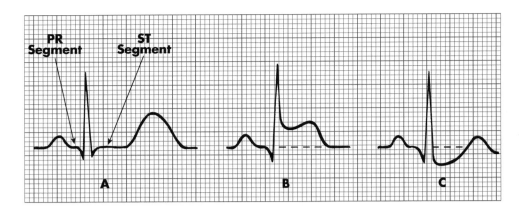

Figure 6-12 ST segment. **A,** PR segment is used as the baseline from which to determine the presence of ST-segment elevation or depression. **B,** ST-segment elevation. **C,** ST-segment depression.

MYOCARDIAL INFARCTION

1. Myocardial infarction is death of myocardial cells due to ischemia
   a. Occurs when there is a sudden decrease or total cessation of blood flow through a coronary artery to an area of the myocardium because of a thrombus
   b. May also occur as a result of:
      (1) Coronary spasm
         (a) Coronary spasm as a primary cause of MI is rare; however, MI as a result of cocaine abuse is frequently thought to be caused by coronary spasm
      (2) Coronary embolism (rare)
2. According to the World Health Organization, diagnosis of MI is based on the presence of at least two of the following three criteria[8]:
   a. Clinical history of ischemic type chest discomfort
   b. Changes on serially obtained ECGs
   c. Rise and fall in serum cardiac markers
3. Terminology related to MI:
   a. Myocardial infarctions are usually classified by size—microscopic (focal necrosis), small (<10% of the left ventricle), medium (10% to 30% of the left ventricle), or large (>30% of the left ventricle)—as well as by location (anterior, lateral, inferior, posterior or septal, or a combination of locations)[9]
   b. In the past, MI was classified according to its location (i.e., anterior, inferior, etc.) and whether it produced Q waves on the ECG (i.e., Q wave vs. non–Q wave MI)
   c. Today, the World Health Organization recommends classification of infarctions as ST-segment elevation or non–ST-segment elevation infarction rather than Q-wave or non–Q-wave infarction

Myocardial Infarction Redefined

According to the Joint European Society of Cardiology/American College of Cardiology Committee for the redefinition of myocardial infarction, the "term *MI* should not be used without further qualifications, whether in clinical practice, in the description of patient cohorts or in population studies. Such qualifications should refer to the amount of myocardial cell loss (infarct size), to the circumstances leading to the infarct (spontaneous or in the setting of a coronary artery diagnostic or therapeutic procedure) and to the timing of the myocardial necrosis relative to the time of the observation (evolving, healing or healed MI)."

Acute MI is 6 hours to 7 days; healing is 7 to 28 days, and healed is 29 days or more.

Definition of MI

Criteria for acute, evolving, or recent MI

Either one of the following criteria satisfies the diagnosis for an acute, evolving, or recent MI:

1. Typical rise and gradual fall (troponin) or more rapid rise and fall (CK-MB) of biochemical markers of myocardial necrosis with at least one of the following:
   a. Ischemic symptoms
   b. Development of pathologic Q waves on the ECG
   c. ECG changes indicative of ischemia (ST-segment elevation or depression)
   d. Coronary artery intervention (e.g., coronary angioplasty)

2. Pathologic findings of an acute MI

Criteria for established MI

Any one of the following criteria satisfies the diagnosis for established MI:

1. Development of new pathologic Q-waves on serial ECGs. The patient may or may not remember previous symptoms. Biochemical markers of myocardial necrosis may have normalized, depending on the length of time that has passed since the infarct developed

2. Pathologic findings of a healed or healing MI

From Myocardial infarction redefined—a consensus document of The Joint European Society of Cardiology/American College of Cardiology Committee for the redefinition of myocardial infarction, *J Am Coll Cardiol* 36(3):959-969, 2000.

Clinical Manifestations

History

1. Precipitating factors
   a. A precipitating factor is usually present in approximately 50% of patients experiencing MI (e.g., unusually vigorous exercise, severe emotional stress, serious illness)[10] (Figure 6-13)
   b. Approximately two thirds of patients describe the new onset of angina or a change in their anginal pattern in the month preceding infarction[11]
   c. Cocaine use may be a factor in an acute coronary syndrome, presumably because of its ability to cause coronary vasospasm and thrombosis in addition to its direct effects on heart rate and arterial pressure and its myocardial toxic properties[7]
      (1) Inquire about the use of cocaine in patients with suspected acute coronary syndromes, particularly in patients <40 years of age

Figure 6-13 Possible triggers of myocardial infarction. (Redrawn from Waxman, S., and Muller, J.E.: Risk factors for an acute ischemic event. *In* Califf, R.M. [vol. ed.]: Acute Myocardial Infarction and Other Acute Ischemic Syndromes. Braunwald, E. [ser. ed]: Atlas of Heart Disease, Vol. 8, Philadelphia, Current Medicine, 1996, p. 2.5; adapted from American Journal of Cardiology, vol 66, Tofler, G.H., Stone, P.H., Maclure, M., and the MILIS Study Group: Analysis of possible triggers of acute myocardial infarction [the MILIS study], pp 22-27, Copyright 1990, with permission from Excerpta Medica Inc.)

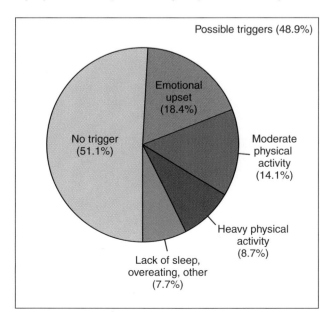

2. Circadian rhythmicity[12]
   a. In the early morning hours:
      (1) Frequency of ischemic episodes increases shortly after awakening; secondary peak may occur in the early evening hours
      (2) Heart rate, blood pressure, and contractility peak, contributing to increased myocardial oxygen demand
      (3) Platelet aggregation greater; intrinsic fibrinolytic activity of the blood lowest
      (4) Levels of plasma norepinephrine and renin activity are increased, contributing to vasoconstriction
   b. Pattern of increased ischemia in the early morning may be amplified by the assumption of an upright posture

Clinical Presentation

1. Chest discomfort suggestive of ischemia present in 75% to 80% of patients with acute MI
   a. Single most common symptom of infarction
   b. Symptoms frequently include chest, epigastric, arm, and wrist or jaw discomfort with exertion or at rest
      (1) Discomfort typically described as heaviness, pressure, squeezing, or tightness in the chest that has persisted for at least 20 minutes but may be shorter in duration
      (2) May begin in the central or left chest and then radiate to the arm, jaw, back or shoulder
      (3) Patient may describe discomfort with a clenched fist held against his or her sternum (Levine's sign)
   c. May be accompanied by unexplained nausea and vomiting, persistent shortness of breath caused by left ventricular failure, and unexplained weakness, dizziness, sweating, anxiety, lightheadedness or syncope, or a combination of these symptoms
      (1) Symptoms may occur with or without associated chest discomfort
   d. Discomfort is usually *not* sharp, worsened by deep inspiration, affected by moving muscles in the area where the discomfort is localized, or positional in nature
   e. Nausea, vomiting, and epigastric pain may result in confusion with GI disturbances (e.g., peptic ulcer, acute cholecystitis, gastritis)—patient may describe symptoms as "heartburn" or "indigestion"
2. Overall mortality rate of patients *without* chest pain is substantially higher than those *with* substernal discomfort[13]
3. Atypical presentation
   a. Chest discomfort is absent in approximately 20% of patients—these patients are more likely to present with dyspnea, palpitations, dysrhythmias ("anginal equivalent" symptoms) or vague, nonspecific complaints
   b. Patients more likely to present in an atypical manner include the elderly, those with diabetes, and women
      (1) Elderly
         (a) Chest pain typical of acute MI is described by only one third of patients >85 years[14]
         (b) Most frequent symptoms of acute MI are shortness of breath, fatigue, abdominal or epigastric discomfort
         (c) Elderly patients are more likely to present with more severe preexisting conditions, such as hypertension, congestive

heart failure, or previous acute MI, are likely to delay longer in seeking treatment as compared with younger patients, and are less likely to have ST-segment elevation on initial ECG[15]

(2) Patients with diabetes may present atypically (because of autonomic dysfunction) with generalized weakness, syncope, lightheadedness, or a change in mental status

(3) Women

    (a) Cardiac-related pain in women may be centered in chest with or without radiation down one or both arms; located in ear, jaw, or neck region; located in back or shoulder region

    (b) Some women may have only vague chest discomfort that tends to come and go with no known aggravating factors and others do not have chest pain but have other signs and symptoms that may include diaphoresis, lightheadedness, shortness of breath, back pain, nausea/vomiting

    (c) Women are twice as likely as men to die in the early weeks after MI and experience reinfarction more frequently; have higher rates of stroke, shock, heart failure, recurrent chest pain, and cardiac rupture than men; and have a higher risk of intracranial hemorrhage with fibrinolytic therapy[14]

4. Symptom recognition

  a. After the onset of ischemic chest pain symptoms, most patients do not seek medical care for 2 hours or more and many wait 12 hours or more. Women often delay longer than men do in seeking hospital medical treatment

    (1) Major advantage of reperfusion therapy is time dependent

    (2) Perfusion therapy has the greatest benefit for eligible patients when initiated at or close to the onset of acute MI symptoms

    (3) Generally, reperfusion therapy beyond 12 hours may offer little benefit

  b. Mortality from acute MI decreases as the interval between symptom onset and initiation of treatment decreases

    (1) According to the National Heart Attack Alert Program, the relationship between time to treatment (i.e., delay) and absolute mortality is about 1% per hour (i.e., each hour of delay = 1% increased mortality)

  c. Components of delay in onset of treatment (Table 6-1)

    (1) Patient delay in seeking medical attention

Table 6-1   Factors Affecting Prehospital Delay in Patients with Signs and Symptoms of Acute Myocardial Infarction

Factors Contributing to Increased Delay	Factors Contributing to Decreased Delay
Older age	Hemodynamic instability
Female gender	Large infarct size
African-American race	Sudden onset of severe chest pain
Low socioeconomic status	Recognition by patient that symptoms are heart-related
Low emotional or somatic awareness	Consulting a friend, coworker, or stranger
History of angina, diabetes, or both	
Consulting a spouse or other relative	
Consulting a physician	
Self-treatment	

From *Educational strategies to prevent prehospital delay in patients at high risk for acute myocardial infarction*, NIH Publication No 97-3787, September, 1997, National Institutes of Health, National Heart, Lung, and Blood Institute.

(2) Prehospital evaluation and transportation
(3) Evaluation and start of treatment in the hospital
d. Efforts of health care professionals must be directed at reducing all components of delay

---

QUICK REVIEW

1. What is the single most common symptom of acute MI?

2. Name three types of patients experiencing an acute coronary syndrome that are likely to present atypically.

3. After the onset of ischemic chest pain symptoms, most patients do not seek medical care for _____ hours or more.

1. Chest discomfort.   2. Elderly, persons with diabetes, women.   3. Two.

Serum Cardiac Markers

1. As myocardial cells die, intracellular substances pass through broken cell membranes and leak substances into the bloodstream. The presence of these substances in the blood can subsequently be measured by means of blood tests to verify the presence of an infarction. These substances (called *cardiac markers* or *serum cardiac markers*) include creatine kinase (CK) MB isoforms, troponin, and myoglobin (Table 6-2)

Table 6-2   Serum Cardiac Markers

	Rises	Peaks	Duration
Troponin I	3-6 hours	20 hours	14 days
CK-MB	4-6 hours	12-24 hours	4-5 days
Myoglobin	1-2 hours	4-6 hours	1-2 days

2. Useful for confirming the diagnosis of MI when patients present without ST-segment elevation, when the diagnosis may be unclear, and when physicians must distinguish patients with unstable angina from those with a non-ST-segment elevation (non–Q-wave) MI. Also useful for confirming the diagnosis of MI for patients with ST-segment elevation
3. CK-MB isoforms
   a. CK-MB exists in only one form in myocardial tissue but in different isoforms (or subforms) in the plasma
   b. An absolute level of CK-MB2 >1 U/L or a ratio of CK-MB2 to CK-MB1 of 1.5 is considered positive for diagnosis of MI
4. Troponins
   a. Troponin T and Troponin I are not normally detected in the blood of healthy individuals
      (1) Elevation (positive test) is highly specific for myocardial necrosis (infarction)
      (2) Troponin I appears to have better specificity for MI than Troponin T

b. Half-life of the troponins is long; not used for diagnosis of reinfarction in the period after an MI

5. Myoglobin

a. Released by necrotic myocardium more rapidly than CK-MB; may be detected as early as 2 hours after MI

b. Also released after injury to skeletal muscle; thus it is not specific to cardiac tissue (cannot distinguish cardiac muscle injury from skeletal muscle injury)

6. For patients presenting within the first 2 or 3 hours of symptom onset, myoglobin and CK-MB subforms are the cardiac markers most appropriate for early diagnosis of acute MI

7. Because there is no tissue death, there is no serum marker release in stable or unstable angina

ECG Changes

The sudden occlusion of a coronary artery by a thrombus may result in ischemia, injury, and/or necrosis of the area of the myocardium supplied by the affected artery. The area supplied by the obstructed artery goes through a characteristic sequence of events that has been identified as involving "zones" of ischemia, injury, and infarction. Each zone is associated with characteristic ECG changes (Figure 6-14).

Non–ST-Segment Elevation Myocardial Infarction

1. In the acute phase of a non–ST-segment elevation MI, the ST segment may be depressed in the leads facing the surface of the infarcted area

a. Non–ST-segment elevation MI can only be diagnosed if ST segment and T wave changes are accompanied by elevations of cardiac serum markers indicative of myocardial necrosis

b. Patients with non–ST-segment elevation acute MI are known to be at higher risk for death, reinfarction, and other morbidity than those with unstable angina

(1) Non–ST-elevation MIs tend to be smaller and have a better *short-term* prognosis than ST-elevation infarctions however, overall prognosis is similar to ST-elevation MIs

(2) Recurrence of the infarct is common in the days to weeks after the patient has been sent home; "completion" of the infarction

2. Recent data suggest the incidence of non–ST-segment elevation MI is increasing as the population of older patients with more advanced disease increases

ST-Segment Elevation Myocardial Infarction

1. Most patients with ST-segment elevation will develop Q-wave MI. Only a minority of patients with ischemic chest discomfort at rest who do *not* have ST-segment elevation will develop Q-wave MI

a. Q-wave MI is diagnosed by the development of abnormal Q waves in serial ECGs. These infarctions tend to be larger than non–Q-wave MIs, reflecting more damage to the left ventricle, and are associated with a more prolonged and complete coronary thrombosis

b. With the exception of leads III and aVR, an abnormal (pathologic) Q-wave is more than 0.04 sec in duration and more than 25% of the amplitude of the following R wave in that lead

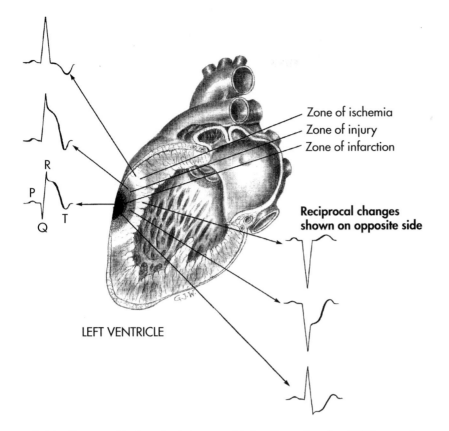

Zone of ischemia
Zone of injury
Zone of infarction

**Reciprocal changes
shown on opposite side**

LEFT VENTRICLE

Figure 6-14   Zones of ischemia, injury, and infarction, showing ECG waveforms and reciprocal waveforms corresponding to each zone.

    (1) An abnormal Q wave indicates presence of dead myocardial tissue and, subsequently, a loss of electrical activity

    (2) Abnormal Q waves can appear within hours after occlusion of a coronary artery but more commonly appear several hours or days after the onset of signs and symptoms of an acute MI

    (3) Q waves do not reflect when an MI occurred, but, when combined with ST segment or T wave changes, their presence suggests a recent (acute) MI

2. Because a pathologic Q wave may take hours to develop to confirm the presence of MI, the patient's signs and symptoms, laboratory tests, and the presence of ST-segment elevation provides the strongest evidence for the early recognition of MI

QUICK REVIEW

1. ST-segment elevation is considered significant when the ST segment is _____ the baseline at a point 0.04 sec (one small box) to the right of the J point.
2. How is death of myocardial tissue manifested on the ECG?

3. With the exception of leads III and aVR, an abnormal (pathologic) Q wave is more than _____ sec in duration and more than _____ % of the amplitude of the following R wave in that lead.

1. ≥ 1 mm above.   2. Abnormal (pathologic) Q waves.   3. 0.04 sec, 25%.

GOALS IN THE IMMEDIATE MANAGEMENT OF ACUTE CORONARY SYNDROMES (ACS)

1. Minimize infarct size
2. Salvage ischemic myocardium
3. Alleviate vasoconstriction
4. Reduce myocardial oxygen demand
5. Prevent and manage complications
6. Improve chances of survival

Prehospital Issues

1. Recommendations for every community[16]
   a. Availability of 9-1-1 access (Class I)
   b. Access to an EMS sytem in which all response units are equipped with defibrillators (Class I)
   c. Access to an EMS system staffed by persons trained to provide ACLS interventions in a timely manner, including intubation and IV medications (Class I)
   d. Prehospital 12-lead ECG (Class I for urban/suburban)
   e. Access to first-responder defibrillation program in a tiered response system (Class IIa)
   f. Availability of EMS able to triage patients with ischemic-type chest discomfort and assess the need to rapidly alert receiving hospital of probable acute coronary syndrome patients (Class IIa)
2. Prehospital fibrinolytic therapy recommended when (Class IIa):
   a. A physician is present in the ambulance/practice site/home
   b. **Or** prehospital transport time is ≥60 minutes
3. Health care providers should educate patients/families about signs and symptoms of acute MI, accessing EMS, and medications
   a. Patients should be taught that not all acute MIs are accompanied by sudden, crushing chest pain and unresponsiveness—symptoms may begin gradually or may be intermittent
   b. Patients who have had a previous MI should be taught that the signs and symptoms of a second MI might differ from those of the first

INITIAL RECOGNITION AND MANAGEMENT OF ACS IN THE FIELD AND EMERGENCY DEPARTMENT

Initial Assessment (Table 6-3)

1. Emergency departments should have an acute MI protocol that yields a targeted clinical examination and a 12-lead ECG within 10 minutes and a door-to-drug time that is less than 30 minutes[17] (Class I)
2. **Immediate** management of all acute coronary syndromes is generally the same
3. Obtain a brief, targeted history/physical examination
   a. Determine age, gender, signs and symptoms (including location of pain, duration, quality, relation to effort, and time of symptom onset), history of CAD, CAD risk factors present? History of Viagra use? (last questions should be asked of men *and* women)
   b. Consider possibility of other potentially lethal conditions that mimic acute MI ("When is an MI not an MI?")—aortic dissection, acute pericarditis, acute myocarditis, pulmonary embolism
4. Definitions[7]
   a. *Possible* acute coronary syndrome
      (1) Recent episode of chest discomfort at rest not entirely typical of ischemia but pain free at time of initial evaluation
      (2) Normal or unchanged ECG
      (3) No serum cardiac marker elevation
      (4) Managed by either observation in Emergency Department, chest pain unit or admitted to monitored hospital bed
   b. *Definite* acute coronary syndrome
      (1) Recent episode of typical ischemic discomfort that is either of new onset or severe or exhibits an accelerating pattern of previous stable angina (especially if it occurs at rest or within 2 weeks of previously documented MI)
      (2) Triage based on 12-lead ECG
5. If findings consistent with possible or definite acute coronary syndrome, perform the following interventions (including obtaining and reviewing 12-lead ECG), within 10 minutes of patient presentation
   a. Targeted history/physical exam, use checklist (yes-no), focus on eligibility for reperfusion therapy
   b. Assess vital signs, determine oxygen saturation
   c. Establish IV access, ECG monitoring
   d. Administer aspirin 162 to 325 mg (chewed) if no reason for exclusion
   e. Obtain baseline serum cardiac marker levels
   f. Obtain 12-lead ECG (physician to review)—categorize patient into one of three groups:
      (1) ST-segment elevation or new or presumably new LBBB
      (2) ST-segment depression/transient ST-segment/T wave changes
      (3) Normal or nondiagnostic ECG
   g. Perform serial ECGs in patients with Hx suggesting MI and nondiagnostic ECG
   h. Obtain lab specimens (CBC, lipid profile, electrolytes)
   i. Obtain portable chest x-ray film, preferably upright (<30 minutes)

Time of symptom onset is defined as the beginning of continuous, persistent discomfort that prompted the patient to seek medical attention.

Table 6-3 Initial Assessment and General Treatment of the Patient with an Acute Coronary Syndrome

PREHOSPITAL	EMERGENCY DEPARTMENT

Initial Assessment (Goal: Targeted Clinical Exam and 12-Lead ECG Within 10 Minutes)

PREHOSPITAL

- Obtain a brief, targeted history/physical exam (determine age, gender; signs/symptoms, pain presentation, including location of pain, duration, quality, relation to effort, time of symptom onset, Hx CAD, CAD risk factors present?) Hx of Viagra use?
- Assess vital signs, determine oxygen saturation

If previous consistent with possible or definite ACS:

- Use checklist (yes-no), focus on eligibility for reperfusion therapy, evaluate contraindications to aspirin and heparin
- Establish IV access, ECG monitoring
- Administer aspirin 162 to 325 mg (chewed) if no reason for exclusion
- Obtain 12-lead ECG (machine interpretation or transmission of ECG to physician)
- Draw blood for initial serum cardiac marker levels (to lab on arrival in Emergency Department)

Consider triage to facility capable of angiography and revascularization if any of the following are present:

- Signs of shock
- Pulmonary edema (rales > halfway up)
- Heart rate ≥100 beats/min and SBP ≤100 mm Hg

EMERGENCY DEPARTMENT

RN triage for rapid care
- Targeted history: determine age, gender, signs/symptoms, pain presentation, including location of pain, duration, quality, relation to effort, time of symptom onset; Hx CAD, CAD risk factors present? Hx of Viagra use?
- Assess vital signs, determine oxygen saturation
- Establish IV access, ECG monitoring
- Obtain 12-lead ECG (present to physician for review)

Physician evaluation
If previous consistent with possible or definite ACS:

- Obtain brief, targeted history/physical exam
- Evaluate eligibility for reperfusion therapy + contra-indications to aspirin and heparin
- Administer aspirin 162 to 325 mg (chewed) if no reason for exclusion
- Administer nitroglycerin as indicated
- Evaluate 12-lead ECG: Categorize patient into one of three groups: ST-elevation or new or presumably new LBBB, ST-depression/transient ST-segment/T wave changes, normal or nondiagnostic ECG
- Obtain serial ECGs in patients with Hx suggesting MI and nondiagnostic ECG
- Obtain baseline serum cardiac marker levels (CK-MB, Troponin T or I, myoglobin)
- Obtain lab specimens (CBC, lipid profile, electrolytes, coagulation studies)
- Obtain portable chest x-ray film
- Evaluate results

Routine Measures

- Oxygen 4 L/min by nasal cannula
- Aspirin-162-325 mg (non-enteric); if the patient is not already receiving aspirin, have him/her chew the first dose to rapidly establish a high blood level. Subsequent doses may be swallowed.
- Nitroglycerin SL or spray. May repeat at 5-minute intervals (max 3 doses). (Ensure IV access, SBP >90 mm Hg, HR >50 beats/min, no RV infarction)
- Morphine 2 to 4 mg IV if pain not relieved with NTG; may repeat every 5 minutes (ensure SBP >90 mm Hg)

Routine Measures: Oxygen, Aspirin, Nitroglycerin, Morphine (MONA)[17]

Studies suggest that oxygen administration may limit ischemic myocardial injury[18] and reduce ST-segment elevation in patients with MI.[19]

1. Oxygen
   a. Give at 4 L/min
   b. Overt pulmonary congestion, arterial oxygen desaturation (SaO_2 <90%) (Class I)
   c. Routine administration to all patients with uncomplicated MI during the first 2 to 3 hours (Class IIa)

2. Aspirin
   a. Initial dose of 162-325 mg of a non-enteric formulation followed by 75-160 mg/day of an enteric or non-enteric formulation. In patients who present with suspected ACS who are not already receiving aspirin, the first dose may be chewed to rapidly establish a high blood level. Sub-sequent doses may be swallowed. May administer via rectal suppository (325 mg) if nausea, vomiting, upper GI disorder present
   b. Other antiplatelet agents such as ticlopidine, or clopidogrel may be substituted if true aspirin allergy is present or if patient is unresponsive to aspirin
3. Nitroglycerin
   a. Pain relief is a priority
      (1) Benefits: Decreases anxiety and pain, may decrease BP and heart rate, decreases myocardial oxygen demand, decreases risk of dysrhythmias
      (2) Possible complications: hypotension
   b. Therapy
      (1) Nitroglycerin SL or spray
          (a) Ensure IV access, systolic BP >90 mm Hg
          (b) Avoid nitroglycerin administration in the presence of marked bradycardia (<50 beats/min)[20] and in patients with suspected right ventricular infarction. "Patients with right ventricular infarction are especially dependent on adequate right ventricular preload to maintain cardiac output and can experience profound hypotension during administration of nitrates."[17,21]
          (c) Avoid nitroglycerin administration if patient has used Viagra within past 24 hours
          (d) Avoid long-acting oral nitrate preparations in the early management of acute MI
      (2) Morphine 2 to 4 mg IV (if discomfort is not relieved with nitroglycerin)—may repeat every 5 minutes (ensure SBP >90 mm Hg) titrated to pain relief
          (a) Respiratory depression secondary to morphine administration is unusual with acute MI;[6] however, if it occurs it can be treated with IV naloxone or nalmefene

---

MONA

MONA is an acronym that may be used to recall medications used in the management of acute coronary syndromes (although not in the order they are administered).

M = morphine

O = oxygen

N = nitroglycerin

A = aspirin

MANAGEMENT OF ST-SEGMENT ELEVATION MI (Table 6-4)

ST-segment elevation on the ECG has a specificity of 91% and a sensitivity of 46% for diagnosing acute MI.[17]

1. Patient presents with signs and/or symptoms consistent with an acute coronary syndrome
2. 12-lead ECG reveals:
   a. ST-segment elevation in two contiguous leads: ≥1 mm in limb leads OR ≥2 mm in precordial leads
   b. **Or** new, or presumably new, LBBB
3. Confirm diagnosis by signs/symptoms, ECG, serum cardiac markers
4. Evaluate candidacy for reperfusion therapy
   a. Goals
      (1) Door-to-drug time <30 minutes[6]
      (2) Door-to-balloon inflation time 90 minutes ± 30 minutes
5. Patients with ST-segment elevation MI should receive[17,22]:
   a. Aspirin (antiplatelet therapy) 162 to 325 mg (chewed) if not already administered (and no contraindications)
   b. Anti-ischemia therapy
      (1) Beta-blockers (in the absence of contraindications)
      (2) Nitroglycerin IV if ongoing ischemia or uncorrected hypertension
         (a) Recommended for the first 24 to 48 hours in patients with acute MI and CHF, large anterior infarction, persistent ischemia, or hypertension (Class I)
         (b) Not recommended/may be harmful in patients with systolic pressure <90 mm Hg or severe bradycardia (<50 bpm) (Class III)
   c. Heparin (antithrombin therapy) if using fibrin-specific lytics
   d. ACE inhibitors (after 6 hours or when stable)—especially with large or anterior MI, heart failure without hypotension (SBP >100 mm Hg), previous MI
6. Patients at high risk for mortality or severe left ventricular (LV) dysfunction with signs of shock, pulmonary congestion, heart rate >100 beats/min,

Table 6-4 Management of ST-Segment Elevation Myocardial Infarction[17,22]

ST-segment elevation in two contiguous leads: ≥1 mm in limb leads OR ≥2 mm in precordial leads

↓

Confirm diagnosis by signs/symptoms, ECG, serum cardiac markers

All patients with ST-segment elevation MI should receive (if no contraindications):

- Antiplatelet therapy—aspirin 162 to 325 mg (chewed)
- Anti-ischemia therapy (beta-blockers, nitroglycerin IV if ongoing ischemia or uncorrected hypertension)
- Antithrombin therapy—heparin (if using fibrin-specific lytics)
- ACE inhibitors (after 6 hours or when stable)—especially with large or anterior MI, heart failure without hypotension (SBP >100 mm Hg), previous MI

Symptom onset ≤12 hours?				Symptom onset >12 hours?	
Patient Eligible for Reperfusion? Goals • Fibrinolytics: Door-to-drug time <30 min • Primary PCI: Door-to-dilation time 90 ± 30 min				Persistent Symptoms ↓	Resolution of Symptoms ↓
Yes ↓		No ↓		Consider reperfusion	Medical management
Signs of cardiogenic shock or contraindications to fibrinolytics?		Persistent or stuttering symptoms or ECG changes?		Medical management	
Yes ↓	No ↓	Yes ↓	No ↓		
PCI medical management	Can cath lab be mobilized within 60 min?	Cardiac cath, medical management	Medical management		
	Yes ↓	No ↓				
	PCI	Fibrinolysis (alteplase, reteplase, streptokinase, anistreplase, or tenecteplase)			

Note: *PCI* = percutaneous coronary intervention (angioplasty ± stent).
[17,22]See chapter references.

and SBP <100 mm Hg should be triaged to facility capable of angiography and rapid revascularization (e.g., PCI, CABG)

7. Determine best reperfusion strategy
   a. Fibrinolytic therapy is considered a Class I intervention for patients who have ST-segment elevation in two or more anatomically contiguous leads (or bundle branch block [obscuring ST-segment analysis] and a history suggesting acute MI), time to therapy is ≤12 hours, and who are <75 years of age[17]
   b. Goals of fibrinolytic therapy: Restoration of blood flow through the infarct-related artery resulting in:
      (1) Improved myocardial oxygenation
      (2) Decreased myocardial ischemia

(3) Improved left ventricular function and cardiac output
(4) Improved arterial perfusion
(5) Decreased incidence of dysrhythmias
(6) Reduced mortality

QUICK REVIEW

1. Fibrinolytic therapy is considered a Class I intervention for patients who have ST-segment _____ in two or more anatomically contiguous leads (or bundle-branch block [obscuring ST-segment analysis] and a history suggesting acute MI), time to therapy is _____ hours, and who are _____ years of age
2. Name three goals of fibrinolytic therapy in acute MI.

3. In the absence of contraindications, patients with ST-segment elevation MI should receive anti-ischemic therapy. Name two medications that may be used for this purpose.

1. Elevation, ≤12 hours, <75. 2. Restoration of blood flow through the infarct-related artery, resulting in improved myocardial oxygenation, decreased myocardial ischemia, improved left ventricular function and cardiac output, improved arterial perfusion, decreased incidence of dysrhythmias, reduced mortality. 3. Beta-blockers, nitroglycerin.

---

c. Fibrinolytic therapy: considerations
  (1) Monitor ECG and BP closely
    (a) Observe for reperfusion dysrhythmias as blood flow is reestablished through the infarct-related artery
    (b) Reocclusion may occur—watch for ST-segment changes and dysrhythmias, hypotension, chest discomfort
  (2) Monitor coagulation studies
  (3) Monitor for neurologic changes
d. Primary (direct) percutaneous coronary intervention (PCI)
  (1) Primary or direct PCI involves angioplasty and possible stent placement
  (2) Indications[17]
    (a) Patients within 36 hours of an acute ST-elevation/or new LBBB MI who develop cardiogenic shock, are <75 years of age, and on whom the procedure can be performed within 18 hours of onset of shock (Class I)
    (b) Alternative to fibrinolytic therapy in patients with ST-segment elevation or new or presumed new LBBB MI if performed within 12 hours of symptom onset (Class I)
    (c) As a reperfusion strategy in candidates for reperfusion who have a contraindication to fibrinolytic therapy (Class IIa)
  (3) Optimum results achieved with PCI when:
    (a) Performed in a timely fashion (balloon inflation within 90 [±30] minutes of admission)
    (b) Performed by persons skilled in the procedure (persons who perform more than 75 percutaneous transluminal coronary angioplasty [PTCA] procedures/year)
    (c) Supported by experienced personnel in an appropriate laboratory environment (centers that perform more than 200 PTCA procedures/year and have cardiac surgical capability)

The major risk of fibrinolytic therapy is intracranial hemorrhage, which usually occurs in the first 24 hours after starting therapy.[23]

Intravenous Thrombolysis in Acute Myocardial Infarction

1. *Fibrinolytic Therapy*
1.1. We recommend that all patients with acute MI who receive fibrinolytic therapy receive aspirin (165 to 325 mg) on arrival to the hospital and daily thereafter (grade 1A).
1.2. We recommend that patients with ischemic symptoms characteristic of acute MI for ≤12 hours who have ST-segment elevation or left bundle branch block on the ECG receive IV fibrinolytic therapy unless they have contraindications (grade 1A).
1.3. For patients with symptoms characteristic of acute MI and duration of 12 to 24 hours who have ST-segment elevation or left bundle branch block on the ECG, we recommend that IV fibrinolytic therapy should be considered (grade 2B).
1.4. We recommend that in patients with prior intracranial hemorrhage, any stroke within the past year, or active bleeding, clinicians do not administer IV fibrinolytic therapy (grade 1B).
1.5. We recommend that all patients with acute MI who are candidates for fibrinolytic therapy receive it within 30 minutes after arrival to the hospital (grade 1A). For patients with symptom duration ≤12 hours, we recommend administration of one of the fibrinolytic agents: streptokinase, anistreplase, or alteplase (all grade 1A in comparison to placebo).
    Remark: r-PA (r-PA = reteplase) is equivalent to streptokinase.
1.6. For patients with symptom duration 6 h, we recommend the administration of alteplase over streptokinase (grade 1A).
    Remark: TNK-tPA (TNK-tPA = tenecteplase) is equivalent to alteplase.
1.7. We recommend that patients with known allergy or sensitivity to streptokinase receive alteplase, TNK-tPA, or r-PA (grade 1C+).

2. *Adjunctive Treatment with Thrombin Inhibitors*
2.1. Heparin
2.1.1. For patients receiving streptokinase, we recommend administration of subcutaneous unfractionated heparin (12,500 U q12hr for 48 hr) (grade 2A).
2.1.2. For patients given streptokinase or anistreplase, we recommend administration of IV unfractionated heparin only if they are at high risk of systemic or venous thromboembolism (anterior MI, existing heart failure, previous embolus, atrial fibrillation, or left ventricular thrombus) (grade 1C).
    Remark: Heparin should be given not earlier than 4 hours after therapy and when the activated partial thromboplastin time (APTT) is <70 seconds. The target APTT should be 50 to 70 seconds, and the infusion should continue for ≥48 hours.
2.1.3. For patients receiving alteplase, r-PA, or TNK-tPA, we recommend administration of IV unfractionated heparin for 48 hours (grade 1B).
2.1.4. For patients receiving IV heparin with alteplase, r-PA, or TNK-tPA, we recommend administration of either standard-dose unfractionated heparin (5000-U bolus followed by 1000 U/hr) (grade 2A) or weight-adjusted dosing (60-U/kg bolus [4000 U maximum] followed by 12 U/kg/hr [1000 U/hr maximum]) (grade 2C), both adjusted to maintain an APTT of 50 to 70 seconds.

2.2. *Direct Thrombin Inhibitors*
2.2.1. For patients with known or suspected heparin-induced thrombocytopenia or thrombosis who are receiving fibrinolytic therapy (either alteplase or streptokinase), we recommend administration of IV hirudin (lepuridin 0.1-mg/kg bolus followed 0.15-mg/h infusion) (grade 2A).

*Recommendations from the American College of Chest Physicians.[23]

MANAGEMENT OF UNSTABLE ANGINA/ NON–ST-SEGMENT ELEVATION MI (Table 6-5)

1. Patient presentation consistent with an acute coronary syndrome
2. 12-lead ECG changes viewed in two or more anatomically contiguous leads:
   a. ST-segment depression >1 mm **or** T wave inversion >1 mm **or**
   b. Transient (<30 min) ST-segment/T wave changes >1 mm with discomfort
3. Confirm diagnosis of possible non–ST-elevation MI or unstable angina by signs/symptoms, ECG, serum cardiac markers
4. Subgroup of patients at high-risk of adverse outcomes
   a. Persistent ("stuttering") symptoms/recurrent ischemia
   b. Left ventricular (LV) dysfunction, CHF
   c. Widespread ECG changes
   d. Previous MI
   e. Positive troponin or CK-MB
5. General management guidelines
   a. Patients with unstable angina/non–ST-segment elevation MI (*and no contraindications*) should receive[6,7,22]:
      (1) Oxygen, IV access, continuous ECG monitoring
      (2) Antiplatelet therapy—aspirin 162 to 325 mg (chewed) if not already administered
      (3) Antithrombin therapy—IV heparin
      (4) Anti-ischemic therapy
         (a) Beta-blockers (e.g., metoprolol, atenolol, esmolol, or propranolol) if patient not previously on beta-blockers or inadequately treated on current dose of beta-blocker (if no contraindications)
         (b) Nitroglycerin sublingual tablet or spray, followed by IV nitroglycerin if symptoms persist despite sublingual nitroglycerin therapy and initiation of beta-blocker therapy (and SBP >90 mm Hg)
         (c) Morphine 2 to 4 mg IV (if discomfort is not relieved or symptoms recur despite anti-ischemic therapy); may repeat every 5 min (ensure SBP >90 mm Hg)
   b. Calcium channel blocker: consider if symptoms persist despite adequate doses of beta-blockers or contraindications to beta-blocker administration exist
6. If patient meets high-risk criteria, give:
   a. Aspirin + glycoprotein IIb/IIIa inhibitors + IV heparin **or** aspirin + glycoprotein IIb/IIIa inhibitors + SC low-molecular-weight heparin
   b. Beta-blockers (e.g., metoprolol, atenolol, esmolol, or propranolol): If patient not previously on beta-blockers or inadequately treated on current dose of beta-blocker (if no contraindications)
   c. IV nitroglycerin for recurrent angina: If symptoms persist despite sublingual nitroglycerin therapy and initiation of beta-blocker therapy (and SBP >90 mm Hg)
   d. Calcium channel blockers: If symptoms persist despite adequate doses of nitrates and beta-blockers or patient cannot tolerate nitrate or beta-blocker therapy (avoid in pulmonary edema, evidence of LV dysfunction)

7. Assess patient's clinical status
   a. If clinically stable, continue in-hospital observation; consider stress testing
   b. If high-risk patient: Perform cardiac cath
      (1) If anatomy suitable for revascularization—PCI, CABG
      (2) If anatomy unsuitable—medical management

Table 6-5 Management of Unstable Angina/Non–ST-Segment Elevation Myocardial Infarction[6,7,22]

ECG Changes in 2 or More Anatomically Contiguous Leads:

ST-segment depression >1 mm **or** T wave inversion >1 mm **or**

Transient (<30 min) ST-segment/T wave changes >1 mm with discomfort

▼

Confirm diagnosis by signs/symptoms, ECG, serum cardiac markers

▼

All patients with unstable angina/non–ST-segment elevation MI should receive (if no contraindications)
- Aspirin 162 to 325 mg (chewed) if not already administered (and no contraindications) (antiplatelet therapy)
- Heparin IV (antithrombin therapy)

▼

If high-risk patient, give:
- Aspirin + glycoprotein IIb/IIIa inhibitors (i.e., Integrilin, Aggrastat, ReoPro) + IV heparin **or**
- Aspirin + glycoprotein IIb/IIIa inhibitors + SC low-molecular-weight heparin (i.e., enoxaparin [Lovenox], dalteparin [Fragmin])

High-Risk Criteria

- Persistent ("stuttering") symptoms/recurrent ischemia; left ventricular (LV) dysfunction, CHF; widespread ECG changes; prior MI, positive troponin or CK-MB

▼

Anti-ischemic therapy:
- Beta-blockers—(e.g., metoprolol, atenolol, esmolol, or propranolol)—if patient not previously on beta-blockers or inadequately treated on current dose of beta-blocker (if no contraindications)
- Nitroglycerin sublingual tablet or spray, followed by intravenous nitroglycerin if symptoms persist despite sublingual nitroglycerin therapy and initiation of beta-blocker therapy (and SBP >90 mm Hg)
- Morphine 2 to 4 mg IV (if discomfort is not relieved or symptoms recur despite anti-ischemic therapy)—may repeat every 5 min (ensure SBP >90 mm Hg)

▼

Assess clinical status: Is patient clinically stable?

Yes	No
• Continue in-hospital observation • Consider stress testing	Cardiac cath • If anatomy suitable for revascularization—PCI, CABG • If anatomy unsuitable—medical management

[6,7,22]See chapter references.

MANAGEMENT OF SUSPECTED ACS AND NONDIAGNOSTIC/NORMAL ECG (Table 6-6)

It is important to note that the ECG is nondiagnostic in approximately 50% of patients with chest discomfort indicative of an acute coronary syndrome (ACS) (Figure 6-15). A normal ECG does not rule out an acute MI, particularly in the early hours of a coronary artery occlusion.

1. Nondiagnostic or normal ECG
   a. ST-segment depression 0.5 to 1.0 mm
   b. T wave inversion or flattening in leads with dominant R waves
   c. Normal ECG
2. Nondiagnostic ECGs are more common in the elderly and patients with previous MI
3. Currently available data do not support routine use of fibrinolytic therapy as a form of reperfusion in patients with ischemic-type chest discomfort and nondiagnostic ECGs
4. General management guidelines
   a. Administer aspirin + other therapy as appropriate (e.g., beta-blockers, nitroglycerin)
   b. Obtain complete history and physical exam
   c. Obtain follow-up serum cardiac marker levels, serial ECG monitoring
   d. Continue evaluation and treatment in Emergency Department, chest pain unit or monitored bed
   e. Consider radionuclide, echocardiography

Table 6-6   Patients with a Suspected Acute Coronary Syndrome and Nondiagnostic/Normal ECG

Nondiagnostic or Normal ECG

▼

Evaluate signs/symptoms, serial ECGs, serum cardiac markers

▼

Aspirin + other therapy as appropriate

▼

- Assess patient's clinical risk of death/nonfatal MI
- History and physical exam
- Obtain follow-up serum cardiac marker levels, serial ECG monitoring
- Continue evaluation and treatment in Emergency Department chest pain unit or monitored bed
- Consider radionuclide, echocardiography

COMPLICATIONS OF MYOCARDIAL INFARCTION

Complications Associated with MI
1. Dysrhythmias (most common)
2. Congestive heart failure, pulmonary edema
3. Cardiogenic shock
4. Systemic or pulmonary thromboembolism
5. Papillary muscle rupture, mitral insufficiency
6. Dressler's syndrome (pericarditis occurring 2 to 4 weeks after MI)
7. Ventricular aneurysm/rupture
8. Ventricular septal defect

Cardiac dysrhythmias are the primary *electrical* complication of acute MI. The primary *mechanical* complications of acute MI are CHF and shock.[24]

Dysrhythmias Associated with Ischemia, Injury, and Infarction

Dysrhythmias are the most common complication in the first few hours following MI.

Atrial fibrillation

1. Atrial fibrillation occurs in approximately 15% of patients with acute MI, most often occurs within the first 24 hours, is usually transient (but may recur), and more commonly occurs in patients with left ventricular failure, large anterior MIs or with AV block, and in the elderly[10]
   a. May also occur in patients with inferior MI
2. If atrial fibrillation with a rapid ventricular rate results in hemodynamic compromise, immediate synchronized cardioversion is warranted with 100 joules (J), 200 J, 300 J, and then 360 J (or equivalent biphasic energy), if the rhythm fails to convert with lower energies
3. In stable patients, medications that may be used to slow the ventricular rate include:
   a. Beta-blockers (in the absence of severe CHF, asthma, or other contraindications)
      (1) Diltiazem may be used if beta-blockers are contraindicated
      (2) Because of their negative effects on myocardial contractility, calcium channel blockers are not recommended as first-line medications in acute MI

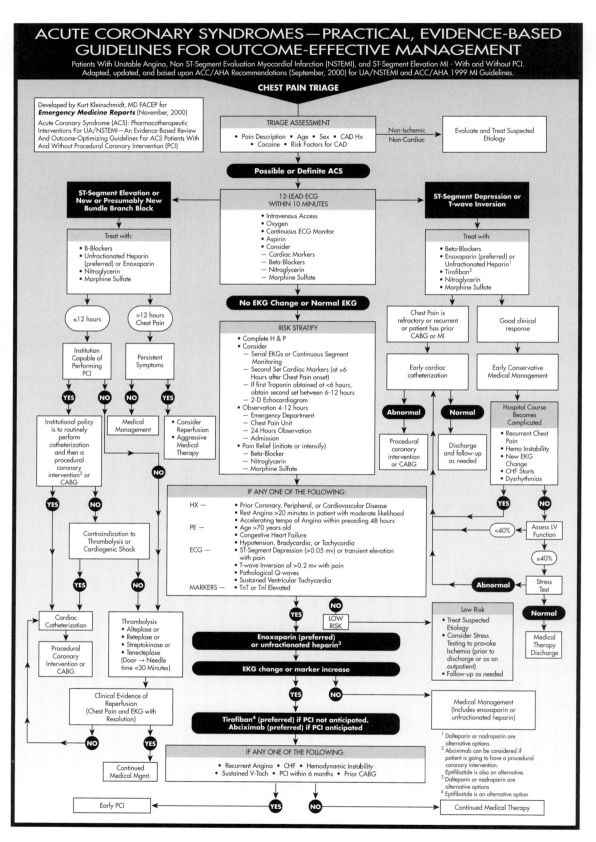

Figure 6-15 Management of acute coronary syndromes (ACS).

    b. Digitalis may be effective, but toxicity poses a concern in the setting of acute ischemia

Ventricular dysrhythmias

1. "Warning" dysrhythmias
    a. For many years, PVCs observed in patients experiencing an acute MI were thought to be "warning" dysrhythmias of impending ventricular fibrillation (VF), particularly multiform PVCs, R-on-T PVCs, couplets, frequent (>6/min) PVCs
        (1) Research has shown that half the patients who have warning dysrhythmias do not develop VF and the majority of patients (80%) who do develop VF have not had previous warning dysrhythmias[25]
        (2) It is considered prudent clinical practice to observe these premature beats (including bigeminy, R-on-T PVCs, multiform PVCs, etc.) closely and consider the reason for their occurrence (e.g., hypoxemia, acid-base disturbance, electrolyte imbalance, heart failure)
        (3) PVCs may accompany sinus tachycardia early in the course of MI, possibly because of increased sympathetic stimulation. Management with beta-blockers decreases mortality, decreases the incidence of VF, and decreases the incidence of sudden death associated with acute MI[25] when administered to patients without contraindications
2. Pulseless ventricular tachycardia (VT)/ventricular fibrillation (VF)
    a. Treat with unsynchronized shocks beginning with 200 J (or equivalent biphasic energy). If unsuccessful, deliver a second shock using 200 to 300 J, and a third shock with 360 J (or equivalent biphasic energy), if necessary
    b. Correct any electrolyte and acid-base disturbances
    c. If a maintenance infusion of an antiarrhythmic is initiated, current recommendations are to continue the infusion for no more than 24 hours and then discontinue it to assess the patient's ongoing need for antiarrhythmic treatment
3. Accelerated idioventricular rhythm (AIVR)
    a. Sometimes called "slow" VT
    b. Occurs frequently during the first 12 to 48 hours of acute MI
    c. May be a reperfusion dysrhythmia
    d. Does not indicate an increased risk of VF
    e. Best managed by observation
4. Ventricular tachycardia (VT)
    a. Most instances of post-MI VT and VF occur within the first 48 hours of MI
    b. If pulseless, treat as VF with unsynchronized shocks beginning with 200 J (or equivalent biphasic energy)
    c. If sustained monomorphic VT with a rate >150 beats/min and associated with signs of hemodynamic compromise, urgent electrical therapy is indicated beginning with 100 J (or equivalent biphasic energy)
    d. Sustained polymorphic VT should be treated as VF; begin electrical therapy with 200 J (or equivalent biphasic energy)

Bradydysrhythmias

Serious signs and symptoms are generally considered to be a heart rate <50 beats/min associated with hypotension, ischemia, or frequent PVCs

1. Sinus bradycardia
   a. Occurs frequently (30% to 40%) in MI, particularly with inferior and posterior infarction[17]
   b. Treatment with atropine is recommended only if serious signs and symptoms are associated with the decreased rate
2. First-degree AV block
   a. Treatment with atropine usually not required
3. Second-degree AV block, type I (Wenckebach, Mobitz I)
   a. Atropine may occasionally be warranted, generally with a heart rate <50 beats/min or hypotension
      (1) When serious rate-related signs and symptoms occur, atropine is administered IV 0.5 to 1.0 mg every 3 to 5 minutes up to a total dose of 0.03 to 0.04 mg/kg
4. Second-degree AV block, type II—avoid atropine, which may increase sinus rate and worsen the block or precipitate third-degree AV block
5. Complete AV block
   a. Narrow-QRS (junctional escape rhythm)—atropine may be helpful because it may improve AV conduction or accelerate the escape rhythm[17]
   b. Wide-QRS (ventricular escape rhythm)—do **NOT** use atropine
      (1) "Do not use atropine for third-degree AV block with a new wide-QRS complex presumed to be due to AMI (acute MI). Administration of lidocaine to these patients may also have the effect of suppressing a slow escape rhythm and in this setting may result in ventricular standstill."[26]
6. Indications for transcutaneous pacing[17]
   a. Sinus bradycardia (rate <50 bpm) with symptoms of hypotension (SBP <80 mm Hg) unresponsive to drug therapy
   b. Second-degree AV block, type II
   c. Third-degree (complete) AV block
   d. Bilateral bundle branch block (alternating BBB, or RBBB and alternating left anterior fascicular block [LAFB], left posterior fascicular block [LPFB]) (irrespective of time of onset)
   e. Newly acquired or age indeterminate LBBB, alternating LBBB and LAFB, alternating RBBB and LPFB
   f. RBBB or LBBB and first-degree AV block

QUICK REVIEW

1. Electrical therapy for sustained polymorphic VT should begin with _____ joules (J).
2. True or False. An accelerated idioventricular rhythm (AIVR) is best managed with lidocaine or amiodarone.
3. True or False. Calcium channel blockers are recommended as first-line medications to slow the ventricular rate of atrial fibrillation in acute MI.
4. True or False. Lidocaine should be avoided in the management of third-degree AV block with new wide-QRS complexes.

1. 200. 2. False. 3. False. 4. True.

Mechanical Complications ("Pump Problems")

1. Pump failure
   a. Caused by acute MI, which may result in decreased cardiac output and may produce signs and symptoms of tissue hypoperfusion or pulmonary congestion
   b. May be primary or secondary
      (1) Causes of primary pump problems: MI, drug overdose/poisoning
      (2) Causes of secondary pump problems: As oxygen, glucose, and ATP (adenosine triphosphate) are depleted, essentially all patients in shock will eventually develop a secondary pump problem
   c. Signs and symptoms of hypoperfusion: hypotension, weak pulse, weakness, skin findings (pallor, sweating), fatigue
   d. Signs and symptoms of pulmonary congestion: tachypnea, labored respirations, jugular venous distention, frothy sputum, cyanosis, dyspnea
   e. Patients in pump failure may require:
      (1) Treatment of a coexisting rate or volume problem
      (2) Correction of underlying problems (hypoglycemia, hypoxia, drug overdose, poisoning)
      (3) Support for failing pump
         (a) Agents to increase contractility (dopamine, dobutamine, etc.)
         (b) Vasodilators to decrease afterload
         (c) Vasodilators, diuretics to decrease preload
         (d) Mechanical assistance (intra-aortic balloon pump)
         (e) Surgery (coronary artery bypass graft, valve, heart transplant)
2. Left ventricular dysfunction/congestive heart failure (CHF)
   a. **Cardiac output** is the amount of blood pumped into the aorta each minute by the heart
      (1) Defined as the stroke volume (amount of blood ejected from a ventricle with each heart beat) × the heart rate
      (2) Cardiac output may be affected by an increase or decrease in heart rate **or** stroke volume
      (3) Stroke volume is affected by preload, afterload, and contractility
         (a) **Preload** is the force exerted on the walls of the ventricles at the end of diastole. The volume of blood returning to the heart influences preload. More blood returning to the right atrium increases preload; less blood returning decreases preload. If the ventricle is stretched beyond its physiological limit, cardiac output may fall because of volume overload and overstretching of the muscle fibers
         (b) **Afterload** is the pressure or resistance against which the ventricles must pump to eject blood. Afterload is influenced by arterial blood pressure, arterial distensibility (ability to become stretched), and arterial resistance. The less the resistance (lower afterload), the more easily blood can be ejected. Increased afterload (increased resistance) results in increased cardiac workload
         (c) **Ejection fraction** is the percentage of total ventricular volume ejected during each myocardial contraction
            (i) Used as a measure of ventricular function

CHF can be defined based on symptom onset, the primary ventricle involved, and the overall cardiac output.

(ii) Normally, the heart empties (ejects) slightly more than half the blood that it contains with each beat thus, a normal ejection fraction is >50%

(iii) Impaired ventricular function = ejection fraction <40%

b. MI may result in left ventricular dysfunction/CHF

  (1) As the heart begins to fail, compensatory mechanisms attempt to maintain adequate perfusion pressure and enhance cardiac output by manipulating one or more of the following—heart rate, stroke volume, preload, contractility, and/or afterload

  (2) Compensatory mechanisms may, over time, worsen the degree of failure

  (a) Tachycardia increases myocardial oxygen demand, decreases time for coronary artery perfusion

  (b) Sodium and water retention leads to overdistention of ventricles and, ultimately, decrease in force of ventricular contraction

  (3) Left ventricular failure is manifested as pulmonary venous congestion and pulmonary edema

  (a) As the left ventricle fails, blood backs up into the pulmonary veins and capillaries. As the pulmonary capillaries become congested, fluid is pushed from the pulmonary capillaries across the alveolar wall into the alveoli, resulting in pulmonary edema.

  (b) Pulmonary edema inhibits gas exchange by impairing the diffusion pathway between the alveolus and capillary (Figure 6-16)

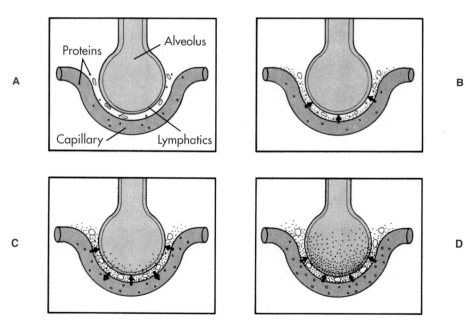

Figure 6-16 As pulmonary edema progresses, it inhibits the exchange of oxygen and carbon dioxide at the alveolar-capillary interface. **A,** Normal relationship. **B,** Increased pulmonary capillary hydrostatic pressure causes fluid to move from the vascular space into the pulmonary interstitial space. **C,** Lymphatic flow increases in an attempt to pull fluid back into the vascular or lymphatic space. **D,** Failure of lymphatic flow and worsening of left ventricular failure results in further movement of fluid into the interstitial space and the alveoli.

  (i) Results in excessive accumulation of fluid in the inter-
      stitial spaces and alveoli of the lungs
  (c) Hypotension develops as cardiac output decreases
  (d) Other signs of LV failure include anxiety, orthopnea, cough
      with frothy sputum, tachypnea, diaphoresis, dyspnea
(4) Right ventricular failure is manifested as systemic venous con-
    gestion and peripheral edema (Figure 6-17)
  (a) Other signs of RV failure include diaphoresis, tachycardia,
      dyspnea, jugular venous distention (Figure 6-18), fatigue,
      dependent edema, weakness, weight gain

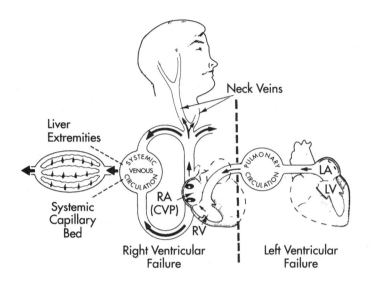

Figure 6-17   Right ventricular failure: pressure changes and effects.

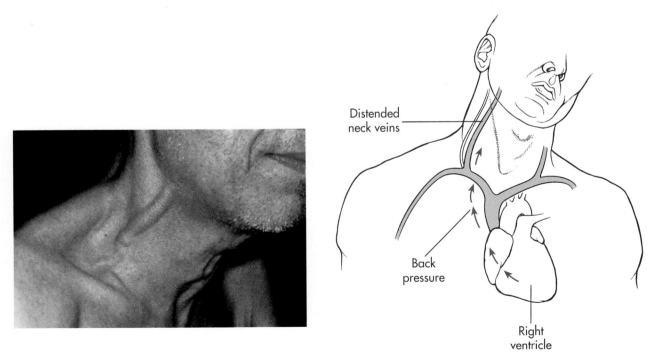

Figure 6-18   Neck vein distention because of right ventricular failure.

c. Management of acute pulmonary edema (Table 6-7)

(1) If feasible and BP permits, place patient in sitting position with feet dependent—increases lung volume and vital capacity, decreases work of respiration, decreases venous return to the heart

(2) Administer oxygen/intubate as needed (obtain arterial blood gas before oxygen administration if possible)

(3) Establish IV access

(4) If systolic BP >100 mm Hg:

Reduces preload and afterload.

(a) Administer sublingual nitroglycerin 1 tablet or spray every 5 minutes (max 3 doses) until IV nitroglycerin or nitroprusside can take effect[27]

Venodilation, then diuresis, mobilizes fluid from the lungs into the circulation.

(b) Administer furosemide 0.5 to 1.0 mg/kg (typically 20 to 40 mg IV). Furosemide causes venodilation. Administer *slowly* IV push. Can repeat in 30 minutes if symptoms persist and BP stable

Reduces preload and afterload, decreases anxiety/tachypnea

(c) Consider morphine IV 2 to 4 mg

Decreases preload, dilates coronary arteries, causing decreased myocardial ischemia.

(d) Consider additional preload/afterload reduction with nitroglycerin or nitroprusside IV, ACE inhibitors[17]

(i) Nitroglycerin—start at 5 mcg/min and increase gradually until mean systolic pressure falls by 10% to 15%; avoid hypotension (SBP <90 mm Hg)[17]

or

Decreases preload and afterload.

(ii) Nitroprusside IV (if SBP >100 mm Hg)—0.1 to 5 mcg/kg/min

(iii) ACE inhibitors—decreases afterload

(5) Evaluate early for:

(a) Readily reversible cause and institute appropriate intervention (e.g., cardiac dysrhythmias, tamponade)

(b) Myocardial ischemia/infarction (institute appropriate intervention—candidate for fibrinolytic therapy? PTCA?)

(6) If patient is refractory to previous therapies or is hypotensive or in cardiogenic shock[27]:

(a) Consider fluid or IV inotropic and/or vasopressor agents (e.g., dobutamine, dopamine, norepinephrine)

(b) Consider pulmonary and systemic arterial catheterization

(c) Obtain echocardiogram to assist in diagnosis, evaluation, and reparability of culprit lesion or condition

(d) Consider need for mechanical circulatory assistance (balloon pump)

Table 6-7 Management of Acute Pulmonary Edema

Perform Primary ABCD Survey (Basic Life Support)

(Correct critical problems IMMEDIATELY as they are identified)
Assess responsiveness, **A**irway, **B**reathing, **C**irculation,
ensure availability of monitor/**D**efibrillator

▼

Perform Secondary ABCD Survey (Advanced Life Support)

(Obtain arterial blood gas before oxygen administration if possible)
Administer oxygen, establish IV access, attach cardiac monitor (O_2, IV, monitor)
Assess vital signs, attach pulse oximeter, and monitor blood pressure
Obtain and review 12-lead ECG, portable chest x-ray film
Perform a focused history and physical exam

▼

If feasible and BP permits, place patient in sitting position with feet dependent
- Increases lung volume and vital capacity
- Decreases work of respiration
- Decreases venous return, decreases preload

If systolic BP >100 mm Hg:
- **Sublingual nitroglycerin:** 1 tablet or spray every 5 minutes (max 3 doses) until IV nitroglycerin or nitroprusside can take effect[27]
- **Furosemide IV:** 0.5 to 1.0 mg/kg (typically 20 to 40 mg), can repeat in 30 minutes if symptoms persist and BP stable
- **Consider morphine IV:** 2 to 4 mg

Consider additional preload/afterload reduction—nitroglycerin or nitroprusside IV, ACE inhibitors:
- **Nitroglycerin IV:** start at 5 mcg/min and increase gradually until mean systolic pressure falls by 10% to 15%, avoid hypotension (SBP <90 mm Hg)[17] **or**
- **Nitroprusside IV** (if SBP >100 mm Hg): 0.1 to 5 mcg/kg/min

Evaluate early for:
- Readily reversible cause (e.g., cardiac dysrhythmias, tamponade) and institute appropriate intervention
- Myocardial ischemia/infarction (institute appropriate intervention—candidate for fibrinolytic therapy? PTCA?)

If patient is refractory to previous therapies, or is hypotensive or in cardiogenic shock[27]:
- Consider fluid or IV inotropic and/or vasopressor agents (e.g., dobutamine, dopamine, norepinephrine)
- Consider pulmonary and systemic arterial catheterization
- Obtain echocardiogram to assist in diagnosis, evaluation, and reparability of culprit lesion or condition
- Consider need for mechanical circulatory assistance (balloon pump)

[17,27]See chapter references.

3. Cardiogenic shock
   a. Definition: Persistent hypotension (SBP <80 mm Hg) for more than 30 minutes in the absence of hypovolemia[28]
   b. Causes[28]
      (1) Myocardial infarction
         (a) Large left ventricular infarction (usually >40% of left ventricle) in 80% of shock patients
         (b) Right ventricular infarction in 10% of shock patients
      (2) Mechanical complications (e.g., ventricular septal defect, acute mitral regurgitation, cardiac tamponade) in 10% of shock patients
   c. Often associated with anuria/oliguria, acidosis, peripheral hypoperfusion, cerebral hypoxia
   d. High-risk patients with cardiogenic shock should be managed in cardiovascular facilities with interventional specialists

> For every patient with shock or hypotension, ask, "Is there a rate problem, a pump problem, a volume problem, or a vascular resistance problem?"

(1) Fibrinolytics have not been shown to consistently improve outcome
(2) Primary PCI is considered by some the treatment of choice

4. Management of hypotension/shock caused by a suspected pump problem (Table 6-8)
  a. Perform primary and secondary ABCD surveys
  b. If pulmonary edema absent, consider fluid challenge of 250- to 500-mL normal saline to ensure adequate ventricular filling pressure
  c. **Marked hypotension/cardiogenic shock**
    (1) Pharmacologic management:[17]
      (a) Administer norepinephrine infusion (0.5 to 30 mcg/min) until SBP 80 mm Hg
      (b) Then attempt to change to dopamine 5 to 15 mcg/kg/min until SBP 90 mm Hg
      (c) IV dobutamine (2 to 20 mcg/kg/min) can be given simultaneously in an attempt to reduce magnitude of dopamine infusion
    (2) Consider balloon pump or patient transfer to a cardiac interventional facility
  d. **Moderate hypotension** (SBP 70 to 90 mm Hg)[29]
    (1) Dopamine 5 to 15 mcg/kg/min until SBP 100 mm Hg
      (a) If BP remains low despite dopamine doses >20 mcg/kg/min, may substitute norepinephrine in doses of 0.5 to 30 mcg/min (norepinephrine has fewer chronotropic effects)
      (b) Once SBP ≥90 mm Hg with dopamine, add dobutamine 2 to 20 mcg/kg/min and attempt to taper off dopamine
  e. **SBP ≥90 mm Hg**[10,27]
    (1) Dobutamine 2 to 20 mcg/kg/min

Hypotension/cardiogenic shock has very high mortality; often a result of a pump **AND** volume problem.

Table 6-8 Management of Hypotension/Shock: Suspected Pump Problem

Perform Primary ABCD Survey (Basic Life Support)

(Correct critical problems IMMEDIATELY as they are identified)

Assess responsiveness, **A**irway, **B**reathing, **C**irculation,
ensure availability of monitor/**D**efibrillator

▼

Perform Secondary ABCD Survey (Advanced Life Support)

Administer oxygen, establish IV access, attach cardiac monitor,
administer fluids as needed (O_2, IV, monitor, fluids)

Assess vital signs, attach pulse oximeter, and monitor blood pressure

Obtain and review 12-lead ECG, portable chest x-ray film

Perform a focused history & physical exam

▼

Hypotension—suspected pump problem

If breath sounds are clear, consider fluid challenge of 250- to 500-mL NS to ensure adequate ventricular filling pressure before vasopressor administration

▼

Marked hypotension (systolic BP <70 mm Hg)/cardiogenic shock

Pharmacologic management[17]:
- Norepinephrine infusion (0.5 to 30 mcg/min) until SBP 80 mm Hg
- Then attempt to change to dopamine 5 to 15 mcg/kg/min until SBP 90 mm Hg
- IV dobutamine (2 to 20 mcg/kg/min) can be given simultaneously in an attempt to reduce magnitude of dopamine infusion

Consider balloon pump or patient transfer to a cardiac interventional facility

Moderate hypotension (systolic BP 70 to 90 mm Hg)[16]

- Dopamine 5 to 15 mcg/kg/min
- If BP remains low despite dopamine doses > 20 mcg/kg/min, may substitute norepinephrine in doses of 0.5 to 30 mcg/min
- Once SBP ≥90 with dopamine, add dobutamine 2 to 20 mcg/kg/min and attempt to taper off dopamine

Systolic BP ≥ 90 mm Hg[10,27]

- Dobutamine 2 to 20 mcg/kg/min

Medication Dosing

Norepinephrine IV	0.5 to 30 mcg/min
Dopamine IV	5 to 15 mcg/kg/min
Dobutamine IV	2 to 20 mcg/kg/min

[10,16,17,27]See chapter references.

5. Management of hypotension/shock caused by suspected volume (or vascular resistance) problem (Table 6-9)
   a. Consider possible causes of volume deficit
      (1) Absolute (actual fluid deficit): Hemorrhage, gastrointestinal loss (vomiting, diarrhea), renal losses (polyuria), insensible losses (perspiration), adrenal insufficiency (aldosterone), phlebotomy, reduced fluid intake because of pain, nausea/vomiting
      (2) Relative (vasodilation from any cause or redistribution of fluid to third spaces): Central nervous system injury, spinal injury, third-space loss, adrenal insufficiency (cortisol), sepsis, medications that alter vascular tone
   b. Management
      (1) Primary and Secondary ABCD surveys
      (2) Generally, first priority = fluid replacement

QUICK REVIEW

1. Define cardiogenic shock.

2. What is the preferred medication (and dose) in the management of a suspected pump problem with a SBP of 70 to 90 mm Hg?

3. True or False. Norepinephrine is the medication of choice in the management of marked hypotension not due to hypovolemia.

1. Persistent hypotension (SBP <80 mm Hg) for more than 30 minutes in the absence of hypovolemia. 2. Dopamine IV infusion at 5 to 15 mcg/kg/min. 3. True.

Table 6-9   Management of Hypotension/Shock: Suspected Volume Problem

Perform Primary ABCD Survey (Basic Life Support)
(Correct critical problems IMMEDIATELY as they are identified)
Assess responsiveness, **A**irway, **B**reathing, **C**irculation, ensure availability of monitor/**D**efibrillator

▼

Perform Secondary ABCD Survey (Advanced Life Support)
Administer oxygen, establish IV access, attach cardiac monitor, administer fluids as needed (O_2, IV, monitor, fluids)
Assess vital signs, attach pulse oximeter, and monitor blood pressure
Obtain and review 12-lead ECG, portable chest x-ray film
Perform a focused history and physical exam

▼

Hypotension: suspected volume (or vascular resistance) problem

▼

Volume replacement

- Fluid challenge (250- to 500-mL IV boluses: reassess)
- Blood transfusion (if appropriate)
- If cause known, institute appropriate intervention (e.g., septic shock, anaphylaxis)
- Consider vasopressors, if indicated, to improve vascular tone if no response to fluid challenge(s)

        (a) Fluid challenge (250- to 500-mL IV boluses: reassess)
        (b) Blood transfusion (if appropriate)
        (c) If cause known, institute appropriate intervention (e.g., septic shock, anaphylaxis)
        (d) Consider vasopressors, if indicated, to improve vascular tone if no response to fluid challenge(s)
   6. Management of hypotension/shock caused by suspected rate problem (Table 6-10)
     a. Rate problem is NOT synonymous with "conduction problem"
       (1) Adequate rate may be present although a conduction defect exists
       (2) Assess patient for possible pump, volume, or vascular resistance problem if hypotensive but rate within normal limits

---

Table 6-10	Management of Hypotension/Shock: Suspected Rate Problem

Perform Primary ABCD Survey (Basic Life Support)

(Correct critical problems IMMEDIATELY as they are identified)

Assess responsiveness, **A**irway, **B**reathing, **C**irculation,
ensure availability of monitor/**D**efibrillator

▼

Perform Secondary ABCD Survey (Advanced Life Support)

Administer oxygen, establish IV access, attach cardiac monitor, administer fluids as needed (O$_2$, IV, monitor, fluids)

Assess vital signs, attach pulse oximeter, and monitor blood pressure

Obtain and review 12-lead ECG, portable chest x-ray

Perform a focused history and physical exam

▼

Hypotension: suspected rate problem

- If rate too slow, use bradycardia algorithm
- If rate too fast, determine width of QRS, then use appropriate tachycardia algorithm

---

  b. If a rate problem exists and it is unclear if significant pump, volume, or vascular resistance problem coexists, correct rate problem first
  c. If a rate problem coexists with suspected pump, volume, or vascular resistance problem, treat simultaneously
  d. Management
     (1) Primary and Secondary ABCD surveys
     (2) If rate too slow, use bradycardia algorithm (see Table 8-12)
     (3) If rate too fast, determine width of QRS, then use appropriate tachycardia algorithm (see Tables 8-13 to 8-16)

QUICK REVIEW

1. Hypotension may occur during an acute MI for several reasons. Name four possible causes of hypotension associated with a rate problem.

2. Cardiogenic shock is most often caused by extensive myocardial infarction, involving approximately _____ % or more of the left ventricle.

1. Rate too fast: sinus tachycardia, atrial fibrillation, atrial flutter, PSVT, ventricular tachycardia; Rate too slow: sinus bradycardia, second-degree AV block, type I; second-degree AV block, type II; complete AV block; pacemaker failure.   2. 40%.

---

7. Right ventricular infarction (RVI)
   a. RVI should be suspected in the patient with an inferior left ventricular MI; unexplained, persistent hypotension; clear lung fields; and jugular venous distention
      (1) During right ventricular infarction, the right ventricle dilates acutely and does not effectively pump blood to the pulmonary system. Jugular venous distention occurs because of the backup of blood into the systemic venous vessels

The combination of hypotension (of varying degrees), clear lung fields, and elevated jugular venous pressure in a patient with inferior MI suggests RV ischemia.

    (2) Signs of pulmonary edema are absent because the right ventricle is unable to effectively pump blood into the pulmonary vasculature. Filling of the left ventricle is subsequently decreased, resulting in decreased cardiac output and, ultimately, hypotension

b. RVI may occur in up to 50% of inferior MIs; an infarction of ONLY the right ventricle is rare

c. Consider presence of RVI if patient with inferior wall MI becomes hypotensive after administration of nitrates

d. Clinical presentation (findings listed are present in only 10% to 15% of patients)
    (1) RV ischemia triad: Hypotension (of varying degrees), clear lung fields, and elevated jugular venous pressure (in a patient with inferior MI)
    (2) Kussmaul's sign (jugular venous distention paradoxically increases with inspiration)

Jugular venous distention may be absent in the volume-depleted patient.

e. ECG findings
    (1) ST-segment elevation in leads II, III, aVF (inferior MI)
    (2) ST-segment elevation $\geq$1 mm in **right** precordial lead V_4R **strongly** suggests RV injury
    (3) Consider these facts[17]
        (a) Approximately half of patients with right ventricular injury show resolution of ST-segment elevation within 10 hours of onset of symptoms
        (b) AV block is common and occurs in approximately half of patients with RVI
        (c) Atrial fibrillation may occur in up to a third of patients—consider prompt cardioversion if patient demonstrates signs of hemodynamic compromise

f. Management
    (1) Avoid use of nitrates and diuretics—may cause reduction in cardiac output and severe hypotension
    (2) Administer IV fluid challenges of 250- to 500-mL as rapidly as possible, then assess response

Reassess breath sounds, BP, etc. after each fluid challenge

        (a) Repeat IV fluid challenges every 15 minutes as needed up to 1 to 2 L
        (b) If BP fails to improve after administration of 1/2 to 1 L of fluid, begin dobutamine infusion (2 to 20 mcg/kg/min)
    (4) *Note:* "Volume loading with normal saline alone often resolves accompanying hypotension and improves cardiac output. In other cases, volume loading further elevates the right-sided filling pressure and RV dilatation, resulting in **decreased** LV output. . . . When LV dysfunction accompanies RV ischemia, the right ventricle is further compromised because of increased RV afterload and reduction in stroke volume. In such circumstances, the use of afterload-reducing agents such as sodium nitroprusside or an intra-aortic counterpulsation device is often necessary to 'unload' the left and subsequently the right ventricle"[17] (emphasis added)
    (5) Reperfusion—fibrinolytics, PCI, CABG if multi-vessel disease

QUICK REVIEW

1. When should you suspect a right ventricular infarction?

2. Can you name the components of the right ventricular ischemia triad?

3. "MONA" is commonly used to recall the medications generally administered to patients experiencing an acute coronary syndrome. Which of these medications should be avoided in the patient experiencing a right ventricular infarction?

1. When the patient has experienced an inferior wall MI of the left ventricle.   2. Hypotension (of varying degrees), clear lung fields, and elevated jugular venous pressure (in a patient with inferior MI).   3. Medications that decrease preload (such as nitroglycerin, morphine, diuretics, etc.) should be avoided because they may cause a reduction in cardiac output and severe hypotension.

12-LEAD ECG

1. Obtaining and reviewing a 12-lead ECG is an important component of the initial assessment of the patient presenting with ischemic chest pain
2. Patients should be rapidly assessed and the 12-lead reviewed to classify them into one of three management categories:
   a. *ST-segment elevation or new-onset left bundle branch block* (possible myocardial injury or ST-elevation MI)
   b. *ST-segment depression or transient ST-segment/T-wave changes* (possible ischemia; high-risk unstable angina/non-ST-elevation MI)
   c. *Nondiagnostic or normal ECG* (possible ischemia; intermediate/low-risk unstable angina)

Layout of the 12-Lead ECG

1. A 12-lead ECG is obtained with a 12-lead monitor that simultaneously records the leads and provides a read-out in a conventional four-column format (Figure 6-19)
2. Each column consists of three rows. Standard limb leads are recorded in the first column, augmented limb leads in the second column, and precordial leads in the third and fourth columns (Table 6-11)

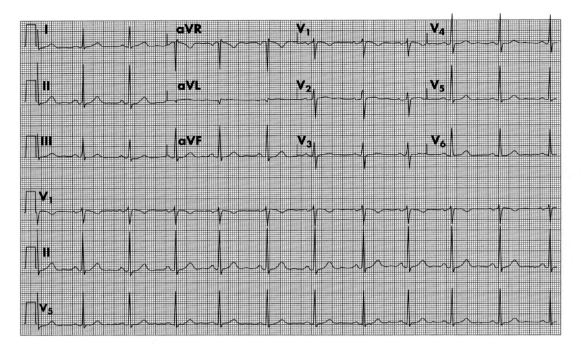

Figure 6-19 Example of a 12-lead ECG. Note the four columns. In this example, continuous recordings of leads V_1, II, and V5 are shown at the bottom.

Table 6-11	**Layout of the Four-Column 12-lead ECG**			
Plane	Frontal	Frontal	Horizontal	Horizontal
Lead type	Bipolar	Unipolar	Unipolar	Unipolar
	Limb Leads		**Precordial Leads**	
	Standard Leads	**Augmented Leads**	V_1-V_3	V_4-V_6
	Column I	Column II	Column III	Column IV
	I – lateral	aVR	V_1 – septum	V_4 – anterior
	II – inferior	aVL – lateral	V_2 – septum	V_5 – lateral
	III – inferior	aVF – inferior	V_3 – anterior	V_6 – lateral

12-lead Changes Indicating Infarction

1. In the standard 12-lead ECG
   a. Leads II, III, and aVF "look" at tissue supplied by the right coronary artery (Figure 6-20)
   b. Eight leads "look" at tissue supplied by the left coronary artery— leads I, aVL, V_1, V_2, V_3, V_4, V_5, and V_6
      (1) When evaluating the extent of infarction produced by a left coronary artery occlusion, determine how many of these leads are showing changes consistent with an acute infarction. The more of these eight leads demonstrating acute changes, the larger the infarction is presumed to be[30]
2. Viewing the right ventricle
   a. Approximately 40% of inferior wall MIs involve the *right* ventricle
   b. To view the right ventricle, use right precordial leads (Figure 6-21). Place them identical to the standard precordial leads except on the

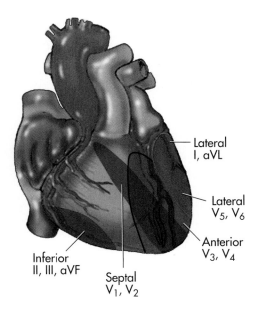

Figure 6-20 Multi-lead assessment of the heart.

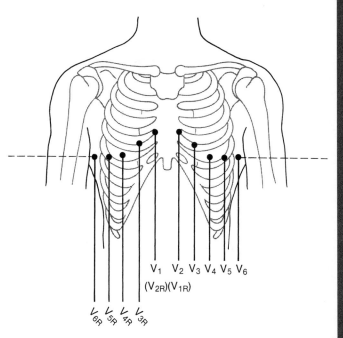

Figure 6-21 Anatomic placement of the left and right precordial leads.

right side of the chest. If time does not permit obtaining all of the right precordial leads, the lead of choice is V_4R

c. A modification of lead V_4R (MC_4R) using a standard 3-lead system may be used to view the right ventricle. The positive electrode is placed in the fifth intercostal space, right midclavicular line. The negative electrode is placed on the left arm and the lead selector on the monitor placed in the lead III position

3. Viewing the heart's posterior surface
   a. No leads of the standard 12-lead ECG directly view the posterior wall of the left ventricle
      (1) Changes in the opposite (anterior) wall of the heart can be viewed as reciprocal changes or additional precordial leads may be used to view the heart's posterior surface
      (2) Leads are placed further left and toward the back. All of the leads are placed on the same horizontal line as V_4 to V_6. Lead V_7 is placed at the posterior axillary line. Lead V_8 is placed at the angle of the scapula (posterior scapular line) and Lead V_9 is placed over the left border of the spine (Figure 6-22)

Modified Chest Leads

1. Modified chest leads (MCL) are bipolar precordial (chest) leads that are variations of the unipolar precordial leads
   a. Each modified chest lead consists of a positive and negative electrode applied to a specific location on the thorax. Accurate placement of the positive electrode is important
   b. Modified chest leads are useful in detecting bundle branch blocks (BBB), differentiating right and left premature beats, and differentiating supraventricular tachycardia (SVT) from ventricular tachycardia (VT)
2. Lead MCL_1
   a. Variation of precordial lead V_1; views ventricular septum

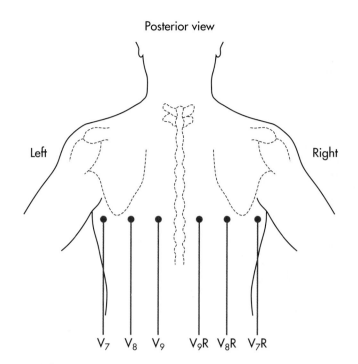

Figure 6-22 Posterior precordial lead placement.

   b. Negative electrode is placed below left clavicle toward left shoulder
   c. Positive electrode is placed to right of sternum in fourth intercostal space (Figure 6-23, *A*)
   d. In this lead, the positive electrode is in a position to the right of the left ventricle. Because the primary wave of depolarization is directed toward the left ventricle, the QRS complex recorded in this lead will normally appear negative (Figure 6-23, *B*)

3. Lead MCL_6
   a. A variation of precordial lead V_6; views low lateral wall of the left ventricle
   b. Negative electrode is placed below the left clavicle toward the left shoulder
   c. Positive electrode is placed at the fifth intercostal space, left midaxillary line (Figure 6-23, *C*)

Localization of a Myocardial Infarction

1. The left ventricle has been divided into four regions where MI may occur—anterior, lateral, inferior, and posterior (Table 6-12). Figure 6-24 shows the coronary artery that supplies blood to each portion of the heart, the site of infarction if one of these vessels is occluded, and the area of the heart viewed by each of the leads in a standard 12-lead ECG
2. MI may not be limited to one region. For example, if the precordial leads indicated ECG changes in leads V_3 and V_4 suggestive of an anterior wall MI and diagnostic changes were also present in V_5 and V_6, the infarction would be called an *anterolateral infarction* or an *anterior infarction with lateral extension*
3. Lateral wall MI
   a. Leads I, aVL, V_5, and V_6 view the lateral wall of the left ventricle
   b. Usually supplied by circumflex branch of LCA. Lateral wall infarctions often occur as extensions of anterior or inferior infarctions

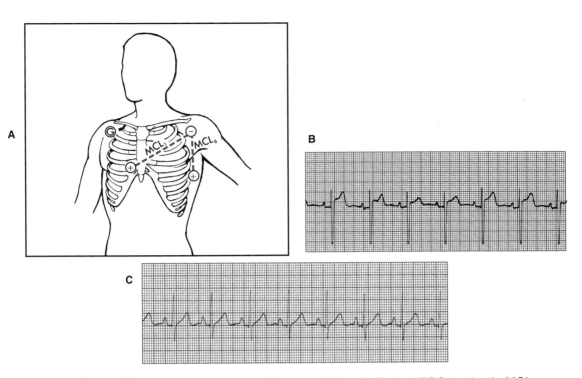

Figure 6-23   A, Electrode placement for MCL$_1$ and MCL$_6$. **B,** Typical ECG tracing in MCL$_1$.
C, Typical ECG tracing in MCL$_6$.

Table 6-12   Localization of a Myocardial Infarction

Location of MI	Indicative Changes (leads facing affected area)	Reciprocal Changes (leads opposite affected area)	Affected Coronary Artery
Lateral	I, aVL, V$_5$, V$_6$	V$_1$-V$_3$	Left coronary artery—circumflex branch
Inferior	II, III, aVF	I, aVL	Right coronary artery—posterior descending branch
Septum	V$_1$, V$_2$	None	Left coronary artery—left anterior descending artery, septal branch
Anterior	V$_3$, V$_4$	II, III, aVF	Left coronary artery—left anterior descending artery, diagonal branch
Posterior	Not visualized	V$_1$, V$_2$, V$_3$, V$_4$	Right coronary artery or left circumflex artery
Right ventricular	V$_1$R-V$_6$R		Right coronary artery—proximal branches

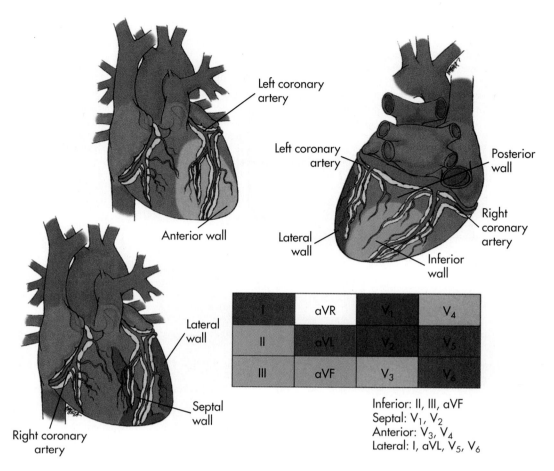

I	aVR	V₁	V₄
II	aVL	V₂	V₅
III	aVF	V₃	V₆

Inferior: II, III, aVF
Septal: V₁, V₂
Anterior: V₃, V₄
Lateral: I, aVL, V₅, V₆

Figure 6-24 Coronary artery anatomy.

    c. In some patients, the AV node is supplied by a branch of the circumflex artery. In these patients, occlusion of this vessel may result in AV blocks

4. Inferior wall MI (Figure 6-25)

    a. Leads II, III, and aVF view the inferior surface of the left ventricle. Reciprocal changes are observed in leads I and aVL. In most individuals, the inferior wall is supplied by the posterior descending branch of the right coronary artery

    b. Parasympathetic hyperactivity is common with inferior wall MIs, resulting in bradydysrhythmias. Conduction delays such as first-degree AV block and second-degree AV block type I are common and usually transient

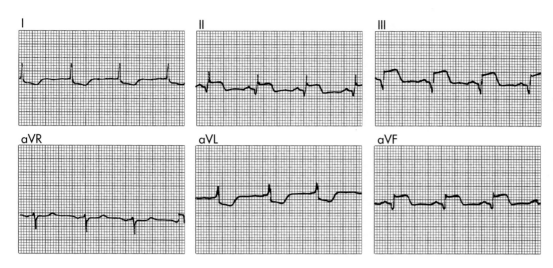

Figure 6-25 Acute inferior wall infarction. Note the ST-segment elevation in leads II, III, and aVF and the reciprocal ST depression in leads I and aVL. Abnormal Q waves are also present in leads II, III, and aVF.

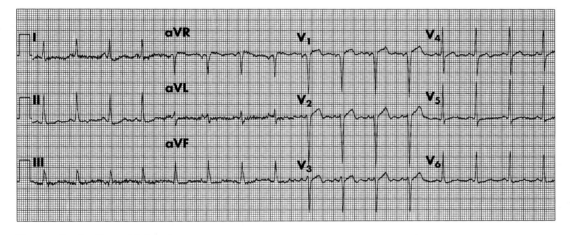

Figure 6-26 Septal infarction.

5. Septal MI (Figure 6-26)
   a. Leads V_1 and V_2 face the septal area of the left ventricle. The septum, which contains the bundle of His and bundle branches, is normally supplied by the left anterior descending artery
   b. If the site of infarction is limited to the septum, ECG changes are seen in V_1 and V_2. If the entire anterior wall is involved, ECG changes will be visible in V_1, V_2, V_3, and V_4
   c. An occlusion in this area may result in both right and left (more common) bundle branch blocks, second-degree AV block type II, and complete AV block
6. Anterior wall MI (Figures 6-27 and 6-28)
   a. Leads V_3 and V_4 face the anterior wall of the left ventricle. Reciprocal changes of injury, such as ST depression, appear in leads II, III, and aVF. This area is normally supplied by the diagonal branch of the left anterior descending artery
   b. Because the left anterior descending artery supplies about 40% of the heart's blood and a critical section of the left ventricle, an occlusion in this area can lead to complications such as left ventricular dysfunction, including congestive heart failure (CHF) and cardiogenic shock

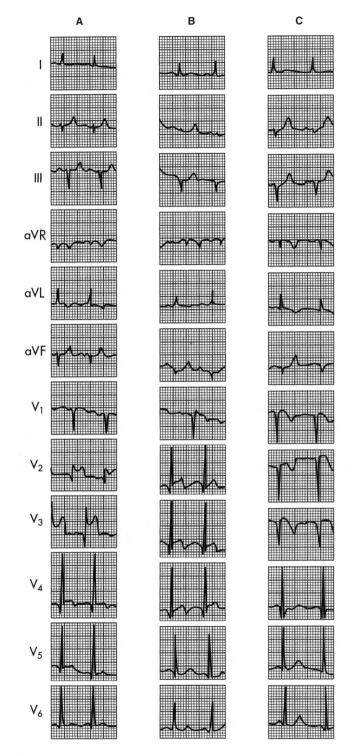

Figure 6-27 Evolutionary changes in anteroseptal myocardial infarction, reflected in leads V_1 to V_2. **A,** At admission, hyperacute phase is reflected by ST segment elevation. **B,** At 24 hours. **C,** At 48 hours, there are abnormal (pathologic) Q waves.

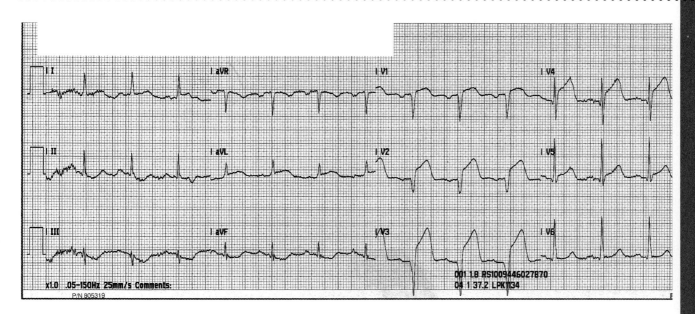

Figure 6-28 Extensive anterior infarction. Reciprocal changes present.

   c. Sympathetic hyperactivity is common with resulting sinus tachycardia and/or hypertension. An anterior wall MI may cause other dysrhythmias, including PVCs, atrial flutter, or atrial fibrillation. Because the bundle branches travel through this area, BBBs may result from injury in this area

7. Posterior wall MI

   a. Posterior wall of the left ventricle is supplied by the left circumflex coronary artery in most patients; however, in some patients it is supplied by the right coronary artery

   b. On the standard 12-lead ECG, no leads directly view the posterior wall of the left ventricle. Changes in the opposite (anterior) wall of the heart can be viewed as reciprocal changes (Figures 6-29 and 6-30). Posterior wall MI usually produces tall R waves and ST-segment depression in leads V_1 through V_4.

   c. "When marked ST-segment depression is confined to leads V_1 through V_4, there is a likelihood that this reflects a posterior current of injury and suggests a circumflex artery occlusion for which thrombolytic therapy would be considered appropriate"[17]

   d. Complications of a posterior wall MI may include left ventricular dysfunction. If the posterior wall is supplied by the right coronary artery, complications may include dysrhythmias involving the SA node, AV node, and bundle of His

To assist in the recognition of ECG changes suggesting a posterior wall MI, the "mirror test" is helpful. Flip over the ECG to the blank side and turn it upside down. When held up to the light, the tall R waves become deep Q waves and ST depression becomes ST elevation—the "classic" ECG changes associated with MI.

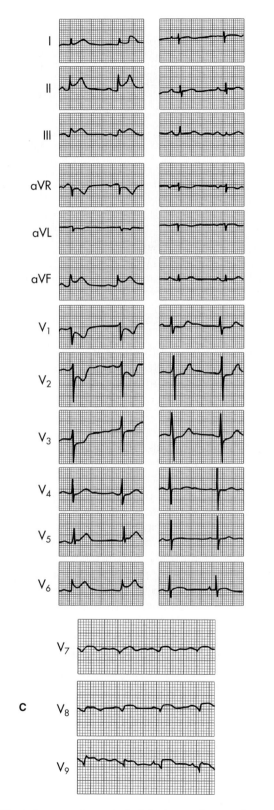

I

II

III

aVR

aVL

aVF

A

V₁

V₂

V₃

V₄

V₅

V₆

B

V₇

C

V₈

V₉

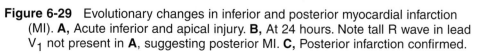

Figure 6-29 Evolutionary changes in inferior and posterior myocardial infarction (MI). **A,** Acute inferior and apical injury. **B,** At 24 hours. Note tall R wave in lead V_1 not present in **A,** suggesting posterior MI. **C,** Posterior infarction confirmed.

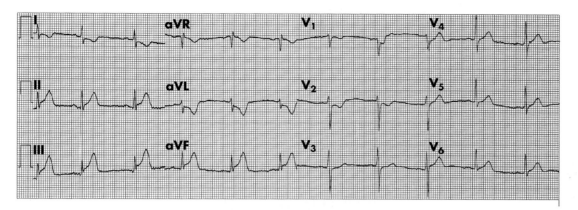

Figure 6-30   Inferior wall infarction with a possible posterior wall infarction. Reciprocal changes present.

8. Right ventricular infarction (RVI)
   a. RVI should be suspected when ECG changes suggesting an acute inferior wall MI (viewed in leads II, III, and aVF) are observed
   b. ST segment elevation of 1 mm or more in lead V_4R has a sensitivity of 70% to 93% and a specificity of 77% to 100%[31]
   c. Complications associated with RVI include hypotension, cardiogenic shock, AV blocks, atrial flutter or fibrillation, and PACs (Figures 6-31 and 6-32)

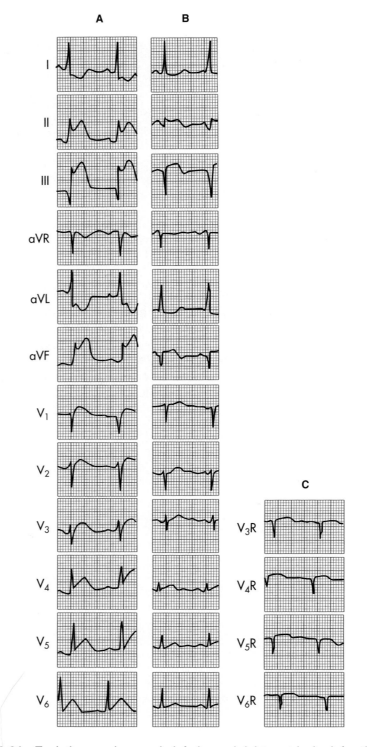

Figure 6-31 Evolutionary changes in inferior and right ventricular infarction. **A,** At admission—acute phase. **B,** At 12 hours. **C,** Right chest leads demonstrating right ventricular infarction.

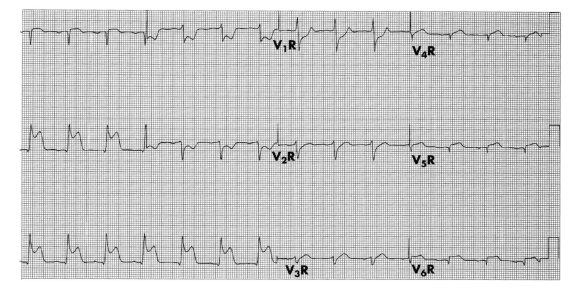

Figure 6-32   A 12-lead ECG obtained using the right-sided precordial leads. Inferior infarction with evidence of right ventricular injury (V_4R).

QUICK REVIEW

1. Which chamber of the heart is most often involved in acute myocardial infarction?

2. Patients who experience a(n) _____ myocardial infarction have a greater incidence of congestive heart failure and cardiogenic shock than those who have MIs affecting other areas of the left ventricle.

3. ST-segment elevation of 1 mm or more in lead V_4R is suggestive of _____ _____ injury.

4. True or False. Leads I, II, and III directly view the posterior wall of the left ventricle.

5. Which leads on a standard 12-lead ECG should be viewed for changes when identifying an inferior wall MI?

1. Left ventricle.   2. Anterior.   3. Right ventricular.   4. False.   5. II, III, aVF.

STOP AND REVIEW

1. Medications administered in the management of acute pulmonary edema without hypotension include:
   a. Furosemide and sublingual nitroglycerin
   b. Nitroglycerin, nitroprusside, and dopamine
   c. Aspirin and dobutamine
   d. Amrinone, aminophylline, and digoxin

2. A myocardial infarction is:
   a. A thin-walled bulge in a necrotic area of the left ventricle that balloons out when the ventricle contracts
   b. Death of myocardial cells because of myocardial ischemia
   c. The inability of the heart to maintain cardiac output adequate to meet the metabolic demands of the body
   d. A gradual process involving obstruction and hardening of the arterial wall

3. *True* or *False*. When right ventricular failure occurs, blood backs up behind the right ventricle, resulting in increased pressure in the right atrium and systemic venous circulation.

4. List the two main branches of the left coronary artery.

   a. _____

   b. _____

5. What is the primary electrical complication of acute myocardial infarction?
   a. Cardiac dysrhythmias
   b. Ventricular aneurysm
   c. Congestive heart failure
   d. Papillary muscle dysfunction

6. The most common cause of an anterior or lateral wall myocardial infarction is occlusion of a branch of the _____ coronary artery.
   a. Left
   b. Right

7. Reducing preload in the management of a normotensive patient with congestive heart failure (CHF) most commonly involves the use of:
   a. Diuretics and antidysrhythmics
   b. Venodilators and vasopressors
   c. Diuretics and venodilators
   d. Antidysrhythmics and vasopressors

Your patient is a 62-year-old male complaining of chest pain. The following questions (8 through 15) refer to the initial assessment and management of this patient.

8. List at least three (3) important questions that should be asked of this patient to determine if he may be experiencing an acute coronary syndrome.

   a. _____

   b. _____

   c. _____

9. The patient states his pain is located in the center of his chest and radiates to his left arm. He was reading the newspaper when his discomfort began about 1½ hours ago. On a 1 to 10 scale, the patient rates his discomfort a "9." He has no significant past medical history, takes no medications regularly, and states he has "never had anything like this before." His father died of a heart attack at the age of 66. The patient is an investment banker and states he is under considerable daily stress. Describe the initial assessment interventions that should be performed for this patient.

   _____

   _____

   _____

   _____

10. *True* or *False*. Decisions regarding this patient's care will primarily be based on his signs and symptoms, oxygen saturation, and presence of cardiac risk factors.

11. The patient's 12-lead ECG reveals 3-mm ST-segment elevation in leads V_3, and V_4. These leads view the _____ surface of the _____ ventricle.
    a. Anterior, left
    b. Inferior, left
    c. Lateral, left
    d. Septal, right

12. The presence of ST-segment elevation on this patient's 12-lead ECG suggests myocardial _____.
    a. Ischemia
    b. Injury
    c. Infarction
    d. Necrosis

13. The patient's BP is 156/88, P 118, R 24. The cardiac monitor reveals sinus tachycardia with occasional uniform PVCs. An IV has been established. Which of the following reflects the appropriate sequence of interventions that should be performed in the immediate general treatment of this patient?
    a. Oxygen, sublingual nitroglycerin, aspirin 162 to 325 mg, and then morphine sulfate 2 to 4 mg IV if pain unrelieved with nitroglycerin
    b. Aspirin 162 to 325 mg, morphine 2 to 4 mg IV, sublingual nitroglycerin, and then oxygen
    c. Sublingual nitroglycerin, aspirin 162 to 325 mg, oxygen, and then morphine 2 to 4 mg IV if pain unrelieved with nitroglycerin
    d. Morphine 2 to 4 mg IV, oxygen, aspirin 162 to 325 mg, and then sublingual nitroglycerin if morphine fails to relieve pain

14. The patient's physician has ordered a beta-blocker for this patient. What is the rationale for administration of a beta-blocker in this situation?
    a. Increase heart rate
    b. Improve ventilation through bronchodilation
    c. Increase myocardial contractility
    d. Decrease myocardial oxygen consumption

15. Based on the information presented, additional interventions that may be considered for this patient include:
    a. Reperfusion therapy
    b. Heparin IV if using fibrin-specific lytics
    c. IV nitroglycerin
    d. All of the above

STOP AND REVIEW ANSWERS

1. a. Furosemide, sublingual nitroglycerin, and morphine may be used in the management of acute pulmonary edema without hypotension

2. b. Myocardial infarction is death of myocardial cells because of myocardial ischemia. MI occurs when there is a sudden decrease or total cessation of blood flow through a coronary artery to an area of the myocardium. Choice "a" describes a ventricular aneurysm, "c" describes congestive heart failure, cardiogenic shock and "d" describes arteriosclerosis.

3. *True.* When right ventricular failure occurs, blood backs up behind the right ventricle, resulting in increased pressure in the right atrium and systemic venous circulation.

4. The two main branches of the left coronary artery are the left anterior descending (LAD) and the left circumflex (LC).

5. a. Cardiac dysrhythmias are the primary **electrical** complication of MI. The primary **mechanical** complications of acute MI are congestive heart failure and shock.

6. a. The most common cause of an anterior or lateral wall myocardial infarction is occlusion of a branch of the left coronary artery. Branches of the left anterior descending (LAD) artery supply blood to the anterior surfaces of both ventricles. The left circumflex (LC) branch supplies blood to the left atrium and lateral wall of the left

ventricle. In some patients, the circumflex artery may also supply the inferior portion of the left ventricle.

7. c. Venodilators and diuretics (e.g., nitroglycerin, morphine, furosemide) are used to reduce preload in the management of the normotensive patient with congestive heart failure (CHF).

8. Questions that should be asked of this patient to determine if he may be experiencing an acute coronary syndrome include his age (already known), signs and symptoms including his pain presentation (location of pain, duration, quality, relation to effort, time of symptom onset), history of coronary artery disease, presence of CAD risk factors, and use of Viagra within the past 24 hours.

9. Based on the information obtained thus far, it appears this patient is experiencing an acute coronary syndrome. At this point, you should obtain a targeted history/physical exam using a checklist to focus on his eligibility for reperfusion therapy, assess vital signs, determine oxygen saturation, establish IV access, connect the patient to the ECG monitor, administer aspirin 162 to 325 mg (chewed) if no reason for exclusion, draw blood for laboratory analysis (baseline serum cardiac marker levels, CBC, lipid profile, electrolytes), obtain a 12-lead ECG and a portable chest x-ray, preferably upright (<30 minutes).

10. *False*. Decisions regarding this patient's care will primarily be based on his signs and symptoms, 12-lead ECG, and serum cardiac markers.

11. a. Leads V_3 and V_4 view the anterior surface of the left ventricle.

12. b. The presence of ST-segment elevation (in a patient experiencing an acute coronary syndrome) suggests myocardial *injury*.

13. a. Immediate general treatment of this patient should include oxygen, sublingual nitroglycerin, aspirin 162 to 325 mg (if not already administered and no contraindications), and then morphine sulfate 2 to 4 mg IV if pain unrelieved with nitroglycerin.

14. d. Beta-blockers are used in acute MI to reduce myocardial oxygen consumption, decrease the incidence of dysrhythmias, lower blood pressure, block catecholamine stimulation, decrease myocardial contractility, and decrease the incidence of VF.

15. d. Based on the information presented, additional interventions that may be considered for this patient include reperfusion therapy, heparin if using fibrin-specific lytics, and the use of IV nitroglycerin as needed.

REFERENCES

1. American Heart Association: *2000 heart and stroke statistical update.* Dallas, Texas, 1999, American Heart Association.
2. Braunwald E, editor: *Heart disease*, Philadelphia, 1997, WB Saunders.
3. Cohen M: Platelet glycoprotein IIb/IIIa receptor inhibitors in coronary artery disease, *Ann Intern Med* 124:843-844, 1996.
4. Lefkovits J: Recent advances in antiplatelet therapy, *Aust Prescr* 19:98-100, 1996.

5. Falk E, Shah PK: Pathology of acute ischemic syndromes. In Braunwald E, senior editor; Califf RM, volume editor: *Atlas of heart diseases: acute myocardial infarction and other acute ischemic syndromes*, Volume VIII, 1996, Singapore, Current Medicine.

6. Goldman L, Braunwald E: *Primary cardiology*, Philadelphia, 1998, WB Saunders.

7. Braunwald E, Antman EM, Beasley JW, Califf RM, Cheitlin MD, Hochman JS, Jones RH, Kereiakes D, Kupersmith J, Levin TN, Pepine CJ, Schaeffer JW, Smith EE III, Steward DE, Theroux P: ACC/AHA guidelines for the management of patients with unstable angina and non–ST-segment elevation myocardial infarction: a report of the American College of Cardiology/American Heart Association Task Force on Practice Guidelines (Committee on the Management of Patients With Unstable Angina), *J Am Coll Cardiol* 36:970-1062, 2000.

8. Pedoe-Tunstall H, Kuulasmaa K, Amouyel P, et al: Myocardial infarction and coronary deaths in the World Health Organization MONICA Project, *Circulation* 90:583, 1994.

9. Alpert JS, Thygesen K, et al: Myocardial infarction redefined—a consensus document of The Joint European Society of Cardiology/American College of Cardiology Committee for the redefinition of myocardial infarction, *J Am Coll Cardiol*, 36(3):959-969, 2000.

10. Braunwald E. Recognition and management of patients with acute myocardial infarction. In Goldman L, Braunwald E: *Primary cardiology*, Philadelphia, 1998, WB Saunders.

11. Kouvaras G, Bacoulas G: Unstable angina as a warning symptom before acute myocardial infarction, *Q J Med* 64:679, 1987.

12. Woods SL, Sivarajan Froelicher ES, Motzer SA: *Cardiac nursing*, ed 4, Philadelphia, 2000, Lippincott, Williams & Wilkins.

13. Fesmire FM, Wears RL: The utility of the presence or absence of chest pain in patients with suspected acute myocardial infarction, *Am J Emerg Med* 7(4):372-377, 1989.

14. Wenger NK: Cardiovascular disease in the elderly and in women. In Goldman L, Braunwald E: *Primary cardiology*, Philadelphia, 1998, WB Saunders.

15. *Educational strategies to prevent prehospital delay in patients at high risk for acute myocardial infarction*, NIH Publication No 97-3787, September, 1997, National Institutes of Health National Heart, Lung, and Blood Institute.

16. The American Heart Association in Collaboration with the International Liaison Committee on Resuscitation (ILCOR): Advanced cardiovascular life support, Part 7: Era of reperfusion, Section 1: Acute coronary syndromes (acute myocardial infarction): a consensus on science, *Circulation* 102 (suppl I):173-176, 2000.

17. Ryan TJ, Antman EM, Brooks NH, Califf RM, Hillis LD, Hiratzka LF, Rapaport E, Riegel B, Russell RO, Smith EE III, Weaver WD. ACC/AHA guidelines for the management of patients with acute myocardial infarction: 1999 update: a report of the American College of Cardiology/American Heart Association Task Force on Practice Guidelines (Committee on Management of Acute Myocardial Infarction).

18. Maroko PR, Radvany P, Braunwald E, Hale SL: Reduction of infarct size by oxygen inhalation following acute coronary occlusion, *Circulation* 52:360-368, 1975.

19. Madias JE, Hood WB Jr: Reduction of precordial ST-segment elevation in patients with anterior myocardial infarction by oxygen breathing, *Circulation* 53(suppl I):198-200, 1976.

20. Come PC, Pitt B: Nitroglycerin-induced severe hypotension and brady-cardia in patients with acute myocardial infarction, *Circulation* 54:624-628, 1976.

21. Kinch JW, Ryan TJ: Right ventricular infarction, *N Engl J Med* 330:1211-1217, 1994.

22. The American Heart Association in Collaboration with the International Liaison Committee on Resuscitation (ILCOR): Advanced cardiovascular life support, Part 7: Era of reperfusion, Section 1: acute coronary syndromes (acute myocardial infarction): a consensus on science, *Circulation* 102 (suppl I):178-192, 2000.

23. Ohman EM, Harrington RA, Cannon CP, Agnelli G, Cairns JA, Kennedy JW: Intravenous thrombolysis in acute myocardial infarction, *Chest* 119(1 Suppl):253S-277S, 2001.

24. Crawford MV, Spence MI: *Common sense approach to coronary care*, ed 6, St Louis, 1995, Mosby.

25. Weil MH, Tang W, editors: *CPR: resuscitation of the arrested heart*, Philadelphia, 1999, WB Saunders.

26. The American Heart Association in Collaboration with the International Liaison Committee on Resuscitation (ILCOR): Advanced cardiovascular life support, Part 7: Era of reperfusion, Section 1: acute coronary syndromes (acute myocardial infarction): a consensus on science, *Circulation* 102 (suppl I):1-195, 2000.

27. Leier CV: Unstable heart failure. In Braundwald E, series editor, Colucci WS, volume editor: *Heart failure: cardiac function and dysfunction, atlas of heart diseases;* Volume IV, Singapore, 1995, Current Medicine.

28. Murphy JG, editor: *Mayo clinic cardiology review*, ed 2, Philadelphia, 2000, Lippincott, Williams & Wilkins.

29. The American Heart Association in Collaboration with the International Liaison Committee on Resuscitation (ILCOR): Advanced cardiovascular life support, Part 7: Era of reperfusion, Section 1: Acute coronary syndromes (acute myocardial infarction): a consensus on science, *Circulation* 102 (suppl I):1-189, 2000.

30. Phalen T: *The 12-lead ECG in acute myocardial infarction*, St Louis, 1996, Mosby.

31. Chou T, Knilans TK: *Electrocardiography in clinical practice: adult and pediatric*, Philadelphia, 1996, WB Saunders.

BIBLIOGRAPHY

The American Heart Association in Collaboration with the International Liaison Committee on Resuscitation (ILCOR): Advanced cardiovascular life support, Part 7: Era of reperfusion, Section 1: Acute coronary syndromes (acute myocardial infarction): a consensus on science, *Circulation* 102 (suppl I):I-172-203, 2000.

Braunwald E, senior editor, Califf RM, volume editor: *Atlas of heart diseases: acute myocardial infarction and other acute ischemic syndromes*, Vol VIII, Singapore, Current Medicine, 1996.

Braunwald E, Antman EM, Beasley JW, Califf RM, Cheitlin MD, Hochman JS, Jones RH, Kereiakes D, Kupersmith J, Levin TN, Pepine CJ, Schaeffer JW, Smith EE III, Steward DE, Theroux P: ACC/AHA guidelines for the management of patients with unstable angina and non–ST-segment elevation myocardial infarction: a report of the American College of Cardiology/American Heart Association Task Force on Practice Guidelines (Committee on the Management of Patients With Unstable Angina), *J Am Coll Cardiol* 36:970-1062, 2000.

Chou T, Knilans TK: *Electrocardiography in clinical practice: adult and pediatric*, Philadelphia, 1996, WB Saunders.

Clochesy JM, Breu C, Cardin S, Whittaker AA, Rudy EB: *Critical care nursing*, ed 2, Philadelphia, 1996, WB Saunders.

Crawford MV, Spence MI: *Common sense approach to coronary care*, ed 6, St Louis, 1995, Mosby.

Driscoll P, Gwinnutt C, Mackway-Jones K, Wardle T, editors: *Advanced cardiac life support: the practical approach*, ed 2, London, 1997, Chapman & Hall Medical.

Goldberger AL: *Clinical electrocardiography: a simplified approach*, ed 6, St Louis, 1999, Mosby.

Goldman L, Braunwald E: *Primary cardiology*, Philadelphia, 1998, WB Saunders.

McCance KL, Huether SE: *Pathophysiology: the biologic basis for disease in adults and children*, ed 2, St Louis, 1994, Mosby.

Murphy JG, editor: *Mayo clinic cardiology review*, ed 2, Philadelphia, 2000, Lippincott Williams & Wilkins.

Padrid PJ, Kowey PR, editors: *Cardiac arrhythmia: mechanisms, diagnosis, and management*, Baltimore, 1995, Williams & Wilkins.

Paradis NA, Halperin HR, Nowak RM, editors: *Cardiac arrest: the science and practice of resuscitation medicine*, Baltimore, 1996, Williams & Wilkins.

Phalen T: *The 12-lead ECG in acute myocardial infarction*, St Louis, 1996, Mosby.

Porth CM: *Pathophysiology: concepts of altered health states*, ed 5, Philadelphia, 1998, Lippincott-Raven Publishers.

Ryan TJ, Antman EM, Brooks NH, Califf RM, Hillis LD, Hiratzka LF, Rapaport E, Riegel B, Russell RO, Smith EE III, Weaver WD: ACC/AHA guidelines for the management of patients with acute myocardial infarction: 1999 update: a report of the American College of Cardiology/American Heart Association Task Force on Practice Guidelines (Committee on Management of Acute Myocardial Infarction).

Thelan LA, Davie JK, Urden LD, Lough ME: *Critical care nursing: diagnosis and management*, ed 2, St Louis, 1994, Mosby.

Thibodeau GA, Patton KT: Anatomy and Physiology, ed 4, St Louis, 1999, Mosby.

Weil MH, Tang W, editors: *CPR: resuscitation of the arrested heart*, Philadelphia, 1999, WB Saunders.

Woods SL, Sivarajan Froelicher ES, Motzer SA: *Cardiac nursing*, ed 4, Philadelphia, 2000, Lippincott Williams & Wilkins.

Cardiovascular Pharmacology

7

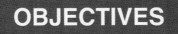

On completion of this chapter, you will be able to:

1. Describe the location and effects of stimulation of α, β, and dopaminergic receptors.
2. Define the following terms:
   a. Afterload
   b. Agonist
   c. Antagonist
   d. Chronotrope
   e. Dromotrope
   f. Inotrope
   g. Parasympatholytic
   h. Preload
   i. Sympathomimetic
3. Identify the primary neurotransmitter for the sympathetic and parasympathetic divisions of the autonomic nervous system.
4. Identify the mechanism of action, indications, dosage, and precautions for each of the following medications:
   a. Medications used in acute coronary syndromes
      (1) Oxygen
      (2) Nitroglycerin
      (3) Morphine sulfate
      (4) Naloxone
      (5) Aspirin
      (6) Glycoprotein IIb/IIIa inhibitors
         (a) Abciximab
         (b) Eptifibatide
         (c) Tirofiban
      (7) Antiplatelet agents
         (a) Ticlopidine
         (b) Clopidogrel
         (c) Dipyridamole
      (8) Fibrinolytic agents
         (a) Alteplase
         (b) Anistreplase
         (c) Reteplase
         (d). Streptokinase
         (e) Tenecteplase
      (9) Heparin
      (10) Low molecular weight heparin
         (a) Enoxaparin
         (b) Dalteparin

(11) Thrombin inhibitors
 (a) Hirudin therapy
(12) ACE inhibitors
b. Medications used to manage cardiac dysrhythmias
 (1) Adenosine
 (2) Amiodarone
 (3) Atropine
 (4) Beta-blockers (e.g., atenolol, esmolol, labetalol, metoprolol, pro-pranolol)
 (5) Calcium channel blockers (e.g., verapamil, diltiazem)
 (6) Digitalis
 (7) Disopyramide
 (8) Epinephrine
 (9) Flecainide
 (10) Ibutilide
 (11) Isoproterenol
 (12) Lidocaine
 (13) Magnesium
 (14) Procainamide
 (15) Propafenone
 (16) Sotalol
c. Medications used to improve cardiac output and blood pressure
 (1) Dopamine
 (2) Norepinephrine
 (3) Dobutamine
 (4) Vasopressin
 (5) Amrinone
 (6) Milrinone
 (7) Calcium chloride
 (8) Sodium nitroprusside
d. Other medications
 (1) Sodium bicarbonate
 (2) Furosemide

Note: Mosby's Drug Consult 2002, was the primary source for medication information used throughout this text unless otherwise noted.

REVIEW OF THE AUTONOMIC NERVOUS SYSTEM

1. The autonomic nervous system (ANS) consists of sympathetic and parasympathetic divisions (Figure 7-1) (Table 7-1)
   a. Sympathetic division mobilizes the body, allowing the body to function under stress ("fight-or-flight" response)
   b. Parasympathetic division is responsible for the conservation and restoration of body resources ("feed-and-breed" or "resting-and-digesting" response)
2. Nerve impulses are carried from the sensory receptors to the brain by means of the vagus and glossopharyngeal nerves (afferent pathways)
   a. Medulla of the brain serves as the integration center and interprets the sensory information received. Determines what body parameters need adjustment (if any) and transmits that information to the heart and blood vessels by means of motor nerves (efferent pathways)
3. Motor pathways of the ANS use two neurons to conduct information from the central nervous system (CNS) to various organs (effectors)

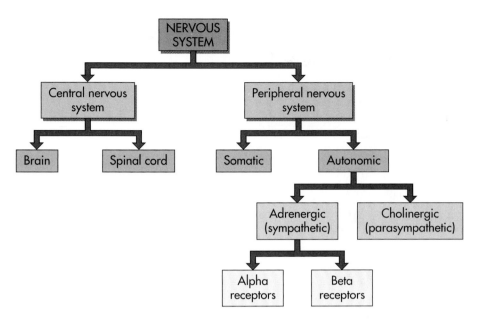

Figure 7-1 Overview of the autonomic nervous system.

Table 7-1 Overview of the Divisions of the Autonomic Nervous System	
Sympathetic Division	**Parasympathetic Division**
"Fight-or-Flight" response	"Feed-and-Breed" or "Resting-and-Digesting" response
• Mobilizes the body	• Conservation of body resources
• Allows the body to function under stress	• Restoration of body resources

     a. The first (preganglionic) neuron conducts impulses from the CNS to the ganglion (cell body) of a second (postganglionic) neuron

     b. The postganglionic neuron extends from the ganglion to the organ (Figure 7-2). The junction between these two neurons is called a **synapse**

4. Sympathetic preganglionic neurons are relatively short, and the postganglionic neurons relatively long

     a. One sympathetic preganglionic neuron may synapse with many postganglionic neurons in many organs. Thus sympathetic effects are often widespread, affecting many organs (see Table 7-3)

5. Parasympathetic preganglionic neurons are relatively long, and the postganglionic neurons relatively short that lead to a single organ. Thus, parasympathetic stimulation often involves a response by only one organ. (Figure 7-3)

6. Preganglionic nerve fibers of both the sympathetic and parasympathetic divisions of the ANS release acetylcholine (Ach), a **neurotransmitter**

     a. However, different neurotransmitters are released from the postganglionic fibers of the sympathetic and parasympathetic divisions of the ANS, resulting in different effects on various body organs

7. Postganglionic fibers that release *norepinephrine* are called *adrenergic* fibers. Those that release *acetylcholine* are called *cholinergic* fibers (Figure 7-4) (see Table 7-4)

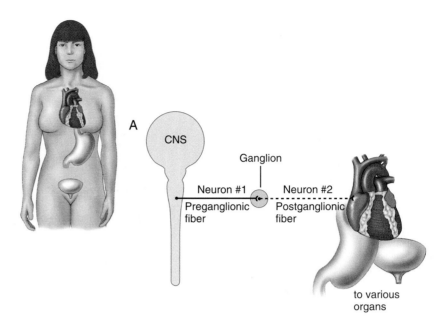

Figure 7-2 The motor pathways of the autonomic nervous system use two neurons to conduct information from the central nervous system to various organs (effectors). The first (preganglionic) neuron conducts impulses from the CNS to the ganglion (cell body) of a second (postganglionic) neuron. The postganglionic neuron extends from the ganglion to the organ.

Sympathetic Division

1. Activation of the sympathetic division of the ANS results in:
   a. Increased blood flow to skeletal muscle
   b. Release of glucose from the liver to ensure an adequate supply of oxygen and nutrients during a time of mental or physical stress
   c. Narrowing of **splanchnic** (internal organ) blood vessels diverts blood into vascular beds in muscles
   d. In the lungs, smooth muscles of the bronchi dilate, allowing an increase in the uptake of alveolar oxygen and tidal volume
   e. In the heart, sympathetic (accelerator) nerve fibers supply the SA node, AV node, atrial muscle, and the ventricular myocardium
2. Stimulation of sympathetic nerve fibers results in the release of norepinephrine. Norepinephrine binds to receptor sites located in the plasma membrane of cells (Figure 7-5)
3. Sympathetic (adrenergic) receptor sites are divided into *alpha*, *beta*, and *dopaminergic* receptors (Table 7-2)
   a. *Dopaminergic* receptor sites are located in the coronary arteries, renal, mesenteric and visceral blood vessels. Stimulation of dopaminergic receptor sites results in dilation
   b. Different body tissues have different proportions of alpha- and beta-receptors. Stimulation of *alpha*-receptor sites results in constriction of blood vessels in the skin, cerebral, and splanchnic circulation
   c. Beta-receptor sites are divided into beta-1 and beta-2. *Beta-1* receptors are found in the heart. Stimulation of beta-1 receptors results in an increased heart rate, contractility, and, ultimately, irritability of cardiac cells (Figure 7-6)
   d. *Beta-2* receptor sites are found in the lungs and blood vessels of skeletal muscle. Stimulation of these receptor sites results in dilation of the smooth muscle of the bronchi and blood vessel dilation

In general, alpha-receptors are more sensitive to norepinephrine, and beta-receptors are more sensitive to epinephrine.

Smooth muscle is located in the walls of many hollow organs including organs of the digestive, urinary, and reproductive tracts. Smooth muscle is also found in blood vessels, the bronchi, hair follicles, and the iris and ciliary muscles of the eye.

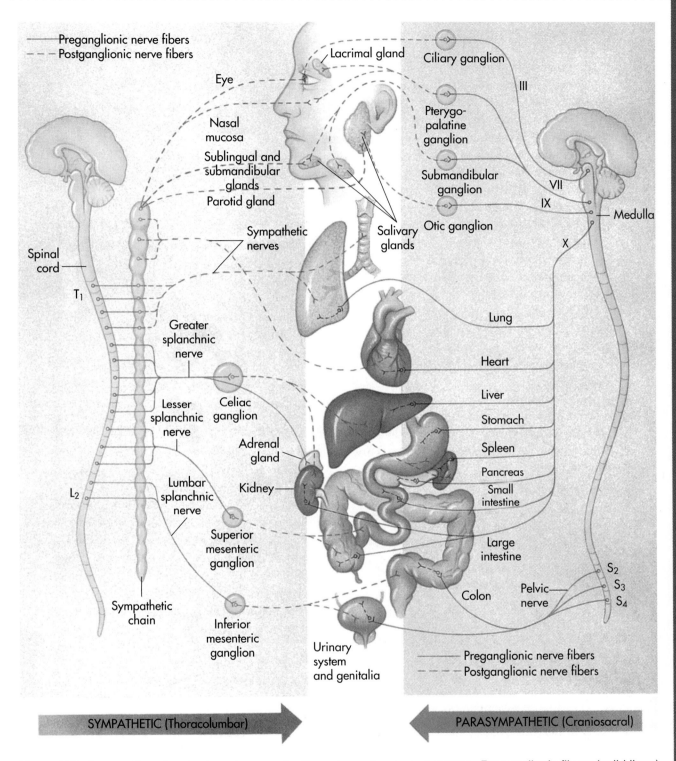

Figure 7-3 Innervation of major target organs by the autonomic nervous system. Preganglionic fibers (solid lines), postganglionic fibers (broken lines).

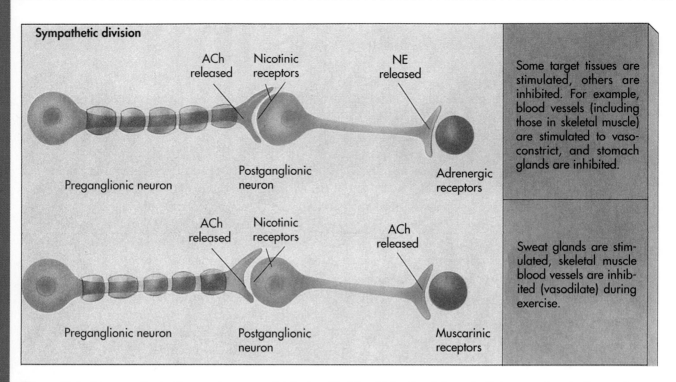

Figure 7-4 Preganglionic fibers release acetylcholine (Ach), which stimulates nicotinic receptors in the postganglionic neuron. Most sympathetic postganglionic fibers secrete norepinephrine (NE), resulting in alpha- or beta-receptor stimulation. A few postganglionic fibers are cholinergic (e.g., sweat glands and some blood vessels), resulting in stimulation of muscarinic receptors.

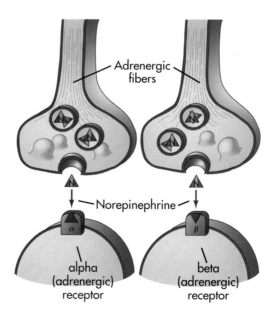
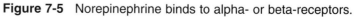

Figure 7-5 Norepinephrine binds to alpha- or beta-receptors.

Table 7-2 Sympathetic (Adrenergic) Receptors

	Alpha-1	Alpha-2	Beta-1	Beta-2	Dopaminergic
Location	Vascular smooth muscle	Skeletal blood vessels	Myocardium	Predominantly in bronchiolar and arterial smooth muscle	Coronary arteries, renal, mesenteric, and visceral blood vessels
Effects of Stimulation	Vasoconstriction increases peripheral vascular resistance	Inhibits norepinephrine release	Increases heart rate Increases myocardial contractility Increases oxygen consumption	Relaxation of bronchial smooth muscle; arteriolar dilation	Dilation

Table 7-3 Organ Responses to Sympathetic and Parasympathetic Stimulation

	Sympathetic	Parasympathetic
Eyes	Pupillary dilation	Accommodation for near vision
Saliva	Decreased secretions; viscous	Increased secretions; watery
Bronchial Smooth Muscle	Dilation	Constriction, increased secretion
Heart	Increased rate and force of contraction (beta-receptors)	Decreased rate Minimal effect on force of contraction
Liver	Glucose release (glycogenolysis) (beta receptors)	No effect
GI Tract	Decreased peristalsis (beta-receptors) Sphincter constriction (alpha-receptors) Decreased blood flow	Increased peristalsis Sphincter relaxation Increased secretion
Bladder	Relaxation (beta-receptors) Sphincter constriction (alpha-receptors)	Contraction Relaxation
Sweat Glands	Increased	No effect
Smooth Muscle of Blood Vessels		
Abdominal	Constriction (alpha-receptors)	No effect
Coronary	Constriction (alpha-receptors) Dilation (beta-receptors)	Dilation
Skeletal muscle	Dilation (beta-receptors)	No effect
Skin	Constriction (alpha-receptors)	No effect

Table 7-4 Autonomic Nervous System Terminology

Neurotransmitter	Norepinephrine	Acetylcholine
Synonymous Terms	Adrenergic, sympathomimetic, catecholamine, anticholinergic, parasympatholytic, cholinergic blocker	Cholinergic, parasympathomimetic, sympathetic blocker, cholinomimetic, sympatholytic, adrenergic blocker
Opposite Terms	Sympatholytic, antiadrenergic, sympathetic blocker, adrenergic blocker	Parasympatholytic, anticholinergic, cholinergic blocker, vagolytic

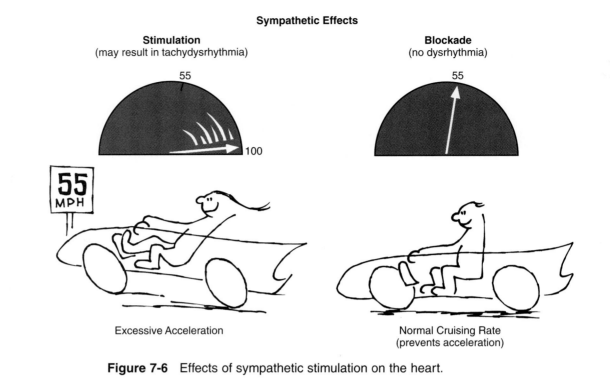

Figure 7-6 Effects of sympathetic stimulation on the heart.

Parasympathetic Division

1. Stimulation results in the release of acetylcholine (Figure 7-7). Acetylcholine binds to parasympathetic receptors. The two main types of cholinergic receptors are *nicotinic* and *muscarinic* receptors

2. Nicotinic receptors are located in skeletal muscle. Muscarinic receptors are located in smooth muscle. When acetylcholine binds to nicotinic receptors, there is an excitatory response. When acetylcholine binds with muscarinic receptors, the result may be excitation or inhibition, depending on the target tissues in which the receptors are found (Figure 7-8)

3. In the heart, parasympathetic (inhibitory) nerve fibers supply the SA node, atrial muscle, and the AV junction by means of the vagus nerves. The net effect of parasympathetic stimulation is slowing of the heart rate (Figure 7-9)

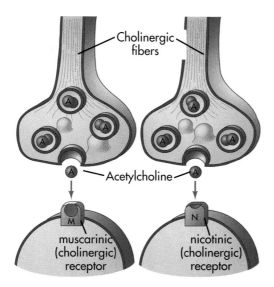

Figure 7-7 Acetylcholine (Ach) is released when parasympathetic nerve fibers are stimulated.

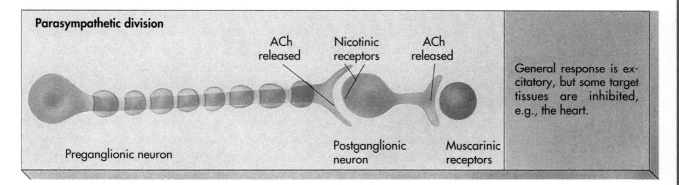

Figure 7-8 Acetylcholine binds to muscarinic or nicotinic receptor sites. When acetylcholine binds to nicotinic receptors, there is an excitatory response. When Ach binds with muscarinic receptors, the result may be excitation or inhibition, depending on the target tissues in which the receptors are found.

Table 7-5 Terms to Commit to Memory

Term	Definition
Chronotrope	Substance that affects the heart rate • Positive chronotrope = ↑ heart rate • Negative chronotrope = ↓ heart rate
Inotrope	Substance that affects myocardial contractility • Positive inotrope = ↑ force of contraction • Negative inotrope = ↓ force of contraction
Dromotrope	Substance that affects AV conduction velocity • Positive dromotrope = ↑ AV conduction velocity • Negative dromotrope = ↓ AV conduction velocity
Preload	Pressure/volume in the left ventricle at the end of diastole
Afterload	Pressure or resistance against which the heart must pump
Agonist	Drug or substance that produces a predictable response (stimulates action)
Antagonist	Agent that exerts an opposite action to another (blocks action)

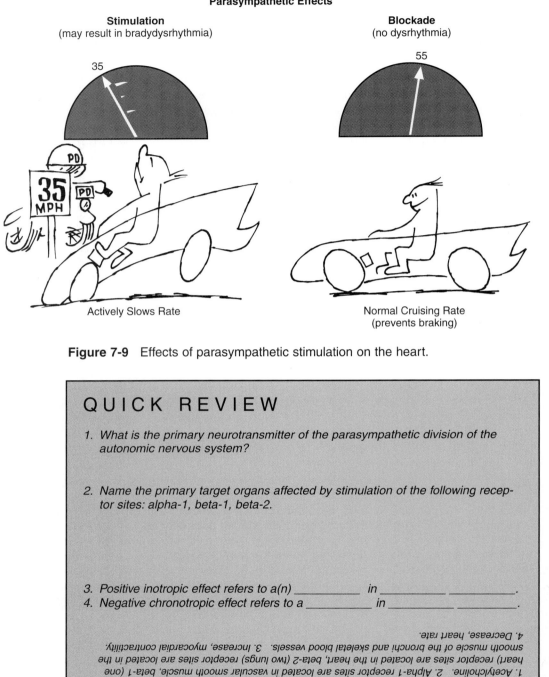

Parasympathetic Effects

Stimulation
(may result in bradydysrhythmia)

Blockade
(no dysrhythmia)

Actively Slows Rate

Normal Cruising Rate
(prevents braking)

Figure 7-9 Effects of parasympathetic stimulation on the heart.

QUICK REVIEW

1. What is the primary neurotransmitter of the parasympathetic division of the autonomic nervous system?

2. Name the primary target organs affected by stimulation of the following receptor sites: alpha-1, beta-1, beta-2.

3. Positive inotropic effect refers to a(n) _____ in _____ _____.
4. Negative chronotropic effect refers to a _____ in _____ _____.

1. Acetylcholine. 2. Alpha-1 receptor sites are located in vascular smooth muscle, beta-1 (one heart) receptor sites are located in the heart, beta-2 (two lungs) receptor sites are located in the smooth muscle of the bronchi and skeletal blood vessels. 3. Increase, myocardial contractility. 4. Decrease, heart rate.

MEDICATIONS USED IN ACUTE CORONARY SYNDROMES

The following medications are used in treating acute coronary syndromes
(ACS) (Tables 7-6 to 7-24).

Table 7-6   Oxygen

Mechanism of Action	• Increases oxygen tension • Increases hemoglobin saturation if ventilation is supported • Improves tissue oxygenation when circulation is maintained
Indications	• Cardiac or pulmonary arrest • Suspected hypoxemia of any cause • Any suspected cardiopulmonary emergency, especially complaints of shortness of breath and/or suspected ischemic chest pain
Dosing	*Spontaneously breathing patient*—best guided by pulse oximetry*—blood gases, and • patient tolerance to oxygen administration device: • Nasal cannula (1 to 6 L/min) • Simple face mask (8 to 10 L/min) • Partial rebreather mask (6 to 10 L/min) • Nonrebreather mask (10 to 15 L/min)
Precautions	Cardiac arrest—ventilation with 100% oxygen by bag-valve device, ET intubation Toxicity possible with prolonged administration of high flow oxygen

* Note: Pulse oximetry is inaccurate in low cardiac output states or with vasoconstriction.

Table 7-7   Nitroglycerin

Generic Name	nitroglycerin
Trade Name(s)	Nitrostat; Nitrobid [SL forms]; Tridil [IV]
Classification	Vasodilator; organic nitrate; antianginal
Pronunciation	nye-troh-GLIH-sir-in
How Supplied	SL tablets: 0.3, 0.4 and 0.6 mg SL spray: 0.4 mg/spray IV: 5 mg/mL in 1 or 10 mL vials. Must be diluted in D5W or NS (0.9%) before IV administration
Mechanism of Action	• Relaxes vascular smooth muscle. Dilates arterial and venous vascular beds, primarily venous. Venous dilation (predominates at low doses—30 to 40 mcg/min) results in peripheral venous pooling, decreased preload, decreased blood pressure. Arteriolar dilation (occurs at high doses[1]—150 to 500 mcg/min) results in decreased systemic vascular resistance decreased arterial pressure, reduction in afterload. These effects result in decreased myocardial oxygen consumption • Redistributes blood flow in the heart, improving circulation to ischemic areas[2]
Indications	• Ischemic chest pain • For the first 24 to 48 hours in patients with acute MI and CHF, large anterior infarction, persistent ischemia, or hypertension • Acute pulmonary edema caused by LV failure (if systolic blood pressure [SBP] >100 mm Hg)
Dosing (adult)	• Sublingual: 0.3 or 0.4 mg (1 tablet) repeated at 5-min intervals to maximum of 3 doses • Nitroglycerin tablets are light-, moisture-, and heat-sensitive. Keep tablets in their original brown glass bottles. Replace metal cap on bottle quickly after opening. Tablets usually lose potency within 3 to 4 months • Sublingual Spray: Spray on or under the tongue for 0.5 to 1.0 sec at 5-min intervals (delivers 0.4 mg/metered dose). *Do not shake* the canister before use. Shaking may produce bubbles within the canister, altering delivery of the medication

Continued

Table 7-7	**Nitroglycerin—cont'd**

	• **IV infusion:** Begin infusion at 5 mcg/min and increase dose in increments of 5 mcg/min every 5 to 10 min to desired hemodynamic or clinical response. Most patients respond to 50 to 200 mcg/min
	• Glass bottles and non–polyvinyl chloride infusion tubing must be used to avoid the loss of half the active drug by adsorption onto plastics
	• When administering to patients with evidence of acute MI, limit the fall in SBP to 10% in normotensive patients and 30% in hypertensive patients. Do not allow SBP to fall below 90 mm Hg
Precautions	Primary side effect is hypotension. Other side effects include tachycardia, bradycardia, headache, palpitations, syncope
Contraindications	• Viagra use within 24 hours
	• Right ventricular infarction
	• Severe bradycardia or tachycardia
	• Uncorrected hypotension
	• Hypovolemia
	• Increased intracranial pressure or intracranial bleeding (nitroglycerin's vasodilatory effect on meningeal blood vessels could increase cerebrospinal fluid pressure)
Special Considerations	• Nitroglycerin can cause hypotension and paradoxical bradycardia (or even asystole) because of triggering of the Bezold-Jarisch reflex. The Bezold-Jarisch reflex (also called the *bradycardia-hypotension syndrome*) is most common in patients with volume depletion or acute inferior MI, especially if the right ventricle is involved. It is likely caused by ventricular underfilling resulting from venodilation, followed by activation of cardiopulmonary receptors that trigger a vagal reflex.[3] Atropine administration may be necessary for management of the bradycardia. Hypotension usually responds to administration of IV fluids.[4] **Establishing an IV before administration of sublingual nitroglycerin is strongly recommended**
	• When administering nitroglycerin for ischemic chest pain, assess the patient's pain, duration, time started, activity being performed, quality, etc. Document the patient's response to the medication
	• Hypotension may exacerbate myocardial ischemia
	• Monitor vital signs and cardiac rhythm closely before, during, and after administration of this medication
Onset of Action	SL: Typically within 1 to 3 min; IV: Immediate—within 1.5 min
Duration	SL: 10 to 30 min; IV: 1 to 10 min after IV discontinued

---

Viagra and Nitrates

The combination of Viagra (sildenafil citrate) and nitrates may result in irreversible hypotension. After patients have taken Viagra, it is unknown when nitrates can be safely administered.

Nitrates are found in many prescription medicines such as nitroglycerin (sprays, ointments, skin patches or pastes, and tablets), isosorbide mononitrate (Imdur), and isosorbide dinitrate (Isordil). Nitrates are also found in recreational drugs such as amyl nitrate or nitrite. Street names for amyl nitrite inhalants include "Amy" and "poppers."

Table 7-8 Morphine Sulfate

Generic Name	morphine sulfate
Trade Name(s)	Duramorph; Infumorph; MS Contin; MSIR; Oramorph; Roxanol
Classification	Narcotic (opioid) analgesic
Pronunciation	MOR-feen
How Supplied	Injection: 0.5 mg/mL, 1 mg/mL, 2 mg/mL, 4 mg/mL, 5 mg/mL, 8 mg/mL, 10 mg/mL, 15 mg/mL, 25 mg/mL, 50 mg/mL
Mechanism of Action	The principal actions of a therapeutic value of morphine are analgesia, sedation, and alterations of mood. Opioids of this class do not usually eliminate pain, but they do reduce the *perception* of pain by the central nervous system. • Reduces pain of ischemia • Reduces anxiety • Increases venous capacitance (venous pooling) and decreases venous return (preload) (sometimes called "chemical phlebotomy") • Decreases systemic vascular resistance (afterload) • Decreases myocardial oxygen demand (Pain ↑ sympathetic response → ↑ heart rate, ↑ systemic vascular resistance, ↑ blood pressure → ↑ myocardial O_2 consumption = reason pain relief is a priority in the management of the patient with an acute coronary syndrome)
Indications	• Analgesia in patients with an acute coronary syndrome • Acute cardiogenic pulmonary edema (SBP >90 mm Hg)
Dosing (adult)	2 to 4 mg (administer in 2-mg increments) slow IV push over 4 to 5 min until desired effect is achieved. May repeat every 5 to 30 min as needed
Precautions	Watch closely for: • Bradycardia • CNS depression • Nausea/vomiting • Respiratory depression (most serious side effect—reversible with naloxone or nalmefene) • Hypotension
Contraindications	• Hypersensitivity to morphine or other opiates • Respiratory depression • CNS depression caused by head injury, overdose, poisoning, etc. • Increased intracranial pressure • Asthma (relative) • Undiagnosed abdominal pain • Hypovolemia • Hypotension
Special Considerations	Ensure naloxone or nalmefene and airway equipment are readily available before administration
Onset of Action	IV: Immediate (peak 20 min)
Duration	IV: 2 to 4 hours

Table 7-9   Naloxone

Generic Name	naloxone hydrochloride
Trade Name(s)	Narcan
Classification	Narcotic antagonist
Pronunciation	nal-OX-ohn
How Supplied	Injection: 0.02 mg/mL, 0.4 mg/mL
Mechanism of Action	While the mechanism of action of naloxone is not fully understood, evidence suggests naloxone antagonizes the effects of opiates by competing for the same receptor sites, thereby preventing or reversing the effects of narcotics, including respiratory depression, sedation, and hypotension
Indications	• Coma of unknown etiology to rule out (or reverse) opiate-induced coma • Opiate induced respiratory depression
Dosing (adult)	• IV, IM, SC–Narcotic Overdose-Known or Suspected: Initial dose 0.4 mg to 2 mg. If the desired degree of counteraction and improvement in respiratory functions is not obtained, it may be repeated at 2 to 3 minute intervals. If no response is observed after 10 mg of naloxone have been administered, reevaluate diagnosis. Intramuscular or subcutaneous administration may be necessary if the intravenous route is not available. • IM or SC: 0.8 mg • Endotracheal dose: 2.0 mg
Precautions	Several instances of hypotension, hypertension, ventricular tachycardia and fibrillation, and pulmonary edema have been reported. These have occurred in postoperative patients most of whom had pre-existing cardiovascular disorders or received other drugs that may have similar adverse cardiovascular effects. Although a direct cause and effect relationship has not been established, naloxone injection should be used with caution in patients with pre-existing cardiac disease or patients who have received potentially cardiotoxic drugs. Abrupt reversal of narcotic depression may result in: • Nausea, vomiting • Sweating • Tachycardia • Increased blood pressure • Tremulousness • Seizures • Cardiac arrest
Contraindications	Known hypersensitivity to the medication
Special Considerations	• Ineffective if respiratory depression is caused by hypnotics, sedatives, anesthetics, or other nonnarcotic CNS depressants • Effects of narcotics are usually longer than those of naloxone; thus, respiratory depression may return when naloxone has worn off. Monitor the patient closely
Onset of Action	IV: 2 min, SC/IM: <5 min
Duration	IV: 45 min, SC/IM: 45 to 60 min

Table 7-10   Acetylsalicylic acid (aspirin)

Generic Name	acetylsalicylic acid
Trade Name(s)	Bufferin; Anacin; APC
Classification	Nonnarcotic analgesic; antipyretic; antiinflammatory
Pronunciation	ah-SEE-till-sal-ih-SILL-ick AH-sid
How Supplied	Tablets: 81 and 325 mg
Mechanism of Action	• When an atherosclerotic plaque ruptures or erodes, within 1 to 5 sec platelets adhere to the damaged lining of the vessel and to each other, forming a plug • "Sticky platelets" secrete several chemicals including thromboxane A_2. These substances stimulate vasoconstriction, reducing blood flow at the site • Aspirin blocks the synthesis of thromboxane A_2, inhibiting platelet aggregation
Indications	• Chest pain or other signs/symptoms suggestive of an acute coronary syndrome (unless hypersensitive to aspirin) • Unstable angina • ECG changes suggestive of acute MI
Dosing (adult)	• Initial dose of 162-325 mg non-enteric formulation followed by 75-160 mg/day of an enteric or a non-enteric formulation.[5] In patients who present with suspected ACS who are not already receiving aspirin, the first dose may be chewed to rapidly establish a high blood level. Subsequent doses may be swallowed. • Consider ticlopidine or clopidogrel is aspirin allergy, intolerant, or ineffective • Rectal suppository may be used for patients who cannot take aspirin orally
Precautions	• Asthma (relative contraindication) • Active ulcer disease (relative contraindication)
Contraindications	• Hypersensitivity to aspirin and/or nonsteroidal antiinflammatory agents • Recent history of GI bleeding • Bleeding disorders (hemophilia)
Onset of Action	20 to 30 min
Duration	4 to 6 hours

QUICK REVIEW

1. In general, a patient experiencing an acute coronary syndrome should receive "MONA." Can you recall each medication and its dosage?

2. Name two indications for administration of morphine sulfate.

1. Oxygen 4L/min, aspirin 162 to 325 mg (chewed), nitroglycerin 0.4 mg SL tablets × 3 (5 min apart), morphine 2 to 4 mg q 5 min.   2. Analgesia in patients with an acute coronary syndrome, acute cardiogenic pulmonary edema (SBP >90 mm Hg).

Glycoprotein IIb/IIIa Inhibitors

Table 7-11   Glycoprotein IIb/IIIa Inhibitors

Generic/Trade Name(s) Abciximab-ReoPro®; Eptifibatide-Integrilin®; Tirofiban-Aggrastat®

Pronunciation Abciximab: ab-SIX-ih-mab; Eptifibatide: ep-tih-FY-beh-tide; Tirofiban: ty-roh-FYE-ban

How Supplied
- Abciximab-Injection: 2 mg/mL; Eptifibatide-Injection: 0.75 mg/mL, 2 mg/mL;
- Tirofiban-Injection: 50 mcg/mL; Injection for solution: 250 mcg/mL

Mechanism of Action Aspirin blocks the synthesis of thromboxane A_2, inhibiting platelet aggregation. Despite the absence of thromboxane A_2, platelets may be induced to aggregate by triggers such as thrombin, subendothelial collagen, or stainless steel from intracoronary stents. Once platelets are activated, glycoprotein IIb/IIIa receptors that are essential for platelet aggregation appear on the surface of the platelet. Fibrinogen molecules bind to these receptors to form bridges ("cross-links") between adjacent platelets, allowing them to aggregate. Glycoprotein IIb/IIIa receptor inhibitors prevent fibrinogen binding and platelet aggregation, regardless of the trigger responsible for platelet aggregation[7]

Indications For use in patients experiencing an MI without ST segment elevation who have some high-risk features and/or refractory ischemia, provided they do not have a contraindication because of a bleeding risks

Dosing (adult) *Abciximab*
- Acute coronary syndromes with planned percutaneous coronary intervention (PCI) within 24 hours: Patients with unstable angina not responding to conventional medical therapy and who are planned to undergo percutaneous coronary intervention within 24 hours may be treated with an abciximab 0.25 mg/kg IV bolus followed by an 18- to 24-hour IV intravenous infusion of 10 mcg/min, concluding 1 hour after the PCI
- PCI only: 0.25 mg/kg intravenous bolus administered 10 to 60 min before the start of PCI, followed by a continuous IV infusion of 0.125 mcg/kg/min (to a maximum of 10 mcg/min) for 12 hours

Eptifibatide
- Acute coronary syndromes: If serum creatinine <2.0 mg/dl, give 180 mcg/kg IV bolus as soon as possible following diagnosis, followed by a continuous infusion of 2 mcg/kg/min until hospital discharge or initiation of CABG surgery, up to 72 hours. If the patient is to undergo a PCI while receiving eptifibatide, the infusion should be continued up to hospital discharge, or for up to 18-24 hours after the procedure, whichever comes first, allowing for up to 96 hours of therapy. Patients weighing more than 121 kg should receive a maximum bolus of 22.6 mg followed by a maximum infusion rate of 15 mg/hour. If serum creatinine between 2.0 and 4.0 mg/dl, give 180 mcg/kg IV bolus as soon as possible following diagnosis, immediately followed by a continuous infusion of 1.0 mcg/kg/min. If serum creatinine is between 2.0 and 4.0 mg/dl and weight is more than 121 kg, the patient should receive a maximum bolus of 22.6 mg followed by a maximum infusion rate of 7.5 mg/hour.
- PCI: If serum creatinine <2.0 mg/dl at the time of PCI, give 180 mcg/kg IV bolus immediately before the initiation of PCI followed by a continuous infusion of 2.0 mcg/kg/min and a second 180 mcg/kg bolus 10 minutes after the first bolus. Infusion should be continued until hospital discharge, or for up to 18-24 hours, whichever comes first. A minimum of 12 hours of infusion is recommended. Patients weighing more than 121 kg should receive a maximum of 22.6 mg per bolus followed by a maximum infusion rate of 15 mg/hour. If serum creatinine between 2.0 and 4.0 mg/dl at the time of PCI, give 180 mcg/kg IV bolus immediately before the initiation of the procedure, immediately followed by a continuous infusion of 1.0 mcg/kg/min and a second 180 mcg/kg bolus administered 10 minutes after the first. If serum creatinine is between 2.0 and 4.0 mg/dl and weight is more than 121 kg, the patient should receive a maximum of 22.6 mg per bolus followed by a maximum infusion rate of 7.5 mg/hour.

Tirofiban
- Acute coronary syndromes or PCI: In most patients, tirofiban should be administered IV at an initial rate of 0.4 mcg/kg/min for 30 min and then continued at 0.1 mcg/kg/min. Patients with severe renal insufficiency (creatinine clearance <30 mL/min) should receive half the usual rate of infusion.

Table 7-11 Glycoprotein IIb/IIIa Inhibitors—cont'd

Precautions

Minimize arterial and venous punctures, IM injections, and use of urinary catheters, nasotracheal intubation, and nasogastric tubes. When establishing IV access, avoid non-compressible sites (e.g., subclavian or jugular veins)

Abciximab
- Initial half-life of less than 10 min, second phase half-life about 30 min
- Intended for use with aspirin and heparin
- Platelet function generally recovers over the course of 48 hours
- Readministration of abciximab may result in allergic or hypersensitivity reactions (including anaphylaxis)
- No incompatibilities have been shown with intravenous infusion fluids or commonly used cardiovascular drugs. Nevertheless, abciximab should be administered in a separate IV line whenever possible and not mixed with other medications
- In the event of serious bleeding that cannot be controlled by compression, abciximab and heparin should be discontinued immediately

Eptifibatide
- Half-life approximately 2 1/2 hours
- Should not be administered through the same IV line as furosemide
- Vials should be stored refrigerated at 36° to 46° F
- Platelet function generally recovers within 4 to 8 hours after discontinuation
- In patients who undergo coronary artery bypass graft surgery, eptifibatide infusion should be discontinued before surgery
- In the clinical trials that showed eptifibatide to be effective, most patients received concomitant aspirin and heparin

Tirofiban
- Half-life approximately 2 1/2 hours
- Platelet function generally recovers within 4 to 8 hours after discontinuation
- In clinical studies, patients receiving tirofiban also received aspirin (unless it was contraindicated) and heparin

QUICK REVIEW

1. How do glycoprotein IIb/IIIa inhibitors work?

2. When are glycoprotein IIb/IIIa inhibitors indicated?

1. Prevent fibrinogen binding and platelet aggregation.   2. For use in patients experiencing an MI without ST-segment elevation who have some high-risk features and/or refractory ischemia, provided they do not have a contraindication because of a bleeding risk.

Antiplatelet Agents

Table 7-12 Ticlopidine

Generic Name	ticlopidine
Trade Name(s)	Ticlid
Classification	Antiplatelet agent
Pronunciation	tie-KLOH-pih-deen
How Supplied	*Tablet:* 250 mg
Mechanism of Action	• Ticlopidine causes a time- and dose-dependent inhibition of both platelet aggregation and release of platelet granule constituents as well as a prolongation of bleeding time
Indications	• To reduce the risk of thrombotic stroke (fatal or nonfatal) in patients who have experienced stroke precursors and in patients who have had a completed thrombotic stroke. Because of the risk of neutropenia or agranulocytosis, use should be reserved for patients intolerant to aspirin therapy
Dosing (adult)	250 mg BID taken with food
Contraindications	• Hypersensitivity to the drug • Presence of hematopoietic disorders, such as neutropenia and thrombocytopenia • Presence of a hemostatic disorder or active pathologic bleeding (e.g., bleeding peptic ulcer or intracranial bleeding) • Patients with severe liver impairment
Special Considerations	• Prolonged bleeding time is normalized within 2 hours after administration of 20 mg methylprednisolone IV. Platelet transfusions may also be used to reverse the effect of ticlopidine HCl on bleeding • In most patients, bleeding time and other platelet function tests return to normal within 2 weeks after discontinuation of the drug • Causes increased serum cholesterol and triglycerides. Serum total cholesterol levels are increased 8% to 10% within 1 month of therapy and persist at that level

Table 7-13 Clopidogrel

Generic Name	clopidogrel
Trade Name(s)	Plavix
Classification	Antiplatelet agent, anticoagulant
Pronunciation	kloh-PID-oh-grel
How Supplied	*Tablet:* 75 mg
Mechanism of Action	• Selectively inhibits the binding of adenosine diphosphate (ADP) to its platelet receptor and subsequent ADP-mediated activation of the glycoprotein GPIIb/IIIa complex, thereby inhibiting platelet aggregation. Also inhibits platelet aggregation induced by agonists other than ADP by blocking amplification of platelet activation by released ADP. • Acts by irreversibly modifying the platelet ADP receptor. Consequently, platelets exposed to clopidogrel are affected for the remainder of their lifespan
Indications	Reduction of MI, stroke, and vascular death in patients with atherosclerosis documented by recent stroke, MI, or established peripheral arterial disease
Dosing (adult)	75 mg once daily with or without food
Contraindications	• Hypersensitivity to the drug substance or any component of the product. • Active pathologic bleeding, such as peptic ulcer or intracranial hemorrhage
Special Considerations	Platelet aggregation and bleeding time gradually return to baseline values after treatment is discontinued, generally in about 5 days

Table 7-14   Dipyridamole

Generic Name	dipyridamole
Trade Name(s)	Persantine
Classification	Platelet adhesion inhibitor; antianginal; coronary vasodilator
Pronunciation	dye-peer-ID-ah-mohl
How Supplied	• Injection: 5 mg/mL • Tablets: 25 mg, 50 mg, 75 mg
Mechanism of Action	Dipyridamole is a platelet adhesion inhibitor although its mechanism of action is not completely clear
Indications	*Oral* • Adjunct to coumarin anticoagulants in the prevention of postoperative thrombo-embolic complications after cardiac valve replacement • With aspirin to reduce the risk of stroke in patients who have previously had a stroke or a TIA *IV* • Alternative to exercise in thallium myocardial perfusion imaging for the evaluation of coronary artery disease in those who cannot exercise adequately
Dosing (adult)	• Adjunct in prophylaxis of thromboembolism after cardiac valve replacement: Tablets 75 to 100 mg QID as adjunct to warfarin therapy • Prevention of thromboembolic complications in other thromboembolic disorders: Tablets 150 to 400 mg/day in combination with another platelet-aggregation inhibitor (e.g., aspirin) or an anticoagulant • Adjunct to thallium myocardial perfusion imaging: IV, adjust dose according to body weight. Recommended dose 0.142 mg/kg/min infused over 4 min. Total dose should not exceed 60 mg
Contraindications	Hypersensitivity to dipyridamole

Fibrinolytic Agents

Table 7-15   Alteplase

Generic Name	alteplase recombinant; tissue plasminogen activator
Trade Name(s)	Activase, tPA
Classification	Fibrinolytic
Pronunciation	AL-teh-playz
How Supplied	Powder for injection: 50 mg, 100 mg
Mechanism of Action	Alteplase recombinant is an enzyme that has the property of fibrin-enhanced conversion of plasminogen to plasmin. It produces limited conversion of plasminogen in the absence of fibrin. When introduced into the systemic circulation, alteplase binds to fibrin in a thrombus and converts the entrapped plasminogen to plasmin. This initiates local fibrinolysis with limited systemic proteolysis
Indications	• Improvement of ventricular function following acute MI, including reducing the incidence of CHF and decreasing mortality • Acute ischemic stroke, after intracranial hemorrhage has been excluded by CT scan or other diagnostic imaging • Acute pulmonary thromboembolism
Dosing (adult)	*Acute MI, accelerated infusion (1.5 hours):* Recommended total dose is based on patient weight, not to exceed 100 mg • *Weight >67 kg (148 lbs):* 15 mg IV bolus, followed by 50 mg infused over the next 30 min, and then by 35 mg infused over the next 60 min • *Weight ≤67 kg (148 lbs):* 15 mg bolus, followed by 0.75 mg/kg over the next 30 min (not to exceed 50 mg), and then 0.50 mg/kg over the next 60 min (not to exceed 35 mg)

Continued

Table 7-15 Alteplase—cont'd

Acute MI, 3-hr infusion

Weight ≥65 kg (143 lbs): 100 mg IV administered over 3 hours as follows:

- *First hour:* 60 mg. Administer 6 to 10 mg within 1 to 2 min by IV bolus. Remaining 50 to 54 mg is given by IV infusion administered over the remainder of the hour. *Second hour:* 20 mg by IV infusion. *Third hour:* 20 mg by IV infusion

Weight <65 kg: 1.25 mg/kg given over 3 hours as follows:

- *First hour:* 60% of the total dose. Initially, 6% to 10% of the dose within 1 to 2 min by IV bolus. The next 50% to 54% of the dose by IV infusion administered over the remainder of the hour. *Second hour:* 20% of the dose by IV infusion. *Third hour:* 20% of the dose by IV infusion
- Patients should receive 162 to 325 mg chewable aspirin as soon as possible
- Begin heparin immediately and continue for 48 hours

Acute pulmonary embolism

- The recommended dose is 100 mg administered by intravenous infusion over 2 hours. Heparin therapy should be instituted or reinstituted near the end of or immediately following the alteplase infusion when the partial thromboplastin time or thrombin time returns to twice normal or less.

Acute ischemic stroke

- 0.9 mg/kg (maximum of 90 mg) by IV infusion (over 60 min), with 10% of the total dose administered as an initial IV loading dose over 1 min
- Doses greater than 0.9 mg/kg may cause an increased incidence of intracranial hemorrhage

Contraindications

Acute MI or pulmonary embolism

- Active internal bleeding
- History of stroke
- Recent (within 2 months) intracranial or intraspinal surgery or trauma
- Intracranial neoplasm, arteriovenous malformation, or aneurysm
- Known bleeding diathesis
- Severe uncontrolled hypertension

Acute ischemic stroke

- Symptoms of intracranial hemorrhage on pretreatment evaluation
- Suspected subarachnoid hemorrhage
- Recent intracranial surgery or serious head trauma
- Recent previous stroke
- History of intracranial hemorrhage
- Uncontrolled hypertension (SBP >185 mm Hg or DBP >110 mm Hg) at time of treatment
- Active internal bleeding
- Seizure at onset of stroke
- Intracranial neoplasm, AV malformation, or aneurysm
- Bleeding diathesis

Special Considerations Pay careful attention to all potential bleeding sites (including catheter insertion sites, arterial and venous puncture sites, cutdown sites, and needle puncture sites)

Duration >50% present in plasma is cleared within 5 min after the infusion has been terminated, and ~80% is cleared within 10 min

Table 7-16 Anistreplase

Generic Name	anistreplase, anisoylated plasminogen streptokinase activator complex (APSAC)
Trade Name(s)	Eminase
Classification	Fibrinolytic, thrombolytic enzyme
Pronunciation	an-ih-STREP-layz
How Supplied	Powder for injection: 30 U
Mechanism of Action	Anistreplase is a complex composed of streptokinase and human lys-plasminogen. Activation of anistreplase occurs with release of the anisoyl group by deacylation, a non-enzymatic process with a half-life in vitro in human blood of about 2 hours. In solution, deacylation of anistreplase starts immediately, and the enzymatically active lys-plasminogen-streptokinase activator complex is progressively formed. The production of plasmin from plasminogen by deacylated anistreplase can take place in the bloodstream or within the thrombus
Indications	• Management of acute myocardial infarction (AMI) in adults • For lysis of thrombi obstructing coronary arteries • Reduction of infarct size • Improvement of ventricular function following AMI • Reduction of mortality associated with AMI
Dosing (adult)	*IV only:* 30 units (U) over 2 to 5 min into an IV line or vein as soon as possible after onset of symptoms. Reconstitute 30 U in 50-mL sterile water or D5W
Precautions	May not be effective if administered more than 5 days after prior anistreplase or streptokinase therapy, particularly between 5 days and 12 months. Increased antistreptokinase antibody levels after anistreplase or streptokinase may also increase the risk of allergic reactions following readministration
Contraindications	• Active internal bleeding • History of cerebrovascular accident • Recent (within 2 months) intracranial or intraspinal surgery or trauma • Intracranial neoplasm, arteriovenous malformation, or aneurysm • Known bleeding diathesis • Severe, uncontrolled hypertension
Special Considerations	• Pay careful attention to all potential bleeding sites (including catheter insertion sites, arterial and venous puncture sites, cutdown sites, and needle puncture sites) • Discard if not administered within 30 min of reconstitution • Patency of occluded arteries and myocardial perfusion usually occurs 45 min following IV administration. Half-life of fibrinolytic activity of circulating anistreplase is 70 to 120 min (mean 94 min); however, fibrinolytic action can persist for 6 hours • Reduces mortality when administered within 6 hours of onset of symptoms of AMI • Use in patients >75 years has not been adequately studied
Drug Interactions	Increased risk of bleeding or hemorrhage if used with heparin, oral anticoagulants, vitamin K antagonists, aspirin, or dipyridamole

Table 7-17   Reteplase

Generic Name	reteplase
Trade Name(s)	Retavase
Classification	Fibrinolytics
Pronunciation	REE-teh-place
How Supplied	Kit: 10.8 U
Mechanism of Action	Reteplase is a recombinant plasminogen activator that catalyzes the cleavage of endogenous plasminogen to generate plasmin. Plasmin in turn degrades the fibrin matrix of the thrombus, thereby exerting its thrombolytic action
Indications	Management of AMI in adults by improving ventricular function following AMI, reduction of the incidence of congestive heart failure, and reduction of mortality associated with AMI. Treatment should be initiated as soon as possible after the onset of AMI symptoms
Dosing (adult)	*IV only* • Two 10-unit boluses, each given over 2 min • Second bolus given 30 min after first • Give flush of normal saline before and after each bolus • Patients should receive chewable aspirin as soon as possible • Begin heparin immediately and continue for 48 hours
Precautions	• Intramuscular injections and nonessential handling of the patient should be avoided during treatment • Monitor for bleeding complications • Perform venipunctures carefully and only when necessary • If arterial puncture is necessary, use an upper extremity that can be manually compressed
Contraindications	• Active internal bleeding • History of stroke • Recent intracranial or intraspinal surgery or trauma • Intracranial neoplasm, arteriovenous malformation, or aneurysm • Known bleeding diathesis • Severe uncontrolled hypertension
Special Considerations	• Pay careful attention to all potential bleeding sites (including catheter insertion sites, arterial and venous puncture sites, cutdown sites, and needle puncture sites) • Do **not** administer heparin and reteplase simultaneously in the same IV line. If reteplase is to be injected through an IV line containing heparin, flush a normal saline or 5% dextrose solution through the line before and after the reteplase injection
Duration	Half-life: 13 to 16 min
Drug Interactions	Use with abciximab, aspirin, dipyridamole, heparin, or vitamin K antagonists may increase risk of bleeding

Table 7-18 Streptokinase

Generic Name	streptokinase
Trade Name(s)	Streptase; Kabikinase
Classification	Fibrinolytic
Pronunciation	strep-toe-KI-nace
How Supplied	Powder for injection: 250,000 IU, 750,000 IU, 1.5 million IU
Mechanism of Action	Streptokinase acts with plasminogen to produce an "activator complex" that converts plasminogen to plasmin. Plasmin then breaks down fibrinogen, fibrin clots, and other plasma proteins, promoting lysis of the insoluble fibrin trapped in intravascular emboli and thrombi
Indications	• Acute evolving MI • Acute pulmonary embolism • Deep vein thrombosis (DVT) • Acute arterial thrombosis and embolism
Dosing (adult)	*Acute MI* • 1.5 million units IV within a 1-hour infusion period *Acute pulmonary embolism, deep vein thrombosis (DVT), or acute arterial thromboembolism:* • Since human exposure to streptococci is common, antibodies to strepto-kinase are prevalent. Thus, a loading dose of streptokinase sufficient to neutralize these antibodies is required. A dose of 250,000 IU of streptokinase infused into a peripheral vein over 30 minutes has been found appropriate in over 90% of patients. This should be followed by 100,000 IU/hour as an IV infusion. Continue the infusion for 72 hours for deep vein thrombosis, 24 hours for pulmonary embolism (72 hours if concurrent DVT is suspected), and 24-72 hours for arterial thromboembolism
Precautions	May not be effective if administered between 5 days and 12 months of prior strepto-kinase or anistreplase administration or streptococcal infections, such as streptococcal pharyngitis, acute rheumatic fever, or acute glomerulonephritis secondary to a streptococcal infection
Contraindications	• Active internal bleeding • Recent (within 2 months) stroke, intracranial or intraspinal surgery • Intracranial neoplasm • Severe uncontrolled hypertension • Patients having experienced severe allergic reaction to the product
Special Considerations	• Pay careful attention to all potential bleeding sites (including catheter insertion sites, arterial and venous puncture sites, cutdown sites, and needle puncture sites) • Hypotension, sometimes severe, not secondary to bleeding or anaphylaxis has been observed during IV streptokinase infusion in 1% to 10% of patients • In acute MI, the greatest benefit in mortality reduction has been observed when streptokinase was administered within 4 hours of symptom onset, but statistically significant benefits have been reported up to 24 hours
Onset of Action	Rapid
Duration	12 hours
Drug Interactions	Increased risk of bleeding when the following are administered concomitantly with streptokinase: anticoagulants, aspirin, heparin, indomethacin, and phenylbutazone

Table 7-19 Tenecteplase

Generic Name	tenecteplase
Trade Name(s)	TNKase
Classification	Fibrinolytic
Pronunciation	ten-eck-teh-place
How Supplied	Powder for injection, lyophilized (recombinant): 50 mg
Mechanism of Action	Initiates fibrinolysis by binding to fibrin and converting plasminogen to plasmin
Indications	Reduce mortality associated with acute MI
Dosing (adult)	Recommended total dose should not exceed 50 mg and is based on weight. Administer as an IV bolus over 5 sec: • <60 kg: 30 mg • >60 to <70 kg: 35 mg • >70 to <80 kg: 40 mg • >80 to <90 kg: 45 mg • >90 kg: 50 mg • Reconstitute using the supplied 10-mL syringe with TwinPak™ Dual Cannula Device and 10 mL sterile water for injection • Incompatible with dextrose solutions. Dextrose-containing lines must be flushed with a saline solution before and after administration • Administer as a single IV bolus over 5 sec
Precautions	• Stop antiplatelet agents and heparin if serious bleeding occurs • Intramuscular injections and nonessential handling of the patient should be avoided during treatment • Monitor for bleeding complications • Perform venipunctures carefully and only when necessary • If arterial puncture is necessary, use an upper extremity that can be manually compressed
Contraindications	• Hypersensitivity to tenecteplase or any component • Active internal bleeding • History of stroke • Intracranial/intraspinal surgery or trauma within 2 months • Intracranial neoplasm, AV malformation, or aneurysm • Known bleeding diathesis • Severe uncontrolled hypertension
Special Considerations	Pay careful attention to all potential bleeding sites (including catheter insertion sites, arterial and venous puncture sites, cutdown sites, and needle puncture sites) If reconstituted and not used immediately, store in refrigerator and use within 8 hours Tenecteplase is also known as TNK-tPA. "TNK" refers to the sites of the tPA molecule that have been modified
Drug Interactions	Use with abciximab, aspirin, dipyridamole, heparin, or vitamin K antagonists may increase risk of bleeding

**Contraindications and Cautions for
Fibrinolytic Use in Myocardial Infarction[5]**

Absolute Contraindications
- Previous hemorrhagic stroke at any time: other strokes or cerebrovascular events within 1 year
- Known intracranial neoplasm
- Active internal bleeding (does not include menses)
- Suspected aortic dissection

Cautions/Relative Contraindications
- Severe uncontrolled hypertension on presentation (blood pressure >180/110 mm Hg) (could be an absolute contraindication in low-risk patients with MI)
- History of prior cerebrovascular accident or known intracerebral pathology not covered in contraindications
- Current use of anticoagulants in therapeutic doses (International Normalized Ratio ≥2-3); known bleeding diathesis
- Recent trauma (within 2 to 4 weeks), including head trauma
- Noncompressible vascular punctures
- Recent (within 2 to 4 weeks) internal bleeding
- For streptokinase/anistreplase: prior exposure (especially within 5 days to 2 years) or prior allergic reaction
- Pregnancy
- Active peptic ulcer
- History of chronic hypertension

Heparin

Table 7-20   Heparin (Unfractionated)

Generic Name	heparin
Trade Name(s)	Sodium Heparin, Liquaemin Sodium
Classification	Anticoagulant
Pronunciation	HEP-ah-rin
How Supplied	Heparin sodium injection: 1000 U/mL, 2000 U/mL, 2500 U/mL, 5000 U/mL, 7500 U/mL, 10,000 U/mL, 20,000 U/mL
Mechanism of Action	Heparin inhibits reactions that lead to blood clotting and formation of fibrin clots. Heparin acts at multiple sites in the normal coagulation system. Small amounts of heparin in combination with antithrombin III (heparin cofactor) can inhibit thrombosis by inactivating activated Factor X and inhibiting the conversion of prothrombin to thrombin. Once active thrombosis has developed, larger amounts of heparin can inhibit further coagulation by inactivating thrombin and preventing the conversion of fibrinogen to fibrin. Heparin also prevents the formation of a stable fibrin clot by inhibiting the activation of the fibrin-stabilizing factor
Indications[5]	**Class I** • Patients undergoing percutaneous or surgical revascularization **Class IIa** • IV in patients undergoing reperfusion therapy with selective fibrinolytics agents (e.g., alteplase, reteplase, tenecteplase) • IV unfractionated heparin (UFH) or low-molecular-weight heparin (LMWH) subcutaneously for patients with non-ST elevation MI • Subcutaneous UFH (e.g., 7,500 U BID.) or LMWH (e.g., enoxaparin 1 mg/kg BID) in all patients not treated with fibrinolytic therapy and who do not have a contraindication to heparin. In patients at high risk for systemic emboli (large or anterior MI, atrial fibrillation, previous embolus, or known left ventricular thrombus), IV heparin is preferred

Continued

Table 7-20   Heparin (Unfractionated)—cont'd

	• IV in patients treated with nonselective fibrinolytic agents (streptokinase, anistreplase) at high risk for systemic emboli (large or anterior MI, atrial fibrillation, previous embolus, or known left ventricular thrombus)
	Class IIb
	• Patients treated with nonselective thrombolytic agents, not at high risk, subcutaneous heparin, 7500 U to 12500 U twice a day until completely ambulatory
	Class III
	• Routine IV heparin within 6 hours to patients receiving a nonselective fibrinolytic agent (streptokinase, anistreplase) who are not at high risk for systemic emboli
Dosing (adult)[5]	**IV dosing in patients undergoing reperfusion therapy**
	• *Bolus dose:* 60 U/kg as an IV bolus (maximum bolus 4000 U) at initiation of fibrinolytic infusion
	• *Maintenance dose:* Approximately 12 U/kg/h (maximum 1000 U/h infusion for patients weighing >70 kg), adjusted to maintain activated partial thromboplastin time (aPTT) at 1.5 to 2.0 times control (50 to 70 sec) for 48 hours or until angiography
	• Continuation of heparin infusion beyond 48 hours should be considered in patients at high risk for systemic or venous thromboembolism
	• Check aPTT at 6, 12, 18, and 24 hours. Follow institutional heparin protocol
Precautions	It has been reported that patients on heparin may develop new thrombus formation in association with thrombocytopenia resulting from irreversible aggregation of platelets induced by the heparin—the so-called "white clot syndrome." The process may lead to severe thromboembolic complications, including skin necrosis, gangrene of the extremities that may lead to amputation, MI, pulmonary embolism, stroke, and possibly death.
	Discontinue heparin administration promptly if a patient develops new thrombosis in association with a reduction in platelet count
Contraindications	Should not be used in patients:
	• With severe thrombocytopenia
	• In whom suitable blood coagulation tests (e.g., the whole-blood clotting time, partial thromboplastin time, etc.) cannot be performed at appropriate intervals (this contraindication refers to full-dose heparin; there is usually no need to monitor coagulation parameters in patients receiving low-dose heparin).
	• With an uncontrollable active bleeding state, except when this is caused by disseminated intravascular coagulation
Special Considerations	Anticoagulants prevent new clots from forming but do not dissolve previously formed clots

Low Molecular Weight Heparin

Table 7-21   Enoxaparin

Generic Name	enoxaparin
Trade Name(s)	Lovenox; Clexane
Classification	Anticoagulant; low-molecular-weight heparin
Pronunciation	ee-nox-ah-PAIR-in
How Supplied	• Injection: Prefilled syringes: 30 mg/0.3 mL, 40 mg/0.4 mL • Injection: Graduated prefilled syringes: 60 mg/0.6 mL, 80 mg/0.8 mL, 100 mg/1 mL
Mechanism of Action	Low-molecular-weight heparin with antithrombotic properties
Indications	In conjunction with aspirin to prevent ischemic complications of unstable angina and non-ST-elevation MI
Dosing (adult)	1 mg/kg SC every 12 hours in conjunction with oral aspirin therapy (100 to 325 mg once daily for a minimum of 2 days). Usual duration for enoxaparin therapy is 2 to 8 days
Precautions	• Should not be mixed with other injections or infusions • Periodic complete blood counts, including platelet count, and stool occult blood tests are recommended during the course of treatment
Contraindications	• Known hypersensitivity to heparin or pork products • Hypersensitivity to enoxaparin • Active major bleeding • Thrombocytopenia associated with a positive in vitro test for anti-platelet antibody in the presence of enoxaparin
Special Considerations	• Cannot be used interchangeably (unit for unit) with unfractionated heparin or other low-molecular-weight heparins • Not intended for intramuscular administration

Table 7-22   Dalteparin

Generic Name	dalteparin
Trade Name(s)	Fragmin
Classification	Anticoagulant, low-molecular-weight heparin
Pronunciation	DAL-tih-pair-in
How Supplied	Injection: 2500 IU/0.2 mL, 5000 IU/0.2 mL, 10,000 IU/mL
Mechanism of Action	Low-molecular-weight heparin with antithrombotic properties
Indications	In conjunction with aspirin to prevent ischemic complications of unstable angina and non–ST-elevation MI
Dosing (adult)	120 IU/kg of body weight, but not more than 10,000 IU, SC every 12 hours with concurrent oral aspirin (75-165 mg once daily) therapy. Treatment should be continued until the patient is clinically stabilized. The usual duration of administration is 5-8 days. Concurrent aspirin therapy is recommended except when contraindicated
Precautions	• Dalteparin sodium should not be mixed with other injections or infusions unless specific compatibility data are available that support such mixing • Periodic complete blood counts, including platelet count, and stool occult blood tests are recommended during the course of treatment
Contraindications	• Known hypersensitivity to heparin or pork products • Hypersensitivity to enoxaparin • Active major bleeding • Thrombocytopenia associated with a positive in vitro test for anti-platelet antibody in the presence of dalteparin sodium
Special Considerations	• Cannot be used interchangeably (unit for unit) with unfractionated heparin or other low-molecular-weight heparins • Not intended for intramuscular administration

Thrombin Inhibitors

Table 7-23 Hirudin Therapy	
Generic/Trade Name(s)	lepirudin (Refludan) bivalirudin (Angioman)
Classification	Anticoagulant
Pronunciation	lepirudin: leh-PEER-you-din; bivalirudin: by-val-ih-ROO-din
How Supplied	lepirudin—50 mg/vial
Mechanism of Action	Lepirudin is recombinant hirudin. Bivalirudin is a synthetic direct thrombin inhibitor. Hirudin is a naturally occurring specific thrombin inhibitor. Hirudin, derived from the saliva of the medicinal leech, is an anticoagulant that binds to thrombin with a very high affinity, rendering it inactive. Hirudin inhibits thrombus-induced platelet activation; heparin does not[8]
Indications	*Lepirudin* • Concomitant use with fibrinolytics *Bivalirudin* • Unstable angina • Adjunct to streptokinase in acute MI • To reduce ischemic complications in postinfarction MI patients undergoing coronary angioplasty
Dosing (adult)	*Lepirudin* **Concomitant use with fibrinolytics** • Initial IV bolus: 0.2 mg/kg slowly over 15 to 20 sec • Continuous IV infusion: 0.1 mg/kg/hr *Bivalirudin* **MI patients undergoing coronary angioplasty** • Initial IV bolus: 1 mg/kg; then 2.5 mg/kg/hr for 4 hr by continuous IV infusion followed by 0.2 mg/kg/hr for 14 to 20 hr. Initiate immediately before angioplasty. Intended for use with aspirin (300-325 mg daily) **Unstable angina** • 0.2 mg/kg/hr by continuous IV infusion for up to 5 days. Use in addition to aspirin, nitrates, or calcium channel blockers **Adjunct to streptokinase in acute MI** • 0.5 mg/kg/hr by IV infusion, decreasing to 0.1 mg/kg/hr after 12 hr. Start infusion immediately before or with streptokinase, 1.5 million units IV over 60 min. Continue infusion until 1 hr before second angiogram (average of 4.7 days). 325 mg aspirin is given before bivalirudin/streptokinase therapy
Contraindications	*Lepirudin* • Known hypersensitivity to hirudins *Bivalirudin* • Cerebral aneurysm • Intracranial hemorrhage • General uncontrollable hemorrhage • Known hypersensitivity to hirudins

Angiotensin Converting Enzyme (ACE) Inhibitors

Table 7-24 ACE Inhibitors

Generic/Trade Names	captopril (Capoten); enalapril (Vasotec); lisinopril (Prinivil, Zestril); ramipril (Altace)
Classification	Antihypertensive, ACE inhibitor
Pronunciation	captopril: KAP-toe-prill; enalapril: en-AL-ah-prill; lisinopril: lie-SIN-oh-prill; ramipril: RAM-ih-prill
How Supplied	• captopril—tablet: 12.5 mg, 25 mg, 50 mg, 100 mg • enalapril—tablet: 2.5 mg, 5 mg, 10 mg, 20 mg; injection: 1.25 mg/mL (as enalaprilat) • lisinopril—tablet: 2.5 mg, 5 mg, 10 mg, 20 mg, 40 mg • ramipril—capsule: 1.25 mg, 2.5 mg, 5 mg, 10 mg
Mechanism of Action	In the body, the hormone angiotensin I is converted to angiotensin II (the active form of angiotensin) by the action of angiotensin-converting enzyme (ACE). Angiotensin II causes vasoconstriction (more potent than norepinephrine) and increased aldosterone secretion from the kidneys. Aldosterone causes the kidneys to retain salt and water and to excrete potassium, leading to an increase in blood volume and blood pressure. ACE inhibitors prevent the conversion of angiotensin I to angiotensin II. As a result, blood vessels relax, reducing the pressure the heart must pump against, and decreasing myocardial workload. By increasing renal blood flow, ACE inhibitors help rid the body of excess sodium and fluid accumulation
Indications[5]	*Class I* • Patients within the first 24 hours of a suspected acute MI with ST-segment elevation in two or more anterior precordial leads or with clinical heart failure in the absence of hypotension (SBP <100 mm Hg) or known contraindications to use of ACE inhibitors • Patients with MI and LV ejection fraction less than 40% or patients with clinical heart failure on the basis of systolic pump dysfunction during and after convalescence from acute MI *Class IIa* • All other patients within the first 24 hours of a suspected or established acute MI, provided significant hypotension or other clear-cut contraindications are absent • Asymptomatic patients with mildly impaired LV function (ejection fraction 40% to 50%) and a history of old MI *Class IIb* • Patients who have recently recovered from MI but have normal or mildly abnormal global LV function
Dosing (adult)	*Captopril* • Left ventricular dysfunction after MI • Initial dose (oral): 6.25 mg; then begin 12.5 mg TID and increase to 25 mg TID over next several days. Target dose is 50 mg TID as tolerated. Aspirin, beta-blockers, fibrinolytics may be used concomitantly *Enalapril* • Oral: Start with a single dose of 2.5 mg. Increase gradually to a dose of 20 mg/day PO given in divided doses. Observe for hypotension for at least 2 hours following first dose and for at least 1 hour following stabilization of BP • IV: 1.25 mg IV every 6 hours. Administer slowly IV over at least 5 min *Lisinopril* • Oral: First dose 5 mg within 24 hours of symptom onset. Then 5 mg after 24 hours, 10 mg after 48 hours, and then 10 mg daily for 6 weeks • Patients with SBP ≤120 mm Hg when treatment is started or within 3 days after MI should receive 2.5 mg. If hypotension occurs (SBP <100 mm Hg), dose may be temporarily reduced to 2.5 mg. Withdraw drug if prolonged hypotension occurs *Ramipril* • Begin with single oral dose of 2.5 mg. Titrate to 5 mg orally BID as tolerated

Continued

Table 7-24 ACE Inhibitors—cont'd

Precautions	• Adjust dose in patients with renal impairment or renal failure • May cause a profound drop in BP following the first dose or if used with diuretics • Persistent nonproductive cough has been reported with all ACE inhibitors, resolving after discontinuation of therapy
Contraindications	• Hypersensitivity to ACE inhibitors (e.g., a patient who has experienced angioedema during therapy with any other ACE inhibitor) • Systolic blood pressure is <100 mm Hg • Presence of clinically relevant renal failure • History of bilateral renal artery stenosis
Special Considerations	When used in pregnancy during the second and third trimesters, ACE inhibitors can cause injury and even death to the developing fetus *Enalapril* • Clinical response usually seen within 15 minutes. Peak effects after the first dose may not occur for up to 4 hours after dosing. The peak effects of the second and subsequent doses may exceed those of the first.

Angiotensin Converting Enzyme Inhibitors: Recommendations[5]

Class I
• Patients within the first 24 hours of a suspected acute MI with ST-segment elevation in two or more anterior precordial leads or with clinical heart failure in the absence of hypotension (systolic blood pressure <100 mm Hg) or known contraindications to use of ACE inhibitors
• Patients with MI and LV ejection fraction less than 40% or patients with clinical heart failure on the basis of systolic pump dysfunction during and after convalescence from acute MI

Class IIa
• All other patients within the first 24 hours of a suspected or established acute MI, provided significant hypotension or other clear-cut contraindications are absent
• Asymptomatic patients with mildly impaired LV function (ejection fraction 40% to 50%) and a history of old MI

Class IIb
• Patients who have recently recovered from MI but have normal or mildly abnormal global LV function

MEDICATIONS USED TO MANAGE CARDIAC DYSRHYTHMIAS

The following medications are used in managing cardiac dysrhythmias (Tables 7-25 to 7-41).

Table 7-25 Classification of Antiarrhythmic Medications

Class	Class I			Class II	Class III	Class IV	
	Class Ia	Class Ib	Class Ic			Class IVa	Class IVb
Major Action	Inhibits fast sodium channels; prolongs repolarization time	Inhibits fast sodium channels, shortens repolarization time	Inhibits fast sodium channels, repolarization time unchanged	Beta-blockers, repolarization time unchanged	Markedly prolongs repolarization time (usually by K^+ channel blockade)	AV node Ca^{++} channel blocker, repolarization time unchanged	Ca^{++} channel openers, repolarization time unchanged
Examples	Quinidine Procainamide Disopyramide	Lidocaine Tocainide Mexiletine	Flecainide Propafenone	Propranolol Esmolol Atenolol	Amiodarone Sotalol Bretylium	Verapamil Diltiazem	Adenosine ATP

Table 7-26 Adenosine

Generic Name	adenosine
Trade Name(s)	Adenocard
Classification	Class IVb antiarrhythmic; endogenous nucleoside
Pronunciation	ah-DEN-oh-seen
How Supplied	3 mg/mL
Mechanism of Action	• Found naturally in all body cells • Rapidly metabolized in the blood vessels • Slows sinus rate • Slows conduction time through AV node • Can interrupt reentry pathways through AV node • Can restore sinus rhythm in PSVT
Indications	First medication for most forms of narrow-QRS supraventricular tachycardia (PSVT)
Dosing (adult)	• *Peripheral IV dose:* 6-mg rapid IV push over 1 to 3 sec. If no response within 1 to 2 min, administer 12 mg. May repeat 12-mg dose once in 1 to 2 min. Follow each dose immediately with a 20-mL normal saline flush. Recommended IV site is the antecubital fossa. • Use the injection port nearest the hub of the IV catheter. **Constant ECG monitoring is essential.**
Precautions	Side effects common but transient and usually resolve within 1 to 2 min • Facial flushing (common) • Coughing/dyspnea, bronchospasm (common) • Nausea • Headache • Hypotension • Chest pressure • Lightheadedness • Paresthesias • Dysrhythmias at time of rhythm conversion • Use with caution in patients with emphysema, bronchitis, asthma • Discontinue in any patient who develops severe respiratory difficulty

Continued

Table 7-26 Adenosine—cont'd

Contraindications	• Poison/drug-induced tachycardia • Asthma • Second- or third-degree AV block • Sick sinus syndrome (except in clients with a functioning artificial pacemaker) • Atrial flutter/atrial fibrillation • Ventricular tachycardia
Special Considerations	• Must be injected into the IV tubing as fast as possible (e.g., over a period of seconds). Failure to do so may result in breakdown of the medication while still in the IV tubing • Adenosine may cause fatal cardiac arrest, sustained ventricular tachycardia requiring resuscitation, and non-fatal MI. Transient or prolonged episodes of asystole have been reported with fatal outcomes in some cases • In a 1993 study,[9] investigators demonstrated that the initial dose of adenosine, if given via the central IV route, should be 3 mg. These data "confirm the hypothesis that lower doses of adenosine are effective when given by a central route." The investigators noted that nearly 80% of the tachycardias terminated after a 3-mg dose
Onset of Action	10 to 40 sec
Duration	1 to 2 min
Drug Interactions	• Use in patients receiving digitalis may rarely be associated with VF • Digoxin and verapamil use may rarely be associated with VF when combined with adenosine because of the potential for additive or synergistic depressant effects on the SA and AV nodes

> *A study published in 1997 evaluated the efficacy of prehospital administration of adenosine, using a 6-mg initial dosing regimen, for the treatment of PSVT. Seventy-four of 102 patients had PSVT as determined by physician analysis of the initial 6-sec electrocardiographic rhythm strip (ECG) recording. Sixty-six of these patients converted their cardiac rhythm from PSVT using adenosine; 46 (70%) converted with the initial 6-mg bolus. Fifteen patients converted after receiving the second dose (12 mg), and five patients required 30 mg.* [10]

Table 7-27 Amiodarone

Generic Name	amiodarone hydrochloride
Trade Name(s)	Cordarone
Classification	Class III antiarrhythmic (Although amiodarone is considered a class III antiarrhythmic, it possesses electrophysiologic characteristics of all four classes of antiarrhythmics. Amiodarone blocks sodium channels [class I action], inhibits sympathetic stimulation [class II action], and blocks potassium channels [class III action] as well as calcium channels [class IV action].)
Pronunciation	am-EE-oh-da-RONE
How Supplied	Injection: 50 mg/mL

Mechanism of Action	• Slows conduction in the His-Purkinje system and in accessory pathway of patients with Wolff-Parkinson-White syndrome
	• Inhibits alpha- and beta-receptors and possesses both vagolytic and calcium channel blocking properties
	• Lengthens the action potential duration and increases the refractory period) in all cardiac tissues, including the SA node, AV node, atrial cells, Purkinje fibers, and in the ventricular myocardium
	• Hemodynamic effects
	  • Coronary and peripheral vasodilator
	  • Mild decrease in myocardial contractility; however, cardiac output may actually increase because of decreased afterload

Table 7-27 Amiodarone—cont'd

	• Suppresses SA node function • Prolongs PR, QRS, and QT intervals • Slows conduction at the AV junction
Indications	• Shock-refractory pulseless VT/VF (Class IIb) • Polymorphic VT, wide-complex tachycardia of uncertain origin (Class IIb) • Stable VT when cardioversion unsuccessful (Class IIb) • Adjunct to electrical cardioversion of SVT/PSVT (Class IIa), atrial tachycardia (Class IIb) • Ectopic or multifocal atrial tachycardia (MAT) with normal LV function (Class IIb) • Pharmacologic conversion of atrial fibrillation (Class IIa) • Rate control of atrial fibrillation or flutter when other therapies ineffective (Class IIb)
Dosing (adult)	*Cardiac arrest: pulseless VT/VF* • Initial bolus—300 mg IV bolus diluted in 20 to 30 mL of NS or D5W • Consider repeat dose (150 mg IV bolus) every 3 to 5 min • If defibrillation successful, follow with 1 mg/min IV infusion for 6 hours (mix 900 mg in 500 mL NS). Then decrease infusion rate to 0.5 mg/min IV infusion for 18 hours. Maximum daily dose 2.0 g IV/24 hours *Other indications* • Loading infusion: 150-mg IV bolus over first 10 min (15 mg/min). Add 3 mL of amiodarone IV (150 mg) to 100 mL D5W and infuse over 10 min. May repeat every 10 min as needed • After conversion: Early ("slow") maintenance infusion—360 mg over next 6 hours (1 mg/min) • Follow with "late" maintenance infusion—540 mg over remaining 18 hours (0.5 mg/min). Decrease rate of early ("slow") loading infusion to 0.5 mg/min • Maximum cumulative dose 2.0 g IV/24 hours
Precautions	• Hypotension most common side effect • Bradycardia and AV block—slow the infusion rate or discontinue if seen. Pacemaker may be required
Contraindications	• Known hypersensitivity • Severe sinus node dysfunction, causing marked sinus bradycardia • Second- and third-degree AV block • Syncope caused by bradycardia (except when used in conjunction with a pacemaker) • Use with caution in patients with uncorrected electrolyte abnormalities, particularly hypokalemia and/or hypomagnesemia, because these conditions may predispose the patient to proarrhythmias
Special Considerations	• Originally developed in Belgium as a coronary vasodilator for treatment of angina. In the United States, approved by FDA for use as an antiarrhythmic December 1985. IV form approved for life-threatening dysrhythmias August 1995 • **Oral** amiodarone: Half-life 26 to 107 days, mean = 53 days. Effects persist for more than 50 days after discontinuing the medication • Forms a precipitate when mixed with sodium bicarbonate or heparin • In therapeutic doses, amiodarone has only a mild negative effect on myocardial contractility, which is why it appears in multiple algorithms involving patients experiencing dysrhythmias but having impaired cardiac function • Infusions lasting more than 2 hours must be administered in polyolefin or glass bottles containing D5W. Use polyvinyl chloride (PVC) tubing during administration. Recommended dosing regimens for amiodarone have considered the amount of amiodarone adsorbed to PVC tubing • Store at room temperature, 59 to 77°F. Does not need to be protected from light during administration. • Amiodarone IV must be delivered by a volumetric infusion pump
Drug Interactions	• Additive effect with other medications that prolong the QT interval (e.g., Class Ia antiarrhythmics, phenothiazines, tricyclic antidepressants, thiazide diuretics, sotalol) • Amiodarone can significantly impair the metabolism of digoxin, theophylline, and warfarin. Dosages of digoxin and warfarin should be decreased by one half when amiodarone therapy is added[11] • Potentiates actions of oral anticoagulants

Table 7-28 Atropine

Generic Name	atropine sulfate
Trade Name(s)	Atropine
Classification	Parasympatholytic; antimuscarinic; anticholinergic; parasympathetic antagonist; parasympathetic blocker
Pronunciation	AH-troh-peen
How Supplied	• Prefilled syringe: 0.5 mg/mL • Multi-dose vial: 0.4 mg/mL
Mechanism of Action	*Cardiovascular* • Increases heart rate (positive chronotropic effect) by accelerating SA node discharge rate and blocking vagus nerve • Increases conduction velocity (positive dromotropic effect) • Little or no effect on force of contraction (inotropic effect) *Respiratory* • Relaxes bronchial smooth muscle (bronchodilation) • Decreases body secretions (lungs, bronchi, GI tract, sweat, saliva) *GI/GU* • Decreases GI motility and secretions • Reduces urinary bladder tone (urinary retention) • Decreases sweat production *Other* • Pupil dilation (mydriasis) • Symptomatic sinus bradycardia (Class I) • Symptomatic AV block at the level of the AV node (Class IIa) • Asystole (after epinephrine) (Class IIb) • Pulseless electrical activity (PEA) (if bradycardic) (Class IIb) • **May** restore cardiac rhythm in asystole or bradycardic pulseless electrical activity (PEA)
Indications	Symptomatic sinus bradycardia
Dosing (adult)	• *Symptomatic bradycardia:* 0.5 to 1.0 mg IV, may repeat every 3 to 5 min, to a total dose of ≤2.5 mg (0.03 to 0.04 mg/kg). 2.5 mg produces complete vagal blockade. The total cumulative dose should not exceed 2.5 mg over 2.5 hours • *Asystole/bradycardic PEA:* 1.0 mg IV, may repeat every 3 to 5 min, to a total dose of ≤2.5 mg (0.03 to 0.04 mg/kg) • Atropine may be administered via ET tube. Adult dose is 2 to 3 mg diluted in 10 mL NS. To administer, use multi-dose atropine vial (0.4 mg/mL). For example, to administer a 2.0-mg adult dose of atropine endotracheally, draw up 5 mL from the 0.4 mg/mL multi-dose vial. Mix the 5 mL of atropine with 5 mL of normal saline. Stop chest compressions and administer medication. Follow with several forceful insufflations of bag-valve device. Resume CPR
Precautions	• Do not push slowly or in smaller than recommended doses. Small doses (under 0.5 mg) produce modest paradoxical cardiac slowing that may last 2 min • May result in tachycardia, palpitations, and ventricular ectopy. • May exacerbate ischemia or induce VT or VF • Use with caution in acute MI; excessive increases in heart rate may further worsen ischemia or increase size of necrotic area • Use with caution in second-degree AV block type II and third-degree AV block with a new wide QRS—may be ineffective or cause paradoxical slowing
Special Considerations	• Denervated transplanted hearts do not respond to atropine. Immediate interventions should include external pacing and/or use of catecholamines • Administer oxygen before administration of atropine • Do not administer unless solution is clear
Onset of Action	IV: 1 min (increased heart rate), 30 min (decreased secretions)
Duration	IV: 2 hours

QUICK REVIEW

1. How is adenosine administered?

2. Name three indications for administration of atropine.

3. How is amiodarone administered in pulseless VT/VF?

1. Because of its extremely short half-life, adenosine should be administered via a large-bore IV line initiated as close to the heart as possible (such as the antecubital vein). When administered via a peripheral vein, the initial bolus is 6-mg RAPID IV bolus over 1 to 3 sec followed by a 20-mL saline flush and elevation of the extremity; may repeat with 12 mg in 1 to 2 min. The 12-mg dose may be repeated once in 1 to 2 min.   2. Symptomatic sinus bradycardia, symptomatic AV block at the level of the AV node, asystole, bradycardic pulseless electrical activity (PEA).   3. Initial bolus—300 mg IV bolus diluted in 20 to 30 mL of NS or D5W. Consider repeat dose (150 mg IV bolus) every 3 to 5 min. If defibrillation successful, follow with 1 mg/min IV infusion for 6 hours (mix 900 mg in 500 mL NS). Then decrease infusion rate to 0.5 mg/min IV infusion for 18 hours.

Table 7-29   Beta-blockers

Generic/Trade Names	atenolol (Tenormin) esmolol (Brevibloc) labetalol (Normodyne, Trandate) metoprolol (Lopressor) propranolol (Inderal)
Classification	Beta-blockers
Pronunciation	atenolol: a-TEN-oh-lol esmolol: EZ-moh-lohl labetalol: lah-BET-ah-lohl metoprolol: meh-TOE-pra-lole propranolol: pro-PRAN-uh-lol
How Supplied	atenolol—Injection: 5 mg/10 mL esmolol—Injection: 100 mg/10 mL single-dose vial labetalol—Injection: 5 mg/mL in 20 mL ampule; 20, 40, 60 mL multi-dose vials metoprolol—Injection: 1 mg/mL in 5 mL ampule propranolol—Injection: 20 mg/5 mL unit-dose containers; 40 mg/5 mL unit-dose containers
Mechanism of Action	• Slows sinus rate • Depresses AV conduction • Reduces blood pressure • Decreases myocardial oxygen consumption • Reduces the incidence of dysrhythmias by decreasing catecholamine levels • Reduces risk of sudden death in patients with an acute coronary syndrome

Continued

Table 7-29   Beta-blockers—cont'd

Indications	• Non–ST-segment elevation MI or unstable angina (Class I)
	• Adjunctive agent with fibrinolytic therapy
	• To reduce incidence of VF in post-MI patients who did not receive fibrinolytics (atenolol, metoprolol, propranolol)
	• To slow the ventricular response in (esmolol):
	  • PSVT (Class I)
	  • Atrial fibrillation or atrial flutter (Class I)
	  • Ectopic atrial tachycardia (Class IIb)
	  • Inappropriate sinus tachycardia (Class IIb)
	  • Polymorphic VT caused by TdP or myocardial ischemia (Class IIb)
	• Control of blood pressure in hypertensive emergencies (labetalol)

Dosing (adult)	*Atenolol* • 5 mg atenolol IV over 5 min followed by another 5 mg IV dose 10 min later. Monitor BP, heart rate, and ECG closely • If patient tolerates full IV dose (10 mg), begin oral atenolol therapy 10 min after last IV dose *Esmolol* • Administer a loading infusion of 500 mcg/kg/min (0.5 mg/kg/min) over 1 min followed by a 4 min maintenance infusion of 50 mcg/kg/min (0.05 mg/kg/min). If an adequate therapeutic effect is observed over the 5 min of drug administration, maintain the maintenance infusion dosage with periodic adjustments up or down as needed. If an adequate therapeutic effect is not observed, the same loading dosage is repeated over 1 min followed by an increased maintenance rate infusion of 100 mcg/kg/min (0.1 mg/kg/min). *Labetalol* • 10 mg slowly IV push over 1-2 min. Additional doses can be given at 10 min intervals as needed to a maximum of 150 mg *Metoprolol* • 5 mg slow IV push over 5 min x 3 as needed to a total dose of 15 mg over 15 min. Closely monitor BP, heart rate, and ECG • In patients who tolerate the full IV dose (15 mg), begin oral metoprolol therapy 15 min after last IV dose *Propranolol* • Usual dose is from 1-3 mg IV administered no faster than 1 mg/min to diminish the possibility of lowering BP and causing cardiac standstill. If necessary, a second dose may be given after 2 min. Thereafter, additional drug should not be given in less than 4 hours. Monitor BP, heart rate, and ECG closely.
Precautions	*Atenolol* • Use with caution in patients with impaired renal function *Esmolol* • In clinical trials 20% to 50% of patients experienced hypotension, SBP <90 mm Hg and/or DBP <50 mm Hg. Monitor patients closely, especially if pretreatment BP low. Decrease of dose or termination of infusion reverses hypotension, usually within 30 min • Infiltration and extravasation may result in skin sloughing and necrosis • Administer with caution in patients with impaired renal function *Labetalol* • Use with caution in patients with impaired hepatic function • Symptomatic postural hypotension (incidence 58%) is likely to occur if patients are tilted or allowed to assume the upright position within 3 hours of receiving IV labetalol *Metoprolol* • Use with caution in patients with impaired hepatic function *Propranolol* • Use with caution in patients with impaired hepatic or renal function

Table 7-29   Beta-blockers—cont'd

Contraindications	• Heart rate <60 beats/min • Hypotension • AV block greater than first degree • Cardiogenic shock • Use with caution in conjunction with medications that slow conduction (e.g., digitalis, calcium channel blockers) and in those that decrease myocardial contractility (e.g., calcium channel blockers)
Special Considerations	• In general, patients with bronchospastic disease should not receive beta-blockers • Beta-blockers may potentiate insulin-induced hypoglycemia and mask some signs and symptoms including tachycardia; however, dizziness and sweating are usually not significantly affected[12] • Labetalol is both an alpha and beta-adrenergic blocker. The ratios of alpha to beta blockade are 1:3 and 1:7 after oral and IV use, respectively

Table 7-30   Calcium Channel Blockers

Generic/Trade Names	verapamil (Calan, Isoptin, Verelan); diltiazem (Cardizem)
Classification	Calcium channel blocker (calcium antagonist)
Pronunciation	verapamil: ver-AP-a-mill; diltiazem: dill-TIE-ah-zem
How Supplied	• verapamil—Injection: 5 mg/2 mL • diltiazem—Injection: 5 mg/mL; monovial: 100 mg freeze-dried diltiazem; Powder for injection: 10 mg, 25 mg
Mechanism of Action	Inhibit movement of calcium ions across cell membranes in the heart and vascular smooth muscle, resulting in: • Depressant effect on the heart's contractile function (negative inotropic effect) • Slowed conduction through the AV node (negative dromotropic effect) • Dilation of coronary arteries and peripheral arterioles • Decreased myocardial oxygen demand
Indications	*PSVT* • Patients with normal LV function (verapamil, diltiazem—Class I) • Patients with impaired LV function (diltiazem—Class IIb) *Atrial tachycardia* • Patients with normal LV function (verapamil, diltiazem—Class IIb) • Patients with impaired LV function (diltiazem—Class IIb) *Atrial flutter/fibrillation: rate control* • Patients with normal LV function (verapamil, diltiazem—Class I) • Patients with impaired LV function (diltiazem—Class IIb) *Pre-excited atrial fibrillation (WPW)* • Patients with normal LV function (verapamil, diltiazem—Class III) *Junctional tachycardia* • Verapamil, diltiazem—Class Indeterminate *Inappropriate sinus tachycardia* • Verapamil, diltiazem—Class Indeterminate
Dosing (adult)	*Verapamil* • 2.5 to 5.0 mg slow IV bolus over 2 min (administer over 3 to 4 min in elderly or if BP is within the lower range of normal). May repeat with 5 to 10 mg in 30 min (if no response and BP remains normal or elevated) • Maximum dose 20 mg *Diltiazem* • Initial dose 0.25 mg/kg IV bolus over 2 min. If needed, follow in 15 min with 0.35 mg/kg over 2 min. Subsequent IV bolus doses should be individualized for each patient. • Maintenance infusion 5 to 15 mg/hr, titrated to heart rate

Continued

Table 7-30 Calcium Channel Blockers—cont'd

Precautions	• Avoid calcium channel blockers in patients with wide-QRS tachycardia unless it is **known with certainty** to be supraventricular in origin (may precipitate VF) • Calcium channel blockers decrease peripheral resistance and can worsen hypotension. These medications should not be administered to patients with a SBP of <90 mm Hg and should be used with caution in patients with mild-to-moderate hypotension. Monitor BP, heart rate, and ECG closely • IV calcium channel blockers and IV beta-blockers should not be administered together or in close proximity (within a few hours)—may cause severe hypotension
Contraindications	• Wide-QRS tachycardia of uncertain origin • Poison/drug-induced tachycardias • Digitalis toxicity (may worsen heart block) • Atrial fibrillation or atrial flutter with an accessory bypass tract (WPW) • Sick sinus syndrome (bradycardia-tachycardia syndrome) except with a functioning ventricular pacemaker • Severe CHF • Second- or third-degree AV block • Hypotension (systolic BP <90 mm Hg) • Cardiogenic shock
Special Considerations	• Diltiazem depresses myocardial contractility to a lesser degree than verapamil and causes less hypotension • During administration, monitor closely for hypotension and AV block
Onset of Action	• Verapamil IV: 2 to 5 min • Diltiazem IV: ½ to 1 hour
Duration	• Verapamil IV: 2 hours • Diltiazem IV: 1 to 3 hours
Drug Interactions	• Beta-blockers may have additive negative inotropic and chronotropic effects • In some cases, coadministration of verapamil or diltiazem may prolong bleeding time • Concurrent use of amiodarone and diltiazem can result in bradycardia and decreased cardiac output by an unknown mechanism • Verapamil has been found to significantly inhibit elimination of alcohol, resulting in elevated blood alcohol concentrations that may prolong the intoxicating effects of alcohol

Table 7-31 Digitalis

Generic Name	digoxin
Trade Name	Lanoxin
Classification	Cardiac glycoside
Pronunciation	dih-JOX-in
How Supplied	0.25 mg/mL in 2-mL ampule
Mechanism of Action	• Inhibits the function of the sodium pump, resulting in an increase in intracellular sodium, accompanied by an increase in cellular calcium[8] • Slows conduction through AV node (prolonging PR interval) • In atrial flutter or fibrillation, decreases number of atrial impulses reaching the ventricles, thus decreasing the ventricular response (– chronotropic effect) • Increases force and velocity of myocardial contraction (+ inotropic effect) • Increases cardiac output
Indications	**Limited use in emergency cardiac care** • Control ventricular response rate in patients with atrial fibrillation or atrial flutter • PSVT • Heart failure caused by poor left ventricular contractility
Dosing (adult)	• 10 to 15 mcg/kg IV loading dose based on lean body weight • Maintenance dose affected by body size and renal function

* Cardiac glycosides are a closely related group of medications that have common specific effects on the heart. *Digitalis* is a term that refers to the entire group of cardiac glycosides.

Table 7-31 Digitalis—cont'd

Precautions	• Toxic-to-therapeutic ratio is narrow • May result in toxicity in patients with hypokalemia or hypomagnesemia, because potassium or magnesium depletion sensitizes the myocardium to digoxin • Hypercalcemia predisposes the patient to digitalis toxicity • May cause severe sinus bradycardia or SA block in patients with pre-existing sinus node disease • May cause complete AV block in patients with pre-existing incomplete AV block • Common adverse effects of chronic digoxin toxicity are visual disturbances and fatigue (95%) followed by weakness (82%), nausea (81%), loss of appetite (80%), abdominal discomfort (65%), psychological complaints (65%), dizziness (59%), abnormal dreams (54%), headache (45%), diarrhea (41%), and vomiting (40%)[13] • Visual disturbances include distorted yellow, red, and green color perception; blurred vision; and halos around solid objects
Contraindications	• Known hypersensitivity • Digitalis toxicity
Special Considerations	• ACE inhibitors have largely replaced digoxin as first-line therapy for CHF caused by systolic dysfunction • In patients with atrial fibrillation or atrial flutter, IV calcium-channel blockers or beta-blockers are generally more effective than digoxin for initial control of ventricular rate • It may be desirable to reduce the dose of digoxin for 1 to 2 days before electrical cardioversion of atrial fibrillation to avoid the induction of ventricular dysrhythmias, but physicians must consider the consequences of increasing the ventricular response if digoxin is withdrawn. If digitalis toxicity is suspected, elective cardioversion should be delayed. If it is not prudent to delay cardioversion, the lowest possible energy level should be selected to avoid provoking ventricular dysrhythmias[12] • After IV digoxin therapy, some patients with paroxysmal atrial fibrillation or flutter and a coexisting accessory AV pathway have developed increased antegrade conduction across the accessory pathway bypassing the AV node, leading to a very rapid ventricular response or ventricular fibrillation. Unless conduction down the accessory pathway has been blocked (either pharmacologically or by surgery), digoxin should not be used in such patients.
Onset of Action	IV: 5 to 30 min
Duration	Several days
Drug Interactions	Simultaneous use with: • Amiodarone, nifedipine, verapamil, flecainide, or quinidine may increase serum digoxin levels, predisposing the patient to toxicity • Medications affecting AV conduction (e.g., procainamide, propranolol, verapamil) may cause additive cardiac effects • Sympathomimetics (e.g., epinephrine) may increase the risk of dysrhythmias • Calcium preparations may cause synergistic effects that precipitate dysrhythmias

QUICK REVIEW

1. Name two indications for the use of diltiazem.

2. What is the recommended dosage range for the administration of verapamil?

3. Does administration of verapamil affect myocardial contractility?

4. Describe the effects of digitalis on heart rate and myocardial contractility.

5. Name three situations in which the use of beta-blockers should generally be avoided.

1. PSVT, atrial tachycardia atrial flutter/fibrillation (rate control); pre-excited atrial fibrillation (WPW), junctional tachycardia, inappropriate sinus tachycardia. 2. 2.5 to 5.0 mg slow IV bolus over 2 min. If no response to the initial dose (and the patient's BP is normal or elevated), repeat with 5 to 10 mg every 15 to 30 min to a maximum dose of 20 mg. Verapamil is a calcium channel blocker and is a negative inotrope (decreases the force of myocardial contraction). 4. Slows heart rate (negative chronotrope), increases myocardial contractility (positive inotrope). 5. Beta-blockers should generally not be administered to patients with hypotension, bradycardia, CHF, second- or third-degree AV block, or a history of bronchospastic disease.

Table 7-32 Disopyramide

Generic Name	disopyramide
Trade Name(s)	Norpace
Classification	Class Ia antiarrhythmic
Pronunciation	dye-soe-PEER-a-mide
How Supplied	IV form not approved for use in the United States
Mechanism of Action	• By inhibiting sodium influx through fast sodium channels in the cell membrane of the myocardium, decreases myocardial conduction velocity, excitability, and contractility and lengthens the recovery period after repolarization • Decreases automaticity in the His-Purkinje system • Decreases conduction velocity in the atria and ventricles
Indications	• For cardioversion of patients with atrial fibrillation/atrial flutter and normal left ventricular function (Class IIb) • Stable ventricular tachycardia (Class IIb)
Dosing (adult)	2 mg/kg IV over 10-15 min, followed by a continuous infusion of 0.4 mg/kg/hr
Precautions	• Reduced dose required in patients with renal dysfunction • Do not use in combination with calcium channel blockers or beta-blockers—additive negative inotropic effects • Quinidine increases disopyramide levels • Monitor QRS and QT interval duration during administration
Contraindications	• Known hypersensitivity to the medication • Severe renal failure • Cardiogenic shock • Preexisting second- or third-degree AV block (if no pacemaker is present) • Congenital Q-T prolongation
Special Considerations	• Pharmacologic action similar to procainamide and quinidine but has significant anticholinergic properties (urinary retention, constipation, worsening of glaucoma) that often limit its use • Has significant negative inotropic and hypotensive effects, precluding its use in patients with poor ventricular function

Table 7-33 Epinephrine

Generic Name	epinephrine
Trade Name(s)	Adrenalin
Classification	Natural catecholamine; sympathomimetic
Pronunciation	ep-ih-NEF-rin
How Supplied	• 1:10,000 solution (1 mg/10 mL) prefilled syringes • 1:1000 solution (1 mg/1 mL) ampule or prefilled syringes • 30 mg/30 mL vial
Mechanism of Action	Stimulates alpha, beta-1, and beta-2 receptors • Alpha-agonist: Constricts arterioles in the skin, mucosa, kidneys, and viscera → increased systemic vascular resistance • Beta-1 agonist: Increases force of contraction (+ inotropic effect), increases heart rate (+ chronotropic effect) → increased myocardial workload and oxygen requirements • Beta-2 agonist: Relaxation of bronchial smooth muscle, dilation of vessels in skeletal muscle; dilation of cerebral, pulmonary, coronary, and hepatic vessels
Indications	• Cardiac arrest: VF, pulseless VT, asystole, pulseless electrical activity (PEA) • Symptomatic bradycardia
Dosing (adult)	*Cardiac arrest* • IV: 1 mg (10 mL) of 1:10,000 solution, follow with 20-mL fluid flush. May repeat 1 mg dose every 3 to 5 min. If 1-mg dose fails, doses of up to 0.2 mg/kg may be used • Endotracheal: 2 to 2.5 mg diluted in 10 mL NS • Continuous infusion during cardiac arrest: Add 30 mg epinephrine (30-mL of 1:1000 solution) to 250 mL NS or D5W to run at 100 mL/hr and titrate to desired hemodynamic response. Central line preferred. Ensure patency of line *Continuous infusion: profound bradycardia* • Dose 2 to 10 mcg/min • To mix, add 1 mg epinephrine to 250 mL NS or D5W for a resulting concentration of 4 mcg/mL. Begin at 1 mcg/min and titrate to desired hemodynamic response
Precautions	• Increases myocardial oxygen demand • Avoid mixing with sodium bicarbonate *Epinephrine infusion* • Ideally, should be administered via central line • Administer via infusion pump • Check IV site frequently for evidence of tissue sloughing
Special Considerations	Should not be administered in the same IV line as alkaline solutions—inactivates epinephrine
Onset of Action	IV: 1 to 2 min
Duration	IV: 5 to 10 min

Table 7-34 Flecainide

Generic Name	flecainide
Trade Name(s)	Tambocor
Classification	Class Ic antiarrhythmic
Pronunciation	fleh-KAY-nyd
How Supplied	Approved in oral form in the United States. **IV form not approved for use in the United States**
Mechanism of Action	• Decreases myocardial contractility (negative inotropic effect) • Slows cardiac conduction in most patients to produce dose-related increases in PR, QRS, and QT intervals
Indications	**In patients without structural heart disease** • To convert atrial fibrillation/flutter <48 hours duration (Class IIa) • To control rate in WPW (Class IIb) • To convert rhythm in WPW <48 hours duration (Class IIb)
Dosing (adult)	2 mg/kg body weight at 10 mg/min slowly IV
Precautions	• May precipitate or worsen heart failure • Must be infused slowly • Side effects include bradycardia, hypotension, oral paresthesias, visual blurring
Contraindications	• Known hypersensitivity to the drug • CHF or left ventricular dysfunction • Should not be used in patients with recent MI • Preexisting second- or third-degree AV block • Cardiogenic shock
Special Considerations	• Not recommended for use in patients with chronic atrial fibrillation • Can cause new or worsened supraventricular or ventricular arrhythmias

QUICK REVIEW

1. Name the adrenergic-receptor sites stimulated by epinephrine.

2. Name four dysrhythmias for which epinephrine may be used.

3. What is the endotracheal dose of epinephrine in cardiac arrest?

4. What is the dose of epinephrine when administered for profound bradycardia?

1. Alpha and beta-adrenergic (beta-1 and beta-2) receptor sites. 2. Pulseless VT, VF, asystole, PEA, symptomatic bradycardia. 3. 2 to 2.5 mg. 4. 2 to 10 mcg/min IV infusion (not IV bolus).

Table 7-35   Ibutilide

Generic Name	ibutilide
Trade Name(s)	Corvert
Classification	Class III antidysrhythmic
Pronunciation	ih-BYOU-tih-lyd
How Supplied	IV solution: 0.1 mg/mL
Mechanism of Action	• Prolongs the duration of the cardiac action potential, resulting in mild slowing of the sinus rate and AV conduction • Converts atrial fibrillation or atrial flutter to a sinus rhythm without altering blood pressure, heart rate, PR interval, or QRS duration
Indications	For rapid conversion of recent onset (duration <48 hours) atrial fibrillation or atrial flutter (Class IIa)
Dosing (adult)	• *Adults weighing ≥60 kg:* 1 mg (1 vial) IV over 10 min. If the dysrhythmia is not terminated within 10 min after the end of the initial infusion, a second 1 mg IV dose may be administered at the same rate • *Adults weighing <60 kg:* 0.01 mg/kg (0.1-mL/kg) IV over 10 min. If the dysrhythmia is not terminated within 10 min after the end of the initial infusion, a second 0.01 mg/kg IV dose may be administered at the same rate
Precautions	• Class Ia antiarrhythmic drugs, such as disopyramide, quinidine, and procainamide, and other class III drugs, such as amiodarone and sotalol, should not be given concomitantly with ibutilide or within 4 hours postinfusion because of their potential to prolong refractoriness • Bradycardia • Breast-feeding • Heart failure • Hypokalemia • Pregnancy • QT prolongation • Ventricular dysrhythmias including VT, torsades de pointes
Contraindications	Hypersensitivity to the drug
Special Considerations	• May cause potentially fatal dysrhythmias, especially sustained polymorphic ventricular tachycardia, usually in association with QT prolongation (TdP) • Like other antiarrhythmic agents, ibutilide can induce or worsen ventricular arrhythmias in some patients. Torsades de pointes may occur because of the effect ibutilide has on cardiac repolarization, but ibutilide can also cause polymorphic VT in the absence of excessive prolongation of the QT interval. In clinical trials of IV ibutilide, patients with a history of CHF or low left ventricular ejection fraction appeared to have a higher incidence of sustained polymorphic VT than those without such underlying conditions • Correct hypokalemia and hypomagnesemia before treatment with ibutilide to reduce the potential for proarrhythmia. Continuously monitor ECG for at least 4 hours following infusion or until QT interval has returned to baseline

Table 7-36   Isoproterenol

Generic Name	isoproterenol
Trade Name(s)	Isuprel
Classification	Sympathomimetic; beta-adrenergic receptor agonist; antiarrhythmic
Pronunciation	eye-so-proh-TER-ih-nohl
How Supplied	Injection: 1 mg/5-mL ampules
Mechanism of Action	• Produces pronounced stimulation of both beta-1 and beta-2 receptors of the heart, bronchi, skeletal muscle vasculature, and the GI tract • *Beta-1 (heart):* Increase in heart rate, increase in rate of discharge of cardiac pacemakers, unchanged stroke volume, increase in ejection velocity • *Beta-2 (lungs and vessels):* Generalized vasodilation results in decreased systemic and pulmonary vascular resistance and an increase in coronary and renal blood flow. • SBP is usually elevated because of increased force of myocardial contraction, although DBP is usually decreased secondary to isoproterenol-induced vasodilation. • Mean arterial BP is usually unchanged or reduced. Produces marked relaxation in the smaller bronchi and may even dilate the trachea and main bronchi past the resting diameter
Indications	• Temporizing measure before pacing for torsades de pointes (Class Indeterminate) • Symptomatic bradycardia when atropine and dopamine or epinephrine have failed and transcutaneous/transvenous pacing is not available (Class IIb) • Temporary bradycardia management in heart transplant patients (denervated heart unresponsive to atropine) • Beta-adrenergic blocker poisoning
Dosing (adult)	Continuous IV infusion: 2 to 10 mcg/min titrated to heart rate and rhythm response. Mix 1 mg isoproterenol in 250-mL for a concentration of 4 mcg/mL or 1 mg in 500 mL for a concentration of 2 mcg/mL
Precautions	• Avoid in drug-induced hemodynamically significant bradycardia (unless caused by beta-blocker poisoning)—use of isoproterenol may induce or aggravate hypotension and ventricular dysrhythmias • If used for symptomatic bradycardia, should be used with extreme caution • Should not be used in hypotensive patients or in cardiac arrest • May cause VT/VF if administered with epinephrine
Contraindications	Tachyarrhythmias, tachycardia, or heart block caused by digitalis toxicity, ventricular dysrhythmias that require inotropic therapy, angina pectoris
Special Considerations	Start at 2 mcg/min and gradually increase if necessary while carefully monitoring the patient
Onset of Action	IV: Immediate
Duration	IV: <1 hour

Table 7-37   Lidocaine hydrochloride

Generic Name	lidocaine hydrochloride
Trade Name(s)	Xylocaine
Classification	Class Ib antiarrhythmic
Pronunciation	LYE-doh-kayn
How Supplied	100 mg/5 mL prefilled syringes (for IV bolus administration) 1 g in 25 mL vials and prefilled syringes (to mix continuous IV infusion) 2 g in 500 mL D5W premixed bags
Mechanism of Action	Lidocaine inhibits the influx of sodium through the fast channels of the myocardial cell membrane and decreases conduction in ischemic cardiac tissue without adversely affecting normal conduction. Clinical studies with lidocaine have demonstrated no change in sinus node recovery time or SA conduction time. AV nodal conduction time is unchanged or shortened. Lidocaine raises the VF threshold. In therapeutic doses, lidocaine does not affect BP, cardiac output, or myocardial contractility. No significant interactions between lidocaine and the autonomic nervous system have been described, and consequently, lidocaine has little or no effect on autonomic tone
Indications	• Monomorphic VT (Class IIb) • Polymorphic VT with normal QT interval (Class IIb) • Polymorphic VT with long QT interval (TdP) (Class Indeterminate) • Pulseless VT/VF that persists after defibrillation and epinephrine administration (Class Indeterminate) • Control of hemodynamically compromising PVCs (Class Indeterminate)
Dosing (adult)	**Monomorphic VT with normal cardiac function, polymorphic VT with normal QT interval, polymorphic VT with long QT interval (Torsades)** • 1 to 1.5 mg/kg initial dose. Repeat dose, ½ initial dose every 5 to 10 min. Maximum total dose 3 mg/kg. Maintenance infusion 1 to 4 mg/min **Monomorphic VT—impaired cardiac function (i.e., signs of shock)** • 0.5 to 0.75 mg/kg IV push. May repeat every 5 to 10 min. Maximum total dose 3 mg/kg **Pulseless VT/VF** • Initial dose: 1 to 1.5 mg/kg IV bolus. Higher (1.5 mg/kg) dose preferred in cardiac arrest. A single dose of 1.5 mg/kg in cardiac arrest is acceptable • Consider repeat dose (0.5 to 0.75 mg/kg) in 5 min[14] • Maximum IV bolus dose 3 mg/kg. • **Only bolus therapy is used in cardiac arrest.** After return of pulse, begin maintenance infusion at 1 to 4 mg/min • Endotracheal dose: 2 to 4 mg/kg
Precautions	• The maintenance infusion of lidocaine is 1 to 4 mg/min. This should be reduced after 24 hours (to 1 to 2 mg/min) or in the setting of altered metabolism (congestive heart failure, hepatic dysfunction, acute MI with hypotension or shock, patients >70 years, poor peripheral perfusion), and as guided by blood level monitoring • These patients should receive the usual bolus dose first, followed by half the usual maintenance infusion • The elimination half-life of lidocaine following an IV bolus injection is typically 1.5 to 2.0 hours. Because of the rapid rate at which lidocaine is metabolized, any condition that affects liver function may alter lidocaine kinetics. The half-life may be prolonged two-fold or more in patients with liver dysfunction[12] • Renal dysfunction does not affect lidocaine kinetics but may increase the accumulation of metabolites • Signs and symptoms of lidocaine toxicity are primarily CNS-related dizziness, drowsiness, mild agitation, tinnitus, slurred speech, hearing impairment, disorientation and confusion, muscle twitching, seizures, and respiratory arrest. These side effects are more common in patients with preexisting neurologic dysfunction and in those of advanced age[15] • In patients with sinus bradycardia or incomplete heart block, administration of IV lidocaine for the elimination of ventricular ectopic beats, without prior acceleration in heart rate (e.g., by atropine or pacing), may promote more frequent and serious ventricular dysrhythmias or complete heart block

Table 7-37 Lidocaine hydrochloride—cont'd

Contraindications	• Hypersensitivity to lidocaine or amide-type local anesthetics • Severe degrees of sinoatrial, atrioventricular, or intraventricular block in the absence of an artificial pacemaker • Stokes-Adams syndrome (sudden recurring episodes of loss of consciousness caused by transient interruption of cardiac output by incomplete or complete heart block) • Wolff-Parkinson-White syndrome
Special Considerations	Routine prophylactic use in uncomplicated myocardial infarction or ischemia without PVCs is no longer recommended Lidocaine may be **lethal** in a bradycardia with a ventricular escape rhythm
Onset of Action	IV: 45 to 90 sec
Duration	IV: 10 to 20 min
Drug Interactions	• Use with caution in patients with digitalis toxicity accompanied by AV block • Concomitant use of beta-blockers or cimetidine (Tagamet) may reduce hepatic blood flow, thereby reducing lidocaine clearance • Lidocaine and tocainide (Tonocard) are pharmacodynamically similar. Concomitant use may cause an increased incidence of adverse reactions, including seizures

---

QUICK REVIEW

1. *Stimulation of beta-adrenergic receptor sites should result in improved myocardial contractility and increased heart rate. Why is isoproterenol not used in the management of cardiac arrest?*

2. *What is the endotracheal dose of lidocaine?*

3. *What is the maximum IV bolus dose of lidocaine?*

1. *Pure beta-adrenergic stimulating agents do increase myocardial contractility and heart rate; however, another effect of beta-receptor stimulation is peripheral vasodilation. In cardiac arrest, vasodilation results in decreased coronary and cerebral perfusion, which offsets any benefit that might be received from improved myocardial contractility and increased heart rate.* 2. *2.2 to 4 mg/kg.* 3. *3 mg/kg.*

Table 7-38 Magnesium sulfate

Generic Name	Magnesium sulfate
Trade Name(s)	N/A
Classification	Antiarrhythmic, electrolyte
Pronunciation	mag-NEE-see-um SUL-fayt
How Supplied	Injection: 50% solution = 1 g/2 mL vials (0.5 g/mL)
Mechanism of Action	Functions of magnesium[12]

- Second most plentiful intracellular cation. Essential for the activity of many enzyme systems and plays an important role with regard to neurochemical transmission and muscular excitability. Deficits are accompanied by a variety of structural and functional disturbances
- Some of the effects of magnesium on the nervous system are similar to those of calcium. An increased concentration of magnesium in the extracellular fluid causes depression of the CNS. Magnesium has a direct depressant effect on skeletal muscle
- Abnormally low concentrations of magnesium in the extracellular fluid result in increased acetylcholine release and increased muscle excitability that can produce tetany
- Magnesium slows the rate of SA nodal impulse formation. Higher concentrations of magnesium (greater than 15 mEq/L) produce cardiac arrest in diastole
- Excess magnesium causes vasodilatation by both a direct action on blood vessels and ganglionic blockade

Evidence exists that magnesium:
- Produces systemic and coronary vasodilatation
- Possesses antiplatelet activity
- Suppresses automaticity in partially depolarized cells
- Protects myocytes against calcium overload under conditions of ischemia by inhibiting calcium influx especially at the time of reperfusion"[5]

Indications

Note: The 2000 International Resuscitation Guidelines recommendations for the use of magnesium sulfate differ from those of the American College of Cardiology (ACC)/American Heart Association (AHA) Guidelines for the Management of Patients with Acute Myocardial Infarction. Both are presented here for comparison and completeness

2000 International Resuscitation Guidelines[16]
- Drug-induced torsades de pointes, even in the absence of magnesium deficiency
- Not recommended in cardiac arrest except when dysrhythmias are suspected to be caused by magnesium deficiency or the monitor displays TdP

ACC/AHA Guidelines for the Management of Patients With Acute Myocardial Infarction

Class IIa
- Correction of documented magnesium (and/or potassium) deficits, especially in patients receiving diuretics before onset of infarction
- Episodes of torsades de pointes–type VT associated with a prolonged QT interval

Class IIb
- Magnesium bolus and infusion in high-risk patients such as the elderly and/or those for whom reperfusion therapy is not suitable

Dosing (adult)

2000 International Resuscitation Guidelines

Drug-induced torsades de pointes, even in the absence of magnesium deficiency
- Loading dose 1 to 2 g mixed in 50 to 100 mL of D5W over 5 to 60 min IV
- Follow with 0.5 to 1 g/hr IV (titrate dose to control TdP)

Cardiac arrest when dysrhythmias are suspected to be caused by magnesium deficiency or monitor displays TdP
- 1 to 2 g (2 to 4 mL of 50% solution) diluted in 10 mL of D5W IV push

Acute MI (If indicated)
- Loading dose 1 to 2 g mixed in 50 to 100 mL of D5W over 5 to 60 min IV
- Follow with 0.5 to 1 g/hr IV (titrate dose to control TdP)

Table 7-38 Magnesium sulfate—cont'd

	• **ACC/AHA Guidelines for the Management of Patients With Acute Myocardial Infarction**[5] *Class IIa* • Correction of documented magnesium (and/or potassium) deficits, especially in patients receiving diuretics before onset of infarction • Episodes of torsades de pointes–type VT associated with a prolonged QT interval should be treated with 1 to 2 g magnesium administered as a bolus over 5 min *Class IIb* • Magnesium bolus and infusion in high-risk patients, such as the elderly and/or those for whom reperfusion therapy is not suitable. Mortality reduction may be seen in high-risk patients, provided magnesium therapy is administered soon after onset of symptoms (preferably <6 hours). Optimum dose has not been established, but an IV bolus of 2 g over 5 to 15 min followed by an infusion of 18 g over 24 hours has been used with success
Precautions	• Caution should be used in patients receiving digitalis • Use with caution in patients with impaired renal function • Use with caution in patients with preexisting heart blocks
Contraindications	• Respiratory depression • Hypocalcemia • Hypermagnesemia
Special Considerations	Signs and symptoms of magnesium overdose include: • Hypotension • Flushing, sweating • Bradycardia, AV block • Respiratory depression • Drowsiness, decreasing level of consciousness • Diminished reflexes or muscle weakness, flaccid paralysis Antidote for magnesium overdose = calcium

Table 7-39 Procainamide

Generic Name	Procainamide
Trade Name(s)	Pronestyl, Procan SR
Classification	Class Ia antiarrhythmic
Pronunciation	proh-KAYN-ah-myd
How Supplied	Injection: 100 mg/mL, 500 mg/mL
Mechanism of Action	• In therapeutic doses, decreases conduction velocity in the atria, ventricles, and His-Purkinje system • Prolongs the effective refractory period of the atria • Shortens the effective refractory period of the AV node • Decreases automaticity in the His-Purkinje system and ectopic pacemakers • Prolongs the PR and QT intervals • Exerts a peripheral vasodilatory effect • In therapeutic doses, myocardial contractility of the undamaged heart is usually not affected • A significant portion of circulating procainamide may be metabolized to N-acetylprocainamide (NAPA), which also has significant antiarrhythmic activity
Indications	• Stable narrow-complex SVT (Class IIa) • Pharmacologic conversion of atrial fibrillation/atrial flutter to sinus rhythm (Class IIa) • Control of rapid ventricular rate in Wolff-Parkinson-White (WPW) syndrome (Class IIb) • Stable wide complex tachycardia of uncertain origin (Class IIb) • Pulseless VT/VF (Class IIb for recurrent pulseless VT/VF; Class Indeterminate for persistent pulseless VT/VF)

Continued

Table 7-39   Procainamide—cont'd

Dosing (adult)	20 mg/min IV infusion until one of the following occurs: • Dysrhythmia resolves • Hypotension • QRS widens by >50% of original width • Total dose of 17 mg/kg administered • Onset of TdP Maintenance infusion: 1 to 4 mg/min
Precautions	• Use with caution with other medications that prolong the QT interval (e.g., phenothiazines, cyclic antidepressants, thiazide diuretics, sotalol) • Conversion of atrial fibrillation to sinus rhythm may cause dislodgement of mural thrombi, leading to embolization • During administration, carefully monitor the patient's ECG and blood pressure. If the blood pressure falls 15 mm Hg or more, procainamide administration should be temporarily discontinued. Observe the ECG closely for increasing PR and QT intervals, widening of the QRS complex, heart block, and/or onset of TdP • Reduce maintenance infusion rate in liver dysfunction (procainamide is metabolized by the liver), renal failure (procainamide is eliminated by the kidneys)
Contraindications	• Complete AV block in the absence of an artificial pacemaker • Patients sensitive to procaine or other ester-type local anesthetics • Lupus erythematosus • Patients with a prolonged QRS duration or QT interval because of the potential for heart block • Pre-existing QT prolongation/torsades de pointes • Digitalis toxicity (procainamide may further depress conduction)
Special Considerations	In conversion of atrial fibrillation to normal sinus rhythm by any means, dislodgement of mural thrombi may lead to embolization, which should be kept in mind
Drug Interactions	• Pharmacologic effects of procainamide may be increased if amiodarone is also administered. Amiodarone may inhibit the hepatic metabolism and renal clearance of procainamide. Elevated procainamide plasma levels can occur with toxicity characterized by GI disturbances, weakness, hypotension, and cardiac disturbances. Anticipate up to a 25% reduction in procainamide dose during concurrent administration of amiodarone • Procainamide has neuromuscular blocking properties that may counteract the action of the cholinergic drugs on skeletal muscle. Taking procainamide and a cholinergic concurrently may exacerbate symptoms of myasthenia gravis • Additive cardiodepressant effects when lidocaine and procainamide are administered concurrently. Additive CNS toxicity has been reported

Table 7-40   Propafenone

Generic Name	propafenone
Trade Name(s)	Rythmol
Classification	Class Ic antiarrhythmic
Pronunciation	proh-pah-FEN-ohn
How Supplied	Approved in oral form in the United States. **IV form not approved for use in the United States**
Mechanism of Action	• Blocks fast sodium channels • Direct stabilizing action on myocardial membranes • Little or no effect on SA node • Prolongs PR interval because of blocking at AV node • Prolongs QRS duration because of prolonged ventricular conduction but has no effect on QT interval • Mild beta-adrenergic blocking effects • Exerts a negative inotropic effect on the myocardium • In patients with WPW, reduces conduction and increases effective refractory period of accessory pathway in both directions
Indications	• To convert atrial fibrillation/atrial flutter of <48 hours duration (normal cardiac function) (Class IIa) • To control rate in WPW (normal cardiac function) (Class IIb) • To convert rhythm in WPW (duration <48 hours) (Class IIb)
Dosing (adult)	1 to 2 mg/kg slowly IV at 10 mg/min (IV form not approved for use in the United States)
Precautions	Negative inotropic effect, can precipitate heart failure
Contraindications	• Heart failure or severe impairment of ventricular function • Disease of the SA node • AV or bundle branch block • Severe bradycardia • Marked hypotension • Cardiogenic shock • Severe COPD
Special Considerations	• May cause bradycardia, hypotension, CHF, or new dysrhythmias • Incidence of proarrhythmias may be less than flecainide
Drug Interactions	Additive negative inotropic effect with beta-blockers or calcium channel blockers

Table 7-41   Sotalol

Generic Name	sotalol
Trade Name(s)	Betapace
Classification	Class III antiarrhythmic
Pronunciation	SOH-tah-lol
How Supplied	Approved in oral form in the United States. **IV form not approved for use in the United States**
Mechanism of Action	Sotalol is a Class III antiarrhythmic with non-selective beta-blockade activity
	• Slows heart rate
	• Decreases AV nodal conduction
	• Increases AV nodal refractoriness
	• Prolongs the effective refractory period of atrial muscle, ventricular muscle, and AV accessory pathways (where present) in both anterograde and retrograde directions
Indications	• Positive inotropic action
	• Narrow-complex supraventricular tachycardia (PSVT) (Class IIa)
	• Monomorphic VT with normal cardiac function (Class IIa)
	• To control rate in WPW (normal cardiac function) (Class IIb)
	• To convert rhythm in WPW (duration <48 hours) (Class IIb)
Dosing (adult)	Polymorphic VT with normal QT interval (Class IIb)
Precautions	• 1 to 1.5 mg/kg IV slowly at a rate of 10 mg/min
	• Because of its effect on cardiac repolarization (QT interval prolongation), TdP is the most common proarrhythmia associated with sotalol, occurring in about 4% of high risk (history of sustained VT/VF) patients. The risk of TdP progressively increases with prolongation of the QT interval and is worsened by reduction in heart rate and reduction in serum potassium. Patients with sustained VT and a history of CHF appear to have the highest risk for serious proarrhythmia
	• Should not be used in patients with hypokalemia or hypomagnesemia (these conditions can exaggerate the degree of QT prolongation and increase the potential for TdP)
	• Bradycardia
	• Hypotension
Contraindications	• Bronchial asthma
	• Sinus bradycardia
	• Second- and third-degree AV block (unless a functioning pacemaker is present)
	• Congenital or acquired long QT syndromes
	• Cardiogenic shock
	• Uncontrolled CHF
	• Previous evidence of hypersensitivity to sotalol

QUICK REVIEW

1. Name four clinical indications of lidocaine toxicity.

2. What is the recommended dose of atropine in the treatment of asystole?

3. Name three indications for IV procainamide administration.

4. When should an infusion of procainamide be discontinued?

5. How is isoproterenol administered?

6. When is ibutilide indicated?

1. Dizziness, drowsiness, mild agitation, hearing impairment, disorientation and confusion, muscle twitching, seizures, respiratory arrest.   2. IV dose 1 mg every 3 to 5 min to max dose of 0.04 mg/kg; ET 2 to 3 mg.   3. Stable narrow-complex SVT, pharmacologic conversion of atrial fibrillation/atrial flutter to sinus rhythm, control of rapid ventricular rate in Wolff-Parkinson-White (WPW) syndrome, stable wide complex tachycardia of uncertain origin, pulseless VT/VF.   4. Procainamide should be discontinued if any of the following occurs: hypotension develops, the dysrhythmia is suppressed, the QRS widens by more than 50% of its original width, a total of 17 mg/kg has been administered, or onset of torsades de pointes.   5. Continuous IV infusion at 2 to 10 mcg/min   6. For rapid conversion of recent onset (duration <48 hours) atrial fibrillation or atrial flutter.

MEDICATIONS USED TO IMPROVE CARDIAC OUTPUT AND BLOOD PRESSURE

The following medications are used to improve cardiac output and blood pressure (Tables 7-42 to 7-49).

Vasoconstrictor Inotropic Agents

Table 7-42   Dopamine

Generic Name	dopamine
Trade Name(s)	Intropin, Dopastat
Classification	Direct- and indirect-acting sympathomimetic; cardiac stimulant and vasopressor, natural catecholamine
Pronunciation	DOH-pah-meen
How Supplied	Injection: 40 mg/mL, 80 mg/mL, 160 mg/mL
Mechanism of Action	• Naturally occurring immediate precursor of norepinephrine in the body • Pharmacologic effects change with increasing dosage • Stimulates dopaminergic, beta-, and alpha-adrenergic receptor sites • Low dose = dopaminergic • Medium dose = beta • High dose = alpha The effects of dopamine are dose related (there is some "overlap" of effects) **Low dose (dopaminergic effects)** *0.5 to 2 mcg/kg/min* • At this dose range, dopaminergic receptors are stimulated, resulting in dilation of the renal, mesenteric, coronary, and intracerebral vascular beds • Diuresis usually occurs in this dose range and renal blood flow increases **Medium dose (beta effects)** *2 to 10 mcg/kg/min ("cardiac dose")* • At this dose range, dopamine acts directly on the beta-1 receptors in the myocardium, resulting in improved myocardial contractility, increased SA rate, and enhanced impulse conduction in the heart. There is little, if any, stimulation of the beta-2 adrenoceptors (peripheral vasodilation) **High dose (alpha effects)** *10 to 20 mcg/kg/min ("pressor dose")* • At this dose range, alpha-1 and alpha-2 receptors are stimulated, BP and systemic vascular resistance increase • Vasoconstrictor effects are first seen in the skeletal muscle vascular beds, but with increasing doses, they are also evident in the renal and mesenteric vessels *>20 mcg/kg/min* • Produces effects similar to norepinephrine • Vasoconstriction may compromise the circulation of the limbs • May increase heart rate and oxygen demand to undesirable limits
Indications	• Hemodynamically significant bradydysrhythmias that have not responded to atropine and/or when external pacing is unavailable • Hypotension that occurs after return of spontaneous circulation • Hemodynamically significant hypotension in the absence of hypovolemia
Dosing (adult)	*Continuous infusion* • Dose range 5 to 20 mcg/kg/min. Begin infusion at 5 mcg/kg/min • Increase infusion rate according to blood pressure and other clinical responses • Various concentrations (800 mcg/mL, 1600 mcg/mL, 3200 mcg/mL) may be used. The less concentrated (800 mcg/mL) solution may be preferred when fluid expansion is not a problem. The more concentrated (1600 mcg/mL or 3200 mcg/mL) solutions may be preferred in patients with fluid retention or when a slower rate of infusion is desired

Table 7-42   Dopamine—cont'd

Precautions	• Dilute before administration (or used premixed bag of IV solution); should not be given as an IV bolus. Should only be infused via an infusion pump. • Volume deficits must be corrected before beginning dopamine therapy for the treatment of hypotension and shock; otherwise, because of poor venous return, cardiac output and renal blood flow would not increase, and excessive vasoconstriction and peripheral necrosis and gangrene could occur[3] • Gradually taper drug before discontinuing the infusion. Monitor blood pressure, ECG, and drip rate closely.
Contraindications	• Hypersensitivity to sulfites or dopamine • Hypovolemia • Pheochromocytoma • Uncorrected tachydysrhythmias or VF • MAO inhibitors (e.g., Marplan, Nardil, Parnate)
Special Considerations	• Patients most likely to respond to dopamine are those whose physiologic parameters (such as urine flow, myocardial function, and blood pressure) have not undergone extreme deterioration[12] • Extravasation into surrounding tissue may cause necrosis and sloughing. Antidote for extravasation = phentolamine (Regitine). Large veins of the antecubital fossa are preferred to veins of the dorsum of the hand. Less suitable infusion sites should be used only when larger veins are unavailable, and the patient's condition requires immediate attention
Onset of Action	2 to 5 min
Duration	5 to 10 min (half-life 2 min); duration may increase to 1 hour if MAO inhibitors are present
Drug Interactions	• Because dopamine is metabolized by monoamine oxidase (MAO), inhibition of this enzyme prolongs and potentiates the effect of dopamine. Patients who have been treated with MAO inhibitors within 2 to 3 weeks before the administration of dopamine should receive initial doses of dopamine no greater than one tenth ($\frac{1}{10}$) the usual dose[12] • Cardiac glycosides (e.g., digitalis) increase inotropic effect • Catecholamines and sympathomimetics increase effects • Cardiac effects of dopamine are antagonized by beta-blockers • Administration of phenytoin to patients receiving dopamine may lead to hypotension and bradycardia • Inactivated in alkaline solutions

1600 mcg/mL Dosing Chart for Dopamine (mL/hr) Infusion Rate

Infusion Rate (mcg/kg/min)	Patient Body Weight (kg)									
	10	20	30	40	50	60	70	80	90	100
2.5	0.9	1.9	2.8	3.8	4.7	5.6	6.6	7.5	8.4	9.4
5	1.9	3.8	5.6	7.5	9.4	11.3	13.1	15	16.9	18.8
10	3.8	7.5	11.3	15	18.8	22.5	26.3	30	33.8	37.5
15	5.6	11.3	16.9	22.5	28.1	33.8	39.4	45	50.6	56.3
20	7.5	15	22.5	30	37.5	45	52.5	60	67.5	75
25	9.4	18.8	28.1	37.5	46.9	56.3	65.6	75	84.4	93.8
30	11.3	22.5	33.8	45	56.3	67.5	78.8	90	101.3	112.5
35	13.1	26.3	39.4	52.5	65.6	78.8	91.9	105	118.1	131.3
40	15	30	45	60	75	90	105	120	135	150
45	16.9	33.8	50.6	67.5	84.4	101.3	118.1	135	151.9	168.8
50	18.8	37.5	56.3	75	93.8	112.5	131.3	150	168.8	187.5

From: *Mosby's GenRx*, ed 10, St. Louis, 2000, Mosby.

Table 7-43   Norepinephrine

Generic Name	norepinephrine
Trade Name(s)	Levophed, Levarterenol
Classification	Direct-acting adrenergic agent
Pronunciation	Nor-ep-ih-NEF-rin
How Supplied	Injection: 1 mg/mL
Mechanism of Action	• Norepinephrine functions as a peripheral vasoconstrictor (alpha-adrenergic action) and as an inotropic stimulator of the heart and dilator of coronary arteries (beta-adrenergic action) • Alpha activity dominant • Increases myocardial oxygen demand
Indications	• Cardiogenic shock • Severe hypotension (systolic BP <70 mm Hg) not caused by hypovolemia
Dosing (adult)	• 0.5 to 1.0 mcg/min IV titrated to improve blood pressure (up to 30 mcg/min) • Administer by continuous IV infusion. A common dilution is 4 mg norepinephrine in 250 mL of D_5W or D_5NS (resulting concentration = 16 mcg/mL). Concentrations of up to 32 mcg/mL have been used in fluid-restricted patients • When discontinuing infusion, taper off gradually
Precautions	• Use with extreme caution in patients receiving monoamine oxidase inhibitors (MAOI) or antidepressants of the triptyline or imipramine types because severe, prolonged hypertension may result • Norepinephrine is a concentrated, potent medication that must be diluted in dextrose containing solutions before infusion
Contraindications	• Hypersensitivity to sulfites or norepinephrine • Hypotension caused by hypovolemia (except in emergencies) • Mesenteric or peripheral vascular thrombosis • Halothane or cyclopropane anesthesia (possibility of fatal dysrhythmias) • Pregnancy (may cause fetal anoxia or hypoxia)

Table 7-43   Norepinephrine—cont'd

Special Considerations	• Should be administered via an infusion pump into a central vein or a large peripheral vein (e.g., antecubital vein) to reduce the risk of necrosis of the overlying skin from prolonged vasoconstriction. Gangrene of the lower extremity has occurred when infusions of norepinephrine were administered via an ankle vein
	• Extravasation into surrounding tissue may cause necrosis and sloughing. Antidote for extravasation = phentolamine (Regitine)
	• Monitor blood pressure every 2 to 3 min until stabilized, then every 5 min. Monitor the patient's ECG continuously
	• Administration in saline solution alone is not recommended
Onset of Action	Immediate
Duration	1 to 2 min
Drug Interactions	• Norepinephrine should be used with extreme caution in patients receiving monoamine oxidase inhibitors or antidepressants of the triptyline or imipramine types because severe, prolonged hypertension may result
	• Use with epinephrine may produce excessive and serious hypertensive episodes and additive CNS stimulation, including agitation, nervousness, ataxia, tremors, and excitability

---

QUICK REVIEW

1. Describe the effects of dopamine administration at 0.5 to 2.0 mcg/kg/min.

2. When is norepinephrine indicated?

3. True or False. Vasopressors should only be infused via an infusion pump.
4. Name two components of the ECG that should be monitored closely during the administration of procainamide.

1. Dilation of the renal, mesenteric, coronary, and intracerebral vascular beds. 2. Cardiogenic shock, severe hypotension (systolic BP <70 mm Hg) not caused by hypovolemia. 3. True. 4. Monitor the ECG closely for increasing PR intervals, increasing QT intervals, widening of the QRS complex.

Catecholamines with Predominant Inotropic Properties with Little Or No Vasoconstriction

Table 7-44	Dobutamine
Generic Name	dobutamine
Trade Name(s)	Dobutrex
Classification	Direct-acting sympathomimetic, cardiac stimulant, adrenergic agonist agent
Pronunciation	doe-BYOO-tah-meen
How Supplied	Injection: 250 mg/20 mL vial
Mechanism of Action	• Stimulates alpha, beta-1, and beta-2 receptors
	• Potent inotropic effect (i.e., increased myocardial contractility, increased stroke volume, increased cardiac output), less chronotropic effect (heart rate), minimal alpha effect (vasoconstriction)
Indications	Short-term management of patients with cardiac decompensation caused by depressed contractility (e.g., CHF, pulmonary congestion)
Dosing (adult)	Continuous IV infusion. Dilute 250 mg (20 mL) in 250 mL D5W or NS. Usual dose is 2 to 20 mcg/kg/min IV, based on patient response
Precautions	• Tachycardia may occur with high dose, although this occurs less commonly than with dopamine
	• Continuously monitor ECG and blood pressure
Contraindications	• Hypersensitivity to sulfites or dobutamine
	• Tachydysrhythmias
	• Severe hypotension
	• Hypertrophic aortic stenosis
Special Considerations	Dobutamine may cause a marked increase in heart rate or blood pressure, especially systolic pressure. Approximately 10% of patients in clinical studies have had rate increases of 30 beats/min or more, and about 7.5% have had a 50 mm Hg or greater increase in systolic pressure. Usually, reduction of dosage promptly reverses these effects. Because dobutamine facilitates AV conduction, patients with atrial fibrillation are at risk of developing rapid ventricular response. Patients with preexisting hypertension appear to face an increased risk of developing an exaggerated pressor response[12] Correct hypovolemia before treatment with dobutamine
Onset of Action	1 to 2 min
Duration	10 to 15 min (half-life 2 min)
Drug Interactions	• Incompatible with sodium bicarbonate
	• Use with tricyclic antidepressants can cause an increased adrenergic effect and possibly result in severe hypertensive crisis or cardiac dysrhythmias

Vasopressin

Table 7-45 Vasopressin	
Generic Name	vasopressin
Trade Name(s)	Pitressin Synthetic
Classification	Pituitary hormone, antidiuretic
Pronunciation	Vay-so-PRESS-in
How Supplied	Injection: 20 U/mL
Mechanism of Action	• Antidiuretic hormone • Vasopressin acts at the tissue level by binding to specific receptors identified as V (vasopressin) receptors. There are two types of V receptors: V1 and V2. There are two subtypes of V1 receptors (V1a and V1b). Stimulation of V1a receptors produces potent vasoconstrictor effects, in contrast to the vasodilator effects of V2-receptor stimulation. Stimulation of V1a receptors in the liver results in glycogenolysis, and in the kidney, stimulation results in inhibition of renin secretion. V1a receptors in the brain appear to be involved in memory, BP regulation, and cerebrospinal fluid production. Stimulation of V1b receptors in the pituitary results in secretion of corticotropin. The V2 receptor is responsible for the antidiuretic effects of vasopressin, its vasodilator effects, its ability to increase factor VIII coagulant activity, and the concentration of von Willebrand factor in plasma[17] • Stimulation of V1 receptors in vascular smooth muscle results in contraction in the coronary, splanchnic, GI, pancreatic, skin, and muscular vascular beds. This effect is particularly prominent in the capillaries, small arterioles, and venules, with less effect on the smooth musculature of large veins **Comparison: vasopressin vs. epinephrine** • Vasopressin exerts a greater vasoconstrictive effect under conditions of hypoxia and acidosis than does epinephrine, and the effects of vasopressin last longer[18,19] • Vasopressin causes a greater increase in arterial tone than does epinephrine, an effect that correlates with greater myocardial perfusion[18,19] • Epinephrine increases myocardial oxygen consumption and lactate production in the arrested heart, and vasopressin does not[20]
Indications	• May be used as an alternative pressor to epinephrine in the treatment of adult shock-refractory pulseless VT/VF (Class IIb) • Hemodynamic support in vasodilatory shock (e.g., septic shock, sepsis syndrome) (Class IIb)
Dosing (adult)	• Adult cardiac arrest caused by pulseless VT/VF • IV/IO: 40 units IV push (One-time dose, if no response, epinephrine may be used after 10 to 20 min)
Precautions	• Because vasopressin can precipitate angina or myocardial infarction, it is not recommended for use in responsive patients with coronary artery disease or peripheral vascular disease • Acute pulmonary edema has been reported in humans after peripheral administration of vasopressin (0.15 U/kg)[21]
Contraindications	Hypersensitivity
Special Considerations	• Vasopressin may be effective in patients with asystole or PEA; however, insufficient data currently exists to support a recommendation for its use in these settings (Class Indeterminate) • Half-life: approximately 10 to 20 min

Phosphodiesterase Inhibitors

Phosphodiesterase inhibitors increase myocardial contractility and have vasodilating properties.

Table 7-46   Amrinone

Generic Name	amrinone (Inamrinone)
Trade Name(s)	Inocor
Classification	Inotropic agent, coronary vasodilator
Pronunciation	AM-rih-nohn/In-AM-rih-nohn
How Supplied	Injection: 5 mg/mL
Mechanism of Action	Phosphodiesterase inhibitor • Positive inotropic agent with vasodilator activity, different in structure and mode of action from either digitalis glycosides or catecholamines • Reduces preload and afterload by its direct relaxant effect on vascular smooth muscle
Indications	**Short-term management of congestive heart failure**
Dosing (adult)	• Initial dose: 0.75 mg/kg as a bolus given slowly over 10 to 15 min. Based on clinical response, an additional loading dose of 0.75 mg/kg may be given 30 min after the initiation of therapy • Maintenance infusion: 5 to 10 mcg/kg/min titrated to desired response. The recommended total daily dose (including loading doses) should not exceed 10 mg/kg; however, up to 18 mg/kg/day has been used in a limited number of patients for short periods
Precautions	Monitor BP and heart rate closely during IV administration. Slow or stop the infusion if the patient shows excessive decreases in BP
Contraindications	• Known hypersensitivity to amrinone • Hypersensitivity to bisulfites

Table 7-46   Amrinone—cont'd

Special Considerations	• Because of medication errors, the generic name for *amrinone* has been changed to *inamrinone*. The name change from *amrinone* to *inamrinone* became effective July 1, 2000, with the *Second Supplement of the United States Pharmacopeia—National Formulary (USP-NF)*. As of March 2000, fourteen medication errors involving amrinone and amiodarone had been reported to the USP Medication Errors Reporting (MER) Program. The consequences of the medication errors included reports of patient injury and death • A chemical interaction occurs slowly over a 24-hour period when the IV amrinone is mixed directly with dextrose-containing solutions. Therefore amrinone should not be diluted with solutions that contain dextrose before injection • Can increase myocardial ischemia
Drug Interactions	• Effective in fully digitalized patients without causing signs of cardiac glycoside toxicity. Its inotropic effects are additive to those of digitalis • In cases of atrial flutter/fibrillation, may increase ventricular response rate because of its slight enhancement of AV conduction • Furosemide should not be administered in intravenous lines containing amrinone (forms precipitate)

Table 7-47   Milrinone

Generic Name	milrinone
Trade Name(s)	Primacor
Classification	Inotropic agent, coronary vasodilator
Pronunciation	MILL-rih-nohn
How Supplied	Injection: 1 mg/mL
Mechanism of Action	Phosphodiesterase inhibitor • Positive inotrope and vasodilator, with little chronotropic activity • Different in structure and mode of action from digitalis glycosides and catecholamines • In addition to increasing myocardial contractility, improves diastolic function as evidenced by improvements in left ventricular diastolic relaxation
Indications	**Short-term treatment of CHF, usually in patients receiving digitalis and diuretics**
Dosing (adult)	• *Loading dose:* 50 mcg/kg: Administer slowly over 10 min • *Maintenance infusion:* Minimum initial IV infusion rate is 0.375 mcg/kg/min (0.59 mg/kg/day) adjusted according to hemodynamic and clinical response. Standard IV infusion rate 0.5 mcg/kg/min (0.77 mg/kg/day); may be titrated up to a maximum infusion rate of 0.75 mcg/kg/min (1.13 mg/kg/day)
Precautions	Administration of milrinone has precipitated supraventricular and ventricular dysrhythmias, including VT
Contraindications	• Hypersensitivity to milrinone • Should not be used in patients with severe obstructive aortic or pulmonic valvular disease in lieu of surgical relief of the obstruction
Special Considerations	Adjust dose in patients with renal failure
Drug Interactions	Favorable inotropic effect in fully digitized patients without causing signs of glycoside toxicity

Other Medications to Improve Cardiac Output and Blood Pressure

Table 7-48   Calcium Chloride

Generic Name	calcium chloride
Trade Name(s)	N/A
Classification	Electrolyte; calcium salt
Pronunciation	KAL-see-um KLOH-ryd
How Supplied	Injection: 10% 100 mg/mL [27.2 mg/mL] (10 mL) (1.4 mEq calcium/mL)
Mechanism of Action	• Fifth most abundant element in the body • Essential for functional integrity of nervous and muscular systems • Necessary for normal cardiac contractility and coagulation of blood • Increases force of cardiac contraction (positive inotropic effect) • Antidote for magnesium sulfate
Indications	• Known or suspected acute hyperkalemia (Class IIb) • Acute hypocalcemia (e.g., after multiple blood transfusions) (Class IIb) • Calcium channel blocker toxicity (Class IIb) • Pretreatment for IV calcium channel blocker administration • Magnesium toxicity • Antidote for toxic effects from beta-blocker toxicity
Dosing (adult)	*Hyperkalemia* • 8 to 16 mg/kg over 10 min. Dosage should be titrated by constant monitoring of ECG changes during administration *Hypocalcemia* • Usual adult dosage ranges from 500 mg to 1 g (5 to 10 mL) at intervals of 1 to 3 days, depending on patient response and/or results of serum calcium determinations. Repeated injections may be required because of rapid excretion of calcium *Calcium channel blocker toxicity or pretreatment for IV calcium channel blocker administration* • 2 to 4 mg/kg **slow** IV push (not to exceed 1 mL/min). May repeat in 10 min if necessary. Stop administration if bradycardia develops *Magnesium toxicity* • 500 mg **slow** IV push. Observe patient for signs of recovery before administering additional doses
Precautions	• Do not administer this medication intramuscularly or subcutaneously; it can cause severe tissue necrosis, sloughing, or abscess formation • Monitor IV site closely. Ensure patency of IV line before administering. Calcium chloride is irritating to veins. Patient may experience pain, burning at the IV site, severe venous thrombosis, and severe tissue necrosis if solution extravasates. Patient may complain of "heat waves," tingling, and/or a metallic taste if administered too rapidly • Calcium chloride administration may be accompanied by peripheral vasodilation, with a moderate fall in blood pressure. • Use with caution in patients taking digitalis—increases ventricular irritability and can precipitate digitalis toxicity
Contraindications	• Hypercalcemia • Concurrent digitalis therapy (relative contraindication) • Renal calculi • VF
Special Considerations	Calcium chloride is preferred over calcium gluceptate or calcium gluconate because calcium chloride produces consistently higher and more predictable levels of ionized calcium in the plasma. A 10% solution of calcium chloride contains 1.36 mEq of calcium/100 mg of salt/mL
Onset of Action	5 to 15 min
Duration	Depends on dose and total body stores of calcium
Drug Interactions	• Incompatible with all medications. Flush line before and after administration • Concurrent administration of sodium bicarbonate and calcium chloride will produce a precipitate, calcium carbonate (chalk)

QUICK REVIEW

1. Name three indications for calcium chloride administration.

2. When should amrinone (Inocor) administration be considered?

3. Name two calcium channel blockers.

1. Hyperkalemia, hypocalcemia, calcium channel blocker toxicity/overdose, pretreatment for calcium channel blocker administration, magnesium toxicity. 2. In patients with severe congestive heart failure refractory to diuretics, vasodilators, and conventional inotropic agents. 3. Diltiazem (Cardizem), verapamil (Isoptin, Calan).

VASODILATORS

Table 7-49   Sodium Nitroprusside

Generic Name	sodium nitroprusside
Trade Name(s)	Nipride; Nitropress
Classification	Vasodilator; antihypertensive
Pronunciation	nye-troh-PRUS-eyed
How Supplied	• Injection: 25 mg/mL • Powder for injection: 50 mg
Mechanism of Action	Direct-acting arterial and venous vasodilator • Relaxes vascular smooth muscle with consequent dilation of peripheral arteries and veins; other smooth muscle (e.g., uterus, duodenum) is not affected • Nitroprusside is more active on veins than on arteries • Venodilation promotes peripheral pooling of blood and decreases venous return to the heart, thereby reducing preload • Arteriolar relaxation reduces systemic vascular resistance (afterload) • Dilates coronary arteries
Indications	**Immediate reduction of blood pressure in a hypertensive emergency or hypertensive urgency**
Dosing (adult)	• Mix 50 or 100 mg in 250 mL D_5W • Wrap solution and tubing in opaque material • Administer via infusion pump • Begin infusion at 0.1 mcg/kg/min and titrate slowly (every 3 to 5 min) upward (to 5 mcg/kg/min) to desired clinical response • Average dose is 3 mcg/kg/min; maximum recommended infusion rate 10 mcg/kg/min • Infusion at the maximum dose rate should never last more than 10 min
Precautions	• Nitroprusside can cause precipitous decreases in BP. In patients not properly monitored, these decreases can lead to irreversible ischemic injuries or death • Monitor for signs of cyanide toxicity • Solution is sensitive to certain wavelengths of light and must be protected from light during clinical use
Contraindications	Hypotension, severe refractory CHF
Onset of Action	1 to 2 min
Duration	Effects stop quickly on discontinuation of infusion
Drug Interactions	• Patients stabilized on diltiazem may require a lower dose of nitroprusside • Severe additive hypotensive reactions have been reported in patients who have been administered clonidine and nitroprusside concurrently

OTHER MEDICATIONS

Alkalinizing Agents/Buffers

Alkalinizing agents/buffers and diuretics are also used in the treatment of cardiovascular conditions (Tables 7-50 and 7-51).

Table 7-50 Sodium bicarbonate	
Generic Name	Sodium bicarbonate
Trade Name(s)	N/A
Classification	Alkalinizing agent, antacid, electrolyte
Pronunciation	SO-dee-um bye-KAR-bon-ayt
How Supplied	Injection: 50 mEq/50 mL prefilled syringes
Mechanism of Action	• Increases plasma bicarbonate • Buffers excess hydrogen ion concentration • Raises blood pH • Reverses clinical manifestations of acidosis
Indications	**Known preexisting hyperkalemia (Class I)** • Sodium bicarbonate is used in hyperkalemia to decrease serum K^+ levels by temporarily shifting potassium into the intracellular fluid. • ECG changes include tall, peaked (tented) T waves; widened QRS complexes; prolonged PR intervals; flattened ST segments; and flattened or absent P waves. Hyperkalemia may lead to ventricular dysrhythmias and asystole if not reversed **Preexisting bicarbonate-responsive acidosis (Class IIa)** • Diabetic ketoacidosis (use of sodium bicarbonate is controversial); severe metabolic acidosis resulting from intoxication by methanol, ethylene glycol, salicylates **Overdose: tricyclic antidepressants, cocaine, diphenhydramine (Class IIa)** • Sodium bicarbonate may be administered in tricyclic antidepressant overdose with QRS prolongation or hypotension. The drug is repeated as needed to maintain the arterial pH between 7.45 and 7.55 **To alkalinize urine in certain overdoses (Class IIa)** • Phenobarbital, aspirin—alkalinization of the urine enhances the renal elimination of these medications **If effective ventilation and long arrest interval (Class IIb)** **On return of spontaneous circulation after a long arrest interval (Class IIb)** **Hypercarbic lactic acidosis (e.g., cardiac arrest without intubation) (Class III)**
Dosing (adult)	• Initial dose 1 mEq/kg IV bolus. Half the initial dose may be repeated every 10 min thereafter • In tricyclic antidepressant overdose, sodium bicarbonate may be administered by continuous IV infusion. Mix 50 mEq of sodium bicarbonate in 250 mL NS or as determined by a physician. Administer as instructed by physician
Precautions	Extravasation may lead to tissue inflammation and necrosis
Contraindications	• Significant metabolic or respiratory alkalosis • Severe pulmonary edema
Onset of Action	2 to 10 min
Duration	30 to 60 min
Drug Interactions	Do not mix with parenteral drugs because of the possibility of drug inactivation or precipitation

Diuretics

Table 7-51 Furosemide	
Generic Name	furosemide
Trade Name(s)	Lasix
Classification	Loop diuretic
Pronunciation	fur-OH-seh-myd
How Supplied	40 mg/4 mL ampule, vial, syringe
Mechanism of Action	• Inhibits the reabsorption of sodium and chloride in the ascending limb of the loop of Henle, resulting in an increase in the urinary excretion of sodium, chloride, and water → profound diuresis • Furosemide increases excretion of potassium, hydrogen, calcium, magnesium, bicarbonate, ammonium, and phosphate • Venodilation—increases venous capacitance, decreases preload (venous return)
Indications	• Adjunctive therapy in acute pulmonary edema (SBP >90 to 100 mm Hg without signs and symptoms of shock) • Hypertensive emergencies • Increased intracranial pressure
Dosing (adult)	• If the patient is not on oral furosemide therapy, the initial dose is 0.5 to 1.0 mg/kg (usually 20 to 40 mg) IV push administered at a rate no faster than 20 mg/min • If the patient is on oral furosemide therapy, consider an initial IV dose that is twice the daily oral dose. Administer slowly IV push at a rate no faster than 20 mg/min

Precautions	• Ototoxicity and resulting transient deafness can occur with rapid administration
	• Do not exceed the recommended rate of infusion
	• Furosemide should be administered cautiously in patients with:
	  • Diabetes mellitus
	  • Dehydration
	  • Severe renal disease
	Patients with sulfonamide hypersensitivity or thiazide diuretic hypersensitivity may also be hypersensitive to furosemide

Contraindications	• Hypersensitivity to furosemide or sulfonamides • Hypovolemia • Electrolyte depletion • Hypotension • Anuria • Hepatic coma
Special Considerations	Can cause excessive fluid loss and dehydration, resulting in hypovolemia and electrolyte imbalance
Onset of Action	• Vasodilation: <5 min; diuresis: within 5 min • Peak effect within ½ hour. Half-life approximately ½ to 1 hour
Duration	• Vasodilation: <2 hours; diuretic effect: approximately 2 hours
Drug Interactions	• Should not be used concomitantly with ethacrynic acid because of the possibility of ototoxicity • May add to or potentiate the therapeutic effect of other antihypertensive drugs • May decrease arterial responsiveness to norepinephrine • Digitalis: digitalis toxicity may be potentiated by loss of potassium • Salicylates: increased risk of salicylate toxicity caused by decreased renal excretion

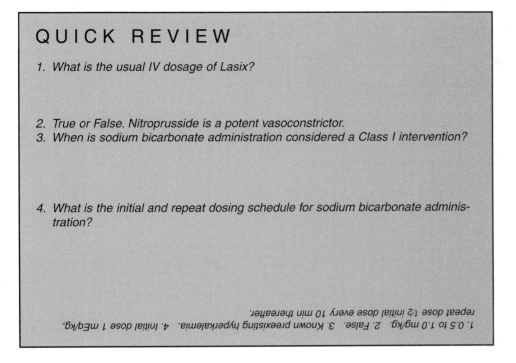

QUICK REVIEW

1. What is the usual IV dosage of Lasix?

2. True or False. Nitroprusside is a potent vasoconstrictor.
3. When is sodium bicarbonate administration considered a Class I intervention?

4. What is the initial and repeat dosing schedule for sodium bicarbonate administration?

1. 0.5 to 1.0 mg/kg. 2. False. 3. Known preexisting hyperkalemia. 4. Initial dose 1 mEq/kg, repeat dose 1/2 initial dose every 10 min thereafter.

STOP AND REVIEW

1. Digitalis:
   a. Increases heart rate
   b. Is contraindicated in persons with asthma
   c. Is a calcium channel blocker
   d. Increases the force of myocardial contraction

2. Bronchodilation and vasodilation are effects that occur with stimulation
   of:
   a. Beta-1 receptors
   b. Beta-2 receptors
   c. Alpha-1 receptors
   d. Dopaminergic receptors

3. Furosemide should be:
   a. Administered as quickly as possible because of its short half-life
   b. Administered at a rate of 20 mg/min
   c. Mixed in 50 mL of D5W and infused over 8-10 min
   d. Mixed in 250 mL of D5W and infused via an infusion pump over a
      24-hour period

4. Your patient is a 62-year-old male complaining of palpitations that came on suddenly after walking up a short flight of stairs. His symptoms have been present for approximately 20 min. He denies chest pain and is not short of breath. His skin is warm and dry, breath sounds are clear. BP 144/88, P 186, R 18. The cardiac monitor reveals sustained monomorphic ventricular tachycardia. The patient has been placed on oxygen, and an IV has been established. Which of the following medications is most appropriate in this situation?
   a. Procainamide
   b. Isoproterenol
   c. Propranolol
   d. Nitroglycerin

5. Norepinephrine:
   a. Is administered slowly IV push over at least 5 min
   b. May be used as an alternative to epinephrine in adult shock-refractory VF
   c. Is a potent vasoconstrictor used in the management of severe cardiogenic shock
   d. Is the drug of choice in cases of known preexisting hyperkalemia

6. Which of the following are calcium channel blockers?
   a. Lidocaine, procainamide
   b. Esmolol, atenolol
   c. Verapamil, diltiazem
   d. Sotalol, amiodarone

7. A 50-year-old female is complaining of substernal chest pain, dizziness, and nausea. On a 1 to 10 scale, she rates her discomfort an 8 and states her symptoms began approximately 3 hours ago. Her BP is 162/94, P 122, R 16. The cardiac monitor shows a sinus tachycardia. An IV has been established, and a 12-lead ECG has been ordered. Which of the following reflects the most reasonable management sequence for this patient?
   a. Oxygen, atropine 1.0 mg IV, sublingual nitroglycerin, and morphine 2 to 4 mg IV
   b. Oxygen, sublingual nitroglycerin, morphine 2 to 4 mg IV, and aspirin 162 to 325 mg (chewed)
   c. Sublingual nitroglycerin, adenosine 6 mg IV, oxygen, and diltiazem 20 mg IV
   d. Vasopressin 20 U IV, lidocaine 1 to 1.5 mg/kg IV, oxygen, procainamide 20 mg/min IV

8. All of the following are endpoints for procainamide administration EXCEPT:
   a. Hypotension develops
   b. Dysrhythmia is suppressed
   c. Total of 3 mg/kg has been administered
   d. QRS widens by 50% of its original width

9. In which of the following situations/conditions should nitroglycerin be AVOIDED?
   a. Viagra use within 24 hours
   b. Bronchospastic disease
   c. Unstable angina
   d. Hypertension

10. *True* or *False*. Glycoprotein IIb/IIIa inhibitors are indicated in acute coronary syndromes (ACS) without ST-segment elevation.

11. Angiotensin-converting enzyme (ACE) inhibitors:
    a. Are anticoagulants that bind to thrombin and render it inactive
    b. Cause blood vessels to relax, reducing the pressure against which the heart must pump, decreasing myocardial workload
    c. Act on beta-1 and beta-2 receptors to slow sinus rate, depress AV conduction, and reduce blood pressure
    d. Block the effects of the vagus nerve, resulting in an increase in the rate of discharge of the SA node

12. Diltiazem may be used to:
    a. Control the ventricular rate in atrial fibrillation and atrial flutter
    b. Convert wide-QRS tachycardia of uncertain origin to a sinus rhythm
    c. Control the ventricular rate in Wolff-Parkinson-White (WPW) syndrome
    d. Increase the ventricular rate in second- or third-degree (complete) AV block

13. Which of the following decrease myocardial oxygen requirements?
    a. Atropine, morphine
    b. Epinephrine, atropine
    c. Nitroglycerin, morphine
    d. Norepinephrine, nitroglycerin

14. The primary side effect of nitroglycerin administration is:
    a. Hypokalemia because of excessive diuresis
    b. Hypotension, which may worsen myocardial ischemia
    c. Vasoconstriction, which may excessively elevate blood pressure
    d. Prolongation of the QT interval, which may precipitate torsades de pointes

15. Dobutamine:
    a. Stimulates dopaminergic receptors
    b. Frequently induces reflex peripheral vasoconstriction
    c. Is a synthetic catecholamine useful in the treatment of heart failure
    d. Has predominant alpha-adrenergic receptor stimulating effects that increase myocardial contractility

16. *True* or *False*. Epinephrine decreases myocardial oxygen demand and should be considered early in the management of patients with ischemic heart disease.

17. Sodium bicarbonate:
    a. Is the antidote used for magnesium sulfate toxicity
    b. May be used to alkalinize the urine in aspirin overdose
    c. Is particularly useful in cardiac arrest without intubation
    d. Should be routinely used in cardiac arrest patients

18. Amiodarone is:
    a. The second-line medication used in the management of symptomatic bradycardia
    b. A positive inotropic agent with vasodilator activity used for short-term management of congestive heart failure
    c. A second-line medication used in the management of asystole and pulseless electrical activity
    d. Useful in the management of many atrial and ventricular tachydysrhythmias

19. Which of the following are used in the management of asystole and bradycardic pulseless electrical activity?
    a. Vasopressin and atropine
    b. Epinephrine and atropine
    c. Lidocaine and amiodarone
    d. Epinephrine and lidocaine

20. In the management of a symptomatic narrow-QRS bradycardia, if the maximum dose of atropine had been administered and a pacemaker was not immediately available, your next course of action would include:
    a. Adenosine 6 mg rapid IV push
    b. Dopamine infusion 5 to 20 mcg/kg/min
    c. Diltiazem 15 to 20 mg IV over 2 min
    d. Atenolol 5 mg slow IV push over 5 min

STOP AND REVIEW ANSWERS

1. d. Digitalis is a cardiac glycoside that slows conduction through AV node (prolonging of the PR interval), increases the force and velocity of myocardial contraction (+ inotropic effect), and increases cardiac output.

2. b. Bronchodilation and vasodilation are effects of beta-2 adrenergic receptor stimulation.

3. b. Furosemide should be administered slowly (at a rate of 20 mg/min) IV push.

4. a. From the information provided, the patient appears to be clinically stable despite the presence of monomorphic VT on the cardiac monitor. Procainamide or sotalol would be appropriate to consider in this situation. The IV form of sotalol is currently not approved for use in the United States.

5. c. Norepinephrine is a potent vasoconstrictor used in the management of severe cardiogenic shock (systolic BP <70 mm Hg). This medication is administered as a continuous IV infusion and not as an IV bolus. Vasopressin may be used as an alternative to epinephrine in adult shock-refractory VF. Sodium bicarbonate is considered a Class I intervention in cases of known preexisting hyperkalemia.

6. c. Verapamil and diltiazem are calcium channel blockers (Class IV antiarrhythmics). Lidocaine and procainamide are Class I anti-arrhythmics. Esmolol and atenolol are beta-blockers (Class II anti-arrhythmics). Sotalol and amiodarone are Class III antiarrhythmics.

7. b. From the information presented, it appears this patient may be experiencing an acute MI. Appropriate interventions in the manage-ment of this patient would include oxygen, IV access, sublingual nitroglycerin, morphine, and aspirin (if no contraindications). The acronym MONA (morphine, oxygen, nitroglycerin, aspirin) is used to help recall the immediate general treatment measures that should be considered for a patient experiencing an acute coronary syndrome.

8. c. Endpoints for procainamide administration include the onset of hypotension, suppression of the dysrhythmia, widening of the QRS by more than 50% of its original width, administration of a maximum dose of 17 mg/kg, and the onset of torsades de pointes (TdP).

9. a. Nitroglycerin is contraindicated if the patient has used Viagra within the past 24 hours or in the presence of right ventricular infarction, severe bradycardia or tachycardia, and/or hypotension.

10. *True.* Glycoprotein IIb/IIIa inhibitors (abciximab [ReoPro], eptifibatide [Integrilin], tirofiban [Aggrastat]) prevent fibrinogen binding and platelet aggregation. These medications are indicated in acute coronary syndromes without ST-segment elevation.

11. b. ACE inhibitors prevent the conversion of angiotensin I to angiotensin II. As a result, blood vessels relax, reducing the pres-sure the heart must pump against, and decreasing myocardial work-load. By increasing renal blood flow, ACE inhibitors help rid the body of excess sodium and fluid accumulation. Thrombin inhibitors are anticoagulants that bind to thrombin with a very high affinity, rendering it inactive. Beta-blockers act on beta-1 and beta-2 recep-tors to slow sinus rate, depress AV conduction, and reduce blood pressure. Atropine is a parasympatholytic that blocks the effects of the vagus nerve. This typically results in an increase in the rate of discharge of the SA node with an increase in AV conduction velocity.

12. a. Diltiazem is a calcium channel blocker that may be used to control the ventricular rate in atrial fibrillation and atrial flutter or to treat PSVT (after adenosine) in patients with an adequate blood pres-sure. Calcium channel blockers should be avoided in patients with wide-QRS tachycardia unless it is known with certainty to be supraventricular in origin—may precipitate VF! Calcium channel blockers should be avoided (Class III—may be harmful) in patients with WPW and are contraindicated in second- or third-degree (complete) AV block.

13. c. Nitroglycerin and morphine decrease myocardial oxygen require-ments. Epinephrine, norepinephrine, and atropine increase myocar-dial oxygen requirements.

14. b. The primary side effect of nitroglycerin administration is hypoten-sion, which may worsen myocardial ischemia.

15. c. Dobutamine is a synthetic catecholamine useful in the treatment of heart failure. It stimulates beta-adrenergic receptors and frequently induces reflex peripheral vasodilation. Beta-stimulation results in increased myocardial contractility.

16. *False.* Epinephrine administration results in many effects, including an increase in heart rate, force of contraction, and blood pressure. Because myocardial oxygen requirements are increased as a result of these effects, epinephrine should be used with caution in patients with ischemic heart disease.

17. b. Sodium bicarbonate may be used to alkalinize the urine in aspirin overdose (Class IIa) and is considered a Class III intervention (not useful or effective) in hypercarbic acidosis (e.g., cardiac arrest without intubation). Routine use of this medication in cardiac arrest is not recommended. Calcium is the antidote used for magnesium sulfate toxicity.

18. d. Amiodarone is useful in the management of many atrial and ventricular tachydysrhythmias; however, it is not used in the management of asystole or pulseless electrical activity (PEA). Dopamine is the second-line medication used in the management of symptomatic bradycardia (after atropine). Amrinone (not amiodarone) is a positive inotropic agent with vasodilator activity used for short-term management of congestive heart failure.

19. b. Epinephrine and atropine are used in the management of asystole and bradycardic pulseless electrical activity.

20. b. In the management of a symptomatic bradycardia, an infusion of dopamine at 5 to 20 mcg/kg/min should be initiated if a pacemaker is unavailable. The other medications listed (adenosine, diltiazem, atenolol) slow heart rate and should be avoided in the management of a bradycardia.

REFERENCES

1. Gonzalez ER, Ornato JP: *Field drug reference for emergency care providers*, Hamilton, IL, 1990, Drug Intelligence Publications.
2. Cleveland L, Aschenbrenner DS, Venable SJ, Yensen JAP: *Nursing management in drug therapy*, Philadelphia, 1999, Lippincott Williams & Wilkins.
3. Messerli, Franz H: *Cardiovascular drug therapy*, ed 2, Philadelphia, 1996, WB Saunders.
4. Weil MH, Tang W, editors: *CPR: resuscitation of the arrested heart*, Philadelphia, 1999, WB Saunders.
5. Braunwald E, Antman EM, Beasley JW, Califf RM, Cheitlin MD, Hochman JS, Jones RH, Kereiakes D, Kupersmith J, Levin TN, Pepine CJ, Schaeffer JW, Smith EE III, Steward DE, Théroux P. ACC/AHA 2002 guideline update for the management of patients with unstable angina and non–ST-segment elevation myocardial infarction: a report of the American College of Cardiology/American Heart Association Task Force on Practice Guidelines (Committee on the Management of Patients With Unstable Angina). 2002.
6. Cohen M. Platelet glycoprotein IIb/IIIa receptor Inhibitors in coronary artery disease, *Ann Intern Med* 124:843-844, 1996.

7. Lefkovits J: Recent advances in antiplatelet therapy, *Aust Prescr* 19;98-100, 1996.

8. Kahn MG: *Cardiac drug therapy*, ed 5, London, 2000, Harcourt Publishers Limited.

9. McIntosh-Yellin NL, et al: Safety and efficacy of central intravenous bolus administration of adenosine for termination of supraventricular tachycardia, *J Am Coll Cardiol* 22:741-745, 1993.

10. Wittwer LK, Muhr MD: Adenosine for the treatment of PSVT in the pre-hospital arena: efficacy of an initial 6 mg dosing regimen, *Prehosp Disaster Med* 12(3):237-239, 1997.

11. Trujillo TC, Nolan PE: Antiarrhythmic agents: drug interactions of clinical significance, *Drug Saf* 23(6):509-532, 2000.

12. *Mosby's Drug Consult*, St Louis, 2002, Mosby.

13. Friedman P: Factors in individual sensitivity to cardiac glycosides and recognition of digitalis intoxication, *Primary Cardiol* 1:13-17, 1988.

14. The American Heart Association in Collaboration with the International Liaison Committee on Resuscitation (ILCOR): Part 6: Advanced cardiovascular life support, Section 5: Pharmacology I: agents for arrhythmias, *Circulation* 102 (suppl I):I-123, 2000.

15. Paradis NA, editor: *Cardiac arrest: the science and practice of resuscitation medicine*, Baltimore, 1996, Williams & Wilkins.

16. The American Heart Association in Collaboration with the International Liaison Committee on Resuscitation (ILCOR): Part 6: Advanced cardiovascular life support, section 5: Pharmacology I: agents for Arrhythmias. *Circulation* 102 (suppl I):I-123-124, 2000.

17. Lightman SL: Molecular insights into diabetes insipidus, Editorial, *New Eng J Med* Vol 328, No 21, 1993.

18. Lindner KH, Brinkmann A, Pfenninger EG, Lurie KG, Goertz A, Lindner IM: Effect of vasopressin on hemodynamic variables, organ blood flow, and acid-base status in a pig model of cardiopulmonary resuscitation, *Anesth Analg* 77:427-435, 1993.

19. Lindner KH, Prengel AW, Pfenninger EG, Lindner IM, Strohmenger HU, Georgieff M, et al: Vasopressin improves vital organ blood flow during closed-chest cardiopulmonary resuscitation in pigs, *Circulation* 91:215-221, 1996.

20. Lindner KH, Prengel AW, Brinkmann A, Strohmenger HU, Lindner IM, Lurie KG: Vasopressin administration in refractory cardiac arrest, *Ann Inter Med* 124:1061-1064, 1996.

21. Borgeat A, Popovic V, Nicole A, et al: Acute pulmonary oedema following administration of ornithine-8-vasopressin, *Br J Anaesth* 65:548-551, 1990.

22. Olson KR, editor: *Poisoning and Drug Overdose*, ed 2, Norwalk, CT, 1994, Appleton & Lange.

BIBLIOGRAPHY

Chernow B (ed): *Essentials of critical care pharmacology*, ed 2, Baltimore, 1994, Williams & Wilkins.

Cleveland L, Aschenbrenner DS, Venable SJ, Yensen JAP. *Nursing management in drug therapy*, Philadelphia, 1999, Lippincott Williams & Wilkins.

Kahn MG: *Cardiac drug therapy*, ed 5, London, 2000, Harcourt Publishers Limited.

Messerli, F H: *Cardiovascular drug therapy*, ed 2, Philadelphia, 1996, WB Saunders.

Mosby's GenRx, ed 10, St Louis, 2000, Mosby.

Paradis NA, Halperin HR, Nowak RM, editors: *Cardiac arrest: the science and practice of resuscitation medicine*, Baltimore, 1996, Williams & Wilkins.

Ryan TJ, Antman EM, Brooks NH, Califf RM, Hillis LD, Hiratzka LF, Rapaport E, Riegel B, Russell RO, Smith EE III, Weaver WD: ACC/AHA guidelines for the management of patients with acute myocardial infarction: 1999 update: a report of the American College of Cardiology/ American Heart Association Task Force on Practice Guidelines (Committee on Management of Acute Myocardial Infarction). Available at http://www.acc.org/clinical/guidelines and http://www.americanheart.org.

Weil MH, Tang W, editors: *CPR: resuscitation of the arrested heart*, Philadelphia, 1999, WB Saunders.

Woods SL, Sivarajan Froelicher ES, Motzer SA: *Cardiac nursing*, ed 4, Philadelphia, 2000, Lippincott Williams & Wilkins.

Putting It All Together

OBJECTIVES

On completion of this chapter, you will be able to:

1. Describe the role of each member of the resuscitation team.
2. Describe the critical actions necessary in caring for the adult patient in cardiac arrest.
3. Identify the immediate goals of postresuscitation care.
4. Given a patient situation, describe the management steps (including mechanical, pharmacologic and electrical interventions where applicable) in each of the following situations:
   a. Cardiac arrest rhythms
      (1) Pulseless ventricular tachycardia (VT)/ventricular fibrillation (VF)
      (2) Asystole
      (3) Pulseless electrical activity
   b. Peri-arrest rhythms
      (1) Bradydysrhythmias
      (2) Narrow QRS tachycardia
      (3) Atrial fibrillation and atrial flutter with a rapid ventricular response
      (4) Monomorphic ventricular tachycardia
      (5) Polymorphic ventricular tachycardia
      (6) Wide QRS tachycardia of unknown origin
   c. Acute coronary syndromes
      (1) ST-segment elevation MI
      (2) Unstable angina/non–ST-elevation MI
      (3) Nondiagnostic/normal ECG
   d. Acute pulmonary edema
   e. Hypotension/shock: suspected pump problem
   f. Hypotension/shock: suspected volume problem
   g. Hypotension/shock: suspected rate problem

THE ACLS ALGORITHMS

ACLS algorithms can be found on the following pages. Knowledge of the algorithms is essential to successful completion of the ACLS course. When studying the algorithms, keep the following points in mind:
1. Algorithms are general guidelines for the management of specific dysrhythmias
2. Change in the rhythm or a change in the pulse changes the algorithm
3. Continually reassess the patient—conditions change

ACLS algorithms are presented in the following sequence:

1. Primary ABCD Survey
2. Secondary ABCD Survey
3. Cardiac Arrest Rhythms
   a. Pulseless Ventricular Tachycardia (VT)/Ventricular Fibrillation (VF)
   b. Non-VF/VT Rhythms
      (1) Asystole
      (2) Pulseless Electrical Activity (PEA)
4. Peri-Arrest Rhythms
   a. Symptomatic Bradycardia
   b. Narrow QRS Tachycardia
   c. Atrial Fibrillation/Atrial Flutter
   d. Wolff-Parkinson-White Syndrome
   e. Ventricular Tachycardia (Monomorphic)
   f. Ventricular Tachycardia (Polymorphic)
   g. Wide QRS Tachycardia of Unknown Origin
5. Acute Coronary Syndromes
   a. Initial Recognition and Management of ACS in the Field and Emergency Department
   b. Management of Patients with ST-Segment Elevation MI
   c. Management of Patients with ST-Depression or T Wave Changes
   d. Management of Patients with a Suspected Acute Coronary Syndrome and Nondiagnostic/Normal ECG
6. Pulmonary Edema/Hypotension/Shock
   a. Management of Acute Pulmonary Edema
   b. Management of Hypotension/Shock: Suspected Pump Problem
   c. Management of Hypotension/Shock: Suspected Volume Problem
   d. Management of Hypotension/Shock: Suspected Rate Problem

---

Although presented in Chapter 1, the classifications for therapeutic interventions are repeated here for ease of reference when reviewing the algorithms on the following pages.[1]

The International Guidelines 2000 for CPR and ECC Recommendations have been classified as follows:
1. *Class I: Definitely recommended. Interventions are always acceptable, proven safe, and definitely useful*
2. *Class IIa: Acceptable and useful. Interventions are acceptable, safe, and useful*

Considered intervention of choice by majority of experts
3. *Class IIb: Acceptable and useful. Interventions are acceptable, safe, and useful*

Considered optional or alternative interventions by majority of experts
4. *Indeterminate: Promising, evidence lacking. Describes treatments of promise but limited evidence*
5. *Class III: May be harmful; no documented benefit. Describes interventions with no evidence of any benefit, or studies suggest or confirm harm*

PRIMARY AND SECONDARY ABCD SURVEYS

Tables 8-1 and 8-2 depict the steps in conducting the Primary and Secondary ABCD Surveys.

Table 8-1   Primary ABCD Survey

Primary ABCD Survey

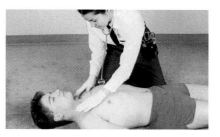

ASSESS RESPONSIVENESS

If responsive, ask patient questions to determine adequacy of airway and breathing

If unresponsive, call for help (9-1-1 "Phone first"), call for defibrillator

Continue Primary ABCD Survey

↓

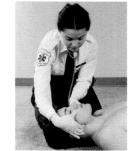

AIRWAY

Open the airway

If the airway is open, evaluate breathing

If the airway is not open, assess for sounds of airway compromise and look in the mouth for blood, broken teeth, loose dentures, gastric contents, and foreign objects

Clear the airway and insert an airway adjunct as needed to maintain an open airway

↓

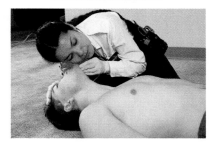

BREATHING

Look, listen, and feel for breathing

If the patient is responsive and breathing is adequate, evaluate circulation

If the unresponsive patient is breathing adequately, place in recovery position if no signs of trauma

If breathing is difficult and the rate is too slow or too fast, provide positive-pressure ventilation with 100% oxygen

If breathing is absent, deliver two slow breaths and ensure the patient's chest rises with each breath. Insert an airway adjunct (if not previously done) and provide positive-pressure ventilation with a pocket mask or bag-valve-mask. Continue the Primary ABCD Survey.

↓

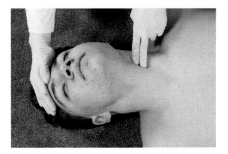

CIRCULATION

Assess for the presence of a pulse

If the patient is unresponsive, assess the carotid pulse on the side of the patient's neck nearest you

If the patient is responsive, assess the radial pulse. If a pulse is present, quickly estimate the rate and determine the quality of the pulse (e.g., fast/slow, regular/irregular, weak/strong), then perform the Secondary ABCD Survey

If there is no pulse, begin chest compressions until an AED or monitor/defibrillator is available

↓

DEFIBRILLATION

Attach AED or monitor/defibrillator when available

If cardiac rhythm is pulseless VT or VF:

Defibrillate up to 3 times in rapid succession pausing only to analyze/verify rhythm ("serial shocks")

Defibrillate with 200 J, 200 to 300 J, 360 J, or equivalent biphasic energy as necessary

If cardiac rhythm is not VT/VF, perform Secondary ABCD Survey

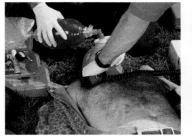
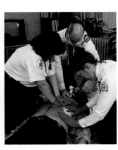

Table 8-2 Secondary ABCD Survey

Secondary ABCD Survey

(ADVANCED) AIRWAY
Reassess the effectiveness of initial airway maneuvers and interventions
Perform endotracheal intubation, if needed

↓

BREATHING
Assess ventilation
Confirm endotracheal tube placement (or other airway device) by at least two methods
Provide positive-pressure ventilation
Evaluate effectiveness of ventilations

↓

CIRCULATION
Establish peripheral intravenous (IV) access
Attach ECG
Administer medications appropriate for cardiac rhythm/clinical situation

↓

DIFFERENTIAL DIAGNOSIS
Consider possible cause(s) of the arrest, rhythm, situation

CARDIAC ARREST RHYTHMS

Resuscitation Team

> *Four Critical Tasks of Resuscitation:*
> - *Airway management*
> - *Chest compressions*
> - *Monitoring and defibrillation*
> - *IV access and medication administration*

Table 8-3 Resuscitation Team: Team Leader Responsibilities

ACLS team leader should:
- Direct team members and assign the four critical resuscitation tasks: airway management, chest compressions, monitoring and defibrillation, IV access and medication administration
- Assess the patient
- Order interventions according to protocols
- Consider reasons for the cardiac arrest and possible reversible causes
- Supervise team members, ensuring each member of the team performs his or her tasks safely and correctly
- Evaluate the adequacy of chest compressions, including hand position, depth of cardiac compressions, proper rate, and ratio of compressions to ventilations
- Ensure the patient is receiving 100% oxygen
- Evaluate the adequacy of ventilation by assessing bilateral, symmetric, chest expansion with each ventilation
- Ensure that defibrillation, when indicated, is performed safely and correctly
- Call for assessment of a pulse following defibrillation
- Ensure the correct choice and placement of IV access
- Confirm proper endotracheal tube position using at least two methods
- Ensure medications administered are appropriate for the clinical situation/dysrhythmia and are given in the correct dose, route, and concentration (if applicable)
- Ensure IV bolus medications are followed with a 20-mL fluid flush
- Ensure the safety of all members of the resuscitation team, especially when procedures such as defibrillation are performed
- Problem-solve, including reevaluating possible causes of the arrest, recognizing malfunctioning equipment and/or misplaced or displaced tubes or lines
- Decide when to terminate resuscitation efforts

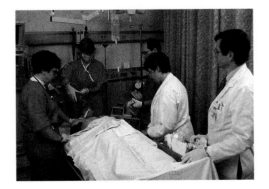

Team leader assigns the four critical resuscitation tasks: (1) airway management, (2) chest compression, (3) monitoring and defibrillation, and (4) IV access and medication administration.

Table 8-4 Resuscitation Team: Airway Management Team Member Responsibilities

ACLS team member responsible for airway management should:
- Be able to perform manual airway maneuvers, including the jaw thrust without head tilt maneuver and head-tilt/chin-lift maneuver
- Be able to correctly size and insert an oropharyngeal airway and nasopharyngeal airway
- Be able to correctly apply and understand the indications, contraindications, advantages, disadvantages, complications, liter flow range, and concentration of delivered oxygen for oxygen delivery devices, including the nasal cannula, simple face mask, pocket mask, nonrebreathing mask, and bag-valve-mask device
- Be able to suction the upper airway by selecting an appropriate suction device, catheter, and technique
- Know how to correctly perform cricoid pressure during endotracheal intubation
- Know the indications, contraindications, advantages, disadvantages, complications, equipment, and technique for (if within his or her scope of practice) endotracheal intubation
- Know how to confirm placement of an endotracheal tube by using at least two methods

Table 8-5 Resuscitation Team: CPR Team Member Responsibilities

ACLS or BLS team member responsible for CPR should:
- Know how to properly perform CPR
- Provide chest compressions of adequate rate, force, and depth in the correct location

Table 8-6 Resuscitation Team: Defibrillation Team Member Responsibilities

ACLS team member responsible for defibrillation should know:
- The difference between defibrillation and synchronized cardioversion, the indications for, and potential complications of these electrical interventions
- The proper placement of conventional defibrillator paddles
- How to perform a "quick-look"
- The safety precautions that must be considered when performing electrical interventions
- The primary clinical indications for and possible complications of transcutaneous pacing
- How to problem-solve equipment failure

Table 8-7 Resuscitation Team: IV Access/Medication Administration Team Member Responsibilities

ACLS team member responsible for IV access and medication administration should know:
- Site(s) of first choice for cannulation if no IV is in place at the time of cardiac arrest
- IV fluids of first choice in cardiac arrest
- Importance of following each IV medication administered in a cardiac arrest with a 20 mL IV fluid bolus
- Routes of administration and appropriate dosages for IV, ET, and IO resuscitation medications

Although not always available, information pertinent to the arrest should be sought including:
- *When and where did the arrest occur?*
- *Was the arrest witnessed?*
- *Was CPR performed? If yes, how long was the patient down before CPR was started?*
- *What was the patient's initial cardiac rhythm? If pulseless VT or VF, when was the first shock delivered?*
- *Are there any special circumstances to consider (e.g., hypothermia, trauma, drug overdose, do-not-attempt-resuscitation orders, etc.)?*
- *What interventions have been performed?*
- *What information is available regarding the patient's past medical history?*

Pulseless Ventricular Tachycardia/Ventricular Fibrillation

Table 8-8 demonstrates ventricular tachycardia (VT) and ventricular fibrillation (VF).

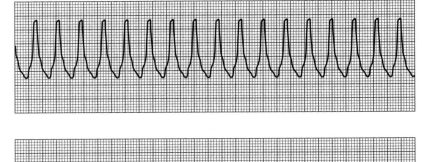

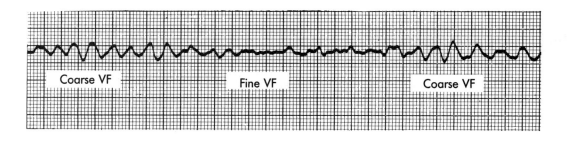

Coarse VF   Fine VF   Coarse VF

Table 8-8   Pulseless Ventricular Tachycardia (VT)/ Ventricular Fibrillation (VF)

Perform Primary ABCD Survey
(Correct critical problems IMMEDIATELY as they are identified)
Assess responsiveness

Basic   Call for help/call for defibrillator
Life   **A**irway—open the airway
Support   **B**reathing—deliver two slow breaths, administer oxygen as soon as it is available
Circulation—perform chest compressions
Ensure availability of monitor/**D**efibrillator
On arrival of AED/monitor/defibrillator, evaluate cardiac rhythm
▼
If PEA or asystole, continue CPR and go to appropriate algorithm.
If pulseless VT/VF, shock up to three times (200 J, 200 to 300 J, 360 J, or equivalent Biphasic energy).
▼

Table 8-8   Pulseless Ventricular Tachycardia (VT)/ Ventricular Fibrillation (VF)—cont'd

▼

Reevaluate cardiac rhythm

- If persistent or recurrent pulse-less VT/VF, continue CPR and perform secondary ABCD Survey

- If PEA or asystole, continue CPR and go to appropriate algorithm

If return of spontaneous circulation (ROSC):
- Assess vital signs
- Maintain open airway
- Provide ventilation
- Administer medications appropriate for rhythm, blood pressure, and heart rate

▼

Perform Secondary ABCD Survey
(ADVANCED) *A*IRWAY
Reassess effectiveness of initial airway maneuvers and interventions
Perform invasive airway management

▼

***B*REATHING**
Assess ventilation

Advanced   Confirm ET tube placement (or other airway device) by at least two methods
Life   Provide positive-pressure ventilation/Evaluate effectiveness of ventilations
Support   Secure airway device in place with commercial tube holder (preferred) or tape

▼

***C*IRCULATION**
Establish IV access and administer appropriate medications

▼

***D*IFFERENTIAL DIAGNOSIS**
Search for and treat reversible causes

▼

Pattern   **Epinephrine** (Class Indeterminate) 1 mg (1:10,000 solution) IV every 3 to 5 min
becomes CPR-   (ET dose 2 to 2.5 mg diluted in 10-mL normal saline or distilled water)
drug-shock or **or**
CPR-drug-   **Vasopressin** (Class IIb) 40 U IV bolus[7] (administer only once)
shock-shock-   (If no response to vasopressin, may resume epinephrine after 10 to 20 min;
shock   epi dose 1 mg every 3 to 5 min)

▼

Defibrillate with 360 J (or equivalent Biphasic energy) within 30 to 60 sec

▼

Consider antiarrhythmics (avoid use of multiple antiarrhythmics because of potential proarrhythmic effects)
- **Amiodarone**[14] (Class IIb): Initial bolus: 300 mg IV bolus diluted in 20 to 30 mL of NS or D5W. Consider repeat dose (150 mg IV bolus) in 3 to 5 min. If defibrillation successful, follow with 1 mg/min IV infusion for 6 hours (mix 900 mg in 500 mL NS), then decrease infusion rate to 0.5 mg/min IV infusion for 18 hours. Maximum daily dose 2.0 g IV/24 hours
- **Lidocaine** (Class Indeterminate): 1 to 1.5 mg/kg IV bolus, consider repeat dose (0.5 to 0.75 mg/kg) in 5 min; maximum IV bolus dose 3 mg/kg. (The 1.5 mg/kg dose is recommended in cardiac arrest). Endotracheal dose: 2 to 4 mg/kg. A single dose of 1.5 mg/kg is acceptable in cardiac arrest
- **Magnesium** (Class IIb if hypomagnesemia present): 1 to 2 g IV (2 to 4 mL of a 50% solution) diluted in 10 mL of D5W if Torsades de Pointes[23,24] or hypomagnesemia[25]
- **Procainamide**[21] (Class IIb for recurrent pulseless VT/VF; Class Indeterminate for persistent pulseless VT/VF): 20 mg/min; maximum total dose 17 mg/kg

Consider **sodium bicarbonate** 1 mEq/kg

14,21,23-25See chapter references.

Non-VF/VT Arrest Rhythms

Asystole

Table 8-9 demonstrates asystole and P-wave asystole.

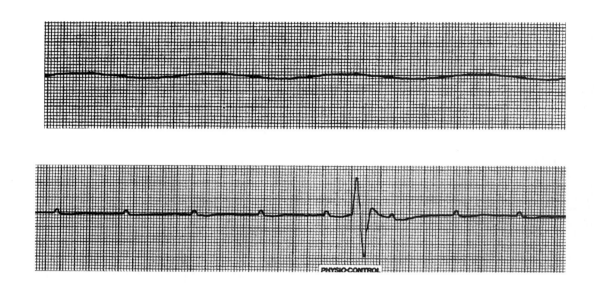

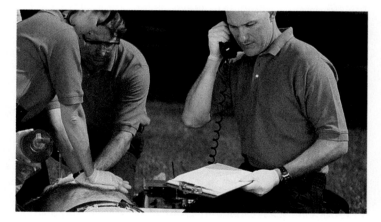

Table 8-9 Asystole

Basic Life Support

Perform Primary ABCD Survey
(Correct critical problems IMMEDIATELY as they are identified)
Assess responsiveness
Call for help/call for defibrillator
Airway—open the airway
Breathing—deliver two slow breaths, administer oxygen as soon as it is available
Circulation—perform chest compressions
Ensure availability of monitor/**D**efibrillator
On arrival of AED/monitor/defibrillator, perform secondary ABCD Survey if rhythm is NOT pulseless VT/VF

▼

Scene Survey—Documentation or other evidence of
Do Not Attempt Resuscitation (DNAR)?
Obvious signs of death? If yes, do not start/attempt resuscitation

▼

Advanced Life Support

Possible causes
of asystole:
PATCH-4-MD

Pulmonary embolism
Acidosis
Tension pneumothorax
Cardiac tamponade
Hypovolemia
Hypoxia
Heat/cold (hypo-/
hyperthermia)
Hypo-/hyperkalemia
(and other electrolytes)
Myocardial infarction
Drug overdose/
accidents (cyclic anti-
depressants, calcium
channel blockers,
beta-blockers, digitalis)

Perform Secondary ABCD Survey
(ADVANCED) *AIRWAY*
Reassess effectiveness of initial airway maneuvers and interventions
Perform invasive airway management

▼

BREATHING
Assess ventilation
Confirm ET tube placement (or other airway device) by at least two methods
Provide positive-pressure ventilation/evaluate effectiveness of ventilations
Secure airway device in place with commercial tube holder (preferred) or tape

▼

CIRCULATION
Confirm presence of asystole
(Check lead/cable connections, ensure power to monitor is on, correct lead is selected,
gain turned up, confirm asystole in second lead)
Establish IV access and administer appropriate medications

▼

DIFFERENTIAL DIAGNOSIS
Search for and treat reversible causes *(PATCH-4-MD)*

▼

Consider immediate transcutaneous pacing

▼

Epinephrine 1 mg (1:10,000 solution) IV every 3 to 5 min
(ET dose 2 to 2.5 mg diluted in 10 mL normal saline or distilled water)

▼

Atropine[27,28] 1 mg IV every 3 to 5 min to maximum 0.04 mg/kg (Class IIb)
(ET dose 2 to 3 mg diluted in 10 mL normal saline or distilled water)

▼

Consider sodium bicarbonate 1 mEq/kg:
- Known preexisting hyperkalemia (Class I)
- Cyclic antidepressant overdose (IIa)
- To alkalinize urine in aspirin or other drug overdoses (IIa)
- Patient that has been intubated + long arrest interval (IIb)
- On return of spontaneous circulation if long arrest interval (IIb)

▼

Consider termination of efforts:
- Evaluate the quality of the resuscitation attempt
- Evaluate the resuscitation for atypical clinical features (e.g., hypothermia, reversible therapeutic or illicit drug use)
- Does support for cease-effort protocols exist?

[27,28]See chapter references.

Pulseless Electrical Activity (PEA)

Tables 8-10 and 8-11 demonstrate pulseless electrical activity (PEA).

1. Pulseless electrical activity (formerly called EMD, electromechanical dissociation) is an organized rhythm on the monitor, other than VT, that does not produce a palpable pulse
   a. The term was changed because research using ultrasonography and indwelling pressure catheters revealed that the electrical activity seen in some of these situations is associated with mechanical contractions—the contractions are simply too weak to produce a palpable pulse or measurable blood pressure
2. Types of PEA include:
   a. Normotensive PEA: Baseline cardiac contractions and shortening of myocardial fibers in the absence of detectable pulses
   b. Pseudo-PEA: Myocardial contractions present but too weak to produce a detectable pulse. The presence of a pulse is measurable by invasive monitoring or echocardiography
   c. True PEA: Myocardial contractions absent
3. In some patients, PEA is not a primary cardiac arrest but a state of severe cardiogenic shock from another cause
   a. Severe hypotension results in decreased coronary perfusion. This impairs cardiac function and results in even greater hypotension
   b. In normotensive PEA, myocardial contractility is normal. As the PEA continues, decreased cardiac contractions occur (pseudo-PEA), eventually resulting in absent cardiac contractions (true PEA)
   c. The cause of many cases of sudden cardiac arrest from PEA is unknown

Pulseless Electrical Activity (PEA)—cont'd

4. **Many ECG rhythms have been associated with PEA (see Figure 8-14) and most can be classified into one of the following categories:**
   a. **Electromechanical dissociation (EMD) rhythms**
      (1) **Organized electrical activity with no clinically detectable pulse**
      (2) **Narrow QRS complex that may be fast or slow**
   b. **Pseudo-EMD rhythms**
      (1) **Organized electrical activity with no clinically detectable pulse; however, pulse detectable by Doppler**
      (2) **Narrow QRS complex that may be fast or slow**
   c. **Idioventricular or ventricular escape rhythms**
      (1) **Organized electrical activity with no clinically detectable pulse**
      (2) **Slow wide QRS complex**
   d. **Bradyasystolic rhythms**
      (1) **"Bradyasystole refers to a cardiac rhythm that has a ventricular rate below 60 beats/min in adults, periods of absent heart rhythm (asystole), or both. Bradyasystolic states are clinical situations during which bradyasystole is the dominant heart rhythm"** [31]
      (2) **Organized electrical activity with no clinically detectable pulse**
      (3) **Profound bradycardia with a wide QRS, often with prolonged periods of asystole**

Table 8-10 Pulseless Electrical Activity (PEA)

Basic Life Support	**Perform Primary ABCD Survey** (Correct critical problems IMMEDIATELY as they are identified) Assess responsiveness Call for help/call for defibrillator **A**irway—open the airway **B**reathing—deliver two slow breaths, administer oxygen as soon as it is available **C**irculation—perform chest compressions Ensure availability of monitor/**D**efibrillator On arrival of AED/monitor/defibrillator, perform secondary ABCD Survey if rhythm is NOT pulseless VT/VF

▼

Perform Secondary ABCD Survey
(ADVANCED) *A*IRWAY
Reassess effectiveness of initial airway maneuvers and interventions
Perform invasive airway management

▼

***B*REATHING**
Assess ventilation
Confirm ET tube placement (or other airway device) by at least two methods
Provide positive-pressure ventilation/evaluate effectiveness of ventilations
Secure airway device in place with commercial tube holder (preferred) or tape

▼

***C*IRCULATION**
Establish IV access
Assess blood flow with Doppler
(If blood flow detected with Doppler, treat using hypotension/shock algorithm)
Administer appropriate medications

▼

***D*IFFERENTIAL DIAGNOSIS**
Search for and treat reversible causes *(PATCH-4-MD)*
(Fast narrow-QRS—consider hypovolemia, tamponade, pulmonary embolism, tension pneumothorax; slow wide QRS—consider cyclic antidepressant overdose, calcium channel blocker, beta-blocker, or digitalis toxicity)

▼

Epinephrine 1 mg (1:10,000 solution) IV every 3 to 5 min
(ET dose 2 to 2.5 mg diluted in 10 mL normal saline or distilled water)

▼

If the rate is slow, atropine 1 mg IV every 3 to 5 min to max 0.04 mg/kg (Class IIb)
(ET dose 2 to 3 mg diluted in 10 mL normal saline or distilled water)

▼

Consider sodium bicarbonate 1 mEq/kg:
* Known preexisting hyperkalemia (Class I)
* Cyclic antidepressant overdose (IIa)
* To alkalinize urine in aspirin or other drug overdoses (IIa)
* Patient that has been intubated + long arrest interval (IIb)
* On return of spontaneous circulation if long arrest interval (IIb)

▼

Consider termination of efforts

Advanced Life Support

Possible causes of PEA:
PATCH-4-MD

Pulmonary embolism
Acidosis
Tension pneumothorax
Cardiac tamponade
Hypovolemia (most common cause)
Hypoxia
Heat/cold (hypo-/hyperthermia)
Hypo-/hyperkalemia (and other electrolytes)
Myocardial infarction
Drug overdose/accidents (cyclic antidepressants, calcium channel blockers, beta-blockers, digitalis)

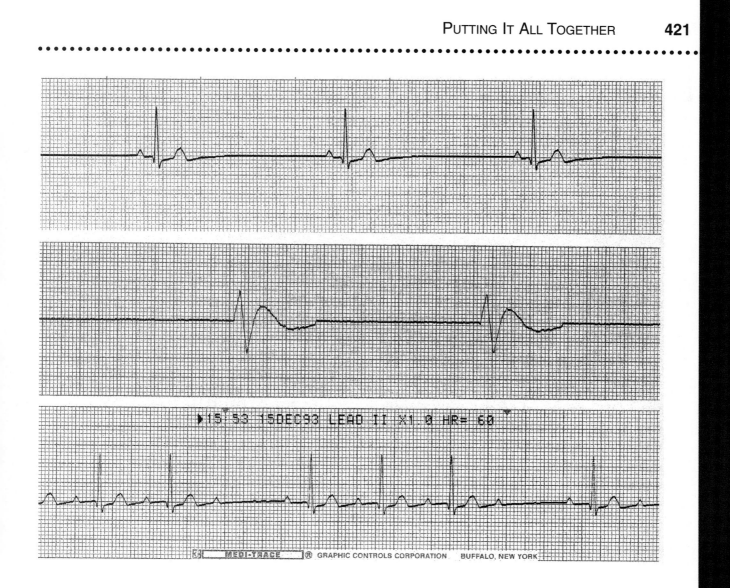

▶15:53 15DEC93 LEAD II X1.0 HR= 60

MEDI-TRACE ® GRAPHIC CONTROLS CORPORATION BUFFALO, NEW YORK

Table 8-11   Pulseless Electrical Activity (PEA): Clinical Signs and Treatment

Cause	Typical ECG Findings	History, Physical Findings	Management
Mechanical Causes			
Tension pneumothorax	Narrow QRS complex, slow rate (because of hypoxia)	History (trauma, asthma, ventilator, COPD), unequal breath sounds, no pulse with CPR, neck vein distention, tracheal deviation, difficult to ventilate patient, hyperresonance to percussion on affected side	Needle decompression—second intercostal space, midclavicular line
Cardiac tamponade	Narrow QRS complex, rapid rate (impending tamponade)—deteriorating to sudden bradycardia as terminal event	History (trauma, renal failure, thoracic malignancy), no pulse with CPR, neck vein distention	Pericardiocentesis
Decreased Preload			
Hypovolemia	Narrow QRS complex, rapid rate	History, flat neck veins	Volume replacement; find source (e.g., bleeding) and manage
Sepsis		History	Volume replacement, antibiotics
Massive pulmonary embolism	Narrow QRS complex, rapid rate	History, no pulse with CPR, neck vein distention, deep vein thrombosis in lower extremities	Pulmonary arteriogram, surgical embolectomy, fibrinolytics
Myocardial Dysfunction			
Massive myocardial infarction	Q waves, ST segment changes, T wave inversion	History, ECG, enzyme levels	Emergency PTCA, if unavailable, fibrinolytics
Drug overdose			
Calcium channel blocker	Slow rate, prolonged PR interval, possible AV block	History of ingestion, empty bottles at the scene, check pupils, neurologic exam	Calcium IV, pacing
Beta-blocker	Slow rate, prolonged PR interval, possible AV block		Glucagon IV, pacing
Cyclic antidepressants	Rapid rate, prolonged QT interval, widening of QRS, ST segment changes		Sodium bicarbonate IV
Digoxin	Slow rate, prolonged PR interval, shortened QT interval, T wave inversion or flattening		Fab antibodies

Table 8-11 Pulseless Electrical Activity (PEA): Clinical Signs and Treatment—cont'd

Cause	Typical ECG Findings	History, Physical Findings	Management
Electrolytes			
Hypokalemia	ST segment depression, T waves flatten, prominent U waves, QRS widens (uncommon in adults)	Prolonged diuretic therapy; administration of K^+ deficient parenteral fluids; severe GI fluid losses from gastric suctioning or lavage; prolonged vomiting or diarrhea, or laxative abuse without K^+ replacement	Rapid, controlled potassium infusion
Hyperkalemia	Rapid rate; tall, narrow, peaked (tented) T waves; QRS widens; flattened or absent P waves; ST segment elevation	History of acute or chronic renal failure; diabetes; dialysis fistulas; medications; severe cell damage such as from burns, trauma, crush injuries	Calcium chloride IV push (immediate); then combination of insulin, glucose, sodium bicarbonate; then sodium polystyrene sulfonate/sorbitol; dialysis (long-term)
Hypocalcemia	Prolonged QT interval and ST segment; VT, TdP	Acute or chronic renal failure, acute pancreatitis	Calcium chloride IV
Hypercalcemia	Shortened QT interval	Excessive intake of Ca^{++} supplements, prolonged immobility, thiazide diuretics	Magnesium sulfate, potassium, diuretics
Hypomagnesemia	Flattened T waves, slightly widened QRS complex, diminished voltage of P waves and QRS complexes, prominent U waves	Severe GI fluid losses from gastric suctioning or lavage, prolonged vomiting or diarrhea, or laxative abuse; administration of IV fluids or TPN without magnesium replacement; cancer chemotherapy	Magnesium sulfate
Hypothermia			
Hypothermia	Initial tachycardia, then progressive bradycardia; J or Osborne waves	History of cold exposure, core body temperature	Rewarming guided by core temperature
Pulmonary Causes			
Severe respiratory insufficiency/arrest resulting in hypoxia	Slow rate because of hypoxia	Cyanosis, blood gas results, airway obstruction	Ventilation
Post-Defibrillation PEA			
After reversal of prolonged VF with electrical countershock			No specific intervention

Medications Used in Pulseless VT/VF

1992 guidelines: Epinephrine, lidocaine, bretylium, magnesium sulfate, procainamide, sodium bicarbonate

2000 guidelines: Epinephrine or vasopressin, consider antidysrhythmics: amiodarone, lidocaine, magnesium sulfate (if hypomagnesemic state), procainamide (for intermittent/recurrent pulseless VT/VF); consider sodium bicarbonate

Epinephrine

Epinephrine has been used in cardiac arrest primarily for its alpha-adrenergic properties (i.e., vasoconstriction), improving coronary and internal carotid artery perfusion. Several studies have compared the effects of high-dose epinephrine with standard-dose epinephrine on the outcome of CPR,[2-5] *none of which showed a statistically significant improvement in the rate of survival to hospital discharge.* These findings were reaffirmed in a more recent study involving 3327 adult patients.[6]

"In patients who reach the point at which epinephrine is used for resuscitation, the rate of survival to hospital discharge is <1%."[7,8]

Vasopressin

Studies regarding the use of vasopressin have shown that:

- Vasopressin exerts a greater vasoconstrictive effect under conditions of hypoxia and acidosis than does epinephrine, and the effects of vasopressin last longer[9,10]
- Vasopressin causes a greater increase in arterial tone than does epinephrine, an effect that correlates with greater myocardial perfusion[9,10]
- Epinephrine increases myocardial oxygen consumption and lactate production in the arrested heart, and vasopressin does not[11]

In a randomized, prospective, double-blind study conducted on 40 patients with out-of-hospital VF resistant to direct-current shocks, a significantly larger proportion of patients initially treated with 40 units of IV vasopressin were resuscitated successfully and survived for 24 hours or more compared with patients treated with 1 mg of IV epinephrine. However, *there was no significant difference in survival to hospital discharge.*

A 1996 report indicates that in pigs, vasopressin produces more severe postresuscitation myocardial dysfunction than epinephrine in the early hours after restoration of spontaneous circulation.[12] Differences in animals treated with epinephrine vs. vasopressin were most pronounced 15 minutes after restoration of spontaneous circulation. In those treated with vasopressin, postresuscitation systemic vascular resistance was twofold greater than that of the epinephrine group with reduced myocardial contractility and less epicardial blood flow.[13] Four hours after CPR, no significant differences were observed between groups.

Amiodarone

The recommendation to include amiodarone in the 2000 Guidelines for pulseless VT/VF was based primarily on the ARREST (Amiodarone in the out-of-hospital Resuscitation of REfractory Sustained ventricular Tachyarrhythmias) study published September 16, 1999 in the *New England Journal of Medicine.*[14,15]

Medications Used in Pulseless VT/VF—cont'd

Amiodarone—cont'd

The ARREST study was a randomized, double blind, placebo-controlled study of IV amiodarone in patients with prehospital cardiac arrest in the Seattle area. Patients who had cardiac arrest with ventricular fibrillation (or pulseless ventricular tachycardia) and who had not been resuscitated after receiving three or more precordial shocks were randomly assigned to receive 300 mg of intravenous amiodarone (246 patients) or placebo (258 patients).

The investigators reported that a single dose of IV amiodarone improved survival to hospital admission (44% of patients in the amiodarone group survived to admission, as compared with 34% of patients in the placebo group). Although there was no statistical difference in long-term survival, more than half of the patients that left the hospital resumed independent living activities or returned to their former employment (55% in the amiodarone group, 50% in the placebo group).

The ALIVE (**A**miodarone versus **L**idocaine **I**n Pre-Hospital Cardiac Arrest Due to **V**entricular Fibrillation **E**valuation) study was conducted by St. Michael's Hospital/University of Toronto and Toronto Emergency Medical System to compare amiodarone with lidocaine in patients with out-of-hospital cardiac arrest due to refractory VF. In this prospective, randomized, controlled, and blinded trial, researchers studied the effectiveness of lidocaine vs. IV amiodarone by following 347 patients that had suffered cardiac arrest and did not respond to three defibrillation shocks. Toronto paramedics administered one of the two drugs to each patient. An initial dose of 5 mg/kg of IV amiodarone or 1.5 mg/kg of IV lidocaine was used. If necessary, a second bolus dose of the study drug was administered (2.5 mg/kg of IV amiodarone or 1.5 mg/kg of IV lidocaine).[59]

The ALIVE trial found that after treatment with amiodarone, 22.8 percent of 180 patients survived to hospital admission, as compared with 12.0 percent of 167 patients treated with lidocaine. Among patients receiving drug treatment within 24 minutes, 27.7 percent of those given amiodarone and 15.3 percent of those given lidocaine survived to hospital admission.

Recent studies have evaluated an aqueous formulation of amiodarone. The standard formulation (Cordarone IV) frequently causes hypotension. Hemodynamic studies have attributed this adverse effect to the solvents employed. A newly developed aqueous formulation (Amio-Aqueous) lacks solvents and thus may not cause hypotension. Researchers at West Los Angeles VA Medical Center in California evaluated the hemodynamic effects of this preparation in a cardiac catheterization laboratory. Two boluses of 150-mg aqueous amiodarone were administered via a peripheral vein to 32 hemodynamically stable patients who underwent cardiac catheterization. Boluses were administered initially over 2 to 5 minutes and in the last 9 patients over 2 minutes. Hemodynamic evaluation was performed and 12-lead ECGs were obtained at baseline, immediately after each bolus, and following 30 minutes of observation. No patient developed hypotension and there were no significant changes in systolic and diastolic blood pressure (BP) following the boluses. These researchers concluded that Amio-Aqueous possesses pharmacodynamic effects that have been attributed to amiodarene, but lacks the hypotensive effect of the standard intravenous amiodarone formulation. Amio-Aqueous appears to be a safer alternative to Cordarone IV when rapid administration is indicated.[60]

Continued

Medications Used in Pulseless VT/VF—cont'd

Amiodarone—cont'd

Another study evaluated the efficacy of water-soluble IV amiodarone versus IV lidocaine for the treatment of shock-resistant VT. In this double-blinded study, patients were randomized to receive up to 2 boluses of either 150 mg IV amiodarone or 2 boluses of 100 mg IV lidocaine followed by a 24-hour infusion. If the first assigned medication failed to terminate VT, the patient was crossed over to the alternative therapy. 29 patients were randomized to the study (18 received amiodarone, 11 received lidocaine). There were no significant differences between groups with regard to baseline characteristics. Immediate VT termination was achieved in 14 patients (78%) with amiodarone versus 3 patients (27%) with lidocaine. After 1 hour, 12 patients (67%) on amiodarone and 1 patient (9%) on lidocaine were alive and free of VT. Amiodarone had a 33% drug failure rate, whereas there was a 91% drug failure rate for lidocaine. The 24-hour survival was 39% on amiodarone and 9% on lidocaine. Drug-related hypotension with aqueous amiodarone was less frequent than with lidocaine.[61]

Lidocaine

In a 1981 clinical trial,[16] drug management of out-of-hospital countershock refractory VF was evaluated by including a 100-mg IV bolus of lidocaine as the only antiarrhythmic option in a protocol for use by paramedics. One hundred-sixteen patients entered the study by failing to convert from VF after the sequence of countershock, sodium bicarbonate, and repeat countershock. Sixty-two patients (53%) received lidocaine during the course of attempted resuscitation (Group I); 54 patients (47%) did not receive lidocaine (Group II). The two groups did not have significant differences in response times, patient profiles, or the use of other drugs or procedures. In Group I, 28 patients (45%) remained in VF on arrival at the hospital, 15 (24%) were admitted to the CCU, and 7 (11%) were ultimately discharged. In Group II, 25 patients (46%) remained in ventricular fibrillation on arrival at the hospital, 8 (17%) survived to hospital admission, and 1 (2%) was ultimately discharged.

In a 1997 retrospective study comparing patients who received lidocaine with those who did not in sustained VF and after conversion to a pulse-generating rhythm,[17] treatment with lidocaine was associated with a higher rate of return of spontaneous circulation and hospitalization *but was not associated with an increased rate of discharge from the hospital.*

Animal studies have shown that lidocaine *increases* the energy necessary to convert VF.[18]

Magnesium

Two prospective, double blind, randomized trials of in-hospital cardiac arrest patients found no benefit from routine treatment with magnesium.[19,20] Magnesium has shown to be effective only in the treatment of known hypomagnesemia and torsades de pointes.

Procainamide

The inclusion of procainamide in the pulseless VT/VF algorithm is supported only by a retrospective comparison study involving 20 patients.[21]

Asystole Management

- Consider transcutaneous pacing (TCP): limited success in asystolic cardiac arrest
- Patients most likely to benefit from pacing:
  - Witnessed asystole
  - "P-wave asystole"
  - Asystolic arrest <10 min duration
- Medications
  - Epinephrine
  - Atropine: In cardiac arrest, the IV dose of atropine is 1.0 mg, which may be repeated every 3 to 5 min to a total dose of ≤2.5 mg (0.03 to 0.04 mg/kg).[26] "The use of atropine in asystole is without proof of benefit, yet anecdotal reports of return of sinus rhythm after atropine may warrant its use when other interventions have failed"[13]
  - Other medications may be appropriate, depending on the cause of the arrest (e.g., sodium bicarbonate)
  - Although vasopressin may be used in pulseless VT/VF, there is currently insufficient data to recommend its use in asystole or PEA
- Defibrillating asystole is not recommended

The Five H's and Five T's[29] is another mnemonic that may be used to recall the causes of PEA and asystole.

Hypovolemia	*Tamponade, cardiac*
Hypoxia	*Tension pneumothorax*
Hypothermia	*Thrombosis: lungs (massive pulmonary embolism)*
Hypo-/hyperkalemia	*Thrombosis: heart (acute coronary syndromes)*
Hydrogen ion (acidosis)	*Tablets/toxins: drug overdose*

Postresuscitation Care

1. **Postresuscitation period:** Interval between restoration of spontaneous circulation and transfer to the intensive care unit
2. Immediate goals of postresuscitation care
   a. Provide cardiorespiratory support to optimize tissue perfusion—especially to the heart, brain, and lungs (the organs most affected by cardiac arrest)
   b. Transport to Emergency Department and then appropriately equipped critical care unit
   c. Attempt to identify the precipitating cause of the arrest and institute specific treatment, if necessary
3. Immediate postresuscitation care: reassess ABCDs
   a. Airway
      (1) Reassess the effectiveness of initial airway maneuvers and interventions
      (2) If not already done, perform endotracheal intubation, if needed
   b. Breathing
      (1) Assess the adequacy of ventilations
      (2) Confirm ETT placement using primary and secondary confirmation methods (bilateral breath sounds/epigastric auscultation + end-tidal CO_2 detector, esophageal detector device, chest x-ray film)
      (3) Provide positive-pressure ventilation with 100% oxygen and assess the effectiveness of ventilations
      (4) Apply pulse oximeter and assess oxygen saturation; order arterial blood gas unless the patient is a candidate for fibrinolytic therapy
      (5) Rule out potential breathing complications from resuscitation (e.g., pneumothorax, rib fractures, sternal fractures, misplaced ETT)
      (6) Mechanical ventilation may be necessary because of absent or inadequate spontaneous respirations
   c. Circulation
      (1) Reassess vital signs, skin color, mental status
      (2) Establish IV access with NS or LR solution if not already done
      (3) Change IV lines that were placed without proper sterile technique
      (4) Perform ECG monitoring (if not already done); order 12-lead ECG

(5) If arrest rhythm was VF or VT and no antidysrhythmic was given:
    (a) Administer a lidocaine bolus
    (b) Follow with a continuous infusion
    (c) CONTRAINDICATED in patients with ventricular escape rhythms
(6) If an antidysrhythmic was used successfully during the resuscitation effort, continue a maintenance infusion of that medication

d. Differential diagnosis
  (1) Consider possible causes of the arrest
    (a) Myocardial infarction (MI)
      (i) Consider fibrinolytic therapy for patients surviving resuscitations of short duration with:
        • ST-segment elevation on postresuscitation 12-lead ECG and
        • No contraindications to fibrinolytic therapy
      (ii) If contraindications to fibrinolytic therapy exist, consider urgent coronary angiography
    (b) Primary dysrhythmias
    (c) Electrolyte disturbances (tall T waves on monitor, etc.)
    (d) Aortic aneurysm (brachial pulses present, femoral pulses absent)

e. Additional actions
  (1) Assess for complications that may have occurred during resuscitation (e.g., rib fracture, hemopneumothorax, pericardial tamponade, intra-abdominal trauma, misplaced ETT)
  (2) Order serum cardiac markers, serum electrolytes (including magnesium and calcium), complete blood count, renal profile, portable chest x-ray film
  (3) Insert a nasogastric tube, Foley catheter—monitor intake and output
  (4) Evaluate IV infusions used during the resuscitation effort
    (a) Are the infusions currently running? Are they still needed?
  (5) Arrange patient transfer to special care unit
    (a) Transfer with oxygen, ECG monitoring, resuscitation equipment
    (b) Have trained personnel accompany the patient
  (6) Ensure family has been updated regarding events
  (7) Finish documentation as needed
  (8) Acknowledge the efforts of the resuscitation team
  (9) Perform post resuscitation critique

PERI-ARREST RHYTHMS

Symptomatic Bradycardia

For rhythm review of symptomatic bradycardia, see Table 8-12 and the following figures.

Table 8-12   Symptomatic Bradycardia

Basic
Life
Support

Perform Primary ABCD Survey
(Correct critical problems IMMEDIATELY as they are identified)
Assess responsiveness, **A**irway, **B**reathing, **C**irculation,
ensure availability of monitor/**D**efibrillator

▼

Advanced
Life
Support

Perform Secondary ABCD Survey
Administer oxygen, establish IV access, attach cardiac monitor,
administer fluids as needed (O2, IV, monitor, fluids)

▼

Assess vital signs, attach pulse oximeter, and monitor blood pressure
Obtain and review 12-lead ECG, portable chest x-ray film
Perform a focused history and physical exam

▼

Identify the Patient's Cardiac Rhythm

▼

Is the patient experiencing serious signs and symptoms because of the bradycardia?

SIGNS	SYMPTOMS
Low blood pressure, shock, pulmonary congestion, congestive heart failure, angina, acute MI, ventricular ectopy	Chest pain, weakness, fatigue, dizziness, lightheadedness, shortness of breath, exercise intolerance, decreased level of responsiveness

- If no serious signs and symptoms, observe
- If serious signs and symptoms are present, further intervention depends on the cardiac rhythm identified

Is the QRS narrow or wide?

NARROW QRS BRADYCARDIA

- **Sinus bradycardia**
- **Junctional rhythm**
- **Second-degree AV block, type I**
- **Third-degree (complete) AV block**

- **Atropine 0.5 to 1.0 mg IV:** May repeat every 3 to 5 min to a total dose of 0.03 to 0.04 mg/kg. Total cumulative dose should not exceed 2.5 mg over 2.5 hours[27]
- **Transcutaneous pacemaker (TCP):** Pacing should not be delayed while waiting for IV access or for atropine to take effect.
- **Dopamine infusion:** 5 to 20 mcg/kg/min
- **Epinephrine infusion:** 2 to 10 mcg/min
- **Isoproterenol infusion:** 2 to 10 mcg/min (low doses)

WIDE QRS BRADYCARDIA

- **Second-degree AV block, type II**
- **Third-degree (complete) AV block**
- **Ventricular escape (idioventricular) rhythm**

- **Transcutaneous pacemaker:** As an interim device until transvenous pacing can be accomplished
- **Dopamine infusion:** 5 to 20 mcg/kg/min
- **Epinephrine infusion:** 2 to 10 mcg/min
- **Isoproterenol infusion:** 2 to 10 mcg/min (low doses)

[26]See chapter references.

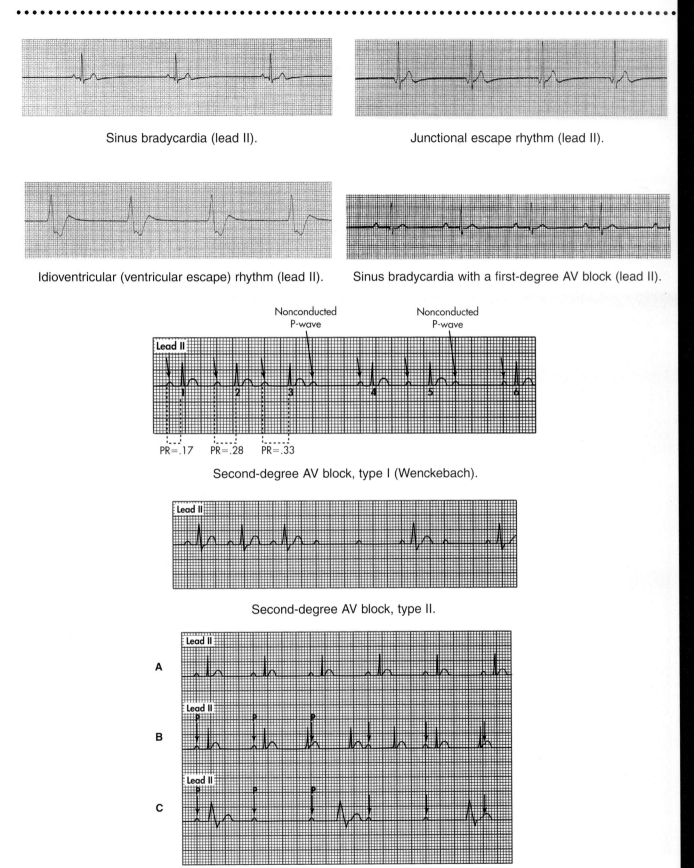

Sinus bradycardia (lead II).

Junctional escape rhythm (lead II).

Idioventricular (ventricular escape) rhythm (lead II).

Sinus bradycardia with a first-degree AV block (lead II).

Nonconducted P-wave

Nonconducted P-wave

Lead II

PR=.17   PR=.28   PR=.33

Second-degree AV block, type I (Wenckebach).

Lead II

Second-degree AV block, type II.

A Lead II

B Lead II

C Lead II

Sequential rhythm strips obtained from an elderly patient with digitalis toxicity.
A, Sinus rhythm at 75 beats/min. **B,** AV dissociation—some P waves are NOT
related to neighboring QRS complexes. **C,** Complete (third-degree) AV block.

- *Absolute bradycardia: Rate <60 beats/min; may be symptomatic or asymptomatic*
- *Relative bradycardia: Rate may be more than 60 beats/min; may occur when hypotensive patients require a tachycardia (i.e., hypovolemia) but the patients are unable to increase their heart rate because of SA node disease or beta-blockers (or other medications)*
- *Treat only when the slow rate causes significant signs and symptoms*

Narrow QRS Tachycardia

Narrow QRS Tachycardia: Overview of the 2000 Guidelines

The stable tachycardia algorithms have undergone the most substantial changes of all of the ACLS algorithms. The 1992 ACLS Guidelines required an immediate determination as to whether the patient presenting with a tachycardia was "stable" or "unstable." In general, patients with serious signs and symptoms because of the tachycardia (typically at a rate of 150 beats/min or more) were managed with electrical therapy. This emphasis has not changed in the 2000 Guidelines.

Substantial changes, however, were made in the treatment recommendations for tachycardic patients not in need of immediate cardioversion.

The International Guidelines 2000 emphasize new concepts including:

1. *Specific identification of the tachycardia*
2. *Recognizing tachycardic patients with significantly impaired cardiac function (ejection fraction <40%; overt signs of heart failure)*
3. *Recognition that all antiarrhythmics are also proarrhythmic (i.e., capable of inducing dysrhythmias). With few exceptions, the 2000 Guidelines recommend the use of only one antiarrhythmic per patient*

Normally, the heart empties (ejects) slightly more than half the blood that it contains with each beat; thus a normal ejection fraction is >50%. Impaired ventricular function = an ejection fraction of <40%. If ventricular function is impaired, the patient will exhibit signs and symptoms of decreased cardiac output. As cardiac output decreases (and tissue perfusion is impaired), the patient's signs and symptoms will become increasingly more severe, consistent with shock.

The 2000 Guidelines Tachycardia Overview Algorithm recommends the following sequence:

1. *Evaluate patient*
   - a. *Stable or unstable?*
   - b. *Serious signs and symptoms present?*
   - c. *Signs and symptoms related to the tachycardia?*
2. *Identify the tachycardia as one of four types:*
   - a. *Atrial fibrillation/atrial flutter*
   - b. *Narrow QRS tachycardia*
   - c. *Stable wide QRS tachycardia: unknown type*
   - d. *Stable monomorphic VT and/or polymorphic VT*

Narrow QRS Tachycardia—cont'd

3. If the rhythm is a narrow complex tachycardia, attempt to establish a specific diagnosis, using a 12-lead ECG, clinical information, vagal maneuvers, and adenosine
   a. Junctional tachycardia
   b. Paroxysmal supraventricular tachycardia (PSVT)
      (1) AV nodal reentrant tachycardia (AVNRT)
      (2) AV reentrant tachycardia (AVRT)
   c. Ectopic atrial tachycardia
   d. Multifocal atrial tachycardia (MAT)
4. If the patient is stable, further interventions require differentiation of "preserved" heart function and "ejection fraction <40%, CHF"

It is the latter concept that has caused confusion among ACLS providers—students and instructors—in both the prehospital and hospital setting because it is simply not possible to determine a patient's ejection fraction without echocardiography or invasive monitoring.

"Treat the patient, not the monitor" is a caveat that has been used for many years in the delivery of ACLS. In the absence of echocardiography or invasive monitoring in the prehospital setting, Emergency Department, or Post-Anesthesia Care Unit (PACU), clinical judgment must suffice.

If the tachycardia does not result in signs and symptoms because of the rapid rate, the patient is considered "stable." If the tachycardia produces serious signs and symptoms such as hypotension, shock, pulmonary congestion, congestive heart failure, acute MI, altered/decreased level of responsiveness, chest pain, or shortness of breath, the patient is considered "unstable." Unstable patients with serious signs and symptoms because of the tachycardia should receive immediate cardioversion, rather than a trial of antiarrhythmics. It is important to note that not all patient situations are so simplistic.

Consider the case of a 55-year-old female complaining of palpitations that have been present for the past 40 minutes. She is awake and alert but anxious. The cardiac monitor reveals PSVT. As the patient converses with you, you note she pauses after every 5 or 6 words to take a breath although she states she does not feel short of breath. Physical examination: BP 114/78, P 170, R 20. She states her normal BP is around 130/80. Breath sounds reveal a few bibasilar rales. Her skin is pink, warm, and moist and her ankles appear swollen. The patient has no pertinent past medical history and takes no medications regularly. Oxygen is being administered, and an IV has been established. Vagal maneuvers were attempted without success. Administration of adenosine failed to convert the rhythm. The patient's condition remains unchanged. What should be done now?

It is at this point that the algorithm appears formidable. Further interventions require a decision regarding the patient's "preserved" or "impaired" cardiac function. Invasive monitoring or echocardiography is not available. The decision regarding how to proceed will depend on the clinician's medical judgment, location and availability of resources, experience and, of course, the patient's condition. In this situation, a reasonable approach would include IV administration of digoxin, amiodarone, or diltiazem.

For rhythm review of narrow QRS tachycardia, see Table 8-13 and Figure 8-1.

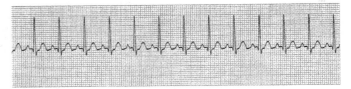

Figure 8-1   Sinus tachycardia (lead II).

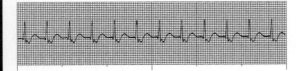

Junctional tachycardia.

Types of supraventricular tachycardias. **A,** Normal sinus rhythm is presented here as a reference. **B,** Atrial tachycardia: a focus (*X*) outside the SA node fires automatically at a rapid rate. **C,** AV nodal reentrant tachycardia (AVNRT): an impulse originates as a wave of excitation that spins around the area of the AV nodal (junctional) area. On the ECG, P waves may be buried in the QRS or appear just before or after the QRS complex because of the nearly simultaneous activation of the atria and ventricles. **D,** AV reentrant tachycardia (AVRT): a similar type of reentrant (circus-movement) mechanism may occur with a bypass tract (*BT*) like that found in Wolff-Parkinson-White syndrome. Note the negative P wave in lead II, after the QRS complex. In lead II, the P wave may be negative, flat, or positive.

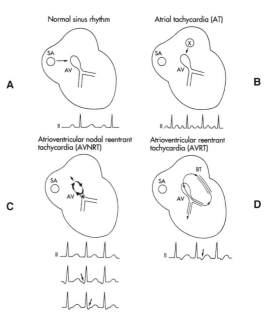

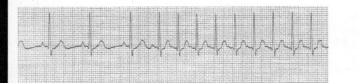

Paroxysmal supraventricular tachycardia (PSVT) (lead II).

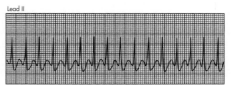

Supraventricular tachycardia.

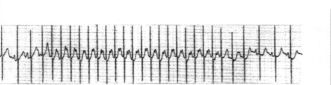

Ectopic atrial tachycardia (lead II), originating near the SA node. P waves, similar in shape to sinus P waves, gradually accelerate and then slow. Note that the P waves merge into the preceding T waves during the first 5 beats. In the subsequent beats, P waves can be seen in the T waves. As the rate slows, the P waves and T waves separate.

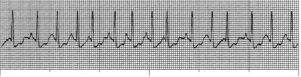

Multifocal atrial tachycardia (MAT).

Table 8-13   Narrow QRS Tachycardia

Perform Primary ABCD Survey (Basic Life Support)
(Correct critical problems IMMEDIATELY as they are identified)
Assess responsiveness, **A**irway, **B**reathing, **C**irculation,
ensure availability of monitor/**D**efibrillator

▼

Perform Secondary ABCD Survey (Advanced Life Support)
Administer oxygen, establish IV access, attach cardiac monitor, administer fluids as needed (O_2, IV, monitor, fluids)
Assess vital signs, attach pulse oximeter, and monitor blood pressure
Obtain and review 12-lead ECG, portable chest x-ray film
Perform a focused history and physical exam

▼

Is the patient stable or unstable?
Is the patient experiencing serious signs and symptoms because of the tachycardia?

▼

Attempt to identify patient's cardiac rhythm using:
- 12-lead ECG, clinical information
- Vagal maneuvers
- Adenosine 6 mg rapid IV bolus over 1 to 3 sec. If needed, administer adenosine 12 mg rapid IV bolus over 1 to 3 sec after 1 to 2 min. May repeat 12 mg dose in 1 to 2 min if needed. Follow each dose immediately with 20 mL IV flush of NS. Use of adenosine is relatively contraindicated in patients with asthma. Decrease dose in patients on dipyridamole (Persantine) or carbamazepine (Tegretol); consider increasing dose in patients taking theophylline or caffeine-containing preparations

▼

Identify the Patient's Cardiac Rhythm

▼

Junctional Tachycardia	Paroxysmal Supraventricular Tachycardia (PSVT) (Includes AVNRT or AVRT)	Ectopic Atrial Tachycardia, Multifocal Atrial Tachycardia (MAT)

Stable Patient		Stable Patient		Stable Patient	
Normal Cardiac Function	Impaired Cardiac Function*	Normal Cardiac Function	Impaired Cardiac Function*	Normal Cardiac Function	Impaired Cardiac Function*
Amiodarone (IIb) **or** Beta-blocker (Indeterminate) or Ca++ channel blocker (Indeterminate) **Cardioversion ineffective**	Amiodarone (IIb) **Cardioversion ineffective**	*Priority order:* Ca++ channel blocker (Class I) Beta-blocker (Class I) Digoxin (IIb) Sync cardioversion	*Priority order:* Sync cardioversion Digoxin (IIb) Amiodarone (IIb) Diltiazem (IIb)	Ca++ channel blocker (IIb) **or** Beta-blocker (IIb) **or** Amiodarone (IIb) **or** Flecainide (IIb) or Propafenone (IIb) **or** Digoxin (Indeterminate) **Cardioversion ineffective**	Amiodarone (IIb) **or** Diltiazem (IIb) **or** Digoxin (Indeterminate) **Cardioversion ineffective**

UNSTABLE PATIENT

If hemodynamically unstable PSVT, perform synchronized cardioversion: 50 J, 100 J, 200 J, 300 J, 360 J, (or equivalent Biphasic energy)

*Impaired cardiac function = ejection fraction <40% or CHF.

Continued

Table 8-13   Narrow QRS Tachycardia—cont'd

Medication Dosing

Amiodarone[34-36]—150 mg IV over 10 min, followed by an infusion of 1 mg/min for 6 hours and then a maintenance infusion of 0.5 mg/min. Repeat supplementary infusions of 150 mg as necessary for recurrent or resistant dysrhythmias. Maximum total daily dose 2.0 g

Beta-blockers—*Atenolol:* 5 mg IV push over 5 min. May give second dose after 10 min. *Esmolol* Loading infusion of 500 mcg/kg/min (0.5 mg/kg/min) over 1 min followed by a 4 min maintenance infusion of 50 mcg/kg/min (0.05 mg/kg/min). If adequate therapeutic effect is not observed, repeat same loading dosage over 1 min followed by an increased maintenance rate infusion of 100 mcg/kg/min (0.1 mg/kg/min) *Metoprolol:* 5 mg IV push over 5 min × 3 for a total of 15 mg over 15 min. *Propranolol:* Usual dose 1-3 mg IV given no faster than 1 mg/min. If necessary, a second dose may be given after 2 min. Thereafter, additional drug should not be given in less than 4 hours.

Calcium channel blockers:[37] *Diltiazem*—0.25 mg/kg over 2 min (e.g., 15 to 20 mg). If ineffective, 0.35 mg/kg over 2 min (e.g., 20 to 25 mg) in 15 min. Maintenance infusion 5 to 15 mg/hr, titrated to heart rate if chemical conversion successful. Calcium chloride (2 to 4 mg/kg) may be given **slow** IV push if borderline hypotension exists before diltiazem administration. *Verapamil*—2.5 to 5.0 mg slow IV bolus over 2 min. May repeat with 5 to 10 mg in 30 min. Maximum dose 20 mg

Digoxin—Loading dose 10 to 15 mcg/kg lean body weight

Flecainide, propafenone—IV form not currently approved for use in the United States

---

[34,35,36,37]See chapter references.

Type of Countershock	Dysrhythmia	Recommended Energy Levels
Defibrillation	Pulseless VT/VF	200 J, 200-300 J, 360 J, or equivalent Biphasic energy
	Sustained polymorphic VT	200 J, 200-300 J, 360 J, or equivalent Biphasic energy
	VT with a pulse	100 J, 200 J, 300 J, 360 J, or equivalent Biphasic energy
	Undue delay in delivery of synchronized countershock	Depends on rhythm
Synchronized Cardioversion	Paroxysmal supraventricular tachycardia (PSVT)	50 J, 100 J, 200 J, 300 J, 360 J, or equivalent Biphasic energy
	Atrial flutter	50 J, 100 J, 200 J, 300 J, 360 J, or equivalent Biphasic energy
	Atrial fibrillation	100 J, 200 J, 300 J, 360 J, or equivalent Biphasic energy
	VT with a pulse	100 J, 200 J, 300 J, 360 J, or equivalent Biphasic energy

Atrial Fibrillation/Atrial Flutter

For rhythm review of atrial fibrillation/atrial flutter, including Wolff-Parkinson-White syndrome, see Tables 8-14 and 8-15 and the following figures.

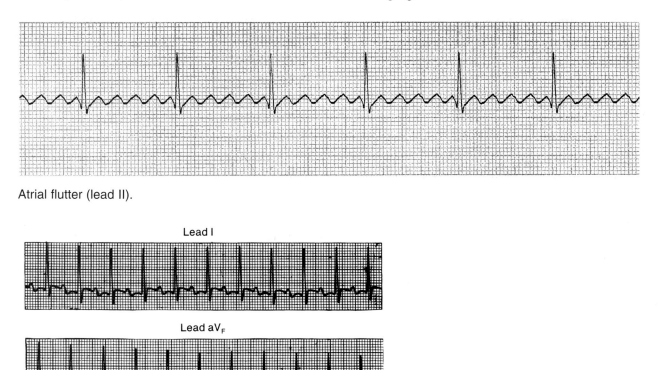

Atrial flutter (lead II).

Lead I

Lead aV$_F$

Simultaneous tracings

Atrial flutter with 2:1 conduction, simultaneous tracings.

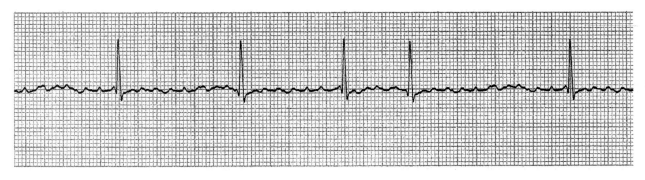

Atrial fibrillation (lead II).

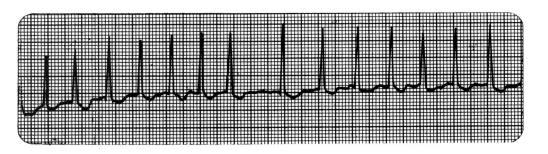

Atrial fibrillation with a rapid ventricular response.

Table 8-14   Atrial Fibrillation/Atrial Flutter Algorithm

Perform Primary ABCD Survey (Basic Life Support)
(Correct critical problems IMMEDIATELY as they are identified)
Assess responsiveness, **A**irway, **B**reathing, **C**irculation, ensure availability of monitor/**D**efibrillator

▼

Perform Secondary ABCD Survey (Advanced Life Support)
Administer oxygen, establish IV access, attach cardiac monitor, administer fluids as needed (O_2, IV, monitor, fluids)
Assess vital signs, attach pulse oximeter, and monitor blood pressure
Obtain and review 12-lead ECG, portable chest x-ray film, perform a focused history and physical exam

▼

Is the patient stable or unstable?
Is the patient's cardiac function normal or impaired?
Is the patient experiencing serious signs and symptoms because of the tachycardia?
Attempt to identify patient's cardiac rhythm using 12-lead ECG, clinical information
Is Wolff-Parkinson-White syndrome (WPW) present? If yes, see WPW algorithm
Has atrial fibrillation/atrial flutter been present for more or less than 48 hours?

▼

STABLE PATIENT

Normal Cardiac Function		Impaired Cardiac Function*	
Onset <48 hours	Onset >48 hours	Onset <48 hours	Onset >48 hours
Control Rate	**Control Rate**	**Control Rate**	**Control Rate**
Calcium channel blocker (Class I) **or** Beta-blocker (Class I) **or** Digoxin (IIb)	Calcium channel blocker (Class I) **or** Beta-blocker (Class I) **or** Digoxin (IIb)	Diltiazem (IIb) **or** Amiodarone (IIb) **or** Digoxin (IIb)	Diltiazem (IIb) **or** Amiodarone (IIb) **or** Digoxin (IIb)
Convert Rhythm	**Convert Rhythm**	**Convert Rhythm**	**Convert Rhythm**
Cardioversion **or** Amiodarone (IIa) **or** Procainamide (IIa) **or** Ibutilide (IIa) **or** Flecainide (IIa) **or** Propafenone (IIa)	Delayed cardioversion **or** Early cardioversion	Cardioversion **or** amiodarone (IIb)	Delayed cardioversion **or** Early cardioversion

Delayed cardioversion: anticoagulation therapy for 3 weeks before cardioversion, for at least 48 hours in conjunction with cardioversion, and for at least 4 weeks after successful cardioversion. **Early cardioversion:** IV heparin immediately, transesophageal echocardiography (TEE) to rule out atrial thrombus, cardioversion within 24 hr, anticoagulation × 4 wks

Unstable Patient

If hemodynamically unstable, perform synchronized cardioversion: Atrial fibrillation: 100 J, 200 J, 300 J, 360 J, or equivalent Biphasic energy. Atrial flutter: 50 J, 100 J, 200 J, 300 J, 360 J, or equivalent Biphasic energy

Medication Dosing

Amiodarone[40,41]—150 mg IV bolus over 10 min followed by an infusion of 1 mg/min for 6 hours and then a maintenance infusion of 0.5 mg/min. Repeat supplementary infusions of 150 mg as necessary for recurrent or resistant dysrhythmias. Maximum total daily dose 2.0 g

Beta-blockers—*Atenolol:* 5 mg IV push over 5 min. May give second dose after 10 min. *Esmolol* Loading infusion of 500 mcg/kg/min (0.5 mg/kg/min) over 1 min followed by a 4 min maintenance infusion of 50 mcg/kg/min (0.05 mg/kg/min). If adequate therapeutic effect is not observed, repeat same loading dosage over 1 min followed by an increased maintenance rate infusion of 100 mcg/kg/min (0.1 mg/kg/min) *Metoprolol:* 5 mg IV push over 5 min × 3 for a total of 15 mg over 15 min. *Propranolol:* Usual dose 1-3 mg IV given no faster than 1 mg/min. If necessary, a second dose may be given after 2 min. Thereafter, additional drug should not be given in less than 4 hours.

Calcium channel blockers:[42,43] *Diltiazem*—0.25 mg/kg over 2 min (e.g., 15 to 20 mg). If ineffective, 0.35 mg/kg over 2 min (e.g., 20 to 25 mg) in 15 min. Maintenance infusion 5 to 15 mg/hr, titrated to heart rate if chemical conversion successful. Calcium chloride (2 to 4 mg/kg) may be given **slow** IV push if borderline hypotension exists before diltiazem administration. *Verapamil*—2.5 to 5.0 mg slow IV bolus over 2 min. May repeat with 5 to 10 mg in 30 min. Maximum dose 20 mg

Ibutilide—Adults ≥60 kg: 1 mg (10 mL) over 10 min. May repeat × 1 in 10 min. Adults <60 kg: 0.01 mg/kg IV over 10 min

Procainamide:[44]—100 mg over 5 min (20 mg/min). Maximum total dose 17 mg/kg. Maintenance infusion 1 to 4 mg/min Flecainide, propafenone, sotalol—IV form not currently approved for use in the United States

*Impaired cardiac function = ejection fraction <40% or CHF
[40-44]See chapter references.

Systemic embolism is the most serious complication of cardioversion and may follow direct current (DC), pharmacologic, and spontaneous cardioversion of AF.[38]

"An association with atrial fibrillation and stroke is well established, with a six-fold higher risk for thromboembolism in patients with nonrheumatic heart disease and atrial fibrillation than in patients in sinus rhythm. The annual risk for stroke in patients with atrial fibrillation may be as high as 4.5%. The embolic risk is greatest at onset of atrial fibrillation, during the first year of atrial fibrillation, and every time the patient is electroconverted back to sinus rhythm. Most embolic accidents occur in the hours after onset of atrial fibrillation, and recurrence of atrial fibrillation includes a renewed risk for embolic stroke."[39]

Anticoagulation for Elective Cardioversion

Because of the risk for thromboembolism in patients presenting with atrial fibrillation, anticoagulation therapy is recommended before cardioversion. The American College of Chest Physicians have made the following recommendations regarding anticoagulation for elective cardioversion.[38]

Atrial Fibrillation (AF)

We recommend that clinicians administer oral anticoagulant therapy (target INR 2.5; range 2.0 to 3.0) for 3 weeks before and at least 4 weeks after elective DC cardioversion of AF patients (grade 1C1).

Alternatively, we recommend that AF patients undergo anticoagulation then undergo transesophageal echocardiography (TEE) and have cardioversion performed without delay if no thrombi are seen (grade 1C). For these patients, adjusted-dose warfarin therapy should still be continued until normal sinus rhythm has been maintained for at least 4 weeks.

Although data are limited, the risk of embolism following cardioversion in patients who have been in AF for <48 hours appears to be low. However, we recommend the use of anticoagulation during the pericardioversion period (grade 2C).

Atrial Flutter and Supraventricular Tachycardia

We recommend that clinicians manage oral anticoagulant therapy at the time of cardioversion in patients with atrial flutter in a manner similar to that used for AF (grade 2C).

In the absence of prior thromboembolism, we do not recommend antithrombotic therapy for cardioversion of supraventricular tachycardia (grade 2C).

Treatment of potential precipitants of AF (i.e., thyrotoxicosis, pneumonia, congestive heart failure) should be completed prior to attempting elective DC cardioversion.

From: Albers GW, Dalen JE, Laupacis A, Manning WJ, Petersen P, Singer DE: Antithrombotic therapy in atrial fibrillation, *Chest* 119(1 Suppl):194S-206S, 2001.

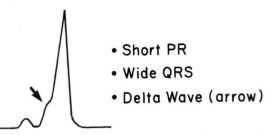

- Short PR
- Wide QRS
- Delta Wave (arrow)

Wolff-Parkinson-White (WPW) syndrome is associated with a triad of ECG findings, including a short PR interval, wide QRS, and delta wave.

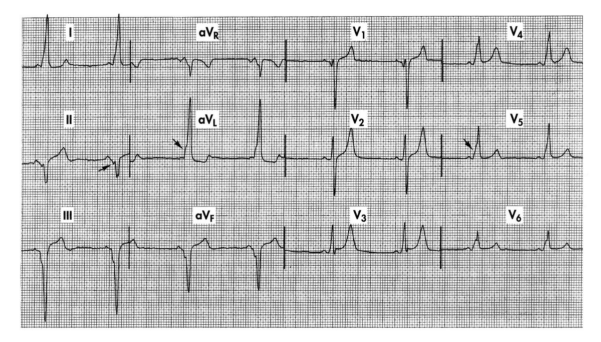

12-lead ECG showing the characteristic triad of the WPW pattern—short PR intervals, wide QRS complexes, and delta waves *(arrows)* that are negative in some leads (e.g., II, III, aVF) and positive in others (aVL, V_4, V_5, V_6). Q waves in leads II, III, and aVF are the result of abnormal ventricular conduction (negative delta waves) rather than an inferior myocardial infarction.

Table 8-15 Wolff-Parkinson-White (WPW) Syndrome Algorithm

Perform Primary ABCD Survey (Basic Life Support)
(Correct critical problems IMMEDIATELY as they are identified)
Assess responsiveness, **A**irway, **B**reathing, **C**irculation, ensure availability of monitor/**D**efibrillator

▼

Perform Secondary ABCD Survey (Advanced Life Support)
Administer oxygen, establish IV access, attach cardiac monitor, administer fluids as needed (O_2, IV, monitor, fluids)
Assess vital signs, attach pulse oximeter, and monitor blood pressure
Obtain and review 12-lead ECG, portable chest x-ray film, perform a focused history and physical exam

▼

Is the patient stable or unstable?
Is the patient experiencing serious signs and symptoms because of the tachycardia?
Is the patient's cardiac function normal or impaired?
Attempt to identify patient's cardiac rhythm using 12-lead ECG, clinical information
Is Wolff-Parkinson-White syndrome (WPW) present? (e.g., young patient, HR >300,
ECG: short PR interval, wide QRS, delta wave)
Has WPW been present for more or less than 48 hours?

▼

Normal Cardiac Function		Impaired Cardiac Function*	
Onset <48 hours	**Onset >48 hours**	**Onset <48 hours**	**Onset >48 hours**
Control Rate	**Control Rate**	**Control Rate**	**Control Rate**
Cardioversion **or** Amiodarone (IIb) **or** Procainamide (IIb) **or** Flecainide (IIb) **or** Propafenone (IIb) **or** Sotalol (IIb)	Use antiarrhythmics with extreme caution because of embolic risk	Cardioversion **or** Amiodarone (IIb)	Use antiarrhythmics with extreme caution because of embolic risk
Convert Rhythm	**Convert Rhythm**	**Convert Rhythm**	**Convert Rhythm**
Cardioversion **or** Amiodarone (IIb) **or** Procainamide (IIb) **or** Flecainide (IIb) **or** Propafenone (IIb) **or** Sotalol (IIb)	Delayed cardioversion **or** Early cardioversion	Cardioversion	Delayed cardioversion **or** Early cardioversion

Delayed cardioversion: Anticoagulation therapy for 3 weeks before cardioversion for at least 48 hours in conjunction with cardioversion and for at least 4 weeks after successful cardioversion. **Early cardioversion:** IV heparin immediately, transesophageal echocardiography (TEE) to rule out atrial thrombus, cardioversion within 24 hr, anticoagulation × 4 weeks

Medication Dosing

Amiodarone:[44]—150 mg IV bolus over 10 min followed by an infusion of 1 mg/min for 6 hours and then a maintenance infusion of 0.5 mg/min. Repeat supplementary infusions of 150 mg as necessary for recurrent or resistant dysrhythmias. Maximum total daily dose 2.0 g
Procainamide—100 mg over 5 min (20 mg/min). Maximum total dose 17 mg/kg. Maintenance infusion 1 to 4 mg/min
Flecainide, propafenone, sotalol—IV form not currently approved for use in the United States

Impaired cardiac function = ejection fraction <40% or CHF.
[44]See chapter references.

Ventricular Tachycardia

For rhythm review of ventricular tachycardia, see Tables 8-16 and 8-17 and the following figures.

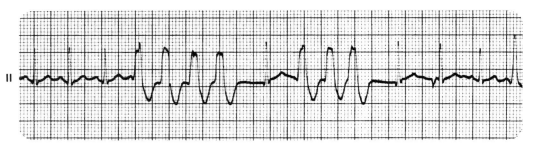

Two "runs," "bursts," or "salvos" of **nonsustained** ventricular tachycardia.

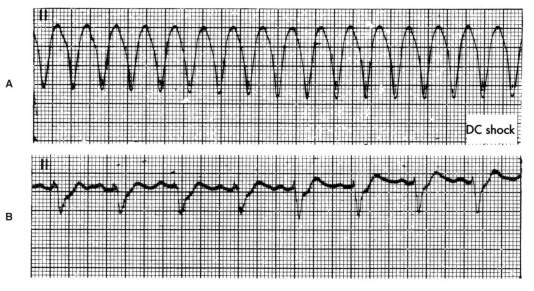

A, Sustained monomorphic ventricular tachycardia. At the end of the rhythm strip, cardioversion was performed. **B,** Sinus rhythm after cardioversion.

Sustained Monomorphic Ventricular Tachycardia

Table 8-16   Sustained Monomorphic Ventricular Tachycardia

Perform Primary ABCD Survey (Basic Life Support)
(Correct critical problems IMMEDIATELY as they are identified)
Assess responsiveness, Airway, Breathing, Circulation, ensure availability of monitor/Defibrillator

▼

Perform Secondary ABCD Survey (Advanced Life Support)
Administer oxygen, establish IV access, attach cardiac monitor, administer fluids as needed (O_2, IV, monitor, fluids)
Assess vital signs, attach pulse oximeter, and monitor blood pressure
Obtain and review 12-lead ECG, portable chest x-ray film, perform a focused history and physical exam

▼

Is the patient stable or unstable?
Is the patient experiencing serious signs and symptoms because of the tachycardia?
Determine if the rhythm is monomorphic or polymorphic VT and determine patient's QT interval

▼

Stable Patient	
Normal Cardiac Function	**Impaired Cardiac Function***

May proceed directly to synchronized cardioversion or use **one** of the following:

• Procainamide (IIa)	• Amiodarone (IIb)
• Sotalol (IIa)	• Lidocaine (Indeterminate)
• Amiodarone (IIb)	
• Lidocaine (IIb)	

▼

If medication therapy ineffective, perform synchronized cardioversion

Unstable VT with a Pulse
If hemodynamically unstable, sync 100 J, 200 J, 300 J, and 360 J, (or equivalent Biphasic energy)
If hypotensive (systolic BP <90), unresponsive, or if severe pulmonary edema exists, defibrillate with same energy

Medication Dosing

Amiodarone:[46-48] 150 mg IV bolus over 10 min. If chemical conversion successful, follow with IV infusion of 1 mg/min for 6 hours and then a maintenance infusion of 0.5 mg/min. Repeat supplementary infusions of 150 mg as necessary for recurrent or resistant dysrhythmias. Maximum total daily dose 2.0 g

Lidocaine:[26,49-51] 1 to 1.5 mg/kg initial dose. Repeat dose is half the initial dose every 5 to 10 min. Maximum total dose 3 mg/kg. If chemical conversion successful, maintenance infusion 1 to 4 mg/min. If impaired cardiac function, dose = 0.5-0.75 mg/kg IV push. May repeat every 5 to 10 min. Maximum total dose 3 mg/kg. If chemical conversion successful, maintenance infusion 1 to 4 mg/min

Procainamide:[52,53] 100 mg over 5 min (20 mg/min). Maximum total dose 17 mg/kg. If chemical conversion successful, maintenance infusion 1 to 4 mg/min

Sotalol:[54] IV form not approved for use in the United States.

Impaired cardiac function = ejection fraction <40% or CHF.
[26,46-54] See chapter references.

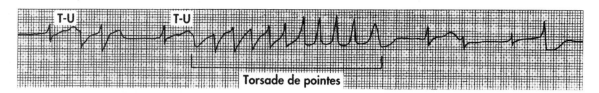

Nonsustained torsade de pointes (TdP). Notice the shifting direction and amplitude of the QRS during the episode of TdP. The QT interval in the underlying sinus beats is prolonged (0.52 sec).

Monitor lead

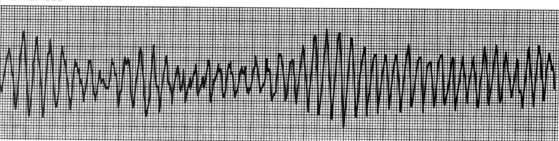

Sustained torsades de pointes.

Table 8-17 Polymorphic Ventricular Tachycardia

Perform Primary ABCD Survey (Basic Life Support)
(Correct critical problems IMMEDIATELY as they are identified)
Assess responsiveness, **A**irway, **B**reathing, **C**irculation, ensure availability of monitor/**D**efibrillator

▼

Perform Secondary ABCD Survey (Advanced Life Support)
Administer oxygen, establish IV access, attach cardiac monitor, administer fluids as needed (O$_2$, IV, monitor, fluids)
Assess vital signs, attach pulse oximeter, and monitor blood pressure
Obtain and review 12-lead ECG, portable chest x-ray film, perform a focused history and physical exam

▼

Is the patient stable or unstable?
Is the patient experiencing serious signs and symptoms because of the tachycardia?
Determine if the rhythm is monomorphic or polymorphic VT and determine patient's QT interval

▼

| **Polymorphic VT**
Normal QT interval | **Polymorphic VT**
Prolonged QT interval
(Suggests torsades de pointes) |

Stable Patient		
Normal Cardiac Function	**Impaired Cardiac Function***	**Impaired Cardiac Function***
Treat ischemia if present Correct electrolyte abnormalities May proceed directly to electrical therapy or use **one** of the following: • Amiodarone (IIb) • Lidocaine (IIb) • Procainamide (IIb) • Sotalol (IIb) • Beta-blockers (Indeterminate)	May proceed directly to electrical therapy or use **one** of the following: • Amiodarone (IIb) • Lidocaine (Indeterminate)	DC meds that prolong QT interval Correct electrolyte abnormalities May proceed directly to electrical therapy or use **one** of the following: • Magnesium (Indeterminate) • Overdrive pacing with or without beta-blocker (Indeterminate) • Isoproterenol (Indeterminate) • Phenytoin (Indeterminate) • Lidocaine (Indeterminate)

If medication therapy ineffective, use electrical therapy

Unstable Patient
Sustained (>30 sec or causing hemodynamic collapse) polymorphic VT should be treated with an unsynchronized shock, using an initial energy of 200 J; if unsuccessful, a second shock of 200 to 300 J should be given and, if necessary, a third shock of 360 J[26]

Medication Dosing

Amiodarone—150 mg IV bolus over 10 min. If chemical conversion successful, follow with IV infusion of 1 mg/min for 6 hours and then a maintenance infusion of 0.5 mg/min. Repeat supplementary infusions of 150 mg as necessary for recurrent or resistant dysrhythmias. Maximum total daily dose 2.0 g

Beta-blockers—*Atenolol:* 5 mg IV push over 5 min. May give second dose after 10 min. *Esmolol* Loading infusion of 500 mcg/kg/min (0.5 mg/kg/min) over 1 min followed by a 4 min maintenance infusion of 50 mcg/kg/min (0.05 mg/kg/min). If adequate therapeutic effect is not observed, repeat same loading dosage over 1 min followed by an increased maintenance rate infusion of 100 mcg/kg/min (0.1 mg/kg/min) *Metoprolol:* 5 mg IV push over 5 min × 3 for a total of 15 mg over 15 min. *Propranolol:* Usual dose 1-3 mg IV given no faster than 1 mg/min. If necessary, a second dose may be given after 2 min. Thereafter, additional drug should not be given in less than 4 hours.

Isoproterenol—Can be used as a temporizing measure until overdrive pacing can be instituted if no evidence of coronary artery disease, ischemic syndromes, or other contraindications. 2 to 10 mcg/min. Mix 1 mg in 500 mL NS or D5W

Lidocaine—1 to 1.5 mg/kg initial dose. Repeat dose half the initial dose every 5 to 10 min. Maximum total dose 3 mg/kg. If chemical conversion successful, maintenance infusion 1 to 4 mg/min. If impaired cardiac function, dose = 0.5 to 0.75 mg/kg IV push. May repeat every 5 to 10 min. Maximum total dose 3 mg/kg. If chemical conversion successful, maintenance infusion 1 to 4 mg/min

Magnesium:[24]—Loading dose of 1 to 2 g mixed in 50 to 100 mL over 5 to 60 min IV. If chemical conversion successful, follow with 0.5 to 1.0 g/hr IV infusion

Phenytoin—250 mg IV at a rate of 25 to 50 mg/min in NS using a central vein

Procainamide—100 mg over 5 min (20 mg/min). Maximum total dose 17 mg/kg. If chemical conversion successful, maintenance infusion 1 to 4 mg/min

Sotalol—IV form not approved for use in the United States.

---

*Impaired cardiac function = ejection fraction <40% or CHF.
24,26See chapter references.

Wide QRS Tachycardia of Unknown Origin

Supraventricular tachycardia with aberrant conduction vs. ventricular tachycardia (Table 8-18):

1. Most wide complex tachycardias are ventricular tachycardia
2. If the patient presents with serious signs and symptoms because of the tachycardia, specific diagnosis of the origin of the tachycardia is irrelevant—the patient needs immediate electrical therapy (cardioversion)
3. Differentiation of supraventricular tachycardia with aberrant conduction and ventricular tachycardia (Figure 8-2)
   a. AV dissociation—presence of independent P waves suggests VT (Figure 8-3)
   b. Precordial concordance (all QRS complexes are either positive or negative in leads V1 to V6) (Figure 8-4)
      (1) Positive concordance: All QRS complexes are positive in V1 through V6, suggesting VT; however, the same pattern may be seen in Wolff-Parkinson-White (WPW) syndrome
      (2) Negative concordance: All QRS complexes are negative in V1 through V6, diagnostic of VT
   c. Left peak ("rabbit ear") of the QRS complex is taller than the right in lead V1 suggests VT
   d. QS or rS configuration in lead V6 suggests VT

See also Figures 8-5 to 8-7 for further examples of differentiating tachycardia.

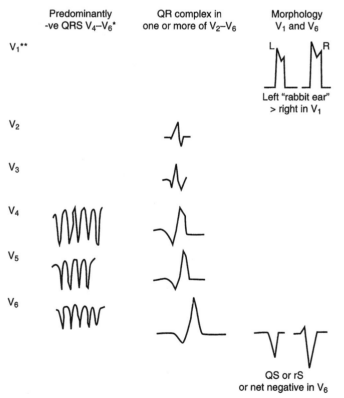

* = or concordant negativity in leads V$_1$ through V$_4$. Positive concordance in leads V$_1$ through V$_6$ can be caused by VT or Wolff-Parkinson-White antidromic (preexcited) tachycardia.

** = it is necessary to study the entire 12-lead tracing with particular emphasis on leads V$_1$ through V$_6$; lead II may be useful for assessment of P waves and AV dissociation.

Figure 8-2 ECG hallmarks of ventricular tachycardia.

Monitor

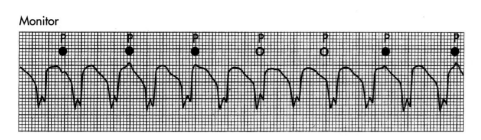

Figure 8-3   Sustained monomorphic ventricular tachycardia with AV dissociation. The ventricular rate is 140 beats/min. The atria are beating independently at a rate of 75 beats/min. Visible sinus P waves are indicated *(dark circle)*. Hidden P waves are also indicated *(clear circle)*.

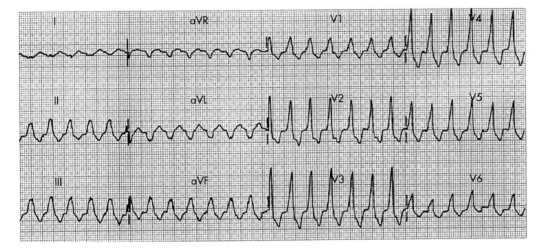

Figure 8-4   Positive concordance (QRS complexes in the same direction) in leads V₁ through V₆, suggesting ventricular tachycardia.

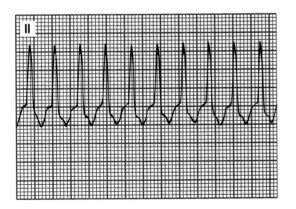

Figure 8-5   Rhythm strip from a 50-year-old male with a history of coronary artery disease. BP 160/100 mm Hg. Patient is aware of a rapid heart beat but denies chest pain. The rhythm is fast and regular at a rate of 210 beats/min. There is no evidence of atrial activity and the QRS does not appear wide.

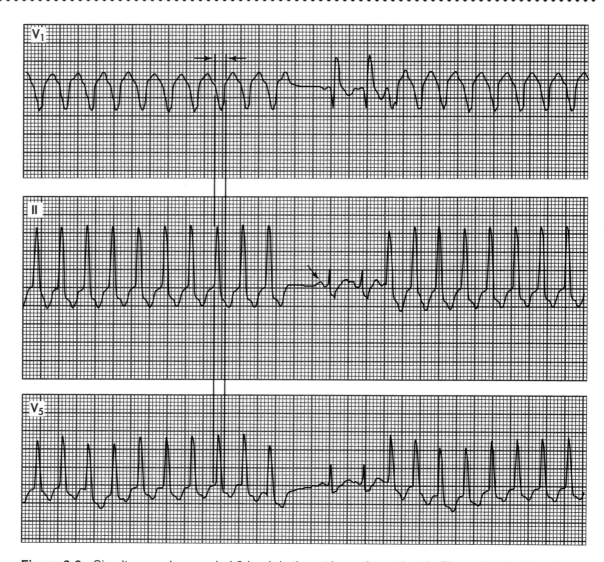

Figure 8-6 Simultaneously recorded 3-lead rhythm strip on the patient in Figure 8-5. Vertical time lines drawn in on the ECG tracing show a portion of the QRS complex in leads II and V_5 lies within what was thought to be the ST segment. The true width of the QRS is seen in lead VI and measures more than 0.12 sec. Thus, the rhythm is actually a wide QRS tachycardia. In the middle of the ECG tracing are two beats that appear to be sinus in origin because each is preceded by an upright P wave *(arrow)*. The QRS morphology for the two sinus beats is consistent with an underlying right BBB (QR complex in V_1, wide terminal S wave in V_5). During the episodes of tachycardia, the shape of the QRS complex is much different from those during the sinus rhythm. This suggests that the rhythm is actually ventricular tachycardia.

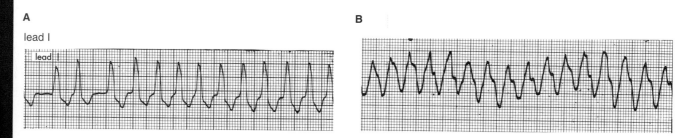

Figure 8-7 **A,** Atrial fibrillation with a rapid ventricular response and left bundle branch block. **B,** Ventricular tachycardia.

Table 8-18 Wide QRS Tachycardia of Unknown Origin[45]

Perform Primary ABCD Survey (Basic Life Support)
(Correct critical problems IMMEDIATELY as they are identified)
Assess responsiveness, **A**irway, **B**reathing, **C**irculation, ensure availability of monitor/**D**efibrillator

▼

Perform Secondary ABCD Survey (Advanced Life Support)
Administer oxygen, establish IV access, attach cardiac monitor
Administer fluids as needed (O_2, IV, monitor, fluids)
Assess vital signs, attach pulse oximeter, and monitor blood pressure
Obtain and review 12-lead ECG, portable chest x-ray film, perform a focused history and physical exam

▼

Is the patient stable or unstable?
Is the patient experiencing serious signs and symptoms because of the tachycardia?

Use 12-lead ECG/clinical information to help clarify rhythm diagnosis

▼

Rhythm confirmed as SVT **Go to narrow-QRS** **tachycardia algorithm**	**Wide-Complex Tachycardia of** **Unknown Origin** **Stable Patient**	**Rhythm confirmed as VT** **Go to VT algorithm**

Normal **Cardiac Function**	**Impaired** **Cardiac Function***
Sync cardioversion **or** Procainamide (IIb) **or** Amiodarone (IIb)	Sync cardioversion **or** Amiodarone (IIb)

▼

If medication therapy ineffective, perform synchronized cardioversion

Unstable Patient

If hemodynamically unstable, sync 100 J, 200 J, 300 J, and 360 J, or equivalent Biphasic energy. If hypotensive (systolic BP <90), unresponsive, or if severe pulmonary edema exists, defibrillate with same energy

Medication Dosing

Amiodarone—150 mg IV bolus over 10 min. If chemical conversion successful, follow with IV infusion of 1 mg/min for 6 hours and then a maintenance infusion of 0.5 mg/min. Repeat supplementary infusions of 150 mg as necessary for recurrent or resistant dysrhythmias. Maximum total daily dose 2.0 g
Procainamide[26]—100 mg over 5 min (20 mg/min). Maximum total dose 17 mg/kg. If chemical conversion successful, maintenance infusion 1 to 4 mg/min

---

Impaired cardiac function = ejection fraction <40% or CHF.
[26,45]See chapter references.

ACUTE CORONARY SYNDROMES

Tables 8-19 to 8-26 demonstrate assessment of an acute coronary syndrome, localization and management of MI, and management of acute pulmonary edema and hypotension/shock.

Table 8-19 Initial Assessment and General Treatment of the Patient with an Acute Coronary Syndrome

PREHOSPITAL	EMERGENCY DEPARTMENT

Initial Assessment (Goal: targeted clinical exam and 12-lead ECG within 10 min)

PREHOSPITAL	EMERGENCY DEPARTMENT
• Obtain a brief, targeted history/physical exam (determine age, gender; signs/symptoms, pain presentation, including location of pain, duration, quality, relation to effort, time of symptom onset; history CAD, CAD risk factors present?) history of Viagra use? • Assess vital signs, determine oxygen saturation If previous consistent with possible or definite ACS: • Use checklist (yes-no); focus on eligibility for reperfusion therapy; evaluate contraindications to aspirin and heparin • Establish IV access, ECG monitoring • Administer aspirin 162 to 325 mg (chewed), if no reason for exclusion • Obtain 12-lead ECG (machine interpretation or transmission of ECG to physician) • Draw blood for initial serum cardiac marker levels (to lab on arrival in Emergency Department) Consider triage to facility capable of angiography and revascularization if any of the following are present: • Signs of shock • Pulmonary edema (rales >halfway up) • Heart rate ≥100 beats/min and SBP ≤100 mm Hg	**RN triage for rapid care** • Targeted history: Determine age, gender, signs/symptoms, pain presentation, including location of pain, duration, quality, relation to effort, time of symptom onset; history CAD, CAD risk factors present? History of Viagra use? • Assess vital signs, determine oxygen saturation • Establish IV access, ECG monitoring • Obtain 12-lead ECG (present to physician for review) **Physician evaluation** If above consistent with possible or definite ACS: • Brief, targeted history/physical exam • Evaluate eligibility for reperfusion therapy + contraindications to aspirin and heparin • Administer aspirin 162 to 325 mg (chewed), if no reason for exclusion • Administer nitroglycerin as indicated • Evaluate 12-lead ECG—Categorize patient into one of three groups: ST-elevation or new or presumably new LBBB; ST-depression/transient ST-segment/T wave changes; normal or nondiagnostic ECG • Obtain serial ECGs in patients with history suggesting MI and nondiagnostic ECG • Obtain baseline serum cardiac marker levels (CK-MB, troponin T or I, myoglobin) • Obtain lab specimens (CBC, lipid profile, electrolytes, coagulation studies) • Obtain portable chest x-ray film • Evaluate results

Routine Measures

- Oxygen 4 L/min by nasal cannula
- Aspirin 162-325 mg (non-enteric); if the patient is not already receiving aspirin, have him/her chew the first dose to rapidly establish a high blood level. Subsequent doses may be swallowed.
- Nitroglycerin SL or spray. May repeat at 5-minute intervals (max 3 doses). (Ensure IV access, SBP >90 mm Hg, HR >50 beats/min, no RV infarction)
- Morphine 2 to 4 mg IV if pain not relieved with NTG; may repeat every 5 min (ensure SBP >90 mm Hg)

Table 8-20   Management of ST-Segment Elevation MI[26,45]

ST-segment elevation in two contiguous leads: ≥1 mm in limb leads
OR ≥2 mm in precordial leads
▼
Confirm diagnosis by signs/symptoms, ECG, serum cardiac markers
▼

All patients with ST-segment elevation MI should receive (if no contraindications):
- Antiplatelet therapy—Aspirin 162 to 325 mg (chewed)
- Anti-ischemia therapy (Beta-blockers, nitroglycerin IV if ongoing ischemia or uncorrected hypertension)
- Antithrombin therapy—Heparin (if using fibrin-specific lytics)
- ACE inhibitors (after 6 hours or when stable)—Especially with large or anterior MI, heart failure without hypotension (SBP >100 mm Hg), previous MI

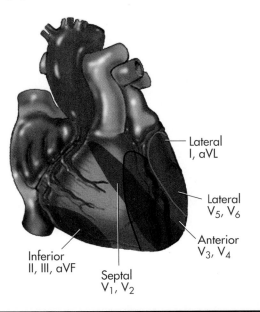

Lateral
I, aVL

Lateral
V₅, V₆

Anterior
V₃, V₄

Septal
V₁, V₂

Inferior
II, III, aVF

Symptom Onset ≤12 Hours?				Symptom Onset >12 Hours?	
Patient Eligible for Reperfusion? Goals— • Fibrinolytics: Door-to-drug time <30 min • Primary PCI: Door-to-dilation time 90 ± 30 min				Persistent symptoms ↓	Resolution of symptoms ↓
Yes ↓		No ↓		Consider reperfusion	Medical management
Signs of cardiogenic shock or contraindications to fibrinolytics?		Persistent or stuttering symptoms or ECG changes?		Medical management	
Yes ↓	No ↓	Yes ↓	No ↓		
PCI, medical management	Can cath lab be mobilized within 60 min?	Cardiac cath, medical management	Medical management		
	Yes ↓ No ↓				
	PCI Fibrinolysis (alteplase, reteplase, streptokinase, anistreplase, **or** tenecteplase)				

*Note: *PCI* = percutaneous coronary intervention (angioplasty ± stent).
[26,45]See chapter references.

Table 8-21 Management of Unstable Angina/Non-ST-Segment Elevation MI[45,55,56]

ECG changes in two or more anatomically contiguous leads:
ST-segment depression >1 mm or T wave inversion >1 mm **or**
Transient (<30 min) ST-segment/T wave changes >1 mm with discomfort

▼

Confirm diagnosis by signs/symptoms, ECG, serum cardiac markers

▼

- Aspirin: 162 to 325 mg (chewed) if not already administered (and no contraindications) (antiplatelet therapy)
- Heparin IV (antithrombin therapy)

▼

All patients with unstable angina/non–ST-segment elevation MI should receive (if no contraindications)

▼

If high-risk patient, give:
- Aspirin + glycoprotein IIb/IIIa inhibitors (i.e., Integrilin, Aggrastat, ReoPro) + IV heparin **or**
- Aspirin + glycoprotein IIb/IIIa inhibitors + SC low-molecular-weight heparin (i.e. enoxaparin [Lovenex], dalteparin [Fragmin])

High-Risk Criteria

▼

- Persistent ("stuttering") symptoms/recurrent ischemia; left ventricular (LV) dysfunction, CHF; widespread ECG changes; prior MI, positive troponin or CK-MB

▼

Anti-ischemic therapy (e.g., metoprolol, atenolol, esmolol, propranolol
- Beta-blockers—If patient not previously on beta-blockers or inadequately treated on current dose of beta-blocker (if no contraindications)
- Nitroglycerin sublingual tablet or spray, followed by IV nitroglycerin: If symptoms persist despite sublingual nitroglycerin therapy and initiation of beta-blocker therapy (and SBP >90 mm Hg)
- Morphine: 2 to 4 mg IV (if discomfort is not relieved or symptoms recur despite anti-ischemic therapy)—May repeat every 5 min (ensure SBP >90 mm Hg)

Assess clinical status: Is patient clinically stable?

Yes	No
- Continue in-hospital observation - Consider stress testing	Cardiac cath: - If anatomy suitable for revascularization; PCI, CABG - If anatomy unsuitable: Medical management

[45,55,56]See chapter references.

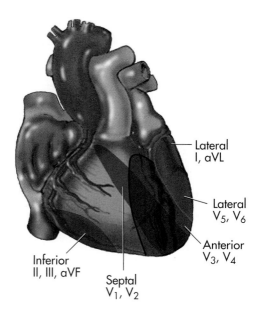

Lateral
I, aVL

Lateral
V₅, V₆

Anterior
V₃, V₄

Inferior
II, III, aVF

Septal
V₁, V₂

Table 8-22   Management of Patient with a Suspected Acute Coronary Syndrome and Nondiagnostic or Normal ECG

Nondiagnostic or Normal ECG

▼

Evaluate signs/symptoms, serial ECGs, serum cardiac markers

▼

Aspirin + other therapy as appropriate

▼

- Assess patient's clinical risk of death/nonfatal MI
- History and physical exam
- Obtain follow-up serum cardiac marker levels, serial ECG monitoring
- Continue evaluation and treatment in Emergency Department, chest pain unit, or monitored bed
- Consider radionuclide, echocardiography

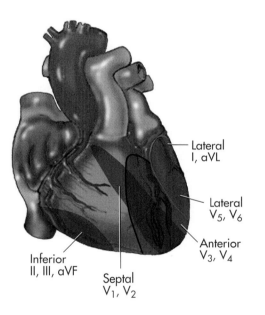

Lateral
I, aVL

Lateral
V₅, V₆

Anterior
V₃, V₄

Inferior
II, III, aVF

Septal
V₁, V₂

Table 8-23   Management of Acute Pulmonary Edema

Perform Primary ABCD Survey (Basic Life Support)

(Correct critical problems IMMEDIATELY as they are identified)
Assess responsiveness, **A**irway, **B**reathing, **C**irculation, ensure availability of monitor/**D**efibrillator

▼

Perform Secondary ABCD Survey (Advanced Life Support)
(Obtain arterial blood gas before oxygen administration if possible)
Administer oxygen, establish IV access, attach cardiac monitor (O_2, IV, monitor)
Assess vital signs, attach pulse oximeter, and monitor blood pressure
Obtain and review 12-lead ECG, portable chest x-ray film
Perform a focused history and physical exam

▼

If feasible and BP permits, place patient in sitting position with feet dependent
- Increases lung volume and vital capacity
- Decreases work of respiration
- Decreases venous return, decreases preload

If systolic BP >100 mm Hg:
- **Sublingual nitroglycerin**—1 tablet or spray every 5 min (max 3 doses) until IV nitroglycerin or nitroprusside can take effect[57]
- **Furosemide IV:** 0.5 to 1.0 mg/kg (typically 20 to 40 mg) (can repeat in 30 minutes if symptoms persist and BP stable)
- **Consider morphine IV** 2 to 4 mg

Consider additional preload/afterload reduction—nitroglycerin or nitroprusside IV, ACE inhibitors (if SBP >100 mm Hg)
- **Nitroglycerin IV**—Start at 5 mcg/min and increase gradually until mean systolic pressure falls by 10% to 15%, avoid hypotension (SBP <90 mm Hg)[26] **or**
- **Nitroprusside IV**—0.1 to 5 mcg/kg/min

Evaluate early for:
- Readily reversible cause: Institute appropriate intervention (e.g., cardiac dysrhythmias, tamponade)
- Myocardial ischemia/infarction (Institute appropriate intervention—candidate for fibrinolytic therapy? PTCA?)

If patient is refractory to previous therapies, hypotensive, or in cardiogenic shock:[57]
- Consider fluid or IV inotropic and/or vasopressor agents (e.g., dobutamine, dopamine, norepinephrine)
- Consider pulmonary and systemic arterial catheterization
- Obtain ECG to assist in diagnosis, evaluation, and reparability of culprit lesion or condition
- Consider need for mechanical circulatory assistance (balloon pump)

[26,57]See chapter references.

Table 8-24   Management of Hypotension/Shock: Suspected Pump Problem

Perform Primary ABCD Survey (Basic Life Support)
(Correct critical problems IMMEDIATELY as they are identified)
Assess responsiveness, **A**irway, **B**reathing, **C**irculation, ensure availability of monitor/**D**efibrillator

▼

Perform Secondary ABCD Survey (Advanced Life Support)
Administer oxygen, establish IV access, attach cardiac monitor, administer fluids as needed
(O_2, IV, monitor, fluids)
Assess vital signs, attach pulse oximeter, and monitor blood pressure
Obtain and review 12-lead ECG, portable chest x-ray film
Perform a focused history and physical exam

▼

Hypotension—Suspected Pump Problem

- If breath sounds are clear, consider fluid challenge of 250 to 500 mL NS to ensure adequate ventricular filling pressure before vasopressor administration

▼

Marked Hypotension (Systolic BP <70 mm Hg)/Cardiogenic Shock

Pharmacologic management:[26]
- Norepinephrine infusion: 0.5 to 30 mcg/min until SBP 80 mm Hg
- Then attempt to change to dopamine: 5 to 15 mcg/kg/min until SBP 90 mm Hg
- IV dobutamine: 2 to 20 mcg/kg/min can be given simultaneously in an attempt to reduce magnitude of dopamine infusion

Consider balloon pump or patient transfer to a cardiac interventional facility

Moderate Hypotension (Systolic BP 70 to 90 mm Hg)[45]

- Dopamine: 5 to 15 mcg/kg/min
- If BP remains low despite dopamine doses >20 mcg/kg/min, may substitute norepinephrine in doses of 0.5 to 30 mcg/min
- Once SBP ≥90 with dopamine, add dobutamine 2 to 20 mcg/kg/min and attempt to taper off dopamine

Systolic BP ≥90 mm Hg[57,58]

- Dobutamine: 2 to 20 mcg/kg/min

Medication Dosing

Norepinephrine IV	0.5 to 30 mcg/min
Dopamine IV	5 to 15 mcg/kg/min
Dobutamine IV	2 to 20 mcg/kg/min

[26,45,57,58]See chapter references.

Table 8-25   Management of Hypotension/Shock: Suspected Volume Problem

Perform Primary ABCD Survey (Basic Life Support)
(Correct critical problems IMMEDIATELY as they are identified)
Assess responsiveness, **A**irway, **B**reathing, **C**irculation, ensure availability of monitor/**D**efibrillator

▼

Perform Secondary ABCD Survey (Advanced Life Support)
Administer oxygen, establish IV access, attach cardiac monitor, administer fluids as needed
(O_2, IV, monitor, fluids)
Assess vital signs, attach pulse oximeter, and monitor blood pressure
Obtain and review 12-lead ECG, portable chest x-ray film
Perform a focused history and physical exam

▼

Hypotension: suspected volume (or vascular resistance) problem

▼

- Volume replacement
- Fluid challenge (250 to 500 mL IV boluses—reassess)
- Blood transfusion (if appropriate)
- If cause known, institute appropriate intervention (e.g., septic shock, anaphylaxis)
- Consider vasopressors, if indicated, to improve vascular tone if no response to fluid challenge(s)

Table 8-26   Management of Hypotension/Shock: Suspected Rate Problem

Perform Primary ABCD Survey (Basic Life Support)
(Correct critical problems IMMEDIATELY as they are identified)
Assess responsiveness, **A**irway, **B**reathing, **C**irculation, ensure availability of monitor/**D**efibrillator

▼

Perform Secondary ABCD Survey (Advanced Life Support)
Administer oxygen, establish IV access, attach cardiac monitor, administer fluids as needed
(O_2, IV, monitor, fluids)
Assess vital signs, attach pulse oximeter, and monitor blood pressure
Obtain and review 12-lead ECG, portable chest x-ray film
Perform a focused history and physical exam

▼

Hypotension: suspected rate problem

▼

- If rate too slow—bradycardia algorithm
- If rate too fast—determine width of QRS, then use appropriate tachycardia algorithm

STOP AND REVIEW

1. The correct dose of epinephrine, when administered by means of an endotracheal tube is:
   a. 0.5 mg
   b. 1.0 mg
   c. 2 to 2.5 mg
   d. 1 to 1.5 mg/kg

2. Lidocaine may be LETHAL if administered for which of the following rhythms?
   a. Monomorphic ventricular tachycardia
   b. Idioventricular (ventricular escape) rhythm
   c. Polymorphic ventricular tachycardia
   d. Sinus tachycardia

3. A 57-year-old male is complaining of chest pain and difficulty breathing. He is disoriented and extremely anxious. Examination reveals bibasilar crackles; a weak carotid pulse, and a blood pressure of 60/30. The cardiac monitor displays SVT at a rate of 210 beats/min. The patient has been placed on oxygen, and an IV has been established. Management of this patient should include:
   a. Administration of sublingual nitroglycerin for pain relief
   b. Administration of 6 mg of adenosine rapid IV bolus and reassessment of the patient
   c. Administration of 2.5 mg of verapamil slow IV bolus and reassessment of the patient
   d. Performing synchronized cardioversion with 50 J and reassessment of the patient

4. A 60-year-old female has suffered a cardiopulmonary arrest. A health care professional trained in endotracheal intubation has intubated the patient. Which of the following findings would indicate inadvertent esophageal intubation?
   a. Subcutaneous emphysema
   b. Jugular vein distention
   c. Gurgling sounds heard over the epigastrium
   d. Breath sounds heard on only one side of the chest

5. You have delivered a synchronized countershock with 50 J to an unstable patient with paroxysmal supraventricular tachycardia (PSVT). The monitor now shows ventricular fibrillation (VF). The patient is pulseless and apneic. Your best course of action will be to:
   a. Administer epinephrine, 1 mg (1:10,000) IV bolus
   b. Administer a synchronized countershock with 100 J
   c. Begin CPR, intubate at once, and establish IV access
   d. Ensure the "sync" control is off and immediately defibrillate with 200 J (or equivalent Biphasic energy)

6. Morphine sulfate may be used in the management of acute pulmonary edema because it:
   a. Causes bronchodilation and increases cardiac output
   b. Increases myocardial contractility
   c. Is a potent, rapid-acting diuretic
   d. Causes vasodilation, reducing preload and afterload

7. Rapid heart rates may produce serious signs and symptoms. The physiologic reason for this is that increases in heart rate result in _____ ventricular filling time, which frequently results in _____ stroke volume.
   a. Decreased, decreased
   b. Decreased, increased
   c. Increased, decreased
   d. Increased, increased

Your patient is a 76-year-old male complaining of chest pressure. The patient is in obvious distress, anxious, and appears short of breath. His symptoms began suddenly while walking from the living room to the kitchen and have lasted about 45 min. The discomfort is located in the center of his chest, and his left arm feels "tingly." The patient states his "pressure" is a 10 on a 1 to 10 scale and does not feel like the pain that he had with his heart attack, 1 month ago. His skin is pale, cool, and clammy, BP 66/40, P 104, R 24. On auscultation, crackles are heard about halfway up his chest.

8. You suspect this patient is most likely suffering from:
   a. Pneumonia
   b. Angina pectoris
   c. Cardiogenic shock
   d. Hypovolemic shock

9. Management of this patient should include:
   a. Sublingual nitroglycerin for relief of the patient's chest pressure
   b. Dobutamine IV to slow the patient's heart rate and increase force of contraction
   c. Furosemide IV for the patient's pulmonary congestion
   d. Norepinephrine IV to increase the patient's blood pressure

10. Dobutamine:
    a. Stimulates alpha, beta-1, and beta-2 receptors
    b. Is recommended in hypotension/shock caused by hypovolemia
    c. May result in bradycardia when administered in high doses
    d. Is administered as a 2- to 20-mcg IV bolus

11. Dopamine, when infused at a dose range of 5 to 10 mcg/kg/min, will most likely produce which of the following effects?
    a. Peripheral vasodilation
    b. Increased cardiac output
    c. Bronchodilation
    d. Renal and mesenteric vasodilation

12. Administration of norepinephrine:
    a. Results in a significant increase in heart rate
    b. May result in tissue sloughing or necrosis if extravasation occurs
    c. Should be abruptly discontinued when the desired hemodynamic response has been achieved
    d. May result in significant hypotension if simultaneously administered with epinephrine

13. A 58-year-old man is complaining of chest pain. Select the question that best evaluates the QUALITY of the patient's pain.
    a. "When did the pain begin?"
    b. "How would you describe your pain?"
    c. "Does anything make the pain better or worse?"
    d. "Where is your discomfort?"

14. A 75-year-old man has suffered a cardiac arrest. A quick-look reveals ventricular fibrillation. Your defibrillator delivers monophasic shocks. You have delivered an initial shock with 200 J and a second shock with 300 J, but there has been no change in the patient's rhythm. Your next action will be to:
    a. Resume CPR
    b. Prepare to intubate
    c. Establish an IV
    d. Defibrillate with 360 J

15. Most myocardial infarctions occur because of:
    a. Coronary artery spasm
    b. Acute volume overload
    c. Acute respiratory failure
    d. Coronary thrombosis

16. You are a paramedic called to a private residence for a "possible code." You find an elderly woman unresponsive on the floor. A quick examination reveals that she is apneic and pulseless. An EMT-Basic has inserted an oropharyngeal airway and is ventilating the patient with a bag-valve-mask. Your partner has begun chest compressions. A quick-look reveals the patient's cardiac rhythm to be asystole. A defibrillator is available that delivers monophasic shocks. Your next action will be to:
    a. Confirm the rhythm in another lead
    b. Defibrillate immediately with 200 J
    c. Establish an IV and administer atropine
    d. Perform synchronized cardioversion immediately with 50 J

17. Select the CORRECT statement regarding adenosine administration:
    a. Adenosine is used for patients with severe congestive heart failure refractory to diuretics, vasodilators, and conventional medications used to increase myocardial contractility
    b. Adenosine is contraindicated in patients with asthma
    c. Adenosine is the medication of choice for atrial fibrillation or atrial flutter with a rapid ventricular response
    d. Because of its long half-life, effects persist for more than 50 days after discontinuing the medication

18. Paramedics are on the scene with a 69-year-old woman who "passed out" at a bowling alley. The patient is lying supine in the lobby of the bowling alley, awake and alert. She states she had just walked into the lobby when she suddenly felt weak and dizzy, as if she were going to "pass out" and quickly sat down on the floor, hoping to relieve her symptoms. She has no chest pain or difficulty breathing, and has no significant past medical history. Her skin is cool and clammy, pulse weak and irregular at a rate of 30 to 40 beats/min, and a blood pressure of 76/54. The cardiac monitor displays a second-degree AV block, type II. Management of this patient should include:
    a. Asking the patient to cough or bear down
    b. Preparations for transcutaneous pacing as quickly as possible
    c. Placement of an IV line, sedation, and then synchronized cardioversion with 50 J
    d. Placement of an IV line and administration of a 1 or 1.5 mg/kg lidocaine bolus

A 77-year-old man is complaining of "pounding in my chest." His symptoms began about 1 hour ago while watching the news. He denies chest pain but repeatedly asks if you think he "might be having a heart attack." Examination reveals the following: BP 144/78, P 140, R 16. There are scattered rales in the bases bilaterally. The remainder of the physical exam is unremarkable. The patient has no significant past medical history. The cardiac monitor reveals a wide complex tachycardia. After briefly consulting with a colleague, you are still uncertain about a more definitive rhythm diagnosis. The patient has been placed on oxygen and an IV established. The patient's condition remains unchanged.

19. Based on the information presented, a reasonable course of action would include:
    a. Cardioversion or administration of procainamide or amiodarone IV
    b. Immediate defibrillation with 200 J
    c. Administration of verapamil slow IV push
    d. Cardioversion or administration of adenosine

20. Which of the following reflects the correct medication and its recommended dosage for this patient situation?
    a. Adenosine: 2.5 to 5 mg slow IV push
    b. Verapamil: 1 to 1.5 mg/kg slow IV push
    c. Procainamide: 20 mg/min IV infusion
    d. Amiodarone: 300 mg IV push

STOP AND REVIEW ANSWERS

1. c. The recommended dose of epinephrine, when administered via an endotracheal tube, is 2 to 2.5 times the IV dose. The medication should be diluted in 10 mL of normal saline or distilled water.

2. b. Lidocaine may be *lethal* if administered for a bradycardia with a ventricular escape rhythm (e.g., idioventricular rhythm, second-degree AV block type II, complete AV block). Lidocaine may be used as an alternative medication in the management of pulseless VT/VF, monomorphic VT, or polymorphic VT.

3. d. This patient is unstable (chest pain, altered level of responsiveness, hypotension, difficulty breathing). Consider sedation, perform synchronized cardioversion with 50 J, and reassess the patient.

4. c. Absence of chest wall expansion and gurgling heard over the epigastrium indicate misplacement of the ETT into the esophagus. If breath sounds were present bilaterally with bag-valve-mask ventilation before placement of an ETT, the presence of breath sounds on only one side of the chest after placement of the tube suggests right mainstem bronchus intubation.

5. d. After ensuring the patient is indeed pulseless and apneic (and a monitoring lead has not become disconnected), defibrillate immediately with 200 J (or equivalent Biphasic energy).

6. d. Medications used in the management of a normotensive patient in acute pulmonary edema include sublingual nitroglycerin, furosemide, and morphine. Morphine reduces anxiety, increases venous capacitance (venous pooling) and decreases venous return (preload) (sometimes called *chemical phlebotomy*), decreases systemic vascular resistance (afterload), and decreases myocardial oxygen demand.

7. a. Rapid heart rates may produce serious signs and symptoms. The physiologic reason for this is that increases in heart rate result in *decreased* ventricular filling time, which frequently results in *decreased* stroke volume.

8. c. Hypotension + pulmonary edema = cardiogenic shock.

9. d. The medication of choice in the management of hypotension/shock (not due to hypovolemia) with a systolic blood pressure <70 mm Hg is norepinephrine. Norepinephrine should be infused at a rate of 0.5 to 1.0 mcg/min, titrated to improve blood pressure (up to 30 mcg/min).

10. a. Dobutamine stimulates alpha, beta-1, and beta-2 receptors and is used for the short-term management of patients with cardiac decompensation caused by depressed contractility (e.g., CHF, pulmonary congestion) with a SBP 70 to 100 mm Hg **and no signs of shock**. Hypovolemia must be corrected before treatment with dobutamine. Dobutamine is administered as a continuous IV infusion at a rate of 2 to 20 mcg/kg/min and may result in tachycardia when administered in high doses.

11. b. When infused at 5 to 10 mcg/kg/min, dopamine acts directly on the beta-1 receptors on the myocardium and indirectly by releasing norepinephrine from its storage sites in sympathetic neurons. These actions increase myocardial contractility and stroke volume, thereby increasing cardiac output. Stimulation of beta-1 receptors also results in an increased SA rate and enhanced impulse conduction in the heart. There is little, if any, stimulation of beta-2 receptors (peripheral vasodilation, bronchodilation).

12. b. Norepinephrine stimulates both alpha (90%) and beta-receptors (10%). As a result, administration of norepinephrine usually results in increased blood pressure with minimal effect on heart rate. Because of its potent alpha effects (vasoconstriction) tissue sloughing or necrosis may result if extravasation occurs. Norepinephrine should be administered via an infusion pump and must be discontinued gradually. Simultaneous administration of epinephrine and norepinephrine may result in excessive and serious hypertensive episodes and additive CNS stimulation including agitation, nervousness, ataxia, tremors, and excitability.

13. b. The quality of the patient's pain may be assessed by asking, "How would you describe your discomfort?" (pressure, pain, crushing, dull, burning, tearing, throbbing, squeezing, stabbing, vise-like). "When did the pain begin?" determines the onset of the patient's symptoms. "Does anything make the pain better or worse?" is asked to determine what provokes the patient's symptoms. "Where is your discomfort?" pinpoints the region/radiation of the patient's symptoms.

14. d. In pulseless VT/VF, three serial unsynchronized shocks are delivered in rapid succession if there is no change in the rhythm. The energies used for the initial shocks are 200 J, 200 to 300 J, and 360 J. In this scenario, two shocks have been delivered. The third shock should be delivered using 360 J.

15. d. Myocardial infarction (MI) most often occurs when there is a sudden decrease or total cessation of blood flow through a coronary artery to an area of the myocardium because of a thrombus. MI may also occur because of coronary spasm. Spasm as a primary cause of MI is rare; however, MI as a result of cocaine abuse is frequently thought to be caused by coronary spasm. MI may also occur because of a coronary embolism (rare).

16. a. A quick-look has revealed what appears to be asystole. It is important to quickly survey the scene and determine if there is documentation or other evidence of a DNAR order. If such as order exists, or if there are obvious signs of death, do not start/attempt resuscitation. For the purposes of this scenario, assume there is no DNAR order and there are no obvious signs of death. It is important to verify the presence of asystole by confirming the rhythm in another lead. Check lead/cable connections, ensure the power to monitor is on, turn the gain up, and then confirm the rhythm in second lead.

17. b. Adenosine is contraindicated in persons with asthma and atrial fibrillation/atrial flutter. Administration may result in many side effects, including dyspnea, coughing, and bronchospasm. *Amrinone* (now known as Inamrinone) is used for patients with severe CHF refractory to diuretics, vasodilators, and conventional medications used to increase myocardial contractility. Because of its very short half-life, adenosine must be injected into the IV tubing as fast as possible (seconds). Failure to do so may result in breakdown of the medication while still in the IV tubing. Oral *amiodarone* has a half-life of 26 to 107 days, mean = 53 days. Effects of amiodarone persist for more than 50 days after discontinuing the medication.

18. b. Second-degree AV block type II may rapidly progress to complete AV block without warning. Transcutaneous pacing should be instituted until transvenous pacemaker insertion can be accomplished. Atropine should be avoided; it may increase the sinus rate and worsen the block or precipitate third-degree AV block.

19. a. The patient appears stable at present. Management of a stable patient with a wide-complex tachycardia of unknown origin may include sedation (the patient is awake and alert with a reasonable BP) and then immediate cardioversion or administration of IV procainamide or IV amiodarone. Calcium channel blockers (e.g., verapamil, diltiazem) are CONTRAINDICATED in wide-complex tachycardias of unknown origin.

20. c. Procainamide is administered via IV infusion at a rate of 20 mg/min until one of the following occurs: the dysrhythmia resolves, hypotension ensues, the QRS widens by >50% of original width, a total dose of 17 mg/kg has been administered, or the rhythm changes to torsades de pointes. (Procainamide is one of many medications that may precipitate torsades). If the dysrhythmia resolves because of procainamide administration, hang a maintenance infusion at 1 to 4 mg/min. Adenosine is not indicated in the management of wide complex tachycardia. It is used for most narrow-QRS tachycardias. The correct dose of adenosine is 6 mg, followed by 12 mg in 1 to 2 min. An additional 12 mg dose may be given in 1 to 2 min if needed ("6-12-12"). Verapamil is *contraindicated* in wide-complex tachycardia. When this medication is used (alternative medication in narrow-QRS PSVT after adenosine), the initial dose is 2.5 to 5.0 mg slow IV push over at least 2 min. Although amiodarone may be used in stable wide complex tachycardia, the dosage listed is that used for the initial dose of this medication in cardiac arrest. In a patient with a pulse, amiodarone is administered initially as a loading infusion of 150 mg IV bolus over 10 min (15 mg/min), and then followed with and "early" and "late" maintenance infusion.

REFERENCES

1. The American Heart Association in Collaboration with the International Liaison Committee on Resuscitation (ILCOR): Part 1: Introduction to the International Guidelines 2000 for CPR and ECC: a consensus on science, *Circulation* 102 (suppl I):1-5, 2000.
2. Lindner K, Ahnefeld F, Bowdler I: Comparison of different doses of epinephrine on myocardial perfusion and resuscitation success during cardiopulmonary resuscitation in a pig model, *Am J Emerg Med* 9:27-31, 1991.
3. Brown CG, Martin DR, Pepe PE, Stueven H, Cummins RO, Gonzalez E, Jastremski M: A comparison of standard-dose and high-dose epinephrine in cardiac arrest outside the hospital, *N Engl J Med* 327:1051-1055, 1992.
4. Callaham M, Madsen CD, Barton CW, Saunders CE, Pointer J: A randomized clinical trial of high-dose epinephrine and norepinephrine vs standard-dose epinephrine in prehospital cardiac arrest, *JAMA* 268(19):2667-2672, 1992.
5. Stiell IG, Hebert PC, Weitzman BN, Wells GA, Raman S, Stark RM, Higginson LA, Ahuja J, Dickinson GE: High-dose epinephrine in adult cardiac arrest, *N Engl J Med* 327(15):1045-1050, 1992.
6. Gueugniaud PY, Mols P, Goldstein P, Pham E, Dubien PY, Deweerdt C, Vergnion M, Petit P, Carli P: European Epinephrine Study Group. A comparison of repeated high doses and repeated standard doses of epinephrine for cardiac arrest outside the hospital [see comments], *N Engl J Med* 339:1595-1601, 1998.
7. Chugh SS, Lurie KG, Lindner KH: Pressor with promise: using vasopressin in cardiopulmonary arrest, *Circulation* 96(7):2453-2454, 1997.
8. Woodhouse SP, Cox S, Boyd P, Case C, Weber M: High dose and standard dose adrenaline do not alter survival, compared with placebo, in cardiac arrest, *Resuscitation* 30:243-249, 1995.
9. Lindner KH, Brinkmann A, Pfenninger EG, Lurie KG, Goertz A, Lindner IM: Effect of vasopressin on hemodynamic variables, organ blood flow, and acid-base status in a pig model of cardiopulmonary resuscitation, *Anesth Analg* 77:427-435, 1993.
10. Lindner KH, Prengel AW, Pfenninger EG, Lindner IM, Strohmenger HU, Georgieff M, et al: Vasopressin improves vital organ blood flow during closed-chest cardiopulmonary resuscitation in pigs, *Circulation* 91:215-221, 1996.
11. Lindner KH, Prengel AW, Brinkmann A, Strohmenger HU, Lindner IM, Lurie KG: Vasopressin administration in refractory cardiac arrest, *Ann Intern Med* 124:1061-1064, 1996.
12. Prengel AW, Lindner KH, Keller A, Lurie KG: Cardiovascular function during the postresuscitation phase after cardiac arrest in pigs: a comparison of epinephrine versus vasopressin, *Crit Care Med* 24(12):2014-2019, 1996.
13. Weil MH, Tang W, editors: *CPR: resuscitation of the arrested heart*, Philadelphia, 1999, WB Saunders.
14. Kudenchuk PJ, Cobb LA, Copass MK, Cummins RO, Doherty AM, Fahrenbruch CE, Hallstrom AP, Murray WA, Olsufka M, Walsh T: Amiodarone for resuscitation after out-of-hospital cardiac arrest due to ventricular fibrillation, *N Engl J Med* 341:871-878, 1999.

15. The American Heart Association in Collaboration with the International Liaison Committee on Resuscitation (ILCOR): Part 6: Advanced cardiovascular life support, Section 1: Introduction to ACLS 2000: Overview of Recommended Changes in ACLS from the Guidelines 2000 Conference, *Circulation* 102 (suppl I):1-87, 2000.

16. Harrison EE: Lidocaine in prehospital countershock refractory ventricular fibrillation, *Ann Emerg Med* 10(8):420-423, 1981.

17. Herlitz J, Ekstrom L, Wennerblom B, Axelsson A, Bang A, Lindkvist J, Persson NG, Holmberg S: Lidocaine in out-of-hospital ventricular fibrillation: does it improve survival? *Resuscitation* 33:199-205, 1997.

18. Ujhelyi MR, Schur M, Frede T, Bottorff MB, Gabel M, Markel ML: Mechanism of antiarrhythmic drug-induced changes in defibrillation threshold: role of potassium and sodium channel conductance, *J Am Coll Cardiol* 27(6):1534-1542, 1996.

19. Thel MC, Armstrong AL, McNulty SE, Califf RM, O'Connor CM, for the Duke Internal Medicine Housestaff: Randomised trial of magnesium in in-hospital cardiac arrest, *Lancet* 350:1272-6.61, 1997.

20. Fatovich DM, Prentice DA, Dobb GJ: Magnesium in cardiac arrest (the magic trial), *Resuscitation* 35:237-241, 1997.

21. Stiell IG, Wells GA, Hebert PC, Laupacis A, Weitzman BN: Association of drug therapy with survival in cardiac arrest: limited role of advanced cardiac life support drugs, *Acad Emerg Med* 2:264-273, 1995.

22. van Walraven C, Stiell IG, Wells GA, Hebert PC, Vandemheen K: Do advanced cardiac life support drugs increase resuscitation rates from in-hospital cardiac arrest? The OTAC Study Group, *Ann Emerg Med* 32(5):544-553, 1998.

23. Tzivoni D, Keren A, Cohen AM, Loebel H, Zahavi I, Chenzbraun A, Stern S: Magnesium therapy for torsades de pointes, *Am J Cardiol* 53:528-530, 1984.

24. Tzivoni D, Banai S, Schuger C, Benhorin J, Keren A, Gottlieb S, Stern S: Treatment of torsade de pointes with magnesium sulfate, *Circulation* 77:392-397, 1988.

25. Cannon LA, Heiselman DE, Dougherty JM, Jones J: Magnesium levels in cardiac arrest victims: relationship between magnesium levels and successful resuscitation, *Ann Emerg Med* 16:1195-1199, 1987.

26. Ryan TJ, Antman EM, Brooks NH, Califf RM, Hillis LD, Hiratzka LF, Rapaport E, Riegel B, Russell RO, Smith EE III, Weaver WD: *ACC/AHA guidelines for the management of patients with acute myocardial infarction: 1999 update: a report of the American College of Cardiology/American Heart Association Task Force on Practice Guidelines (Committee on Management of Acute Myocardial Infarction).* Available at http://www.acc.org/clinical/guidelines and http://www.americanheart.org. (Accessed on 1/31/01).

27. Brown DC, Lewis AJ, Criley JM: Asystole and its treatment: the possible role of the parasympathetic nervous system in cardiac arrest, *JACEP* 8:448-452, 1979.

28. Coon GA, Clinton JE, Ruiz E: Use of atropine for brady-asystolic prehospital cardiac arrest, *Ann Emerg Med* 10:462-467, 1981.

29. Cummins RO, Graves JR: *ACLS scenarios: core concepts for case-based learning*, St Louis, 1996, Mosby.

30. Aufderheide TP: Etiology, electrophysiology, and myocardial mechanics of pulseless electrical activity, *In* Paradis NA, Halperin HR, Nowak RM, editors: *Cardiac arrest: the science and practice of resuscitation medicine*, Baltimore, 1996, Williams & Wilkins.

31. Ornato JP, Peberdy MA: The mystery of bradyasystole during cardiac arrest, *Ann Emerg Med* 27:576-587, 1996.

32. Dauchot P, Gravenstein JS: Bradycardia after myocardial ischemia and its treatment with atropine, *Anesthesiology* 44:501-518, 1976.

33. The American Heart Association in Collaboration with the International Liaison Committee on Resuscitation (ILCOR): Part 6: Advanced cardio-vascular life support, Section 7: Algorithm approach to ACLS emergencies, 7D: The tachycardia algorithms, *Circulation* 102 (suppl I):1-158-165, 2000.

34. Mehta AV, Sanchez GR, Sacks EJ, Casta A, Dunn JM, Donner RM: Ectopic automatic atrial tachycardia in children: clinical characteristics, management and follow-up, *J Am Coll Cardiol* 11:379-385, 1988.

35. Holt P, Crick JC, Davies DW, Curry P: Intravenous amiodarone in the acute termination of supraventricular arrhythmias, *Int J Cardiol* 8:67-79, 1985.

36. Kouvaras G, Cokkinos DV, Halal G, Chronopoulos G, Ioannou N: The effective treatment of multifocal atrial tachycardia with amiodarone, *Jpn Heart J* 30:301-312, 1989.

37. Garratt C, Linker N, Griffith M, Ward D, Camm AJ: Comparison of adenosine and verapamil for termination of paroxysmal junctional tachycardia, *Am J Cardiol* 64:1310-1316, 1989.

38. Albers GW, Dalen JE, Laupacis A, Manning WJ, Petersen P, Singer DE: Antithrombotic therapy in atrial fibrillation, *Chest* 119(1 Suppl):194S-206S, 2001.

39. Camm AJ: *Safety of antiarrhythmic agents: the final frontier in treating atrial fibrillation?* http://www.medscape.com/Medscape/cardiology/TreatmentUpdate/2000/tu03/public/toc-tu03.html (Accessed on 2/19/01).

40. Cotter G, Blatt A, Kaluski E, Metzkor-Cotter E, Koren M, Litinski I, Simantov R, Moshkovitz Y, Zaidenstein R, Peleg E, Vered Z, Golik A: Conversion of recent onset paroxysmal atrial fibrillation to normal sinus rhythm: the effect of no treatment and high-dose amiodarone: a randomized, placebo-controlled study [see comments], *Eur Heart J* 20:1833-1842, 1999.

41. Clemo HF, Wood MA, Gilligan DM, Ellenbogen KA: Intravenous amiodarone for acute heart rate control in the critically ill patient with atrial tachyarrhythmias, *Am J Cardiol* 81:594-598, 1998.

42. Ellenbogen KA, Dias VC, Plumb VJ, Heywood JR, Mirvis DM: A placebo-controlled trial of continuous intravenous diltiazem infusion for 24-hour heart rate control during atrial fibrillation and atrial flutter: a multicenter study, *J Am Coll Cardiol* 18:891-897, 1991.

43. Salerno DM, Dias VC, Kleiger RE, et al: Efficacy and safety of intravenous diltiazem for treatment of atrial fibrillation and atrial flutter, *Am J Cardiol* 63:1046-1051, 1989.

44. Chapman MJ, Moran JL, O'Fathartaigh MS, Peisach AR, Cunningham DN: Management of atrial tachyarrhythmias in the critically ill: a comparison of intravenous procainamide and amiodarone, *Intensive Care Med* 19:48-52, 1993.

45. The American Heart Association in Collaboration with the International Liaison Committee on Resuscitation (ILCOR): Part 7: Era of reperfusion, Section 1: Acute coronary syndromes (acute myocardial infarction): a consensus on science, *Circulation* 102 (suppl I):1-163, 2000.

46. Maury P, Zimmermann M, Metzger J, Reynard C, Dorsaz P, Adamec R: Amiodarone therapy for sustained ventricular tachycardia after myocardial infarction: long-term follow-up, risk assessment and predictive value of programmed ventricular stimulation, *Int J Cardiol* 76(2-3):199-210, 2000.

47. Leak D: Intravenous amiodarone in the treatment of refractory life-threatening cardiac arrhythmias in the critically ill patient, *Am Heart J* 111:456-462, 1986.

48. Remme WJ, Kruyssen HA, Look MP, van Hoogenhuyze DC, Krauss XH: Hemodynamic effects and tolerability of intravenous amiodarone in patients with impaired left ventricular function, *Am Heart J* 122:96–103, 1991.

49. Nasir N Jr, Taylor A, Doyle TK, Pacifico A: Evaluation of intravenous lidocaine for the termination of sustained monomorphic ventricular tachycardia in patients with coronary artery disease with or without healed myocardial infarction, *Am J Cardiol* 74:1183-1186, 1994.

50. Gorgels AP, van den Dool A, Hofs A, Mulleneers R, Smeets JL, Vos MA, Wellens HJ: Comparison of procainamide and lidocaine in terminating sustained monomorphic ventricular tachycardia, *Am J Cardiol* 78:43-46, 1996.

51. Akhtar M, Shenasa M, Jazayeri M, Caceres J, Tchou PJ: Wide QRS complex tachycardia: reappraisal of a common problem, *Ann Intern Med* 109:905-912, 1988.

52. Pinter A, Dorian P: Intravenous antiarrhythmic agents, *Curr Opin Cardiol* 16(1):17-22, 2001.

53. Callans DJ, Marchlinski FE: Dissociation of termination and prevention of inducibility of sustained ventricular tachycardia with infusion of procainamide: evidence for distinct mechanisms, *J Am Coll Cardiol* 19:111-117, 1992.

54. Ho DS, Zecchin RP, Richards DA, Uther JB, Ross DL: Double-blind trial of lignocaine versus sotalol for acute termination of spontaneous sustained ventricular tachycardia [see comments], *Lancet* 344:18–23, 1994.

55. Goldman L, Braunwald E: *Primary cardiology*, Philadelphia, 1998, WB Saunders.

56. Braunwald E, Antman EM, Beasley JW, Califf RM, Cheitlin MD, Hochman JS, Jones RH, Kereiakes D, Kupersmith J, Levin TN, Pepine CJ, Schaeffer JW, Smith EE III, Steward DE, Theroux P: ACC/AHA guidelines for the management of patients with unstable angina and non–ST-segment elevation myocardial infarction: a report of the American College of Cardiology/American Heart Association Task Force on Practice Guidelines (Committee on the Management of Patients With Unstable Angina), *J Am Coll Cardiol* 36:970-1062, 2000.

57. Leier CV: Unstable heart failure. In Braundwald E, senior editor; Colucci WS, volume editor: *Heart failure: cardiac function and dysfunction, atlas of heart diseases*, Vol IV, Singapore, 1995, Current Medicine.

58. Braunwald E: Recognition and management of patients with acute myocardial infarction. In Goldman L, Braunwald E: *Primary Cardiology*, Philadelphia, 1998. WB Saunders.

REFERENCES

Albers GW, Dalen JE, Laupacis A, Manning WJ, Petersen P, Singer DE: Antithrombotic therapy in atrial fibrillation, *Chest* 119(1 suppl):194S-206S, 2001.

The American Heart Association in Collaboration with the International Liaison Committee on Resuscitation (ILCOR): Part 6: Advanced cardiovascular life support, Section 7: Algorithm approach to ACLS emergencies, *Circulation* 102 (suppl I):1-136-171, 2000.

Berne RM, Levy MN: *Cardiovascular physiology*, ed 7, St Louis, 1997, Mosby.

Braunwauld E, Scheinman M, editors: *Arrhythmias: electrophysiologic principles*, Vol IX, Singapore, 1996, Current Medicine.

Braunwald E, senior editor; Califf RM, volume editor: *Atlas of heart diseases: acute myocardial infarction and other acute ischemic syndromes*, Vol VIII, Singapore, 1996, Current Medicine.

Chou T, Knilans TK: *Electrocardiography in clinical practice: adult and pediatric*, Philadelphia, 1996, WB Saunders.

Crawford MV, Spence MI: *Common sense approach to coronary care*, ed 6, St Louis, 1995, Mosby.

Driscoll P, Gwinnutt C, Mackway-Jones K, Wardle T, editors: *Advanced cardiac life support: the practical approach*, ed 2, London, 1997, Chapman & Hall Medical.

Goldberger AL: *Clinical electrocardiography: a simplified approach*, ed 6, St Louis, 1999, Mosby.

Goldman L, Braunwald E: *Primary cardiology*, Philadelphia, 1998, WB Saunders.

Innerarity SA, Stark JL: *Springhouse notes: fluids and electrolytes*, ed 3. Springhouse, PA, 1997, Springhouse Corporation.

Kahn MG: *Rapid ECG interpretation*, Philadelphia, 1997, WB Saunders.

Marriott HJL, Conover MB: *Advanced concepts in arrhythmias*, ed 3, St Louis, 1998, Mosby.

Murphy JG: *Mayo clinical cardiology review*, ed 2, Philadelphia, 2000, Lippincott, Williams & Wilkins.

Padrid PJ, Kowey PR, editors: *Cardiac arrhythmia: mechanisms, diagnosis, and management*, Baltimore, 1995, Williams & Wilkins.

Paradis NA, Halperin HR, Nowak RM, editors: *Cardiac arrest: the science and practice of resuscitation medicine*, Baltimore, 1996, Williams & Wilkins.

Phalen T: *The 12-lead ECG in acute myocardial infarction*, St Louis, 1996, Mosby.

Ryan TJ, Antman EM, Brooks NH, Califf RM, Hillis LD, Hiratzka LF, Rapaport E, Riegel B, Russell RO, Smith EE III, Weaver WD: *ACC/AHA guidelines for the management of patients with acute myocardial infarction: 1999 update: a report of the American College of Cardiology/ American Heart Association Task Force on Practice Guidelines (Committee on Management of Acute Myocardial Infarction)*. Available at http://www.acc.org/clinical/guidelines and http://www.americanheart.org. Accessed on 1/31/01.

Sanders MJ: *Mosby's paramedic textbook*, ed 2, St Louis, 2000, Mosby.

Weil MH, Tang W, editors: *CPR: resuscitation of the arrested heart*, Philadelphia, 1999, WB Saunders.

Willerson JT, Cohn JN, editors: *Cardiovascular medicine*, New York, 1995, Churchill-Livingstone.

Woods SL, Sivarajan Froelicher ES, Motzer SA: Cardiac nursing, ed 4, Philadelphia, 2000, Lippincott, Williams & Wilkins.

Acute Ischemic Stroke

OBJECTIVES

On completion of this chapter, you will be able to:

1. Explain the etiology of stroke, including the two major types of stroke.
2. Describe the sequence of events that occurs during a stroke.
3. Gain insight into why stroke must be treated within the first 3 hours of symptom onset.
4. Identify the signs and symptoms of stroke and list the common dispatch complaints for stroke.
5. Understand the importance of a transient ischemic attack (TIA).
6. Discuss the components of the stroke Chain of Recovery.
7. Understand the importance of determining the time of symptom onset, including asking family or bystanders when the possible stroke patient was last at baseline neurologic function.
8. Explain the components of the initial assessment and general treatment for the patient with a suspected stroke.

WHY DO WE CARE ABOUT STROKE?

1. **Stroke:** any acute clinical event related to diseases of the cerebral circulation that lasts more than 24 hours[1,2]
2. Stroke facts
   a. Third leading cause of death, after heart disease and cancer
   b. Every minute in the United States, someone experiences a stroke and every 3.3 minutes someone dies of one
   c. Stroke kills more than twice as many American women every year than breast cancer
   d. Approximately one third of all stroke survivors will have another stroke within 5 years
   e. Approximately 600,000 people suffer a new or recurrent stroke each year. Of these, about 500,000 are first attacks, and 100,000 are recurrent attacks
   f. "Stroke belt"[3]
      (1) Twelve contiguous states and the District of Columbia have stroke death rates consistently >10% higher than the rest of the country: Virginia, North Carolina, South Carolina, Georgia, Florida, Alabama, Mississippi, Louisiana, Arkansas, Tennessee, Kentucky, Indiana, and Washington, DC
      (2) Higher incidence and mortality may be linked to a number of factors, including a higher than average population of African-Americans, higher than average population of older adults, and dietary factors

3. Risk factors
   a. Non-modifiable: older age, gender, race/ethnicity (higher rates in African-Americans than in whites), family history of stroke
   b. Modifiable: hypertension, smoking, diabetes, atrial fibrillation
4. Early diagnosis
   a. Trauma: "Golden Hour"
   b. Acute MI: "Time is Muscle"
   c. Stroke: "Time is Neurons," "Time is Brain"
5. National Institute of Neurological Disorders and Stroke (NINDS)
   a. Has published study of tissue plasminogen activator (tPA) for acute stroke management
   b. Responsible for reorienting focus of health care practitioners regarding the urgency of managing stroke
6. Stroke also called a *brain attack*
   a. Origination of the term *brain attack* and its application to stroke are credited to Vladimir C. Hachinski, MD, and John Norris, MD, neurologists from Canada
   b. The National Stroke Association (NSA) began using the term in 1990 because it characterizes the medical condition and communicates the actual event more clearly to the public than does the word *stroke*
   c. The earlier the intervention, the better the results
      (1) The later it is in the time course of the stroke, the higher the risk of bleeding complications following fibrinolytic therapy

> Stroke happens in the brain rather than the heart.

CLASSIFICATION OF STROKE

Two Major Types of Stroke

1. Ischemic stroke
   a. Blood vessel supplying the brain is occluded
   b. Can be life-threatening but rarely leads to death within the first hour
2. Hemorrhagic stroke
   a. Cerebral artery ruptures
   b. Can be fatal at onset

Ischemic Stroke

1. Accounts for approximately 85% of strokes
   a. Results from complete occlusion of an artery that deprives the brain of essential nutrients
2. Thrombotic strokes (Figure 9-1)
   a. Most common cause of stroke
   b. Atherosclerosis of large cerebral vessels causes progressive narrowing and platelet adhesion, leading to progressive levels of deficits
   c. Blood clots develop within the brain artery itself (cerebral thrombosis)
   d. **Lacunar strokes** are small areas of infarction and necrosis associated with thrombosis of small arteries of the deep white matter in the brain
      (1) Eclampsia, arteritis, drug-induced

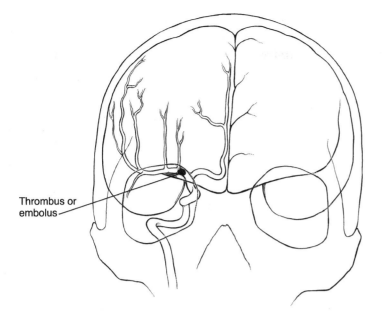

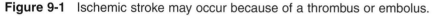

Thrombus or
embolus

Figure 9-1   Ischemic stroke may occur because of a thrombus or embolus.

3. Embolic strokes
   a. Clots arise elsewhere in the body and then migrate to the brain
      (cerebral embolism)
      (1) Become lodged at bifurcations of arteries where blood flow is
          most turbulent
      (2) Fragments may become lodged in smaller vessels
   b. Cardiac sources of clots
      (1) Mural thrombi, secondary to MI and dysrhythmias, particularly
          atrial fibrillation
      (2) Valvular disease/prosthetic valves with resultant thrombus for-
          mation, ventricular septal defects with thrombus formation, and
          cardiac tumors
      (3) Clots from cardiac sources lodge in the:
          (a) Middle cerebral artery or its branches in 80% of cases
              (Figure 9-2)
          (b) Posterior cerebral artery or its branches in 10% of cases
          (c) Vertebral artery or its branches in the remaining 10% of
              cases
   c. Other sources of emboli
      (1) Fat emboli secondary to long bone fractures (rare), particulate
          emboli from IV drug abusers (rare), or septic emboli secondary
          to endocarditis (rare)
4. Evolution of an ischemic stroke
   a. Complete occlusion of an artery may lead to death of an area of
      cells in the brain because of obstruction of blood flow (ischemic
      infarction)
   b. Evolution of the thrombosis may take place in a few minutes, hours,
      or even days
      (1) *Progressive stroke* is a term used to describe a stroke that is
          actively progressing because of increasing occlusion and
          ischemia (progressive development of a deficit over time)
      (2) Large blood vessels, such as the carotid, middle cerebral, and
          basilar arteries, can take longer to become occluded than
          smaller vessels

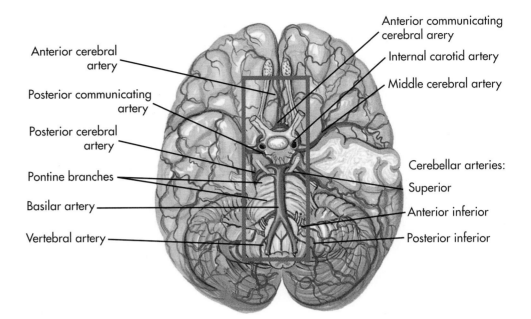

Figure 9-2 Arterial blood supply to the brain.

(a) Warning signs of impending occlusion may be present—a **transient ischemic attack (TIA)** is one of the most important
  (i) TIA is a reversible episode of focal neurologic dysfunction that typically lasts a few minutes to a few hours, resolving within 24 hours
  (ii) Significant indicator of stroke risk
  (iii) Approximately one fourth of patients presenting with stroke have had a previous TIA
  (iv) Approximately 5% of patients with a TIA will develop a completed stroke within 1 month if untreated
  (v) TIA should be treated with the same urgency as a completed stroke
  (vi) **Reversible ischemic neurologic deficit (RIND)** is a neurologic deficit that last more than 24 hours but leaves little or no neurologic deficit
(3) Cerebral damage may occur as a result of the infarction as well as an excessive accumulation of fluid in the brain (cerebral edema)
  (a) As brain tissue dies, fluid begins to accumulate, resulting in swelling
  (b) Because the cranium is a rigid container, as swelling increases, nearby brain tissue is compressed (e.g., neurons, nerve tracts, and cerebral arteries), and intracranial pressure (ICP) increases
  (c) Sustained increase in pressure causes continued ischemia, irreparable damage to brain cells, and potentially death
  (d) Cerebral edema usually peaks 2 to 5 days after the onset of the stroke
  (e) Fluid accumulation then stabilizes and may begin to decrease
c. Zones of injury
  (1) Core zone of ischemia
    (a) Area of severe ischemia (blood flow below 10% to 25%)
    (b) Loss of inadequate supply of oxygen and glucose results in rapid depletion of energy stores

Most TIAs last only about 15 to 20 minutes.

(c) Without neuroprotective agents, nerve cells in this area will be irreversibly damaged within a few minutes

(2) Ischemic penumbra *(transitional zone)*

    (a) A rim of cerebral tissue that surrounds the core zone of ischemia

        (i) Size of this area depends on the number and patency of collateral arteries

    (b) Although cerebral blood flow in this area is diminished (between 20% and 50% of normal), it is not absent

        (i) Cells are not yet irreversibly damaged and may remain viable for several hours

        (ii) Ischemic penumbra is supplied with blood by collateral arteries that connect with branches of the occluded vessel

        (iii) Because the collateral blood supply is inadequate to maintain the brain's demand for oxygen and glucose indefinitely, brain cells in the this area may live or die depending on how quickly perfusion is restored in the early hours of a stroke

d. Pharmacologic interventions are most likely to be effective in the penumbra, but salvage of brain cells within the core zone of ischemia may also be possible

(1) At the time of this writing, the only medication that has received approval from the Federal Food and Drug Administration (FDA) for acute ischemic stroke treatment is a recombinant form of tPA (tissue plasminogen activator)

(2) Window of opportunity to use tPA to treat ischemic stroke patients is 3 hours

    (a) To be evaluated and receive treatment, patients need to be at a hospital within 60 minutes of symptom onset

    (b) Unfortunately, stroke victims and their family members usually either cannot seek or fail to seek medical attention fast enough, precluding the use of tPA

Classification of Stroke by Anatomic Location

1. 80% of blood flow to the brain is supplied by the carotid arteries; 20% is supplied through the vertebrobasilar system
2. Strokes involving the carotid artery are called *anterior circulation strokes* or *carotid territory strokes* and usually involve the cerebral hemispheres
3. Strokes affecting the vertebrobasilar artery are called *posterior circulation strokes* or *vertebrobasilar territory strokes* and usually affect the brain stem or cerebellum (Figures 9-3 and 9-4)
4. Clinical manifestations of stroke are presented in Table 9-1

Table 9-1   Clinical Manifestations of Stroke

Affected Artery	Structures Supplied by Affected Vessel	Signs and Symptoms of Occlusion
Anterior cerebral	Supplies medial surfaces and upper portions of frontal and parietal lobes and medial surface of hemisphere	• Emotional lability • Confusion • Weakness, numbness on affected side • Paralysis of contralateral foot and leg • Impaired mobility, with sensation greater in lower extremities than in upper • Urinary incontinence • Loss of coordination • Personality changes • Impaired sensory function
Middle cerebral (Most commonly occluded vessel in stroke) (Largest branch of the internal carotid artery)	Supplies a portion of the frontal lobe and lateral surface of the temporal and parietal lobes, including the primary motor and sensory areas of the face, throat, hand and arm, and, in the dominant hemisphere, the areas for speech	Alterations in communication, cognition, mobility, and sensation including: • Aphasia • Dysphasia • Reading difficulty (dyslexia) • Inability to write (dysgraphia) • Visual field deficits • Contralateral sensory deficit • Contralateral hemiparesis (more severe in the face and hand than in the leg) • Altered level of responsiveness
Posterior cerebral	Supplies medial and inferior temporal lobes, medial occipital lobe, thalamus, posterior hypothalamus, visual receptive area	• Hemiplegia • Receptive aphasia • Sensory impairment • Dyslexia • Coma • Visual field deficits • Cortical blindness from ischemia
Internal carotid	Supplies the cerebral hemispheres and diencephalon	• Headaches • Altered level of responsiveness • Bruits over the carotid artery • Profound aphasia • Ptosis • Weakness, paralysis, numbness, sensory changes, and visual deficits (e.g., blurring) on the affected side • Unilateral blindness
Vertebral or basilar	Supplies brainstem and cerebellum	*Incomplete occlusion* • Transient ischemic attacks • Unilateral and bilateral weakness of extremities • Visual deficits on affected side (e.g., diplopia, color blindness, lack of depth perception) • Nausea, vertigo, tinnitus • Headache • Dysarthria • Numbness • Dysphagia • "Locked-in" syndrome—no movement except eyelids; sensation and consciousness preserved *Complete occlusion or hemorrhage* • Coma • Decerebrate rigidity • Respiratory and circulatory abnormalities

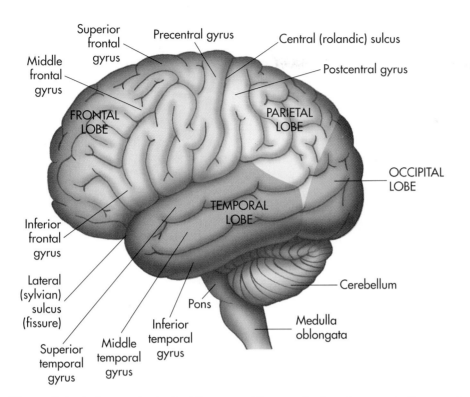

Figure 9-3   Lobes and principal fissures of the cerebral cortex, cerebellum, and brainstem.

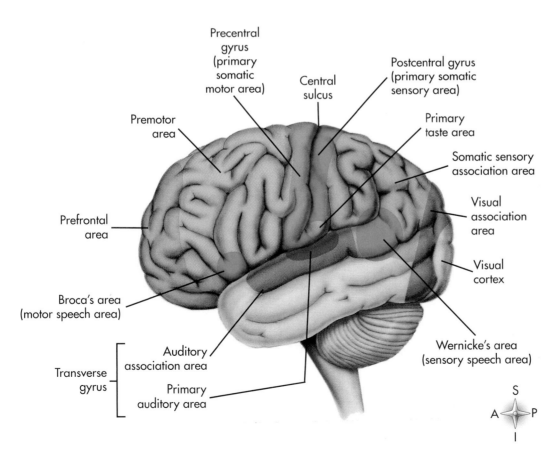

Figure 9-4   Functional subdivisions of the cerebral cortex.

Hemorrhagic Stroke

1. Caused by either rupture of an artery with bleeding onto the surface of the brain (subarachnoid hemorrhage) or bleeding into the brain (intracerebral hemorrhage) (Figure 9-5)
2. Subarachnoid hemorrhage (SAH)
   a. Aneurysm most common cause
   b. Sudden onset of "the worst headache of my life" is a classic description of subarachnoid hemorrhage
   c. AV malformations account for approximately 5% of all subarachnoid hemorrhages
   d. Initial mortality is high
   e. Rebleeding is common
      (1) Mortality from rebleeding is also high
      (2) Rebleeding most commonly occurs during the first day, usually within 12 hours after the initial hemorrhage
3. Intracerebral hemorrhage (IH)
   a. Most intracerebral hemorrhages are associated with chronic hypertension
   b. Small vessels within the brain are damaged by long-standing hypertension and eventually rupture and bleed
   c. May require neurosurgical involvement

Common Signs and Symptoms of Stroke

- Sudden numbness or weakness of the face, arm or leg, especially on one side of the body
- Sudden severe headache with no known cause
- Sudden dimness or loss of vision, particularly in one eye
- Sudden confusion, difficulty speaking, or trouble understanding speech
- Unexplained dizziness, unsteadiness, or sudden falls, especially with any of the other signs

---

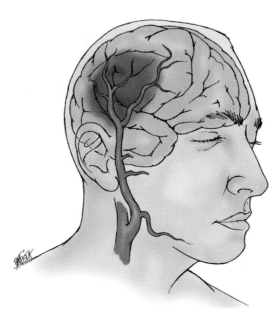

Figure 9-5 Hemorrhagic stroke.

STROKE: CHAIN OF RECOVERY

Like the Sequence of Survival used to describe the sequence of events needed to survive sudden cardiac death, the Chain of Recovery is a metaphor for the series of events that must occur in the emergency care of the possible stroke patient to optimize his or her chances of full recovery (Figure 9-6). The critical links in the chain include[7]:

1. Identification of stroke signs and symptoms by the patient or bystanders
2. Immediate EMS system activation and appropriate dispatch with prearrival instructions
3. Rapid EMS response, assessment, evacuation, and appropriate prehospital care
4. Forewarning of the receiving stroke center for resource preparation and immobilization
5. Rapid definitive diagnosis by experienced specialists at the stroke center

The Chain of Recovery has been modified in the American Heart Association publications and is called *The Stroke Chain of Survival and Recovery.*[28,9] The chain consists of seven links:

1. *Detection* of the onset of stroke signs and symptoms
2. *Dispatch* through activation of the EMS system and prompt EMS response
3. *Delivery* of the victim to the receiving hospital while providing appropriate prehospital assessment and care and prearrival notification
4. *Door* (emergency department triage)
5. *Data* (emergency department evaluation, including computed tomography [CT])
6. *Decision* about potential therapies
7. *Drug* therapy

Components of The Stroke Chain of Survival and Recovery

1. **Detection:** Early Recognition
   a. Recognition of stroke signs and symptoms by patient or bystanders
   b. Need for public and patient education
      (1) In 1996, the Gallup Organization conducted a survey regarding stroke awareness for the National Stroke Association.[3] In a survey of adults age 50 or older:
         (a) 38% did not know where in the body a stroke occurs
         (b) 19% were unaware that there are things you can do to help prevent a stroke
         (c) Only 40% would call 9-1-1 immediately if they were having a stroke
         (d) Two thirds were unaware of the short time frame in which a person must seek treatment
         (e) 91% of older Americans could not identify sudden blurred or decreased vision in one or both eyes as a symptom of stroke

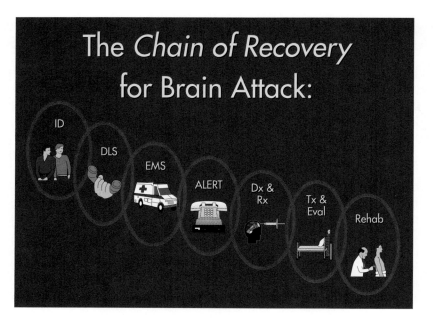

Figure 9-6 Chain of Recovery for acute ischemic stroke patients. *ID*, Identification of symptoms by the patient or bystanders; *DLS*, dispatch life support. *EMS*, emergency medical services; *ALERT*, forewarning of receiving facility of impending arrival of stroke patient; *Dx & Rx*, diagnosis and medication; *Tx & eval*, treatment and evaluation; *Rehab*, rehabilitation.

> The National Stroke Association's web site *(http://www.stroke.org)* is an excellent resource of information for health care professionals.

(f) 85% could not identify loss of balance or coordination (a major sign when accompanied by another symptom) as a symptom of stroke

(g) 68% could not identify difficulty in speaking or understanding simple statements as a stroke symptom

(h) 42% could not identify weakness, numbness, paralysis in face, arm, or leg as a stroke symptom

(i) 17% were unable to name any symptoms at all

2. **Dispatch:** Early EMS Activation and Dispatch Instructions

a. Stroke victims and their families must be taught to activate EMS system immediately on recognition of brain attack signs and symptoms

(1) The Three R's of stroke: Reduce risk, Recognize symptoms, Respond by calling 9-1-1

b. Currently, only half of stroke victims use the EMS system

3. **Delivery:** Prehospital Transport and Management

a. Primary and Secondary ABCD Surveys

(1) Stroke recognition

(a) Common dispatch complaints/presenting chief complaints include can't walk, arm and leg weak, face twisted, ill person, talking funny, possible heart attack, found down

(b) Identify presence of aphasia, dysphasia, unilateral weakness

(2) Differentiate possible stroke from other common causes of stroke symptoms (e.g., hypoglycemia, drug or alcohol intoxication)

(a) **Determine blood glucose**

(b) Give 50% dextrose if hypoglycemic

(c) Give 100 mg thiamine if malnourished, alcoholic

(3) Monitor respiratory efforts and ensure patency of airway
    (a) Be prepared to assist ventilations
    (b) If inadequate breathing occurs, proceed with intubation
    (c) If pulse oximetry is available, administer oxygen as needed to maintain oxygen saturation at (at least) 95% but consider hypoventilation as a possible complication
(4) IV catheter placement and 12-lead ECG preferred; however, do not delay transport to definitive care facilities
    (a) Establish IV access with a saline lock or an IV line containing normal saline or lactated Ringer's solution to run at a keep-open rate
(5) Perform neurologic evaluation
    (a) Cincinnati Prehospital Stroke Scale
    (b) Los Angeles Prehospital Stroke Screen (LAPSS) (Figure 9-7)

Cincinnati Prehospital Stroke Scale

1. If any one of the following signs is abnormal, stroke probability = 72%
2. *Facial droop/weakness:* Ask patient to "Show me your teeth" or "Smile for me"
    a. *Normal:* Both sides of face move equally well
    b. *Abnormal:* One side of face does not move at all
3. *Motor weakness (arm drift):* With eyes closed, ask patient to extend arms out in front of him or her 90 degrees (if sitting) or 45 degrees (if supine)
    a. *Normal:* Both arms move the same OR both arms do not move at all
    b. *Abnormal:* One arm either does not move OR one arm drifts down compared to the other
    c. Drift is scored if the arm falls before 10 sec
4. *Aphasia (speech):* Ask patient to say "You can't teach an old dog new tricks," "The sky is blue in Cincinnati," or similar phase
    a. *Normal:* Phrase is repeated clearly and correctly
    b. *Abnormal:* Words are slurred (dysarthria) or abnormal (aphasia), or patient is mute

---

Differential Diagnosis of Acute Stroke

- *Trauma (e.g., subdural hematoma)*
- *Hemorrhagic stroke (e.g., subarachnoid hemorrhage, intracranial hemorrhage)*
- *Transient ischemic events that have not resolved at presentation*
- *Meningitis/encephalitis*
- *Hypertensive encephalopathy*
- *Intracranial mass*
- *Spinal cord, peripheral nerve disease*
- *Brain abscess*
- *Seizures/Todd's paralysis*
- *Infections*
- *Complex migraines*
- *Metabolic abnormalities (e.g., hypo-/hyperglycemia, drug overdose)*
- *Bell's palsy*

Los Angeles Prehospital Stroke Screen (LAPSS)

1. Patient Name: _____ _____
   (Last Name)   (First Name)
2. Information/History from:
   [   ] Patient
   [   ] Family Member _____ _____
   [   ] Patient   (Name)   (Phone)
3. Last known time patient was at baseline or deficit free and awake:

   _____   _____
   (Military Time)   (Date)

SCREENING CRITERIA

	YES	**UNKNOWN**	**NO**
4. Age >45	[ ]	[ ]	[ ]
5. History of seizures or epilepsy **absent**	[ ]	[ ]	[ ]
6. Symptom duration less than 24 hours	[ ]	[ ]	[ ]
7. At baseline, patient is not wheelchair bound or bedridden	[ ]	[ ]	[ ]

	YES	**NO**
8. Blood glucose between 60 and 400	[ ]	[ ]

9. Exam: **LOOK FOR OBVIOUS ASYMMETRY**

	Normal	**Right**	**Left**
Facial smile/grimace	[ ]	[ ] Droop	[ ] Droop
Grip	[ ]	[ ] Weak grip	[ ] Weak grip
Arm strength	[ ]	[ ] No grip	[ ] No grip
		[ ] Drifts down	[ ] Drifts down
		[ ] Falls rapidly	[ ] Falls rapidly

Based on exam, patient has only unilateral (and not bilateral) weakness:

	YES	**NO**
	[ ]	[ ]

10. Items 4, 5, 6, 7, 8, 9 all YES's (or unknown) – LAPSS screening criteria met:

	YES	**NO**
	[ ]	[ ]

11. If LAPSS criteria for stroke met, call receiving hospital with a "code stroke." If not, then return to the appropriate treatment protocol. (Note: the patient may still be experiencing a stroke even if the LAPSS criteria are not met.)

Figure 9-7 Los Angeles Prehospital Stroke Screen (LAPSS).

b. History
   (1) Does patient have altered mental status, loss of speech, decreased sensation, or loss of motor function without suspected trauma? Past history of stroke?
   (2) Determine and document
      (a) Time of symptom onset
      (b) Time the call for help was received
      (c) Time the first EMS unit arrived on the scene
      (d) Time that transport to the hospital began and ended
   (3) Encourage family members or bystanders to accompany the patient to the hospital so they can provide historical information to the treating team and provide support to the patient. If they cannot go to the hospital, obtain a telephone number where they can be contacted
   (4) Collect and/or document all medications (particularly aspirin, warfarin, insulin, and antihypertensives)
c. Assess and support vital signs
   (1) In general, hypertension should not be treated in the prehospital setting
   (2) Hypotension should be treated aggressively (in accordance with the underlying etiology for the hypotension)
d. Prearrival notification of emergency department (ED)
e. Rapid transport to ED
   (1) In areas with multiple medical facilities, bypass facilities not capable of providing appropriate care for the stroke patient (transport patient to designated Stroke Center)
   (2) In areas without nearby definitive stroke care capabilities, transport patient to closest appropriate emergency facility where rapid evaluation and transfer (if appropriate) can be performed
   (3) In remote areas without nearby facilities, direct on-scene rescue by air medical services can be considered if (a) the closest emergency facility is more than an hour away, (b) the closest facility is not capable of providing definitive diagnosis and care, and (c) the patient can reach the definitive care facility within the agreed-on therapeutic time window for stroke
4. **Door:** Emergency Department Triage
   a. NINDS-Recommended Stroke Evaluation Targets for Potential Fibrinolytic Candidates (Table 9-2)
      (1) Physician evaluation of stroke patient within 10 minutes of arrival at the ED doors (door to doctor)

Table 9-2	NINDS-Recommended Stroke Evaluation Targets for Potential Fibrinolytic Candidates	
ACTIVITY	**TARGET**	
Door to physician evaluation	10 min	
Door to access to neurologic expertise (in person or by phone)	15 min	
Door to CT completion	25 min	
Door to CT read	45 min	
Door to drug/intervention	60 min	
Door to neurosurgical availability (on-site or by transport)	2 hours	
Door to admission to monitored bed	3 hours	

(2) Physician with expertise in stroke management should be available or notified within 15 minutes of patient arrival. Depending on the protocol established, this might be accomplished by activating a stroke team (access to neurologic expertise)

(3) Begin CT scan of the head within 25 minutes of arrival (door to CT completion)

(4) Read CT within 45 minutes of arrival (door to CT read)

(5) Treatment should be initiated within 60 minutes of arrival at ED doors (door to treatment)

(6) Neurosurgical availability on-site or by transport within 2 hours

(7) Time from patient arrival at the ED to placement in a monitored bed should not exceed 3 hours (door to monitored bed)

b. Immediate general assessment (perform within 10 minutes of patient arrival)

(1) Perform Primary and Secondary ABCD Surveys, vital signs, oxygen saturation

(a) Administer oxygen by nasal cannula

(b) Establish IV access, obtain blood samples (complete blood cell count with differential and platelet count, electrolytes, BUN, creatinine, coagulation profile)

(i) Avoid D5W and excessive fluid loading

(c) Evaluate blood pressure in both upper extremities, assess symmetry of pulses, and assess for signs of trauma

(d) Check blood sugar, treat if indicated

(i) **Determine immediately**

(ii) Give 50% dextrose if hypoglycemic; give insulin if >300 mg%

(iii) Give 100 mg thiamine if malnourished, alcoholic

(e) In general, avoid treatment of hypertension if possible

(i) BP elevation common in acute phase of a stroke

(ii) May be a compensatory mechanism for reduced cerebral blood flow in the ischemic penumbra

(iii) Impaired cerebral autoregulation of BP may last for several weeks but often resolves spontaneously within a few days after the stroke

(iv) Any treatment given should be based on multiple measurements taken 10 to 20 minutes apart, *never* on a single BP reading

(v) Aggressive BP control may be provided if hemorrhagic stroke is present or fibrinolytic therapy has been administered

(2) Obtain 12-lead ECG; assess for dysrhythmias

(3) Perform general neurologic screening assessment

c. Stroke Team alerted: neurologist, radiologist, CT technician

d. Immediate neurologic assessment (<25 min from arrival)

(1) Review patient history

(a) History of present illness

(i) Establish onset (<3 hours required for fibrinolytics)

a) When was the last time the patient was known to be without symptoms?

(ii) What was the patient doing when the symptoms began?

(iii) Did the patient complain of a headache? Did he or she have a seizure? Has there been a change in the level of responsiveness? Is there a history of any recent trauma?

Consider stroke team drills similar to mock codes currently used in many hospitals. Drills should review the criteria for proper patient identification, the required tests/procedures to be taken, and preferred communications systems.

      (b) Past medical history

         (i) Determine presence of stroke risk factors: age, hypertension, past history of stroke/TIA, presence of carotid bruit, diabetes, smoking, atrial fibrillation, obesity, hyperlipidemia, heart valve problem, illicit drug use

      (c) Determine medications the patient is currently taking, especially warfarin

      (d) Determine patient's allergies to medications

  (2) Perform physical exam

  (3) Perform neurologic exam

      (a) Scales are used in order to give quantifiable information to other members of the stroke team

      (b) Use Glasgow Coma Scale (Table 9-3) to determine level of responsiveness

         (i) Measures impairment

         (ii) Of limited use in the intubated patient or patient with orbital trauma

      (c) Use NIH Stroke Scale to determine the severity of the stroke

         (i) Developed for the NINDS r-tPA Stroke Trial and is used to assess neurologic outcome and degree of recovery

         (ii) Allows a standardized way to assess outcome and compare outcomes with other centers

         (iii) An 11 item, 42-point standardized scale. Scores of 0 or 1 indicate a normal or near-normal examination. Scores of 1 to 4 indicate minor strokes, a score of 5 to 15 a moderate stroke, 15 to 20 a moderately severe stroke, and a score of more than 20 a severe stroke

e. Order emergent noncontrast computed tomography (CT) scan of brain

  (1) Goal to CT scan performed <25 minutes from arrival

  (2) Goal to read CT scan <45 minutes from arrival

  (3) Purpose of the scan is to rule out other potential mimics of an ischemic event such as an intracranial tumor, abscess, or hemorrhage

  (4) CT scan may not detect an ischemic stroke for 6 to 72 hours after the initial infarction

  (5) Perform lateral cervical spine x-ray if patient comatose/history of trauma

5. **Data:** Emergency Department evaluation and management

  a. Emergency neurologic stroke assessment

    (1) Level of responsiveness

    (2) Type of stroke (hemorrhagic vs. nonhemorrhagic)

    (3) Location of stroke (carotid/vertebrobasilar)

    (4) Severity of stroke

6. **Decision:** About potential therapies

7. **Drugs:** Fibrinolytic therapy for ischemic stroke

Approximately 5% of patients with acute ischemic stroke present with a seizure and up to 30% have a headache.[10]

Table 9-3 Glasgow Coma Scale

Eye Opening	Characteristics	E-Score
Spontaneous	Eyes open (does not imply intact awareness)	4
To speech	Eyes open in response to speech or shout (does not imply patient obeys command to open eyes)	3
To pain	Eyes open in response to painful stimulus	2
No response	Eyes always closed; not attributable to ocular swelling	1

Best Verbal Response	Characteristics	V-Score
Oriented	Normal orientation to time, place, person; appropriate conversation	5
Confused	Responds to questions in conversational manner but responses indicate varying degrees of disorientation and confusion	4
Inappropriate	Intelligible words but not in a meaningful exchange (e.g., shouting, swearing; no meaningful conversation)	3
Incomprehensible	Moaning, groaning, grunting; incomprehensible	2
No response	No sounds	1

Best Motor Response	Characteristics	M-Score
Obeys commands	Follows simple commands	6
Localizes pain	Attempt made to remove stimulus (e.g., hand moves above chin toward supraocular stimulus)	5
Withdrawal	Normal flexor withdrawal; no localizing attempt to remove stimulus	4
Abnormal flexion	Includes preceding extension, stereotyped flexion posture, extreme wrist flexion, abduction of upper arm, flexion of fingers over thumb	3
Extension	Extension at elbow	2
No response	No motor response to pain	1
	Score: E + V + M	**15**

Record findings as "E4V3M5 = GCS 12"

From: Instructions for Scoring the Glasgow Coma Scale From the Head Trauma Research Project, New York University Medical Center Institute of Rehabilitation Medicine, http://www.biact.org/infartcl/glasgow.html (accessed 12/29/00).

FIBRINOLYTIC THERAPY

Fibrinolytic (Thrombolytic) Therapy: Recommendations from the American College of Chest Physicians[14]

1. Acute Ischemic Stroke

1.1. Thrombolytic Therapy

Acute Ischemic Stroke Treatment Within 3 Hours of Symptom Onset

1.1.1. We recommend administration of IV tPA in a dose of 0.9 mg/kg (maximum of 90 mg), with 10% of the total dose given as an initial bolus and the remainder infused over 60 min for eligible patients (see inclusion and exclusion criteria listed below), provided that treatment is initiated within 3 hours of clearly defined symptom onset (grade 1A).

1.1.2. We recommend strict adherence to eligibility criteria for the use of IV tPA based on the NINDS trial protocol (see below for inclusion and exclusion criteria). Therapy should be initiated as soon as possible to optimize benefits (grade 1C1).

Remarks
Inclusion Criteria: Age ≥18 years, clinical diagnosis of stroke with a clinically meaningful neurologic deficit, clearly defined time of onset of <180 min before treatment, and a baseline CT showing no evidence of intracranial hemorrhage.

Exclusion Criteria: Minor or rapidly improving symptoms or signs, CT signs of intracranial hemorrhage, a history of intracranial hemorrhage, seizure at stroke onset, stroke or serious head injury within 3 months, major surgery or serious trauma within 2 weeks, GI or urinary tract hemorrhage within 3 weeks, systolic BP >185 mm Hg, diastolic BP >110 mm Hg, aggressive treatment required to lower BP, glucose level <50 mg/dL or >400 mg/dL, symptoms of subarachnoid hemorrhage, arterial puncture at a noncompressible site or lumbar puncture within 1 week, platelet count <100,000 platelets/mL, heparin therapy within 48 hours associated with elevated activated partial thromboplastin time, clinical presentation suggesting post-MI pericarditis, pregnant or lactating women, current use of oral anticoagulants (International Normalized Ratio [INR] >1.7).

1.1.3. We recommend thrombolytic therapy almost always be withheld in patients with evidence of major early infarct signs (clear evidence of extensive early edema/mass effect) on the pretreatment CT scan (grade 1B).

Remarks: Treatment should be supervised by physicians with expertise in stroke management and CT scan interpretation, and tPA treatment is not recommended if the time of symptom onset is uncertain or if symptoms have been present for >3 hours. Some experts recommend that, if possible, efforts should be made to demonstrate a large artery intracranial occlusion using modern neuroimaging techniques prior to administration of tPA. Treatment should not be unduly delayed in order to facilitate vascular imaging. Adequate hospital facilities and personnel are required for administration of thrombolytic therapy as well as for monitoring and managing potential complications. Following tPA administration, BP should be closely monitored and kept <180/105 mm Hg; antithrombotic agents should be avoided for 24 hours.

Acute Stroke Treatment Within 3 to 6 Hours of Symptom Onset

1.1.4. We do not recommend use of IV tPA for treatment of acute ischemic stroke of >3 hours but <6 hours in unselected patients (grade 2B). This treatment remains investigational.

1.1.5. We do not recommend that clinicians use streptokinase for the treatment of acute ischemic stroke except within the confines of a clinical trial (grade 1A).

1.1.6. In carefully selected patients with angiographically demonstrated MCA occlusion and no signs of major early infarction on the baseline CT scan who can be treated within 6 hours of symptom onset, we recommend the use of intra-arterial thrombolytic therapy for ischemic stroke (grade 2B).

1.2. Patients Not Eligible for Thrombolysis

Remarks: To our knowledge, no trial has adequately evaluated full dose anticoagulation in hyperacute (<12 hours) stroke patients. Clinical trials evaluating IV heparin for stroke treatment are inconclusive with heterogeneous results. In general, trials of subcutaneous heparin and low-molecular-weight heparins or heparinoids have demonstrated an increase in the risk of major bleeding without any clear benefits.

1.2.1. We do not recommend full-dose anticoagulation for treatment of unselected patients with ischemic stroke (grade 2B).

1.2.2. Clinicians may consider early anticoagulation for treatment of acute cardioembolic and large artery ischemic strokes and for progressing stroke when the suspected mechanism is ongoing thromboembolism (grade 2B).

Remarks: Clinical trials have not adequately evaluated anticoagulation in specific stroke subtypes.

For patients with cardioembolic stroke, early anticoagulation is most likely to be beneficial for patients who are at high risk for early recurrent embolism (i.e., patients with mechanical heart valves, an established intracardiac thrombus, atrial fibrillation associated with significant valvular disease, or severe congestive heart failure).

1.2.3. A brain imaging study should be performed prior to initiation of acute anticoagulation to exclude hemorrhage and estimate the size of the infarct. When potential contraindications to anticoagulation are present, such as a large infarction (based on clinical syndrome or brain imaging findings), uncontrolled hypertension, or other bleeding conditions, we recommend that clinicians avoid early anticoagulation (grade 1C).

1.2.4. We recommend early aspirin therapy (160 to 325 mg/day) for patients with ischemic stroke who are not receiving thrombolysis or anticoagulation (grade 1A). Aspirin therapy should be started within 48 hours of stroke onset and may be used safely in combination with low doses of subcutaneous heparin for DVT prophylaxis.

1.2.5. *DVT/PE Prophylaxis:* Because of the increased risk of PE and DVT among ischemic stroke patients, particularly in those with deficits leading to immobility, measures to reduce the risk of DVT and PE are required.

1.2.5.1. For acute stroke patients with restricted mobility, we recommend that clinicians use prophylactic low dose subcutaneous heparin or low-molecular-weight heparins or the heparinoid danaparoid, as long as there are no contraindications to anticoagulation (grade 1A).

1.2.5.2 In patients with an intracerebral hematoma, we recommend that clinicians use low-dose subcutaneous heparin as early as the second day after the onset of the hemorrhage for the prevention of thromboembolic complications (grade 2C).

1.2.5.3. We recommend that clinicians use intermittent pneumatic compression devices or elastic stockings for patients who have contraindications to anticoagulants (grade 1C).

From: Albers GW, Amarenco P, Easton JD, Sacco RL, Teal P: Antithrombotic and thrombolytic therapy for ischemic stroke, *Chest* 119(1 suppl):300S-320S, 2001.

> *If a patient has stroke on awakening from sleep or if the onset of symptoms is not known, then stroke onset is determined from time patient was last seen as "normal" (e.g., when he or she went to bed).[11]*

---

1. Use of intravenous tPA in acute ischemic stroke
   a. Obtain and review stat CT scan of the brain
   b. Establish peripheral IV access (two separate sites)
   c. Obtain CBC, chemistry panel, PT and PTT, type and screen, and urinalysis
   d. Review inclusion and exclusion criteria
   e. Determine patient's weight
   f. Administer tPA
      (1) Intravenous tPA (0.9 mg/kg; maximum of 90 mg), with 10% of the dose given as a bolus, followed by an infusion lasting 60 min, is recommended treatment within 3 hours of onset of ischemic stroke[15]   *Dose is lower than that typically given to treat acute MI*
         (a) If time of symptom onset is uncertain, *do not give tPA*
   g. Monitor for bleeding and neurologic deterioration
   h. Admit to ICU for 24 hours
   i. Monitor BP
      (1) Monitor BP every 15 min for 2 hours after start of infusion; then every 30 min for 6 hours; then every hour, from the 8th hour until 24 hours after the start of tPA; then per routine
   j. Do not give antiplatelet or anticoagulant therapies for 24 hours
   k. Do not perform arterial punctures, invasive procedures, or IM injections for 24 hours
   l. Obtain CT scan of brain 24 hours postinfusion or sooner if neurologic deterioration occurs
2. Complications of tPA therapy
   a. Signs of complications
      (1) Intracranial hemorrhage
      (2) Severe headache
      (3) Vomiting

   (4) Deterioration in neurologic function
  b. Patient should be monitored in ICU
  c. CT should be ordered if hemorrhage suspected
  d. Management of bleeding complications

   (1) "Before using thrombolytic therapy, the following should be considered. Thrombolytic therapy should not be used unless the treatment facility is staffed and equipped to handle bleeding complications. Bleeding is the most feared complication and can be fatal. Hemorrhagic events generally are divided into those that directly affect the central nervous system and those that involve other organs. The treatment of thrombolysis-related bleeding is guided by (a) the location and size of the hematoma, (b) the likelihood that the bleeding can be controlled mechanically, (c) the risk of neurologic worsening or death, (d) the interval between administration of the drug and the onset of hemorrhage, and (e) the thrombolytic drug used. Information necessary to guide recommendations about treatment of hemorrhagic complications of thrombolytic therapy is scarce

   (2) If bleeding is suspected, blood should be drawn to measure the patient's hematocrit, hemoglobin, partial thromboplastin time, prothrombin time (INR), platelet count, and fibrinogen. Blood should be typed and cross-matched if transfusions are needed (at least 4 units of packed red blood cells, 4 to 6 units of cryoprecipitate or fresh frozen plasma, and 1 unit of single donor platelets)

   (3) Thrombolytic therapy should not be used unless facilities to handle bleeding complications are readily available

   (4) Bleeding should be considered the likely cause of neurologic worsening following use of a thrombolytic drug until a CT is available. The study should be obtained on an emergent basis whenever neurologic worsening follows administration of r-tPA

   (5) Any life-threatening hemorrhagic complication, including intracranial bleeding, should lead to the following sequential steps:
    (a) Discontinue infusion of thrombolytic drug if still being given
    (b) Obtain blood samples for coagulation tests (see previously)
    (c) Obtain surgical consultation, as necessary"[15]

Use of Fibrinolytics in the Treatment of Acute Ischemic Stroke

Controversy exists about the use of fibrinolytics in the management of acute ischemic stroke. Administration of tPA is associated with an increased risk of intracranial hemorrhage that can be severe or fatal. The Canadian Association of Emergency Physicians (CAEP) recently released a position statement on thrombolytic therapy for acute ischemic stroke. The abstract from that position paper is provided below:

ABSTRACT

"Current evidence suggests that, in a small subset of acute stroke patients who can be treated within 3 hours of symptom onset, the administration of tissue plasminogen activator (tPA) confers a modest outcome benefit, but that this benefit is associated with an increased risk of intracranial hemorrhage that can be severe or fatal. The data show that tPA therapy must be limited to carefully selected patients within established protocols. Further evidence is necessary to support the widespread application of stroke thrombolysis outside research settings. Until it is clear that the benefits of this therapy outweigh the risks, thrombolytic therapy for acute stroke should be restricted to use within formal research protocols or in monitored practice protocols that adhere to the NINDS eligibility criteria. All data on protocol compliance and patient outcomes should be collated in a central Canadian registry for the purposes of tracking safety and efficacy.

Stroke thrombolysis should be limited to centers with appropriate neurological and neuro-imaging resources that are capable of administering treatment within 3 hours. In such centers, emergency physicians should identify eligible patients, initiate low risk interventions, and facilitate prompt CT scanning. Only physicians with demonstrated expertise in neuroradiology should interpret head CT scans used to determine whether to administer thrombolytic agents to stroke patients. Neurologists should be directly involved prior to the thrombolytic administration."[46]

To view the entire document, visit the CAEP web site at: *http://www.caep.ca*.

STOP AND REVIEW

1. What is the most common cause of a stroke?
   a. Cerebral hemorrhage
   b. Thrombus formation
   c. Dissecting cerebral aneurysm
   d. Cerebral vasospasm

2. Why should the serum glucose level be determined during the initial management of a possible stroke patient?

   _____

   _____

   _____

3. A patient is experiencing signs and symptoms consistent with a possible stroke. Which of the following is a CONTRAINDICATION to fibrinolytic therapy for this patient?
   a. Patient's symptoms began 30 minutes ago
   b. Patient has a history of a myocardial infarction in 1996
   c. Patient is 43 years of age
   d. Patient had a laparoscopic cholecystectomy 2 weeks ago

4. A transient ischemic attack (TIA) is:
   a. A reversible episode of focal neurologic dysfunction that typically lasts a few minutes to a few hours, resolving within 24 hours
   b. A temporary alteration in behavior or consciousness caused by abnormal electrical activity of one or more groups of neurons in the brain
   c. Two or more seizures without an intervening period of consciousness
   d. A neurologic deficit that lasts more than 24 hours but leaves little or no neurologic deficit

5. Current stroke protocols recommend that a possible stroke patient presenting to the Emergency Department should be seen by a physician within _____ of his/her arrival and a CT scan should be completed within _____.
   a. 5 min, 15 min
   b. 10 min, 25 min
   c. 30 min, 45 min
   d. 45 min, 60 min

6. Select the CORRECT statement regarding ischemic strokes:
   a. AV malformations are the cause of most ischemic strokes
   b. Ischemic strokes often lead to death within 1 hour of symptom onset
   c. Ischemic strokes account for the majority of all strokes
   d. Hypertension is the most common cause of an ischemic stroke

7. Which of the following cardiac dysrhythmias is most likely to precipitate a stroke?
   a. Sinus bradycardia
   b. Atrial fibrillation
   c. Sinus tachycardia with occasional PVCs
   d. Idioventricular (ventricular escape) rhythm

8. The "window of opportunity" to use tPA to treat ischemic stroke patients is currently:
   a. 1 hour
   b. 3 hours
   c. 12 hours
   d. 24 hours

9. Most of the blood flow to the brain is supplied by the _____ arteries.
   a. Femoral
   b. Brachial
   c. Vertebral
   d. Carotid

10. During a stroke, the vessel most often involved is the:
    a. Internal carotid artery
    b. Middle cerebral artery
    c. Anterior cerebral artery
    d. Posterior cerebral artery

STOP AND REVIEW ANSWERS

1. b. Most strokes are the result of occlusions caused by blood clots that develop within the brain artery itself (cerebral thrombosis) or clots that arise elsewhere in the body and then migrate to the brain (cerebral embolism).

2. The serum glucose level should be determined during the initial management of a possible stroke patient because hypoglycemia can mimic the signs and symptoms of a stroke. The glucose test is performed to rule out hypoglycemia before proceeding with stroke treatment.

3. d. The patient's history of a cholecystectomy 2 weeks ago is a contraindication for fibrinolytic therapy.

4. a. A transient ischemia attack (TIA) is a reversible episode of focal neurologic dysfunction that typically lasts a few minutes to a few hours, resolving within 24 hours. A seizure is a temporary alteration in behavior or consciousness caused by abnormal electrical activity of one or more groups of neurons in the brain. Status epilepticus is two or more seizures without an intervening period of consciousness. A reversible ischemic neurologic deficit (RIND) is a neurologic deficit that lasts more than 24 hours but leaves little or no neurologic deficit.

5. b. Current stroke protocols recommend that a possible stroke patient presenting to the Emergency Department be seen by a physician within *10 minutes* of his/her arrival. A noncontrast CT scan should be completed within *25 minutes* and read within *45 minutes* of the patient's arrival.

6. c. Ischemic strokes account for the majority of all strokes. They rarely lead to death within the first hour of symptom onset. Hemorrhagic strokes can be fatal at onset. AV malformations account for approximately 5% of all subarachnoid hemorrhages. Hypertension is the most common cause of intracerebral hemorrhage.

7. b. Patients experiencing atrial fibrillation may develop intra-atrial emboli because the atria are not contracting and blood stagnates in the atrial chambers. This predisposes the patient to systemic emboli, particularly stroke, if the clots dislodge spontaneously or because of conversion to a sinus rhythm. It is estimated that 15% to 20% of strokes in patients without rheumatic heart disease are caused by atrial fibrillation, and the incidence is even higher for those with rheumatic heart disease.[17]

8. b. The "window of opportunity" to use tPA to treat ischemic stroke patients is currently 3 hours (Class I). Administration between 3 and 6 hours of symptom onset is rated Class Indeterminate. Patients with occlusion of the middle cerebral artery may benefit from intra-arterial fibrinolysis if performed within 3 to 6 hours of symptom onset (Class IIb).

9. d. 80% of blood flow to the brain is supplied by the carotid arteries. 20% is supplied through the vertebrobasilar system.

10. b. The middle cerebral artery is the largest branch of the internal carotid artery and the most commonly occluded vessel in stroke.

REFERENCES

1. Scheinberg P: The biological basis for the treatment of acute stroke, *Neurology* 41:1867, 1991.
2. Pessin MS, Adams HP, Adams RJ, et al: Acute interventions, *Stroke* 28:1518, 1997.
3. National Stroke Association: *http://www.stroke.org/brain_stat.cfm* (accessed 12/29/00).
4. Williams GR, Jiang JG, Matchar DB, Samsa GP: Incidence and occurrence of total (first-ever and recurrent) stroke, *Stroke* 30:2523-2528, 1999.
5. Kistler JP, et al: In Braunwald E, et al editors: Harrison's principles of internal medicine, New York, 1994, McGraw-Hill.
6. Feinberg WM, Albers GW, Barnett HJM, et al: Guidelines for the management of transient ischemic attacks, *Stroke* 25:1320, 1994.
7. Pepe PE: Overview: prehospital emergency medical care systems. The initial links in the chain of recovery for brain attack—access, prehospital care, notification, and transport. In Marler JR, Winters Jones P, Emr M, editors: *Proceedings of a National Symposium on Rapid Identification and Treatment of Acute Stroke*, Bethesda, MD, 1997, The National Institute of Neurological Disorders and Stroke, National Institutes of Health.
8. Hazinski MF: Demystifying recognition and management of stroke, *Curr Emerg Cardiac Care* 7:8, 1996.
9. Cummins RO, editor: *Textbook of advanced cardiac life support*, Dallas, 1997, American Heart Association.
10. Lewandowski CA, Libman R: Acute presentation of stroke, *J Stroke Cerebrovasc Dis* 8:117-126, 1999.
11. Schneck MJ: Acute stroke: an aggressive approach to intervention and prevention, *Hosp Med* 34(1):11-12, 17-20, 25-26, 28, 1998.
12. Plantz SH, Adler JN, editors: *National medical series for independent study: emergency medicine*, Baltimore, 1998, Williams & Wilkins.
13. Kidwell CS, Starkman S, Eckstein M, Weems K, Saver JL: Identifying stroke in the field: prospective validation of the Los Angeles prehospital stroke screen (LAPSS), *Stroke* 31:71-76, 2000.
14. Albers GW, Amarenco P, Easton JD, Sacco RL, Teal P: Antithrombotic and thrombolytic therapy for ischemic stroke, *Chest* 119(1 Suppl):300S-320S, 2001.
15. Quality Standards Subcommittee of the American Academy of Neurology: Practice advisory: thrombolytic therapy for acute ischemic stroke, *Neurology* 47(3):835-839, 1996.
16. The CAEP Committee on Thrombolytic Therapy for Acute Ischemic Stroke: *http://www.caep.ca* (accessed 2/15/01).
17. Goldman L, Braunwald E: *Primary Cardiology*, Philadelphia, 1998, WB Saunders.

BIBLIOGRAPHY

Albers GW, Amarenco P, Easton JD, Sacco RL, Teal P: Antithrombotic and thrombolytic therapy for ischemic stroke, *Chest* 119(1 Suppl):300S-320S, 2001.

American Heart Association: *2000 heart and stroke statistical update*, Dallas, 1999, American Heart Association.

The American Heart Association in Collaboration with the International Liaison Committee on Resuscitation (ILCOR): Part 7: The era of reperfusion, Section 2: Acute stroke, *Circulation* 102 (suppl I):204-216, 2000.

Marler JR, Winters Jones P, Emr M, editors: *Proceedings of a National Symposium on Rapid Identification and Treatment of Acute Stroke*, Bethesda, MD, 1997, The National Institute of Neurological Disorders and Stroke, National Institutes of Health.

Plantz SH, Adler JN, editors: *National medical series for independent study: emergency medicine*, Baltimore, 1998, Williams & Wilkins.

PART II
Case Presentations

Case Presentations

CASE 1: RESPIRATORY ARREST

Objective

Given a patient situation, describe the management steps (including manual and mechanical maneuvers where applicable) for a patient that has experienced a respiratory arrest.

Skills to Master

1. Primary and Secondary ABCD Surveys
2. Recognition of a patient with respiratory compromise/arrest
3. Manual airway maneuvers: head-tilt/chin-lift, jaw thrust without head-tilt
4. Noninvasive airway techniques
   a. Pocket mask
   b. Bag-valve-mask (1 and 2 rescuer technique)
   c. Supplemental oxygen delivery devices: nasal cannula, simple face mask, nonrebreather mask
   d. Suctioning
5. Invasive airway techniques: Endotracheal intubation + $ETCO_2$ detector, esophageal detector device
6. Intravenous access

Rhythms to Master

1. Sinus bradycardia
2. Sinus rhythm

Medications to Master

1. Oxygen

Related Text Chapters

Chapter 1: ABCDs of Emergency Cardiovascular Care
Chapter 2: Airway Management: Oxygenation and Ventilation
Chapter 3: Vascular Access

Case 1: Questions

Time: 8:28 AM. You are a paramedic called to a private residence for a 78-year-old female complaining of difficulty breathing. The patient is found supine in bed. Home oxygen is in place by nasal cannula at 2 L/min. An anxious neighbor on the scene states she thinks the patient stopped breathing 5 minutes before your arrival. You have two EMT-Basics and another paramedic to assist you. Emergency equipment is immediately available.

Patient History
(available from neighbor)

Allergies	No known allergies
Medications	Adalat, hydrochlorothiazide, Atrovent, cephalexin
Past Medical History	COPD, hypertension, hospitalized 2 weeks ago for pneumonia
Last Oral Intake	Unknown
Events Prior	Per neighbor, patient has been having difficulty breathing since last evening around 10 PM

1. What acronym is used to evaluate responsiveness?

2. The patient is unresponsive. What should be done next?

3. How will you open the patient's airway?

4. The patient's airway is now open. What should be done now?

5. Name four possible causes of an airway obstruction.

6. The airway is clear. What should be done now?

7. The patient is apneic. How should you proceed?

8. Name four possible causes of respiratory arrest.

9. How will you determine the proper size oropharyngeal airway (OPA) for this patient?

10. Describe two methods for insertion of an oropharyngeal airway in the adult patient.

11. Name two possible complications of oropharyngeal airway (OPA) insertion.

12. An oropharyngeal airway has been inserted. The patient remains apneic. Should a nasal cannula be considered at this point?

13. When use of a nasal cannula is indicated, what is the liter flow recommended for use with this device? What is the approximate oxygen concentration that can be delivered with this device?

14. Should a simple face mask be considered at this point?

15. When use of a simple face mask is indicated, what is the liter flow recommended for use with this device? What is the approximate oxygen concentration that can be delivered with this device?

16. A pocket mask and bag-valve-mask are available to provide positive pressure ventilation. Name four advantages of ventilating a patient with a pocket mask.

17. At 10 L/min, what oxygen concentration can be delivered with a pocket mask?

18. During cardiac arrest, a bag-valve-mask device should not have a pop-off (pressure-release) valve. What is the reason for this?

19. If oxygen is available, what is the preferred tidal volume and inspiratory time for ventilating this patient with a bag-valve device?

20. What percentage of oxygen can be delivered with a bag-valve device?

21. Name three advantages of bag-valve device ventilation.

22. What is the most common problem associated with the use of the bag-valve-mask?

23. An oropharyngeal airway has been inserted and the patient is being ventilated by a bag-valve-mask. There are no spontaneous respirations. How would you like to proceed?

24. A carotid pulse is present. The rate is slow, weak, and regular. What should be done now?

25. The patient remains apneic. Since additional help is available, instruct your partner to obtain baseline breath sounds, prepare intubation equipment, and intubate the patient while you establish IV access. Name three indications for endotracheal intubation.

26. Name four advantages of endotracheal intubation.

27. Name the medications that can be administered via the endotracheal route in the adult patient.

28. What is the maximum length of time ventilation should be interrupted for an intubation attempt? At what point does this time interval begin and end?

29. What is the average endotracheal tube size for an adult male? An adult female?

30. Breath sounds are present bilaterally with bag-valve-mask ventilation. As your partner prepares to intubate the patient, a stylet is inserted into the endotracheal tube. What is the purpose of a stylet?

31. Where should the tip of the laryngoscope blade be placed?

32. What is the Sellick maneuver and what is its purpose?

33. While your partner attempts to intubate the patient, an EMT is applying cricoid pressure. At what point should cricoid pressure be released?

34. How far should the endotracheal tube be advanced into the patient's airway?

35. How will you confirm placement of the endotracheal tube?

36. Name five possible complications of endotracheal intubation.

37. After placement of the tube, breath sounds are heard over the right chest, but none are present on the left. What do you suspect?

38. What is the maximum length of time for a suctioning attempt?

39. The endotracheal tube has been successfully placed and secured. An IV has been established with normal saline and the patient has been connected to a cardiac monitor, which reveals the following rhythm.

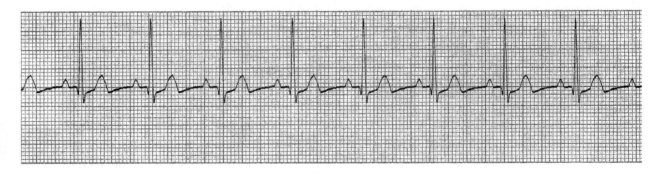

Rhythm identification: _____

40. Palpation reveals a strong, regular carotid pulse at 78/min. What should be done now?

Vital signs now: BP 112/74, P 72, R 12/min via bag-valve-mask; SaO$_2$ 95%.

Case 1 Answers

1. The acronym used to evaluate responsiveness is AVPU. A = Alert, V = responds to Verbal stimulation, P = responds to Pain, U = Unresponsive

2. Primary ABCD Survey: *A* = *A*irway, *B* = *B*reathing, *C* = *C*irculation, *D* = *D*efibrillation, if necessary.

3. Open the airway with a head-tilt/chin-lift (or jaw thrust without head-tilt if the scene suggests possible trauma).

4. Assess for sounds of airway compromise (snoring, gurgling, stridor) and look in the mouth for blood, broken teeth or loose dentures, gastric contents, and foreign objects.

5. Tongue, presence of a foreign body, altered level of responsiveness/ loss of gag reflex, direct injury from trauma, edema formation (e.g., anaphylaxis, thermal/chemical burns, disease process), facial trauma (e.g., fractures, oral bleeding), soft tissue trauma to neck, viral and bacterial infections, vomitus/secretions.

6. Look, listen, and feel for breathing.

7. Insert an airway adjunct, provide positive pressure ventilation, and continue the Primary ABCD Survey.

8. Coma from any cause, drug overdose, electrocution, epiglottitis, foreign body airway obstruction, lightning strike, myocardial infarction, smoke inhalation, stroke, submersion/near-drowning, suffocation, traumatic injury.

9. Proper airway size is determined by holding the device against the side of the patient's face and selecting an airway that extends from the corner of the mouth to the tip of the earlobe or the angle of the jaw.

10. *Method #1:* Hold the device at its flange end and insert it into the mouth with the tip pointing toward the roof of the patient's mouth. Advance the airway along the roof of the mouth. When the distal end reaches the posterior wall of the pharynx, rotate the airway 180 degrees so that it is positioned over the tongue. *Method #2:* Requires the use of a tongue blade to depress the tongue. If this method is used, the OPA is inserted with the tip of the OPA facing the floor of the patient's mouth (curved side down). Using the tongue blade to depress the tongue, the OPA is gently advanced into place over the tongue.

11. Trauma/bleeding of oropharynx, bradycardia because of stimulation of gag reflex. Insertion in a responsive or semiresponsive patient may stimulate vomiting or laryngospasm. If the OPA is improperly positioned, the tongue may be pushed back into the posterior pharynx, causing an airway obstruction. If the airway is too long, it may press the epiglottis against the entrance of the larynx, resulting in a complete airway obstruction. If the airway is too short, it will not displace the tongue and may advance out of the mouth.

12. No. A nasal cannula is used only in spontaneously breathing patients with adequate ventilation.

13. 1 to 6 L/min, 25% to 45% (actual amount of inspired O_2 depends on respiratory rate and depth).

14. No. A simple face mask is used only in spontaneously breathing patients with adequate ventilation.

15. At 6 to 10 L/min, the simple face mask can provide an inspired oxygen concentration of approximately 40% to 60%, the recommended flow rate is 8 to 10 L/min. The patient's actual inspired oxygen concentration will vary because the amount of air that mixes with supplemental oxygen depends on the patient's inspiratory flow rate.

16. Aesthetically more acceptable than mouth-to-mouth ventilation; easy to teach and learn; physical barrier between rescuer and patient's nose, mouth, and secretions; if patient resumes spontaneous breathing, can be used as a simple face mask; greater tidal volume can be delivered with mouth-to-mask ventilation than with a bag-value-mask (BVM); rescuer can feel compliance of patient's lungs.

17. Inspired oxygen concentration: Exhaled air (mouth-to-mask) = 16%; room air = 21%; 10 L/min = 50%.

18. Higher than usual airway pressures are often needed to properly ventilate a patient in cardiac arrest. The pressure needed to overcome the increase in airway resistance may exceed the limits of the pop-off valve, thus preventing delivery of adequate tidal volume.

19. If oxygen is available, lower tidal volumes are recommended—a tidal volume of approximately 6 to 7 mL/kg (400 to 600 mL) given over 1 to 2 seconds until the chest rises.

20. Without supplemental oxygen—21% (room air); 12 to 15 L/min supplemental oxygen but no reservoir—40% to 60%; 12 to 15 L/min supplemental oxygen and reservoir—90% to 100%

21. Provides a means for delivery of an oxygen enriched mixture to the patient, conveys a sense of compliance of patient's lungs to the BVM operator, provides a means for immediate ventilatory support, can be used with the spontaneously breathing patient as well as the apneic patient.

22. The most frequent problem with the bag-valve-mask device is the inability to provide adequate ventilatory volumes. This is caused by the difficulty in providing a leak proof seal to the face while simultaneously maintaining an open airway.

23. Assess for a pulse and other signals of circulation for up to 10 seconds.

24. Assess the need for a defibrillator. The patient has a pulse. A defibrillator is not necessary at present. Perform the Secondary ABCD Survey.

25. Inability of the patient to protect his or her own airway because of the absence of protective reflexes (e.g., coma, respiratory and/or cardiac arrest), inability of the rescuer to ventilate the unresponsive patient with less invasive methods, when prolonged ventilatory support is required, present or impending airway obstruction/respiratory failure (e.g., inhalation injury, severe asthma, exacerbation of COPD, severe pulmonary edema, severe flail chest or pulmonary contusion).

26. Isolates the airway, keeps the airway patent, reduces the risk of aspiration, ensures delivery of a high concentration of oxygen, permits suctioning of the trachea, provides a route for administration of some medications, ensures delivery of a selected tidal volume to maintain lung inflation.

27. ALONE: Atropine, Lidocaine, Oxygen, Naloxone, Epinephrine.

28. 30 seconds. The 30-second interval begins when ventilation of the patient ceases to allow insertion of the laryngoscope blade into the patient's mouth and ends when the patient is reventilated on placement of the endotracheal tube.

29. *Adult male:* 8.0-8.5. *Adult female:* 7.0-8.0. *Emergency rule:* 7.5 will fit.

30. A stylet is a flexible plastic-coated wire inserted into an ET tube that is used for molding and maintaining the shape of the tube. When a stylet is used, the tip of the stylet must be recessed 1/2 inch from the end of the ET tube to avoid trauma to the airway structures.

31. Straight blade—inserted under epiglottis; curved blade—inserted into vallecula.

32. Cricoid pressure (the Sellick maneuver) compresses and occludes the esophagus between the cricoid cartilage and the fifth and sixth cervical vertebrae. This minimizes gastric distention and aspiration during positive pressure ventilation. Cricoid pressure is not intended to facilitate visualization of the vocal cords during intubation.
33. Pressure should be maintained until the cuff of the ET tube is inflated. If the patient vomits while cricoid pressure is being applied, release pressure to avoid rupture of the stomach or esophagus.
34. The black marker on the ET tube should be at the level of the vocal cords. Advance the ET tube until the proximal end of the cuff lies ½ to 1 inch beyond the cords. When the ET tube has been properly placed, the cm markings on the side of the tube should be observed and recorded. This value is typically between the 19 and 23 cm mark at the front teeth. Average tube depth in males is 23 cm at the lips, 22 cm at the teeth; average tube depth in women is 22 cm at the lips, 21 cm at the teeth.
35. Attach a ventilation device to the ET tube and ventilate the patient. Confirm proper placement of the tube by first auscultating over the epigastrium (should be silent) and then in the midaxillary and anterior chest line on the right and left sides of the patient's chest. Observe the patient's chest for full movement with ventilation. Secondary means of confirmation of tube placement include $ETCO_2$ detector, esophageal detector. Once placement is confirmed, note and record the depth (cm marking) of the tube at the patient's teeth.
36. Bleeding, laryngospasm, vocal cord damage, mucosal necrosis, barotrauma, aspiration, cuff leak, esophageal intubation, right mainstem intubation, occlusion caused by patient biting tube or secretions, laryngeal or tracheal edema, tube occlusion, inability to talk, hypoxia caused by prolonged or unsuccessful intubation, dysrhythmias; increased intracranial pressure; trauma to lips, teeth, tongue or soft tissues of oropharynx
37. If breath sounds are diminished or absent on the left after intubation but present on the right, assume right mainstem bronchus intubation. Deflate the ET cuff, pull back the ETT slightly, reinflate the cuff, and reevaluate breath sounds.
38. In an adult, suction should not be applied for more than 10 to 15 seconds.
39. The monitor shows a sinus rhythm at approximately 75 beats/min.
40. Obtain vital signs. Attempt to determine possible causes of the respiratory arrest (view the scene for possible clues, talk with neighbor who placed initial call to 9-1-1). Transport patient for definitive care.

Case 1: Essential Actions

1. Use personal protective equipment
2. Perform Primary ABCD Survey
   a. Assess level of responsiveness, call for help
   b. Open airway and assess breathing
   c. If patient is not breathing, insert oropharyngeal airway and begin rescue breathing with bag-valve-mask
   d. Assess pulse. If present, continue ventilations and continue survey
3. Perform Secondary ABCD Survey
   a. Reassess effectiveness of initial airway maneuvers and interventions

  b. Perform endotracheal intubation, confirm tube placement by primary (visualization, rise and fall of chest, presence of bilateral breath sounds) and secondary (ETCO$_2$ detector, esophageal detector device) means
  c. Establish IV access, connect ECG monitor, administer medications if appropriate
  d. Consider possible causes of the event
4. Transfer patient for definitive care

Case 1: Unacceptable Actions

1. Failure to use personal protective equipment
2. Failure to adequately assess the patient
3. Performing chest compressions or defibrillation before assessing pulses
4. Insertion of an airway adjunct in a manner that would cause patient injury
5. Administration of oxygen by a means other than positive pressure ventilation (e.g., nasal cannula, simple face mask, nonrebreather mask)
6. Failure to ventilate patient at appropriate rate
7. Failure to provide adequate tidal volume/ventilation
8. Failure to preoxygenate patient before intubation
9. Failure to confirm endotracheal tube placement by primary and secondary means
10. Failure to properly secure the endotracheal tube
11. Failure to recognize right mainstem or esophageal intubation
12. Interruption of ventilations for more than 30 seconds at any time
13. Failure to hyperventilate patient between intubation attempts

CASE 2: VENTRICULAR TACHYCARDIA/VENTRICULAR FIBRILLATION WITH AN AED

Objective

Given a patient situation, describe the management steps for a patient in pulseless ventricular tachycardia (VT)/ventricular fibrillation (VF) when an automated external defibrillator (AED) is available.

Skills to Master

1. Primary and Secondary ABCD Surveys
2. Cardiopulmonary resuscitation
3. Oropharyngeal/nasopharyngeal airway insertion
4. Bag-valve-mask ventilation (1 and 2 rescuer technique)
5. Suctioning
6. Operation of an automated external defibrillator (AED)

Rhythms to Master

None

Medications to Master

Oxygen

Related Text Chapters

Chapter 1: ABCDs of Emergency Cardiovascular Care
Chapter 5: Electrical Therapy

Case 2: Questions

Time: 7:45 AM You are a nurse at a freestanding surgery center. The receptionist rushes to tell you that a patient has collapsed in the front lobby. When you arrive, you find a 79-year-old male supine on the lobby floor. You recognize him as a patient scheduled for cataract surgery this morning. Another nurse has arrived to assist you. She has brought an automated external defibrillator (AED) and emergency oxygen kit with her.

Patient History
(obtained from prescreening done via phone yesterday afternoon)
Allergies   No known allergies
Medications   Lopressor
Past Medical History   Hypertension
Last Oral Intake   Unknown
Events Prior   Per bystander in lobby, patient suddenly clutched his
                         chest and collapsed to the floor

1. The patient is supine on the lobby floor. How should you proceed?

2. The patient is unresponsive. What should be done now?

3. The patient's airway is open. What should be done now?

4. The patient is apneic. How would you like to proceed?

5. Positive pressure ventilation is being provided. What should be done now?

6. The patient is pulseless. How would you like to proceed?

7. What is an AED?

8. What is the purpose of defibrillation?

9. When should an AED be used?

10. What is a semi-automated external defibrillator (SAED)?

11. Two additional nurses have arrived to assist you. You have applied the AED to the patient. Instruct your assistants to clear the patient and press the analyze button. The AED advises a shock. Before delivering a shock to the patient, should you ask your assistants to secure the patient's airway and/or establish vascular access? Why or why not?

12. Could an AED be used if this patient had a permanent pacemaker or implantable cardioverter-defibrillator (ICD) in place?

13. You have confirmed everyone is clear of the patient and pressed the shock button. As you press the analyze button for the second time, you see the fire department pull up in front of the lobby doors. The AED advises a shock. You clear the area and press the shock button for the second time. After pressing the analyze button for the third time, the machine states, "No shock advised. Check pulse." An assistant checks the patient's pulse and reports that a carotid pulse is present. Paramedics are now at your side. What should be done now?

14. The oropharyngeal airway is in place. Although a pulse is present, the patient is not breathing. A paramedic has assumed responsibility for ventilating the patient with a bag-valve-mask while another prepares the intubation equipment. A carotid pulse is present. Rate 80/min, weak, regular. BP 90/54. What should be done now?

Case 2: Answers

1. Assess responsiveness.
2. Call for additional help. Instruct receptionist to call 9-1-1. Perform the Primary ABCD Survey. Open airway using jaw thrust without head-tilt. Size and insert oropharyngeal airway.
3. Look, listen, and feel for breathing.
4. Instruct an assistant to begin ventilating patient with a bag-valve-mask connected to oxygen at 15 L/min; attach a reservoir to the bag. Ventilate at a rate of 12/min. Tidal volume delivered should be approximately 6 to 7 mL/kg over 1 to 2 sec.
5. Check for a pulse and other signals of circulation for up to 10 seconds.
6. Instruct an assistant to begin chest compressions while you prepare the AED. Apply the AED pads to the patient's chest and turn the power on to the machine.
7. An AED is an external defibrillator with a computerized cardiac rhythm analysis system. The patient's cardiac rhythm is analyzed by a microprocessor in the defibrillator that uses an algorithm to distinguish rhythms that should be shocked from those that do not require defibrillation.
8. The purpose of defibrillation (unsynchronized countershock) is to produce momentary asystole. The shock attempts to completely depolarize the myocardium at once and provide an opportunity for the natural pacemaker centers of the heart to resume normal activity.
9. AEDs should be used **only** on patients who are apneic, pulseless, and ≥8 years of age (approximately >25 kg body weight).
10. SAEDs require operator intervention at specific points in the treatment sequence, depending on the brand of AED. Some AEDs require the

operator to press an "analyze" control to initiate rhythm analysis, while others automatically begin analyzing the patient's cardiac rhythm when the electrode pads are attached to the patient's chest.

11. No. Defibrillation is the definitive treatment and single most important factor in surviving cardiac arrest caused by pulseless VT or VF. Do not delay defibrillation to perform endotracheal intubation, establish an IV, or other interventions.

12. If the patient has a pacemaker or ICD, the AED may be used, but the adhesive AED pads should be placed at least 1 inch from the implanted device. If an ICD is in the process of delivering shocks to the patient, allow it approximately 30 to 60 seconds to complete its cycle.

13. Perform the Secondary ABCD Survey.

14. Establish vascular access and connect the patient to an ECG monitor. Evaluate the patient's rhythm and administer appropriate medications. Because the arrest rhythm was VF or VT and no antiarrhythmic treatment was given, consider administration of a lidocaine bolus followed by maintenance infusion unless contraindicated (e.g., idioventricular rhythm, AV block with new wide-QRS). Consider possible causes of the arrest.

Case 2: Essential Actions

1. Use personal protective equipment
2. Perform Primary and Secondary ABCD Surveys
   a. Assess level of responsiveness, call for help
   b. Open airway and assess breathing
   c. If patient is not breathing, insert oropharyngeal airway and begin rescue breathing with bag-valve-mask
   d. Assess pulse. If present, continue ventilations and continue survey. If pulseless, begin CPR until arrival of defibrillator
   e. On arrival of AED, attach pads to patient's chest, turn power on to machine, and analyze rhythm
   f. Use proper safety technique when operating defibrillator (i.e., ensure all team members are clear of patient before pressing shock control)
   g. After delivery of three sequential shocks, or when advised by AED, check pulse. If a pulse is present, assess blood pressure and respirations
   h. Reassess effectiveness of initial airway maneuvers and interventions. Maintain airway and provide ventilatory support during immediate postresuscitation period
   i. Perform endotracheal intubation, confirm tube placement by primary (visualization, rise and fall of chest, presence of bilateral breath sounds) and secondary (ETCO$_2$ detector, esophageal detector device) means
   j. Establish IV access, connect ECG monitor, administer medications if appropriate
   k. Consider possible causes of the event
3. Transfer patient for definitive care
4. Facilitate family presence during resuscitative efforts according to agency/institution protocol
5. Be familiar with advance directives and how to respond to them
6. Be familiar with the indications for when to not start resuscitation efforts and when to stop

Case 2: Unacceptable Actions

1. Failure to use personal protective equipment
2. Failure to adequately assess the patient
3. Performing chest compressions or defibrillation before assessing pulses
4. Failure to begin CPR
5. Administration of oxygen by a means other than positive pressure ventilation (e.g., nasal cannula, simple face mask, nonrebreather mask)
6. Ordering intubation, IV access, medications, or performing defibrillation before assessing for presence of VF
7. Unsafe operation of AED (failure to clear self or others before shocking)
8. Failure to check for a pulse after defibrillation series

CASE 3: PULSELESS VENTRICULAR TACHYCARDIA/ VENTRICULAR FIBRILLATION

Objective

Given a patient situation, describe the management steps (including mechanical, pharmacologic, and electrical interventions where applicable) for a patient in pulseless ventricular tachycardia (VT)/ventricular fibrillation (VF).

Skills to Master

1. Primary and Secondary ABCD Surveys
2. Cardiopulmonary resuscitation (1 and 2 rescuer)
3. Oropharyngeal/nasopharyngeal airway insertion
4. Bag-valve-mask ventilation (1 and 2 rescuer technique)
5. Suctioning
6. Operation of a conventional defibrillator
7. Performing a "quick-look"
8. Defibrillation
9. Attachment and use of ECG monitoring leads
10. Endotracheal intubation + ETCO$_2$, esophageal detector device
11. Intravenous (IV) /intraosseous (IO) access
12. IV/IO medication administration

Rhythms to Master

1. Ventricular tachycardia
2. Ventricular fibrillation

Medications to Master

1. Oxygen
2. Epinephrine
3. Vasopressin
4. Amiodarone
5. Lidocaine
6. Magnesium sulfate
7. Procainamide
8. Sodium bicarbonate

Related Text Chapters

Chapter 1: ABCDs of Emergency Cardiovascular Care
Chapter 2: Airway Management: Oxygenation and Ventilation
Chapter 3: Vascular Access
Chapter 4: Dysrhythmia Recognition
Chapter 5: Electrical Therapy
Chapter 7: Cardiovascular Pharmacology
Chapter 8: Putting It All Together

Case 3: Questions

Time: 9:06 AM. You are a paramedic called to a motel for a "possible code." You arrive to find two staff persons performing CPR on the floor. They found the patient (approximately 40 years of age) unresponsive in the bathroom 10 minutes ago. You have two motel staff persons, two EMT-Basics, and a paramedic to assist you. You have a fully stocked drug box, conventional monophasic defibrillator, and other emergency equipment available to you.

Patient History

Allergies	Unknown
Medications	Unknown
Past Medical History	Unknown
Last Oral Intake	Unknown
Events Prior	Unknown

1. What is the first thing you would like to do?

2. The patient is unresponsive, apneic, and pulseless. What should be done now?

3. Should the patient be intubated at this point? Why or why not?

4. How will you determine the patient's cardiac rhythm?

5. The cardiac monitor reveals the following rhythm following.

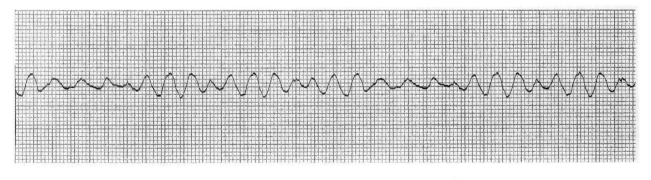

Rhythm identification: _____.

6. You have applied gel to the defibrillator paddles. Where should the paddles be placed on the patient's chest?

7. Your defibrillator is capable of delivering monophasic shocks. Assuming the cardiac rhythm remains unchanged during your electrical interventions for this patient, describe how you will deliver this therapy, including the number of shocks that should be delivered and the corresponding energy level(s).

8. The electrical therapy thus far has been unsuccessful. What should be done now?

9. The patient remains unresponsive, apneic, and pulseless. How would you like to proceed?

10. You have established an IV of NS in the patient's left antecubital fossa. List the medications that may be used in the management of pulseless VT/VF and their order of administration.

11. You administer 1 mg epinephrine (1:10,000 solution) IV bolus and flush the dose with 20 mL of NS. While an EMT circulates the drug with CPR for 30 to 60 seconds, your partner tells you the intubation was successful and tube placement has been confirmed. You assess the patient's pulse and note there is no pulse without CPR. The monitor is unchanged. What should be done now?

12. The patient's cardiac rhythm is unchanged. The EMTs resume CPR. What should be done now?

13. What is the first antiarrhythmic administered in pulseless VT/VF? Indicate the initial and repeat dose of this medication.

14. You choose to administer a 1.5 mg/kg dose of lidocaine IV bolus, followed by a 20 mL flush of NS. If IV access was not available and you chose to administer lidocaine via the ET tube, what would the correct dose be?

15. While the EMT circulates the lidocaine with CPR, you assess the effectiveness of his chest compressions by palpating for a pulse. A pulse is present with CPR. When you ask the EMT to stop compressions, you note there is no pulse. The rhythm on the monitor is unchanged. What should be done now?

16. After your intervention in the preceding question, you observe the following rhythm on the cardiac monitor.

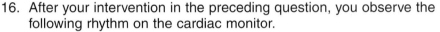

Rhythm identification: _____

17. What should be done now?

18. A carotid pulse is present. You instruct an EMT to check the patient's BP and note the patient is not breathing. You instruct an EMT to continue ventilating the patient. The patient's BP is 94/70. What should be done now?

Case 3: Answers

1. Stop CPR and quickly perform the Primary ABCD Survey.
2. Instruct an EMT to size and insert an oropharyngeal airway and begin ventilating patient with a bag-valve-mask connected to oxygen at 15 L/min (attach a reservoir to the bag). Ventilate at a rate of 12/min. Tidal volume delivered should be approximately 6 to 7 mL/kg over 1 to 2 sec. Instruct the second EMT to begin chest compressions while you prepare the defibrillator. Compression to ventilation ratio should be 15:2 with a compression rate of approximately 100/min.

3. No. The patient can be ventilated with the bag-valve-mask device for now. It is important to determine the patient's cardiac rhythm at this point. If the rhythm is VT or VF, prompt defibrillation is essential.
4. Perform a quick-look. Do not take the time to apply electrodes and cables now.
5. The rhythm is coarse ventricular fibrillation.
6. The anterior paddle (sternum paddle) is placed to the right of the upper sternum below the clavicle. The other (apex paddle) is placed to the left of the patient's left nipple with the center of the paddle in the left midaxillary line.
7. Place the paddles on the patient's chest, charge the paddles to 200 J, call "Clear!" and look 360 degrees to be sure everyone is clear, then deliver the shock. Leave the paddles in place on the chest and do not permit anyone to move toward the patient at this time. Check the rhythm on the monitor. (It is unchanged.) Charge the paddles again, this time to either 200 or 300 J. Call "Clear!"—look, and then deliver the shock. Leaving the paddles in place on the chest, look again at the rhythm on the monitor. (There has been no change.) Charge the paddles to 360 J, call "Clear!"—look, and then deliver the shock. Look again at the rhythm on the monitor. (There is no change.) Remove the paddles from the patient's chest.
8. Perform the Secondary ABCD Survey.
9. Instruct the EMTs to resume CPR. Instruct your paramedic partner to prepare his intubation equipment and intubate the patient while you establish IV access.
10. Vasopressin or epinephrine, amiodarone or lidocaine, magnesium (if hypomagnesemia present), procainamide, sodium bicarbonate.
11. Place the paddles on the patient's chest and charge to 360 J. Call "Clear!" and verify your team is clear of the patient, then deliver the shock.
12. At this point, you can consider administration of an antiarrhythmic.
13. You can administer either amiodarone or lidocaine. *Amiodarone:* Initial bolus—300 mg IV, bolus diluted in 20 to 30 mL of NS or D5W, consider repeat dose (150 mg IV bolus) every 3 to 5 minutes. *Lidocaine:* 1 to 1.5 mg/kg IV bolus, consider repeat dose (0.5 to 0.75 mg/kg) in 5 minutes, maximum IV bolus dose 3 mg/kg. The 1.5 mg/kg dose is recommended in cardiac arrest.
14. The endotracheal dose of lidocaine is 2 to 4 mg/kg.
15. Place the paddles on the patient's chest and charge to 360 J. Call "Clear!" and verify your team is clear of the patient, then deliver the shock.
16. Sinus tachycardia at 120 beats/min.
17. Since it is possible to have an organized rhythm on the monitor, yet no palpable pulse (pulseless electrical activity), determine if a carotid pulse is present.
18. Since a bolus of an antiarrhythmic was administered during the arrest, it is reasonable to continue a maintenance infusion of that agent. The antiarrhythmic used was lidocaine, so you will hang a lidocaine drip and prepare the patient for transport. Reassess the patient's vital signs and ECG rhythm at least every 5 minutes en route.

Case 3: Essential Actions

1. Use personal protective equipment
2. Perform Primary and Secondary ABCD Surveys
   a. Assess level of responsiveness, call for help
   b. Open airway and assess breathing. If patient is not breathing, insert oropharyngeal airway and begin rescue breathing with bag-valve-mask
   c. Assess pulse. If pulseless, begin CPR until arrival of defibrillator. On arrival of the defibrillator, assess rhythm
   d. Use proper safety technique when operating defibrillator (i.e., ensure all team members are clear of patient before pressing shock control)
   e. Correctly identify ventricular fibrillation and ventricular tachycardia
   f. Ensure shocks are delivered in correct sequence
   g. Reassess effectiveness of initial airway maneuvers and interventions. Maintain airway and provide ventilatory support during immediate postresuscitation period
   h. Perform endotracheal intubation, confirm tube placement by primary (visualization, rise and fall of chest, presence of bilateral breath sounds) and secondary ($ETCO_2$ detector, esophageal detector device) means
   i. Establish IV access and administer medications appropriate for dysrhythmia/clinical situation in proper sequence
3. Ensure medications are followed by a 20-mL flush of IV solution
4. Facilitate family presence during resuscitative efforts according to agency/institution protocol
5. Be familiar with advance directives and how to respond to them
6. Be familiar with the indications for when to not start resuscitation efforts and when to stop
7. Consider possible causes of the event
8. Transfer patient for definitive care

Case 3: Unacceptable Actions

1. Failure to use personal protective equipment
2. Failure to adequately assess the patient
3. Performing chest compressions or defibrillation before assessing pulses
4. Failure to begin CPR
5. Administration of oxygen by a means other than positive pressure ventilation (e.g., nasal cannula, simple face mask, nonrebreather mask)
6. Ordering intubation, IV access, medications, or performing defibrillation before assessing for presence of VF
7. Unsafe operation of defibrillator (failure to clear self or others before shocking)
8. Failure to check for a pulse after defibrillation series
9. Failure to recognize rhythm change
10. Medication errors

CASE 4: ASYSTOLE

Objective

Given a patient situation, describe the management steps (including mechanical, pharmacologic, and electrical interventions where applicable) for asystole.

Skills to Master

1. Primary and Secondary ABCD Surveys
2. Cardiopulmonary resuscitation
3. Oropharyngeal/nasopharyngeal airway insertion
4. Bag-valve-mask ventilation (1 and 2 rescuer technique)
5. Suctioning
6. Performing a quick-look
7. Attachment and use of ECG monitoring leads
8. Operation of a transcutaneous pacemaker
9. Endotracheal intubation + $ETCO_2$, esophageal detector device
10. Intravenous (IV)/intraosseous (IO) access
11. IV/IO medication administration
12. Differential diagnosis of asystole

Rhythms to Master

Asystole

Medications to Master

1. Oxygen
2. Epinephrine
3. Atropine
4. Sodium bicarbonate

Related Text Chapters

Chapter 1: ABCDs of Emergency Cardiovascular Care
Chapter 2: Airway Management: Oxygenation and Ventilation
Chapter 3: Vascular Access
Chapter 4: Dysrhythmia Recognition
Chapter 5: Electrical Therapy
Chapter 7: Cardiovascular Pharmacology
Chapter 8: Putting It All Together

Case 4: Questions

Time: 10:00 PM. You are on duty in the Emergency Department when paramedics arrive with a 62-year-old male. The paramedics state the patient was reading in bed when he complained to his wife of chest pain and collapsed. The patient's wife called 9-1-1. On arrival at the scene, paramedics state the patient was responsive to verbal stimuli. The cardiac monitor revealed a complete AV block at a rate of 30. Vital signs 3 minutes ago revealed a blood pressure of 68/42, pulse 30, respiratory rate 14. The paramedics have placed the patient on oxygen by nonrebreather mask and established an IV. As you move the patient to the stretcher, you hear the patient gasp, then he is quiet.

Patient History

Allergies	No known allergies
Medications	Lanoxin, Lasix, nitroglycerin, K-Dur
Past Medical History	CABG 1996
Last Oral Intake	Unknown
Events Prior	Reading in bed when he complained of chest pain and then collapsed

1. What should be done now?

2. The patient is unresponsive, apneic, and pulseless. What are the four critical tasks to be assigned at the start of a resuscitation effort?

3. Before proceeding with this resuscitation effort, what factors should be considered?

4. You are the team leader of this resuscitation effort. How would you like to proceed?

5. How will you determine the patient's cardiac rhythm?

6. The cardiac monitor reveals the following rhythm.

Rhythm identification: _____

7. Name three possible causes of a flat line on the cardiac monitor.

8. How would you like to proceed?

9. A flat line appears in multiple leads. Should you proceed with defibrillation?

10. CPR is ongoing. You instruct a team member to attach monitoring leads to the patient. What should be done now?

11. Name five possible causes of asystole.

12. An IV is in place and the patient has been successfully intubated. Transcutaneous pacer pads are in place. Name two medications indicated in the management of asystole and their dosages.

13. Each IV bolus medication administered during a cardiac arrest should be followed with a 10- to 20-mL flush of normal saline. What is the rationale for this action?

14. When is transcutaneous pacing indicated?

15. Indicate the appropriate transcutaneous pacemaker rate and output (mA) settings for this situation.

16. The rate on the pacemaker has been set and the current is being increased steadily. A change in the patient's rhythm is noted when the current reaches 85 mA. The following rhythm is observed on the monitor.

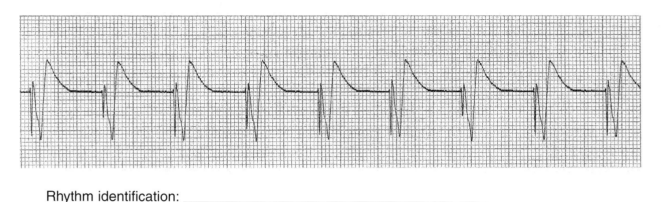

Rhythm identification: _____

17. How will you assess mechanical capture?

18. Pulses are present at a rate consistent with the monitor. The patient is attempting to breathe at a rate of 8 breaths/min. BP 78/40. Breath sounds are clear bilaterally with bagging. You instruct a team member to continue assisting the patient's respirations with the bag-valve-mask until a ventilator arrives. What should be done now?

Case 4: Answers

1. Assess responsiveness and begin the Primary ABCD Survey.
2. Four critical tasks of resuscitation: airway management, chest compressions, monitoring and defibrillation, IV access and medication administration.
3. Factors to consider before beginning a resuscitation effort: documentation or other evidence of DNAR? Obvious signs of death? (Not applicable in this situation.) If yes, do not start/attempt resuscitation. The patient's wife states a DNAR order does not exist.
4. Remove the nonrebreather mask. Instruct a team member to size and insert an OPA and begin ventilating patient with a bag-valve-mask connected to oxygen at 15 L/min (attach a reservoir to the bag). Ventilate at a rate of 12/min. Tidal volume delivered should be approximately 6 to 7 mL/kg over 1 to 2 sec. Instruct a second team member to begin chest compressions while another prepares the defibrillator. Compression to ventilation ratio should be 15:2 with a compression rate of approximately 100/min.
5. Perform a quick-look. Do not take the time to apply electrodes and cables now.
6. The rhythm is asystole.
7. Possibilities include no power, loose leads, true asystole, no connection to the patient, no connection to the defibrillator/monitor.

8. Check lead/cable connections, ensure power to monitor is on, ensure correct lead is selected, turn up the gain, confirm asystole in a second lead.
9. No. Defibrillating asystole is not recommended.
10. Instruct a team member to intubate the patient. An IV is already in place. Direct another to place the transcutaneous pacemaker pads on the patient's chest and prepare for pacing. Review the patient's history and consider possible causes of the arrest.
11. PATCH-4-MD: *P*ulmonary embolism, *A*cidosis, *T*ension pneumothorax, *C*ardiac tamponade, *H*ypovolemia (most common cause), *H*ypoxia, *H*eat/cold (hypo-/hyperthermia), *H*ypo-/hyperkalemia (and other electrolytes), *M*yocardial infarction, *D*rug overdose/accidents.
12. Epinephrine 1 mg (1:10,000 solution) IV every 3 to 5 minutes. Atropine 1 mg IV every 3 to 5 minutes to maximum 0.04 mg/kg. Sodium bicarbonate and other medications may be used, depending on the cause of the arrest.
13. During cardiac arrest, administer IV medications rapidly by bolus injection and follow each medication with a 10- to 20-mL bolus of IV fluid to aid delivery of the medication(s) to the central circulation.
14. Symptomatic bradycardia unresponsive to atropine or when atropine is not immediately available and some cases of asystolic cardiac arrest. Patients in asystole who are most likely to benefit from pacing: Witnessed asystole, "P-wave asystole" (ventricular asystole), asystolic arrest <10 min/duration.
15. Connect the pacing cable to adhesive electrodes on the patient. Turn on the pacemaker generator. Set the pacing rate. In a pulseless patient, set the rate at 80 to 100 beats/min Next, set the output (mA). In asystole, turn the current to maximum output and decrease if capture is achieved.
16. The rhythm is a 100% ventricular paced rhythm. Electrical capture is usually evidenced by a wide QRS and broad T wave.
17. Mechanical capture is evaluated by assessing the patient's right upper extremity or right femoral pulses. Assessment of pulses on the patient's left side should be avoided to help minimize confusion between the presence of an actual pulse and skeletal muscle contractions caused by the pacemaker. Once capture is achieved, continue pacing at an output level slightly higher (approximately 2 mA) than the threshold of initial electrical capture.
18. Consider possible causes of the arrest. In this scenario, possible causes that should be aggressively considered are myocardial infarction and an electrolyte imbalance.

Case 4: Essential Actions

1. Perform the Primary and Secondary ABCD Surveys
2. Begin CPR
3. Identify asystole and confirm the rhythm in at least one other lead. (Check lead/cable connections, ensure power to monitor is on, correct lead is selected, gain turned up)
4. Facilitate family presence during resuscitative efforts according to agency/institution protocol
5. Be familiar with advance directives and how to respond to them
6. Be familiar with the indications for when to not start resuscitation efforts and when to stop

7. Recognize the role of ventilation in acid-base balance
8. Recognize that transcutaneous pacing is not always indicated in an asystolic arrest; however, when considered, it must be performed early and simultaneously with medication administration to be effective.
9. Recognize that a change in the rhythm necessitates a pulse check. If a pulse is present, assess BP and respirations.
10. Recognize the possible causes of asystole and the treatment for each
11. Provide respectful, effective information when "telling the living" about the resuscitation attempt

Case 4: Unacceptable Actions

1. Failure to use personal protective equipment
2. Failure to adequately assess the patient
3. Performing chest compressions before assessing pulses
4. Failure to begin CPR
5. Administration of oxygen by a means other than positive pressure ventilation (e.g., nasal cannula, simple face mask, nonrebreather mask)
6. Ordering intubation, IV access, medications, or performing defibrillation before assessing for presence of VF
7. Failure to recognize rhythm change
8. Medication errors
9. Confirming asystole in only one lead
10. Use of transcutaneous pacing late or without simultaneous administration of medications

CASE 5: PULSELESS ELECTRICAL ACTIVITY (PEA)

Objective

Given a patient situation, describe the management steps (including mechanical, pharmacologic, and electrical interventions where applicable) for a patient in pulseless electrical activity (PEA).

Skills to Master

1. Primary and Secondary ABCD Surveys
2. Cardiopulmonary resuscitation
3. Oropharyngeal/nasopharyngeal airway insertion
4. Bag-valve-mask ventilation (1 and 2 rescuer technique)
5. Suctioning
6. Performing a quick-look
7. Attachment and use of ECG monitoring leads
8. Endotracheal intubation + $ETCO_2$, esophageal detector device
9. Intravenous (IV) /intraosseous (IO) access
10. IV/IO medication administration
11. Differential diagnosis of PEA
12. Fluid resuscitation
13. Needle thoracostomy (chest decompression)

Rhythms to Master

1. Junctional escape rhythm
2. Idioventricular (ventricular escape) rhythm
3. Sinus tachycardia
4. Sinus bradycardia

Medications to Master

1. Oxygen
2. Epinephrine
3. Atropine
4. Sodium bicarbonate

Related Text Chapters

Chapter 1: ABCDs of Emergency Cardiovascular Care
Chapter 2: Airway Management: Oxygenation and Ventilation
Chapter 3: Vascular Access
Chapter 4: Dysrhythmia Recognition
Chapter 5: Electrical Therapy
Chapter 7: Cardiovascular Pharmacology
Chapter 8: Putting It All Together

Case 5: Questions

Time: 8:08 AM. You are working on the medical/surgical floor of a local hospital. A laboratory technician can be heard calling for help down the hall. When you arrive in the room, the technician is standing in the bathroom and informs you she found the patient unresponsive on the floor. The patient, a 33-year-old male, was admitted yesterday for abdominal pain and was last seen 30 minutes ago. A respiratory therapist has arrived to assist you. A bag-valve-mask, oxygen, and cardiac board are the only emergency equipment immediately available.

Patient History
Allergies	Codeine
Medications	Tagamet
Past Medical History	Ulcers
Last Oral Intake	Unknown
Events Prior	Last seen 30 minutes ago

1. You quickly perform the Primary ABCD Survey and find the patient is unresponsive, apneic, and pulseless. What should be done now?

2. The emergency cart has arrived in the room with two nurses to assist you. You place defib pads on the patient's chest, perform a quick-look, and see the rhythm following (lead I).

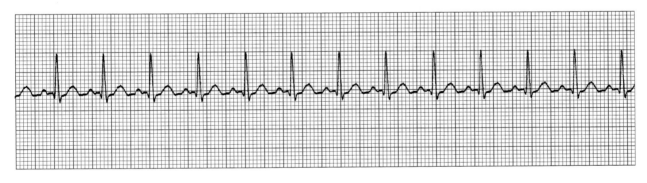

Rhythm identification: _____

3. Despite the presence of an organized rhythm on the cardiac monitor, you are unable to palpate pulses. What is the name given to this clinical situation?

4. Should this patient be defibrillated? Why or why not?

5. A physician has arrived in the room. After you quickly explain what has transpired thus far, he assumes responsibility as the team leader of this resuscitation effort. He instructs the respiratory therapist to continue bag-valve-mask ventilation and instructs the lab technician to resume chest compressions. The physician prepares to intubate the patient and asks you to establish an IV. Where should you start the IV?

6. The lab technician suddenly recalls seeing a large amount of black-appearing stool in the bathroom toilet when she found the patient. Because of its odor, she flushed the toilet and did not think much of it until now. The patient has been successfully intubated. Tube placement has been confirmed and the endotracheal tube secured in place. An IV of normal saline has been established. Based on the information available thus far, what do you suspect is the most likely cause of this arrest?

7. You are instructed to establish a second IV of NS and administer IV fluids at a rapid rate. The physician instructs another team member to administer a 1-mg IV bolus of epinephrine (1:10,000 solution). You know that epinephrine increases heart rate and the force of myocardial contraction and recall that the cardiac monitor revealed a narrow-QRS rhythm with a rapid rate. Why is epinephrine being ordered for this patient?

8. If IV access was unsuccessful, epinephrine could be administered via the endotracheal tube. What is the endotracheal dose of epinephrine?

9. If the rhythm on the cardiac monitor was slow, another medication could have been used. Name this medication and the correct dosage for administration.

10. After 1 L of NS and 1 mg of epinephrine, assessment reveals the patient has pulses consistent with the rhythm on the monitor. What should be done now?

The patient's blood pressure is 96/74, pulse 120, respiratory rate 4/min. Continue ventilation with the bag-valve-mask device and transfer the patient for definitive care.

Case 5: Answers

1. Call for additional help, call for a defibrillator. Instruct the respiratory therapist to insert an OPA and begin ventilating the patient with a bag-value-mask connected to oxygen at 15 L/min; attach a reservoir to bag. Ventilate at a rate of 12/min. Tidal volume delivered should be approximately 6 to 7 mL/kg over 1 to 2 sec. Instruct the lab technician to begin CPR while you prepare the defibrillator. Compression to ventilation ratio should be 15:2 with a compression rate of approximately 100/min.
2. Sinus tachycardia (lead I).
3. Pulseless electrical activity (PEA).
4. No. Defibrillation is the therapeutic delivery of unsynchronized electrical current through the myocardium over a very brief period to terminate a cardiac dysrhythmia. The pacemaker with the highest degree of automaticity should then assume responsibility for pacing the heart. In PEA, an organized rhythm is present on the cardiac monitor. Defibrillation is NOT indicated in PEA.
5. During circulatory collapse or cardiac arrest, the preferred vascular access site is the largest, most accessible vein that does not require the interruption of resuscitation efforts. If no IV is in place before the arrest, establish IV access using a peripheral vein, preferably the antecubital or external jugular vein.
6. Based on the patient's past medical history of ulcers, admission complaint of abdominal pain, and the lab technician's description of her findings in the bathroom at the time of the patient's collapse, hypovolemia is the most likely cause of the patient's situation.
7. The primary beneficial effects of epinephrine administration in cardiac arrest are the result of its alpha-adrenergic receptor stimulating action, resulting in peripheral vasoconstriction. Increased peripheral vasoconstriction improves cerebral and coronary blood flow.
8. The endotracheal dose of epinephrine is 2 to 2.5 times IV dose. Recommended volume = 10 mL. Use 1:1000 solution (2 mg dose = 2 mL of epi + 8 mL NS). Stop chest compressions, administer the medication, follow with several forceful insufflations of the bag-valve device, and then resume CPR.
9. Atropine 1 mg IV every 3 to 5 minutes, maximum dose 0.04 mg/kg. Endotracheal dose 2 to 3 mg diluted in 10 mL normal saline or distilled water.
10. In a resuscitation effort, it is important to recognize that a change in the rhythm necessitates a pulse check. In this situation, the rhythm has not changed, but the patient now has a pulse. If a pulse is present, assess the patient's blood pressure and respirations.

Case 5: Essential Actions

1. Perform the Primary and Secondary ABCD Surveys
2. Begin CPR
3. Properly attach and operate the monitor, correctly recognizing the clinical situation as pulseless electrical activity (PEA)
4. Intubate and establish IV access; administer epinephrine and other medications as indicated
5. Recognize the possible causes of pulseless electrical activity and the treatment for each
6. Recognize the role of ventilation in acid-base balance

7. Recognize that a change in the rhythm necessitates a pulse check. If a pulse is present, assess BP and respirations
8. Provide respectful, effective information when "telling the living" about the resuscitation attempt
9. Facilitate family presence during resuscitative efforts according to agency/institution protocol
10. Be familiar with advance directives and how to respond to them
11. Be familiar with the indications for when to not start resuscitation efforts and when to stop

Case 5: Unacceptable Actions

1. Failure to use personal protective equipment
2. Failure to adequately assess the patient
3. Performing chest compressions or defibrillation before assessing pulses
4. Failure to begin CPR
5. Administration of oxygen by a means other than positive pressure ventilation (e.g., nasal cannula, simple face mask, nonrebreather mask)
6. Ordering intubation, IV access, medications, or performing defibrillation before assessing for presence of VF
7. Failure to recognize rhythm change
8. Medication errors
9. Failure to consider the possible causes of PEA
10. Defibrillating PEA
11. Failure to consider a fluid challenge and/or treating only with epinephrine

CASE 6: ACUTE CORONARY SYNDROMES

Objective

Given a patient situation, describe the management steps (including mechanical, pharmacologic, and electrical interventions where applicable) for a patient experiencing an acute coronary syndrome.

Skills to Master

1. Primary and Secondary ABCD Surveys
2. Supplemental oxygen delivery devices
3. Attachment and use of ECG monitoring leads
4. Intravenous (IV) access
5. IV medication administration
6. Learn the ECG criteria for myocardial ischemia, injury, and infarction
7. Recognize clinical signs and symptoms of right and left ventricular failure

Rhythms to Master

1. Sinus rhythm, sinus bradycardia, sinus tachycardia
2. AV blocks: First-degree, second-degree type I, second-degree type II, complete (third-degree)
3. Premature atrial complexes
4. Premature ventricular complexes
5. Ventricular fibrillation, ventricular tachycardia

Medications to Master

1. Oxygen
2. Nitroglycerin
3. Morphine sulfate
4. Aspirin
5. Fibrinolytic agents
6. Beta-blockers
7. Heparin
8. Glycoprotein IIb/IIIa inhibitors
9. ACE inhibitors
10. Furosemide
11. Dopamine
12. Dobutamine
13. Norepinephrine
14. Nitroprusside

Related Text Chapters

Chapter 1: ABCDs of Emergency Cardiovascular Care
Chapter 2: Airway Management: Oxygenation and Ventilation
Chapter 3: Vascular Access
Chapter 4: Dysrhythmia Recognition
Chapter 5: Electrical Therapy
Chapter 6: Myocardial Ischemia, Injury, and Infarction
Chapter 7: Cardiovascular Pharmacology
Chapter 8: Putting It All Together

Case 6: Questions

Time: 08:01 AM. A 46-year-old male is experiencing "chest pressure." He has driven himself to the Emergency Department where you are the triage nurse on duty.

Patient History

Allergies	No known allergies
Medications	Metoprolol
Past Medical History	Asthma as a child; hypertension
Last Oral Intake	5:30 AM today—coffee
Events Prior	Substernal chest "pressure" began about 6 AM

1. The patient is awake and alert. His airway is patent, breathing adequate, and pulses are strong and equal bilaterally. What questions should you ask of this patient to help ascertain whether he is experiencing an acute coronary syndrome?

2. The patient states he was watching the news this morning when his symptoms began. His discomfort began as a "pressure" sensation that is now pain in the center of his chest. The pain radiates down his left arm. On a 1 to 10 scale, he rates his pain a 9. The patient has a history of hypertension and smokes 2 packs of cigarettes per day. He states he has never used Viagra. What are the goals in the immediate management of an acute coronary syndrome?

3. How is the time of symptom onset defined?

4. Name three potentially lethal conditions that mimic acute MI.

5. The patient's initial vital signs are: BP 178/118, P 80, R 20. Breath sounds are clear bilaterally. Describe your initial interventions for this patient.

6. Oxygen is being administered by nasal cannula at 4 L/min, and an IV has been established. A 12-lead ECG has been obtained. A physician will review the 12-lead and categorize the patient into one of three groups. Can you name them?

7. The diagnosis of an acute MI is based on the presence of at least two of three criteria. List all three criteria.

8. How are changes suggestive of myocardial ischemia or injury identified on an ECG?

9. The patient's 12-lead ECG follows. Are there any significant findings on this 12-lead ECG?

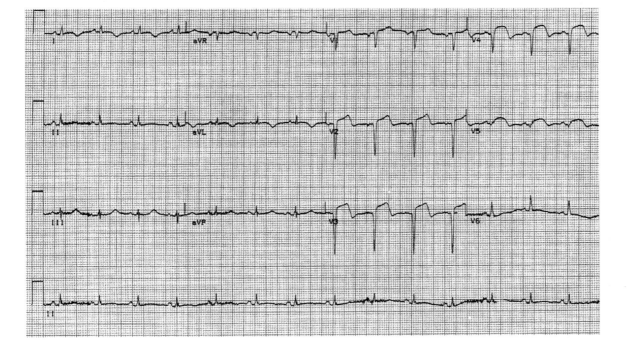

10. What routine measures should be performed for this patient at this time?

11. The patient's serum cardiac markers, ECG, and clinical signs and symptoms suggest an acute MI. What additional interventions should be considered for this patient?

Case 6: Answers

1. Determine age, gender, signs and symptoms (including location of pain, duration, quality, relation to effort, and time of symptom onset), history of CAD. CAD risk factors present? History of Viagra use? (Question should be asked of men and women.)

2. Minimize infarct size, salvage ischemic myocardium, alleviate vasoconstriction, reduce myocardial oxygen demand, prevent and manage complications, improve chances of survival.

3. Time of symptom onset is defined as the beginning of continuous, persistent discomfort that prompted the patient to seek medical attention.

4. Aortic dissection, acute pericarditis, acute myocarditis, pulmonary embolism.

5. Targeted history/physical exam; use checklist (yes-no); focus on eligibility for reperfusion therapy; assess vital signs, determine oxygen saturation, establish IV access, ECG monitoring, administer aspirin 162 to 325 mg (chewed) if no reason for exclusion; obtain baseline serum cardiac marker levels; obtain 12-lead ECG (physician to review); serial ECGs in patients with Hx suggesting MI and nondiagnostic ECG; obtain lab specimens (CBC, lipid profile, electrolytes); portable chest x-ray film, preferably upright (<30 min)

6. The 12-lead ECG will be reviewed and the patient categorized into one of three groups:
(a) ST-segment elevation or new or presumably new LBBB, (b) ST-segment depression/transient ST-segment/T wave changes, (c) normal or nondiagnostic ECG.

7. Clinical history of ischemic type chest discomfort, changes on serially obtained ECGs, rise and fall in serum cardiac markers.

8. On the ECG, changes suggestive of myocardial *ischemia* include ST-segment *depression* in the leads facing the affected area. Changes suggestive of myocardial *injury* include ST-segment *elevation* in the leads facing the affected area.

9. The 12-lead ECG shows significant ST-segment elevation in leads V_2, V_3, V_4, and V_5. These findings are suggestive of an anterior MI.

10. Administer aspirin (if not already done), SL nitroglycerin, and morphine if the patient's pain is not relieved with nitroglycerin. Reassess the patient's vital signs after each dose of nitroglycerin and morphine.

11. Use checklist to determine patient's eligibility for fibrinolytic therapy. Reconfirm time of symptom onset. Consider adjunctive treatments— beta-blockers, heparin, nitrates as indicated.

Case 6: Essential Actions

1. Use personal protective equipment
2. Perform Primary and Secondary ABCD Surveys
3. Obtain a history and perform a physical examination; focus on eligibility for fibrinolytic therapy
4. Assess vital signs, oxygen saturation
5. Review 12-lead ECG for evidence of myocardial ischemia, injury, or infarction
6. Know the actions, indications, dosages, side effects, and contraindications for the medications used in the management of acute coronary syndromes
7. Administer oxygen and appropriate pharmacologic therapy based on patient presentation, vital signs, ECG, and related available data
8. Know the inclusion and exclusion criteria for fibrinolytic therapy

Case 6: Unacceptable Actions

1. Failure to use personal protective equipment
2. Failure to adequately assess the patient
3. Medication errors
4. Failure to administer oxygen and/or other medications appropriate for patients with chest pain suggestive of ischemia
5. Failure to establish IV access
6. Unfamiliarity with exclusion criteria for use of fibrinolytic agents
7. Failure to attempt to control a patient's chest pain

CASE 7: SYMPTOMATIC BRADYCARDIA

Objective

Given a patient situation, describe the management steps (including mechanical, pharmacologic, and electrical interventions where applicable) of a patient with a symptomatic bradycardia.

Skills to Master

1. Primary and Secondary ABCD Surveys
2. Supplemental oxygen delivery devices
3. Attachment and use of ECG monitoring leads
4. Operation of a transcutaneous pacemaker
5. Intravenous (IV) access
6. IV medication administration

Rhythms to Master

1. Sinus rhythm, sinus bradycardia
2. Junctional rhythm
3. Idioventricular (ventricular escape) rhythm
4. AV blocks—first-degree, second-degree type I, second-degree type II, complete (third-degree)
5. Pacemaker rhythm

Medications to Master

1. Oxygen
2. Atropine
3. Dopamine
4. Epinephrine
5. Isoproterenol

Related Text Chapters

Chapter 1: ABCDs of Emergency Cardiovascular Care
Chapter 2: Airway Management: Oxygenation and Ventilation
Chapter 3: Vascular Access
Chapter 4: Dysrhythmia Recognition
Chapter 5: Electrical Therapy
Chapter 7: Cardiovascular Pharmacology
Chapter 8: Putting It All Together

Case 7: Questions

Time: 10:12 PM. A 53-year-old male is complaining of weakness. You have two other advanced life support personnel to assist you. Emergency equipment is immediately available.

Patient History

Allergies	Bactrim
Medications	Lopressor, verapamil, Lasix, procainamide, warfarin, potassium
Past Medical History	Angioplasty/stent 4 months ago
Last Oral Intake	9:30 PM today—diet soft drink
Events Prior	Patient states he had taken a walk about 30 minutes ago and, on his return home, suddenly felt weak and fell to the ground. Denies chest pain or shortness of breath.

1. The patient is awake, alert, and complaining of weakness. His airway is patent, breathing adequate, and a weak radial pulse is present. His color is pale. Breath sounds are clear bilaterally. How would you like to proceed?

2. Oxygen is being administered by nasal cannula at 4 L/min, an IV has been established, and the pulse oximeter is attached. The cardiac monitor reveals the following rhythm.

   Rhythm identification: _____

3. What is meant by the terms *absolute* and *relative* bradycardia?

4. A bradycardia is treated only when it causes signs and symptoms. List signs and symptoms that, if present, would warrant intervention.

5. The patient's blood pressure is 78/44, pulse 34, respirations 16. Should atropine be administered to this patient?

6. The patient's level of responsiveness is decreasing. His blood pressure is now 66/40. His cardiac rhythm is unchanged. How would you like to proceed?

7. You begin preparations for transcutaneous pacing. Where should the pacer pads be placed?

8. At what rate and output (mA) setting should you set the pacer?

9. If a pacemaker was not available, what other interventions could you consider for this patient?

10. The effects of a dopamine infusion are "dose-related." What does this term mean?

11. Explain why epinephrine may be useful in the management of a symptomatic bradycardia.

12. State the dose for each medication that may be used in the management of a symptomatic bradycardia.

13. Identify the following rhythm.

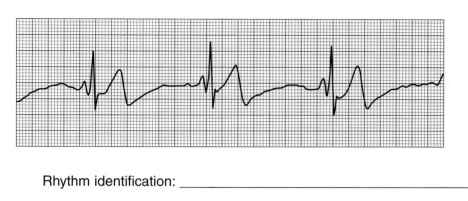

Rhythm identification: _____

14. Identify the following rhythm.

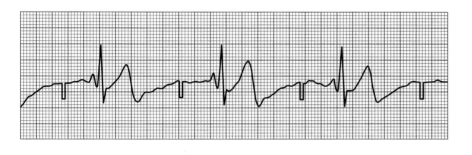

Rhythm identification: _____

15. Identify the following rhythm.

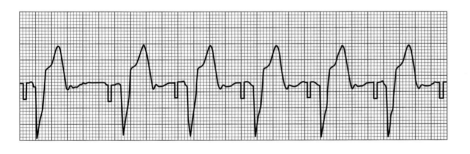

Rhythm identification: _____

Case 7: Answers

1. Administer oxygen, establish IV access, obtain vital signs, attach pulse oximeter, connect the patient to the cardiac monitor, obtain 12-lead ECG.
2. Second-degree AV block, type II.
3. *Absolute bradycardia* = rate <60 beats/min; may be symptomatic or asymptomatic; *relative bradycardia* = rate may be more than 60 beats/min; may occur when hypotensive patients require a tachycardia (i.e., hypovolemia) but are unable to increase their heart rate because of SA node disease or beta-blockers (or other medications).

4. *Signs:* Low blood pressure, shock, pulmonary congestion, congestive heart failure, angina, acute MI, ventricular ectopy. *Symptoms:* Chest pain, weakness, fatigue, dizziness, lightheadedness, shortness of breath, exercise intolerance, decreased level of responsiveness.

5. No. Atropine is indicated for use in symptomatic **narrow-QRS** bradycardias. The QRS associated with this patient's rhythm is wide. Atropine should **not** be used for wide-QRS bradycardias.

6. Consider a fluid challenge of 200 to 250 mL and prepare a transcutaneous pacemaker immediately until a transvenous pacemaker can be inserted.

7. Place the anterior chest electrode to the left of the sternum, halfway between the xiphoid process and left nipple. In female patients, the anterior electrode should be positioned under the left breast. Place the posterior electrode on the left posterior thorax directly behind the anterior electrode.

8. *Initial settings:* Rate: start at 60 to 80 beats/min. *Output:* Start at minimal energy setting; gradually increase until capture. Rate of increasing energy will depend on patient's stability. Assess electrical and mechanical capture.

9. Dopamine infusion (or) epinephrine infusion (or) isoproterenol infusion.

10. Dopamine stimulates different adrenergic receptor sites, depending on its rate of infusion.
    Low dose = dopaminergic; medium dose = beta; high dose = alpha.

11. Epinephrine (a) constricts peripheral blood vessels, increasing blood pressure (vasopressor), (b) increases heart rate (chronotropic effect), (c) increases force of contraction (inotropic effect).

12. Atropine 0.5 to 1.0 mg IV. May repeat every 3 to 5 minutes to a total dose of ≤2.5 mg (0.03 to 0.04 mg/kg). Total cumulative dose should not exceed 2.5 mg over 2.5 hours. Dopamine infusion 5 to 20 mcg/kg/min. Epinephrine infusion 2 to 10 mcg/min. Isoproterenol infusion 2 to 10 mcg/min.

13. Sinus bradycardia at 41 beats/min. No pacing.

14. Sinus bradycardia at 41 beats/min. Pacing stimulus (pulse) markers are visible, but there is no electrical capture. The pacemaker output (current) is set at 35 mA.

15. 100% ventricular-paced rhythm. A pacing stimulus (pulse) marker precedes each wide QRS complex. The pacemaker output (current) is set at 60 mA.

Case 7: Essential Actions

1. Use personal protective equipment
2. Recognize first-degree, second-degree type I, second-degree type II, and complete (third-degree) AV blocks
3. Obtain a history and perform a physical examination, including vital signs, recognizing signs and symptoms of bradycardia
4. Obtain a 12-lead ECG
5. Administer oxygen, establish IV access, and administer medications as indicated
6. Perform transcutaneous pacing as indicated
7. Consider fibrinolytic agents if the patient's presentation is consistent with an acute coronary syndrome, and there are no reasons for exclusion
8. Recognize signs and symptoms caused by bradycardia by appropriate assessment of history and physical examination

Case 7: Unacceptable Actions

1. Failure to use personal protective equipment
2. Failure to adequately assess the patient
3. Medication errors
4. Failure to correctly identify an AV block
5. Failure to prepare the transcutaneous or transvenous pacemaker while trying atropine
6. Failure to establish IV access
7. Administering lidocaine for ventricular escape rhythms
8. Treating an asymptomatic bradycardia

CASES 8 AND 9: STABLE AND UNSTABLE TACHYCARDIAS

Objective

Given a patient situation, describe the management steps (including mechanical, pharmacologic, and electrical interventions where applicable) of a patient with a symptomatic narrow- or wide-QRS tachycardia.

Skills to Master

1. Primary and Secondary ABCD Surveys
2. Supplemental oxygen delivery devices
3. Attachment and use of ECG monitoring leads
4. Vagal maneuvers
5. Operation of a conventional defibrillator
6. Synchronized cardioversion
7. Intravenous (IV) access
8. IV medication administration

Rhythms to Master

1. Sinus tachycardia
2. Paroxysmal supraventricular tachycardia (PSVT)
3. Atrial fibrillation
4. Atrial flutter
5. Wolff-Parkinson-White syndrome
6. Junctional tachycardia
7. Multifocal tachycardia
8. Monomorphic ventricular tachycardia
9. Polymorphic ventricular tachycardia
10. Wide-complex tachycardia of unknown origin

Medications to Master

1. Oxygen
2. Adenosine
3. Amiodarone
4. Beta-blockers
5. Digitalis
6. Diltiazem
7. Isoproterenol
8. Lidocaine
9. Procainamide
10. Verapamil

Related Text Chapters

Chapter 1: ABCDs of Emergency Cardiovascular Care
Chapter 2: Airway Management: Oxygenation and Ventilation
Chapter 3: Vascular Access
Chapter 4: Dysrhythmia Recognition
Chapter 5: Electrical Therapy
Chapter 6: Myocardial Ischemia, Injury, and Infarction

Chapter 7: Cardiovascular Pharmacology
Chapter 8: Putting It All Together

Case 8: Questions

Time: 12:25 PM. A 67-year-old male is complaining of palpitations. You have two other advanced life support personnel to assist you. Emergency equipment is immediately available.

Patient History

Allergies	Darvon, codeine
Medications	Albuterol, Valium p.r.n.
Past Medical History	Asthma, hypertension
Last Oral Intake	20 minutes ago
Events Prior	Was reading newspaper when his heart "started racing"

1. The patient is awake, alert, and oriented. His airway is patent, breathing adequate, and pulses are present and equal bilaterally. Breath sounds are clear. The patient denies chest pain or shortness of breath but states his heart is "racing." He is extremely anxious and tells you he thinks he is going to die. What interventions should be performed at this time?

2. Oxygen is being administered by nasal cannula at 4 L/min, an IV has been established, and the pulse oximeter is attached. The cardiac monitor reveals the following rhythm. Identify the following rhythm.

Rhythm identification: _____

3. Based on the patient's clinical presentation, name three antiarrhythmics that may be used in the management of this patient and the dosages for each.

4. As you are preparing the antiarrhythmic medication, the patient tells you he feels he is "fading" and quickly becomes unresponsive. The cardiac monitor remains unchanged. What should be done now?

5. The patient is unresponsive. He is breathing at a rate of 4 to 6/min. A weak carotid pulse is present at a rate consistent with the monitor. An assistant tells you the patient's blood pressure is 52/38. The patient's cardiac rhythm remains unchanged. You instruct an assistant to prepare to shock the patient. Your defibrillator is capable of delivering monophasic shocks. Should the shocks delivered be synchronized or unsynchronized? What energy level should be used?

Case 8: Answers

1. Administer oxygen, establish IV access, obtain vital signs, attach pulse oximeter, connect the patient to the cardiac monitor, and obtain 12-lead ECG.
2. Monomorphic ventricular tachycardia.
3. *Procainamide:* 100 mg over 5 min (20 mg/min). Maximum total dose 17 mg/kg. Maintenance infusion 1 to 4 mg/min. *Amiodarone:* 150 mg IV bolus over 10 min, followed by an infusion of 1 mg/min for 6 hours and then a maintenance infusion of 0.5 mg/min. Repeat supplementary infusions of 150 mg as necessary for recurrent or resistant dysrhythmias. Maximum total daily dose 2.0 g. *Lidocaine:* Normal cardiac function: 1 to 1.5 mg/kg initial dose. Repeat dose is half the initial dose every 5 to 10 min. Maximum total dose 3 mg/kg. If chemical conversion is successful, maintenance infusion 1 to 4 mg/min. Impaired cardiac function dose: 0.5-0.75 mg/kg IV push. May repeat every 5 to 10 min. Maximum total dose 3 mg/kg. If chemical conversion successful, maintenance infusion 1 to 4 mg/min.
4. Quickly perform a Primary ABCD Survey.
5. In the management of the hemodynamically unstable patient in VT with a pulse, synchronized shocks are delivered with 100 J and, if unsuccessful, 200 J, 300 J, and 360 J (or equivalent biphasic energy) as needed. However, if the patient is hypotensive (systolic BP <90), unresponsive, or if severe pulmonary edema exists, the patient should be defibrillated with the same energy. This patient is hypotensive and unresponsive. He should be defibrillated starting with 100 J.

Case 8: Essential Actions

1. Use personal protective equipment
2. Recognize sinus tachycardia, PSVT, atrial fibrillation, atrial flutter, Wolff-Parkinson-White syndrome, junctional tachycardia, multifocal tachycardia, monomorphic ventricular tachycardia, polymorphic ventricular tachycardia, wide-complex tachycardia of unknown origin
3. Obtain a history and perform a physical examination, including vital signs and recognizing signs and symptoms of bradycardia
4. Obtain a 12-lead ECG

5. Administer oxygen, establish IV access, and administer medications as indicated
6. Perform synchronized cardioversion or defibrillation as indicated
7. Recognize the need to change from synchronized cardioversion to defibrillation if the patient goes into VF or if there is a delay in synchronization
8. Demonstrate safe operation of the defibrillator
9. Recognize signs and symptoms caused by tachycardia by appropriate assessment of history and physical examination
10. Deliver the correct type (sync vs. unsync) of energy and the correct energy level for the specific dysrhythmia

Case 8: Unacceptable Actions

1. Failure to use personal protective equipment
2. Failure to adequately assess the patient
3. Medication errors
4. Failure to correctly identify the dysrhythmia
5. Inability to quickly determine if the patient is stable or unstable
6. Failure to hit the sync control after delivery of an initial synchronized shock in order to deliver additional synchronized shocks
7. Failure to establish IV access
8. Unfamiliarity with exclusion criteria for use of fibrinolytic agents

Case 9: Questions

Time: 11:15 AM. A 43-year-old female is complaining of a "rapid heartbeat." You have two other advanced life support personnel to assist you. Emergency equipment is immediately available.

Patient History

Allergies	No known allergies
Medications	Birth control pills
Past Medical History	Nothing pertinent
Last Oral Intake	8:00 AM—coffee with breakfast
Events Prior	Patient states she was sitting down and had a sudden onset of a rapid heartbeat. Her symptoms started 2 hours ago. She denies chest pain and is not short of breath. She said she stood up to call 9-1-1 and felt lightheaded.

1. The patient is awake, alert, and oriented. Her airway is patent, breathing adequate, and pulses are present and equal bilaterally. Breath sounds are clear. The patient denies chest pain or shortness of breath but states her heart is "racing." What interventions should be performed at this time?

2. Oxygen is being administered by nasal cannula at 4 L/min, an IV has been established, and the pulse oximeter is attached. The patient's blood pressure is 152/94, pulse 180, respirations 24. The cardiac monitor reveals the following rhythm. Identify the rhythm.

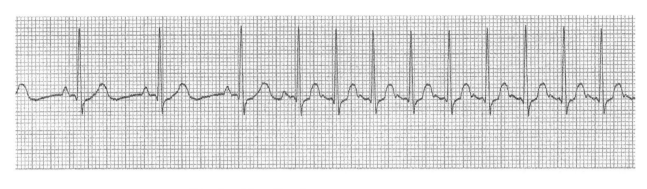

Rhythm identification: _____

3. The patient's heart rate persists at a rate of 180 beats/min. A vagal maneuver should be attempted. What is the purpose of a vagal maneuver?

4. Name four examples of vagal maneuvers.

5. Vagal maneuvers were unsuccessful. Assuming the patient's condition remains unchanged and the cardiac monitor shows a sustained narrow-QRS tachycardia, name three medications (and their dosages) that may be used in the management of this patient.

Case 9: Answers

1. Administer oxygen, establish IV access, obtain vital signs, attach pulse oximeter, connect the patient to the cardiac monitor, and obtain 12-lead ECG.
2. Sinus rhythm to PSVT.
3. Vagal maneuvers (a) increase parasympathetic tone, and (b) slow conduction through the AV node.
4. Bearing down, breath holding, coughing, gagging, carotid sinus pressure, nasogastric tube placement, facial immersion in ice water.
5. *Adenosine:* 6 mg rapid IV bolus over 1 to 3 sec. If needed, administer adenosine 12 mg rapid IV bolus over 1 to 3 sec after 1 to 2 min. May repeat 12 mg dose in 1 to 2 min if needed. Follow each dose immediately with 20 mL IV flush of NS. Use of adenosine is relatively contraindicated in asthmatic patients. Decrease dose in patients on dipyridamole (Persantine) or carbamazepine (Tegretol); consider increasing dose in patients taking theophylline or caffeine-containing preparations.

Diltiazem: 0.25 mg/kg over 2 min (e.g., 15 to 20 mg). If ineffective, 0.35 mg/kg over 2 min (e.g., 20 to 25 mg) in 15 min. Maintenance infusion 5 to 15 mg/hr, titrated to heart rate if chemical conversion successful. Calcium chloride (2 to 4 mg/kg) may be given slow IV push if borderline hypotension exists before diltiazem administration. *Verapamil:* 2.5 to 5.0 mg slow IV push over 2 min. May repeat with 5 to 10 mg in 15 to 30 min. Maximum dose 20 mg. *Esmolol:* 0.5 mg/kg over 1 min followed by a maintenance infusion at 50 mcg/kg/min for 4 min. If inadequate response, administer a second bolus of 0.5 mg/kg over 1 min and increase maintenance infusion to 100 mcg/kg/min. The bolus dose (0.5 mg/kg) and titration of the maintenance infusion (addition of 50 mcg/kg/min) can be repeated every 4 min to a maximum infusion of 300 mcg/kg/min. *Metoprolol:* 5 mg slow IV push over 5 min × 3 as needed to a total dose of 15 mg over 15 min.

Case 9: Essential Actions

1. Use personal protective equipment
2. Recognize sinus tachycardia, PSVT, atrial fibrillation, atrial flutter, Wolff-Parkinson-White syndrome, junctional tachycardia, multifocal tachycardia, monomorphic ventricular tachycardia, polymorphic ventricular tachycardia, wide-complex tachycardia of unknown origin
3. Obtain a history and perform a physical examination, including vital signs, recognizing signs and symptoms of bradycardia
4. Obtain a 12-lead ECG
5. Administer oxygen, establish IV access, and administer medications as indicated
6. Know what a vagal maneuver is, types, and when they are performed
7. Recognize signs and symptoms caused by tachycardia by appropriate assessment of history and physical examination

Case 9: Unacceptable Actions

1. Failure to use personal protective equipment
2. Failure to adequately assess the patient
3. Medication errors
4. Failure to administer oxygen and/or other medications appropriate for patients with chest pain suggestive of ischemia
5. Failure to establish IV access
6. Failure to correctly identify rhythm
7. Failure to listen for a carotid bruit before carotid massage

CASE 10: ACUTE ISCHEMIC STROKE

Objective

Given a patient situation, describe the management steps (including mechanical, pharmacologic, and electrical interventions where applicable) for a patient experiencing an acute ischemic stroke.

Skills to Master

1. Primary and Secondary ABCD Surveys
2. Supplemental oxygen delivery devices
3. Attachment and use of ECG monitoring leads
4. Suctioning
5. Blood glucose determination
6. Intravenous (IV) access
7. IV medication administration

Rhythms to Master

There are no new rhythms to master

Medications to Master

1. Oxygen
2. Fibrinolytic agents

Related Text Chapters

Chapter 1: ABCDs of Emergency Cardiovascular Care
Chapter 2: Airway Management: Oxygenation and Ventilation
Chapter 3: Vascular Access
Chapter 4: Dysrhythmia Recognition and Management
Chapter 7: Cardiovascular Pharmacology
Chapter 9: Acute Ischemic Stroke

Case 10: Questions

Time: 6:13 PM. A 58-year-old woman is exhibiting signs of a possible stroke. You have two other advanced life support personnel to assist you. Emergency equipment is immediately available.

Patient History

Allergies	Yes, but husband does not know what they are
Medications	Coumadin
Past Medical History	Valve replacement 2 years ago
Last Oral Intake	15 minutes ago with lunch
Events Prior	Patient had just finished eating when spouse noted she had a right-sided facial droop and was suddenly incontinent of urine and stool. Patient unable to speak

1. The patient is awake but unable to speak. Her airway is patent, breathing is adequate, and pulses are present and equal bilaterally, although irregular. Breath sounds are clear. What initial interventions should be performed at this time?

2. Oxygen is being administered by nasal cannula at 4 L/min, an IV has been established, and the pulse oximeter is attached. The patient's blood pressure is 162/88, respirations 16. Her blood glucose is 120. The cardiac monitor reveals the following rhythm. Identify the rhythm.

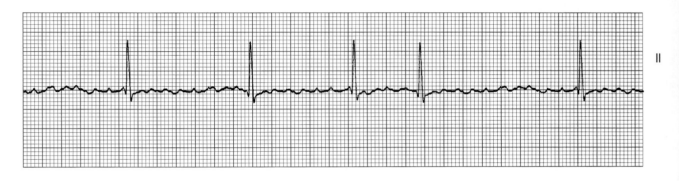

II

Rhythm identification: _____

3. A stroke is also called a *brain attack*. Why is this term recommended when teaching our patients, family, and friends about the signs and symptoms of a stroke?

4. What are the two major types of strokes?

5. Which type of stroke is most common?

6. What are the *3 R's* of stroke?

7. Why is it essential to determine the blood glucose level of a patient with a suspected stroke?

8. List four conditions to consider in the differential diagnosis of stroke.

9. List three questions you should ask when obtaining the history of a patient presenting with signs and symptoms of an acute stroke.

10. If a patient with signs and symptoms consistent with an acute ischemic stroke meets the criteria for administration of fibrinolytic therapy, what is the recommended dose of tPA?

Case 10: Answers

1. Administer oxygen, establish IV access, obtain vital signs, attach pulse oximeter, connect the patient to the cardiac monitor, check blood glucose, and obtain 12-lead ECG.
2. Atrial fibrillation.
3. *Brain attack* characterizes the medical condition and communicates the actual event more clearly to the public than does the word *stroke*.
4. *Ischemic stroke:* A blood vessel supplying the brain is occluded, can be life-threatening, but rarely leads to death within the first hour. *Hemorrhagic stroke:* A cerebral artery ruptures; can be fatal at onset.
5. Ischemic strokes account for approximately 85% of strokes. They are most commonly caused by a thrombus.
6. The three R's of stroke: *R*educe risk, *R*ecognize symptoms, *R*espond by calling 9-1-1
7. It is essential to differentiate a possible stroke from other common causes of stroke symptoms (e.g., hypoglycemia, drug or alcohol intoxication)
8. Trauma (e.g., subdural hematoma), hemorrhagic stroke (e.g., subarachnoid hemorrhage, intracranial hemorrhage), transient ischemic events that have not resolved at presentation, meningitis/encephalitis, hypertensive encephalopathy, intracranial mass, spinal cord or peripheral nerve disease, brain abscess, seizures/Todd's paralysis, infections, complex migraines, metabolic abnormalities (e.g., hypo-/hyperglycemia, drug overdose), Bell's palsy.
9. When was the last time the patient was known to be without symptoms? What was the patient doing when the symptoms began? Did the patient complain of a headache? Did he/she have a seizure? Has there been a change in his level of responsiveness? Is there a history of any recent trauma?
10. tPA is administered in an IV dose of 0.9 mg/kg (maximum of 90 mg), with 10% of the total dose given as an initial bolus and the remainder infused over 60 min for eligible patients, provided that treatment is initiated within 3 hours of clearly defined symptom onset. Administration of t-PA is associated with an increased risk of intracranial hemorrhage that can be severe or fatal.

Case 10: Essential Actions

1. Use personal protective equipment
2. Primary and Secondary ABCD Surveys
3. Administer oxygen by nasal cannula
4. Obtain a history and perform a physical examination, including vital signs and recognizing signs and symptoms of possible stroke
5. Determine time of symptom onset, realizing that <3 hours is required for fibrinolytic therapy
6. Obtain a 12-lead ECG, blood work
7. Perform general neurologic screening assessment
8. Administer oxygen, establish IV access, and administer medications as indicated
9. Order urgent noncontrast CT scan (CT done within 25 min of arrival; read with 45 min)
10. Consider fibrinolytic agents if the patient's presentation is consistent with acute ischemic stroke verified by CT scan, and there are no reasons for exclusion
11. Know inclusion and exclusion criteria for fibrinolytic use in acute ischemic stroke

Case 10: Unacceptable Actions

1. Failure to use personal protective equipment
2. Failure to adequately assess the patient
3. Medication errors
4. Failure to administer oxygen and/or other medications appropriate for patients with acute ischemic stroke
5. Failure to establish IV access
6. Unfamiliarity with exclusion criteria for use of fibrinolytic agents

Posttest

1. Which of the following statements regarding myocardial infarction is INCORRECT?
   a. The most common complication of myocardial infarction is cardiac dysrhythmias
   b. Aspirin is of no value in improving mortality when used within 24 hours of onset of chest pain
   c. Fibrinolytic therapy is of greatest benefit if given as soon as possible after onset of symptoms
   d. Most heart attacks occur in people under age 65

2. *True* or *False*. The term *unsynchronized countershock* is synonymous with defibrillation.

3. Atropine:
   a. May be helpful in sinus tachycardia and asystolic cardiac arrest
   b. Is the drug of choice in cardiac arrest
   c. May be helpful in symptomatic sinus bradycardia and AV block at the level of the AV node
   d. Is the drug of choice for paroxysmal supraventricular tachydysrhythmias

4. *True* or *False*. Complications associated with an inferior wall myocardial infarction often include bradydysrhythmias.

5. Which of the following is recommended for a patient in a wide complex tachycardia with impaired heart function?
   a. Procainamide
   b. Amiodarone
   c. Lidocaine
   d. Adenosine

6. A 72-year-old male is complaining of severe chest pain and weakness that has been present for approximately 3 hours. On a 1 to 10 scale, he rates his pain a 10. He is pale, cool, and diaphoretic. His blood pressure is 62/40. The cardiac monitor reveals a sinus rhythm at 98 beats/min without ectopy. Rales are heard three fourths of the way up both sides of his chest. He has a long history of cardiovascular disease. He has not been compliant with his prescribed medications. Your initial management of this patient should include:
   a. Oxygen administration, dopamine infusion, lidocaine bolus, and infusion
   b. Oxygen administration and a norepinephrine infusion
   c. Oxygen administration, SL nitroglycerin, and morphine 2 to 4 mg every 5 min titrated to pain relief
   d. Oxygen administration, nitroglycerin infusion, a lidocaine bolus and infusion

7. Diltiazem is a:
   a. Ventricular antidysrhythmic
   b. Calcium channel blocker
   c. Natural catecholamine
   d. Beta-blocker

8. A 51-year-old male is complaining of chest pain. The monitor reveals a second-degree AV block, type II. His BP is 70/40 with a heart rate of 46. Which one of the following should be immediately administered to the patient?
   a. Atropine
   b. External pacing
   c. Dopamine infusion
   d. Isoproterenol infusion

9. Nitroprusside:
   a. Is an arterial and venous vasodilator
   b. Is used to increase blood pressure in cases of severe hypotension
   c. Increases preload
   d. Increases afterload

10. In an adult, the maximum length of time for a suctioning attempt is:
    a. 10 to 15 sec
    b. 15 to 20 sec
    c. 20 to 25 sec
    d. 25 to 30 sec

11. List the potential causes of pulseless electrical activity (PEA) or asystole:

    _____

    _____

    _____

12. Leads V_1 and V_2 view the _____ of the heart.
   a. Inferior wall
   b. Anterior wall
   c. Septum
   d. Lateral wall

13. When providing a fluid challenge during resuscitation, which IV solution should be used?
   a. 5% dextrose
   b. 50% dextrose
   c. Any hypotonic solution
   d. Normal saline or Ringer's lactate

14. *True* or *False*. Patients who have denervated transplanted hearts will respond to atropine administration similarly to those who do not have transplanted hearts.

15. Identify the rhythm strip below:

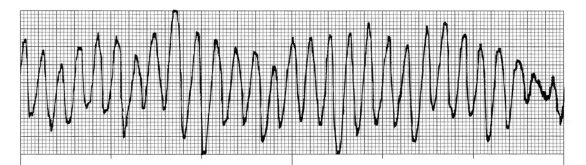

   a. Ventricular fibrillation
   b. Ventricular tachycardia
   c. Torsades de pointes
   d. Multiform PVCs

16. Based on the limited information provided in each patient situation below, select the patient in whom fibrinolytic therapy appears to be indicated (assuming there are no reasons for exclusion):
   a. 57-year-old male. Chest pain suggestive of acute MI present for 6 hours. ST-segment depression (3 mm) present in leads II, III, and aVF
   b. 65-year-old female. Chest pain suggestive of acute MI present for 2 days. ST-segment elevation (2 mm) present in leads V_2, V_3, and V_4
   c. 70-year-old male. Chest pain suggestive of acute MI present for 8 hours. ST-segment elevation (3 mm) present in leads I and III
   d. 72-year-old female. Chest pain suggestive of acute MI present for 4 hours. ST-segment elevation (2 mm) present in leads V_1, V_2, V_3, and V_4

17. *True* or *False*. Simultaneous, bilateral carotid massage should be attempted in the stable patient with PSVT before medication administration.

18. The patient with the rhythm below is a 65-year-old male complaining of palpitations. He denies chest pain or shortness of breath. His blood pressure is 160/90, respiratory rate 18. Breath sounds are clear bilaterally. Identify the rhythm and describe how you will manage this patient.

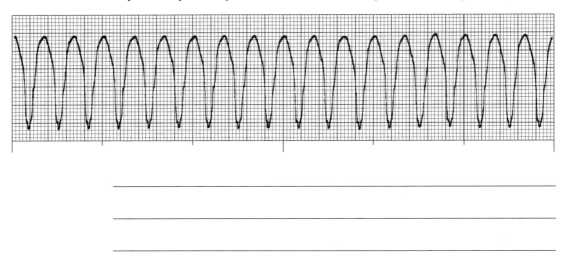

_____

_____

_____

19. The dysrhythmia in the rhythm strip below is Wolff-Parkinson-White syndrome:

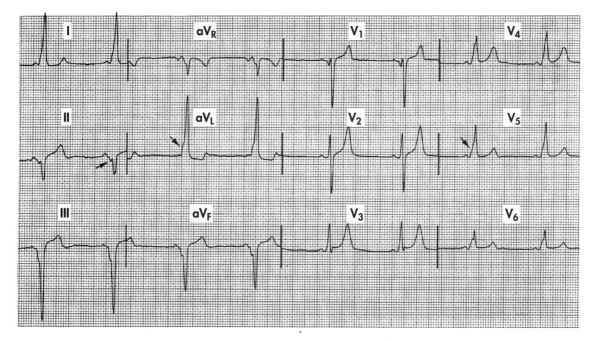

List three ECG features that are characteristic of this dysrhythmia.

a. _____

b. _____

c. _____

20. The lower airway is BEST protected by:
    a. Frequent suctioning
    b. Endotracheal tube
    c. Cuffed oropharyngeal airway (COPA)
    d. Laryngeal mask airway (LMA)

21. The approximate percentage of oxygen delivered by a simple face mask at 6 to 10 L/min is:
    a. 20% to 40%
    b. 40% to 60%
    c. 60% to 80%
    d. 80% to 100%

22. Your patient is a 38-year-old female complaining of "fluttering" in her chest accompanied by chest pressure that has been present for the past hour when the fluttering began. She rates her level of discomfort a 9 on a 1 to 10 scale. Her BP was initially 148/88 but has since decreased steadily during your examination. She now responds only by loudly calling her name. Her skin is pale, cool, and dry. Breath sounds are clear bilaterally. BP 88/64, R 12. Identify the rhythm below and indicate your management of this patient.

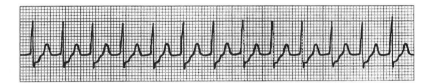

_____

_____

_____

23. Your patient has 12-lead ECG changes consistent with an acute inferior wall MI. Physical examination reveals jugular venous distention. His blood pressure is 80/52, pulse 78, R 14. Breath sounds are clear. You suspect a possible right ventricular infarction. What action(s) could you take at this time to confirm your suspicions?

_____

_____

_____

24. A 73-year-old male has experienced a cardiopulmonary arrest. The cardiac monitor reveals VF. Your defibrillator delivers monophasic shocks. The patient has been defibrillated with 200 joules (J) without success. A second shock is delivered with 300 J. The monitor now reveals a sinus rhythm at 70 beats/min. A palpable pulse is present. As a member of the resuscitation team prepares to assess the patient's blood pressure, you note the monitor again reveals VF. You prepare to defibrillate the patient immediately. What energy level should be used for this defibrillation attempt?
    a. Try using a lower energy level this time—100 J
    b. Start over again using 200 J
    c. Defibrillate with the last successful energy level—300 J
    d. Charge the defibrillator to 360 J and defibrillate

25. A 53-year-old female is unresponsive. BP 50/P, RR 10. The cardiac monitor displays a narrow-QRS tachycardia at 220 beats/min. Oxygen therapy was initiated, and an IV established before the patient's collapse. You promptly deliver a synchronized countershock; however, reassessment reveals the patient is pulseless and apneic. The cardiac monitor now reveals VF. What course of action should you take at this time?
    a. Perform CPR for 1 minute while readying the defibrillator for discharge
    b. Defibrillate immediately with 200 J
    c. Deliver a second synchronized countershock
    d. Place an endotracheal tube and administer epinephrine or vasopressin

26. *True* or *False*. In acute ischemic stroke, fibrinolytics should be considered if the patient is 18 years of age or more and the time from symptom onset is 8 hours or less.

27. Select the INCORRECTLY matched patient situation and rhythm with the recommended energy settings:
    a. Polymorphic VT: unsynchronized countershock with 200, 200-300, 360 J
    b. Ventricular fibrillation: unsynchronized countershock with 200, 200-300, 360 J
    c. Atrial fibrillation with a rapid ventricular response, unstable patient: synchronized countershock with 100, 200, 300, 360 J
    d. Atrial flutter with a rapid ventricular response, unstable patient: unsynchronized countershock with 100, 200, 300, 360 J

28. *True* or *False*. CPR should be briefly halted when administering a medication via the endotracheal tube.

29. During resuscitation of ventricular fibrillation, a 90 kg patient requires procainamide. What is the maximum amount of procainamide you should administer to this patient?
    a. 500 mg
    b. 1.0 g
    c. 1.5 g
    d. 2.0 g

30. Which of the following is NOT a desirable feature of a bag-valve device?
    a. Non-rebreathing valve
    b. Compressible, self-refilling bag
    c. Pop-off (pressure release) valve
    d. Availability in adult and pediatric sizes

31. *True or False.* The "periarrest" period includes the interval preceding a cardiac arrest and the immediate postresuscitation interval.

32. Which of the following memory aids may be used when evaluating a patient's level of responsiveness?
    a. ABCD
    b. AVPU
    c. OPQRST
    d. ALONE

33. List the four critical tasks performed in a resuscitation effort:

    a. _____

    b. _____

    c. _____

    d. _____

34. The "D" in the Primary ABCD Survey stands for:
    a. Disability
    b. Decision
    c. Defibrillation
    d. Differential diagnosis

35. *True or False.* An advance directive is a written document recording an individual's decisions concerning medical treatment that is to be applied (or not applied) in the event of physical or mental inability to communicate these wishes.

36. Select the CORRECT statement regarding ischemic strokes:
    a. AV malformations are the cause of most ischemic strokes
    b. Ischemic strokes often lead to death within 1 hour of symptom onset
    c. Ischemic strokes account for the majority of all strokes
    d. Hypertension is the most common cause of an ischemic stroke

37. *True or False.* A 70-year-old female has suffered a cardiopulmonary arrest. Endotracheal intubation should be performed as the initial step in the management of this patient's airway.

38. Select the INCORRECT statement regarding a complete (third-degree) AV block:
    a. In complete AV block, the atrial rate is greater than the ventricular rate
    b. In complete AV block, the atria and ventricles beat independently of each other
    c. In complete AV block, the ventricular rhythm is essentially regular although the P waves occur irregularly
    d. In complete AV block, the QRS may be either wide or narrow, depending on the origin of the escape pacemaker

39. The difference between second-degree type I and type II AV block is that with:
    a. Type I, the P waves occur irregularly
    b. Type I, the ventricular rhythm is regular
    c. Type II, the PR interval is always less than 0.12 sec in duration
    d. Type I, the PR interval becomes progressively longer until a P wave appears without a QRS complex

40. Acute coronary syndromes include three (3) conditions. Please list them below:

    1. _____

    2. _____

    3. _____

41. Your patient is experiencing an acute anterior wall MI. His BP is 156/88, P 118, R 24. The cardiac monitor reveals sinus tachycardia with occasional uniform PVCs. An IV has been established. Which of the following reflects the appropriate sequence of interventions that should be performed in the immediate general treatment of this patient?
    a. Oxygen, sublingual nitroglycerin, aspirin 162 to 325 mg, and then morphine sulfate 2 to 4 mg IV if pain unrelieved with nitroglycerin
    b. Aspirin 162 to 325 mg, morphine 2 to 4 mg IV, sublingual nitroglycerin, and then oxygen
    c. Sublingual nitroglycerin, aspirin 162 to 325 mg, oxygen, and then morphine 2 to 4 mg IV if pain unrelieved with nitroglycerin
    d. Morphine 2 to 4 mg IV, oxygen, aspirin 162 to 325 mg, and then sublingual nitroglycerin if morphine fails to relieve pain

42. List at least three (3) important questions that should be asked of a patient to determine if he/she may be experiencing an acute coronary syndrome.

    1. _____

    2. _____

    3. _____

43. *True* or *False.* The most common cause of an anterior or lateral wall myocardial infarction is occlusion of a branch of the right coronary artery.

44. A 60-year-old female has suffered a cardiopulmonary arrest. A health care professional trained in endotracheal intubation has intubated the patient. Which of the following findings would indicate inadvertent intubation of the right mainstem bronchus?
    a. Subcutaneous emphysema
    b. Jugular vein distention
    c. Breath sounds heard on only one side of the chest
    d. Gurgling sounds heard over the epigastrium

45. Calcium chloride is NOT routinely indicated in the management of:
    a. Hypocalcemia
    b. Hyperkalemia
    c. Calcium channel blocker toxicity
    d. Symptomatic bradycardia

46. *True* or *False*. A transient ischemic attack (TIA) is an important forecaster of ischemic stroke.

47. The three (3) components measured with the Glasgow Coma Scale are:
    a. Eye opening, verbal response, and motor response
    b. Vital signs, eye opening, and decorticate posturing
    c. Level of consciousness, vital signs, and respiratory pattern
    d. Decorticate and decerebrate posturing and level of consciousness

48. By definition, a transient ischemic attack (TIA) lasts:
    a. 30 to 60 sec
    b. 30 min to 1 hour
    c. No more than four hours
    d. Several minutes or up to 24 hours

49. In the presence of acute myocardial damage or severe ischemia, susceptibility to dysrhythmias is greatest during the _____ of symptom onset.
    a. First 2 weeks
    b. First 3 days
    c. First 4 to 6 min
    d. First several hours

50. Select the INCORRECT statement regarding furosemide:
    a. Furosemide may cause dehydration
    b. Furosemide administration may result in diuresis
    c. Furosemide venodilating effects begin approximately 45 to 60 min after administration
    d. Furosemide administration may result in hypokalemia, with subsequent cardiac dysrhythmias

ANSWERS AND RATIONALES

1. d. Most heart attacks occur in people over age 65.

2. True. The term *unsynchronized countershock* is synonymous with defibrillation.

3. c. Atropine may be helpful in symptomatic sinus bradycardia, AV block at the level of the AV node, asystolic cardiac arrest, and bradycardic pulseless electrical activity.

4. True. Bradydysrhythmias, including second-degree AV block type I (Wenckebach) are common complications of an inferior wall MI.

5. b. Amiodarone is recommended for a patient in a wide complex tachycardia with impaired heart function. Procainamide or amiodarone may be used for this dysrhythmia if the patient has normal heart function.

6. b. This patient's signs and symptoms are consistent with cardiogenic shock. Because his systolic BP is <70 mm Hg, management should include oxygen administration and a norepinephrine infusion.

7. b. Diltiazem is a calcium channel blocker.

8. b. Second-degree AV block type II can progress to a complete (third-degree) AV block without warning. An external pacemaker should be applied immediately. Atropine should be use with caution in second-degree AV block type II and third-degree AV block with a new wide QRS; it may be ineffective or cause paradoxical slowing.

9. a. Nitroprusside is an arterial and venous vasodilator that is more active on veins than on arteries. Venodilation promotes peripheral pooling of blood and decreases venous return to the heart, thereby reducing preload. Arteriolar relaxation reduces systemic vascular resistance (afterload). Nitroprusside is used for immediate reduction of blood pressure of patients in hypertensive crises.

10. a. In an adult, the maximum length of time for a suctioning attempt is 10 to 15 sec.

11. Potential causes for PEA or asystole are **PATCH-4-MD**
    Pulmonary embolism
    Acidosis
    Tension pneumothorax
    Cardiac tamponade
    Hypovolemia
    Hypoxia
    Heat/cold (hypo-/hyperthermia)
    Hypo-/hyperkalemia (and other electrolytes)
    Myocardial infarction
    Drug overdose/accidents (tricyclic antidepressants, calcium channel blockers, beta-blockers, digitalis)

The "Five H's and Five T's"[1] is another mnemonic that may be used to recall the causes of PEA and asystole:

Hypovolemia	Tamponade, cardiac
Hypoxia	Tension pneumothorax
Hypothermia	Thrombosis: lungs (massive pulmonary
Hypo-/hyperkalemia	embolism)
Hydrogen ion (acidosis)	Thrombosis: heart (acute coronary
	syndromes)
	Tablets/toxins: drug overdose

12. c. Leads V_1 and V_2 view the septum of the heart.

13. d. When providing a fluid challenge during resuscitation, normal saline or Ringer's lactate should be used. Both are isotonic IV solutions.

14. False. Patients who have denervated transplanted hearts will not respond to atropine administration. These patients often require a catecholamine infusion.

15. c. The rhythm shown is torsades de pointes (a type of polymorphic VT).

16. d. Based on the limited information provided in each patient situation listed, the patient in whom fibrinolytic therapy appears to be indicated (assuming there are no reasons for exclusion) is the 72-year-old female. Her chest pain suggestive of acute MI has been present for 4 hours. ST-segment elevation (2 mm) present in leads V_1, V_2, V_3, and V_4 suggests an anteroseptal MI.

17. False. Simultaneous, bilateral carotid massage should NEVER be attempted in any patient.

18. The rhythm is monomorphic ventricular tachycardia. The patient is stable. Perform the primary and secondary ABCD surveys. Administer oxygen, establish an IV, and place the patient on a monitor (already done). Management includes multiple options, including going directly to cardioversion. If medication therapy is preferred and the patient has normal cardiac function (no signs of CHF/shock), procainamide (Class IIa) may be administered (20 mg/min IV infusion) or sotalol (IIa) (IV form not approved for use in the United States). If the patient has impaired cardiac function (ejection fraction <40%, CHF), amiodarone 50 mg IV bolus over 10 min (Class IIb) OR lidocaine 0.5 to 0.75 mg/kg IV push (Class Indeterminate) may be used, then synchronized cardioversion.

19. Triad of the WPW pattern: short PR intervals, wide QRS complexes, and delta waves.

20. b. The lower airway is best protected by an endotracheal tube. The laryngeal mask airway (LMA) and cuffed oropharyngeal airway (COPA) do NOT protect the lower airway from aspiration.

21. b. At 6 to 10 L/min, the simple face mask can provide an inspired oxygen concentration of approximately 40% to 60%. The recommended flow rate is 8 to 10 L/min. The patient's actual inspired oxygen concentration will vary because the amount of air that mixes with supplemental oxygen depends on the patient's inspiratory flow rate. When using a simple face mask, the oxygen flow rate must be higher than 5 L/min to flush the accumulation of the patient's exhaled carbon dioxide from the mask.

22. The rhythm shown is supraventricular tachycardia (SVT). The patient is unstable (altered mental status, hypotension, chest pressure). Administer oxygen, establish IV access, and perform synchronized cardioversion beginning with 50 J. If the first shock is unsuccessful and the rhythm is unchanged, verify the rhythm on the monitor, charge the paddles to 100 J (be sure the "sync" button is on), and deliver the shock. The remaining energy levels that may be used are 200, 300, and 360 J. Thus, the shock sequence for unstable PSVT is 50, 100, 200, 300, and 360 J (or equivalent biphasic energy).

23. Obtain a right precordial lead ECG. If obtaining all of the right precordial leads is not feasible, lead V_4R is the most sensitive. ST-segment elevation viewed in lead V_5R is suggestive of right ventricular injury.

24. c. Defibrillate the patient with 300 J—the last energy level that successfully converted him out of the rhythm.

25. b. Take a moment to confirm that the patient is indeed apneic and pulseless. Once confirmed, defibrillate immediately with 200 J.

26. False. In acute ischemic stroke, fibrinolytics should be considered if the patient is 18 years of age or more, and the time from symptom onset is 3 hours or less.

27. d. An unstable patient in atrial flutter with a rapid ventricular response should receive *synchronized* cardioversion beginning with 50 J, then 100, 200, 300, 360 J (or equivalent biphasic energy) as needed.

28. True. CPR should be briefly halted when administering a medication via the endotracheal tube. The patient should receive several (4 to 5) forceful insufflations with the bag-valve-mask to disperse the medication, and CPR should be resumed.

29. c. The maximum dose of procainamide is 17 mg/kg. The patient weighs 90 kg. 90 kg × 17 mg/kg = 1530 mg. Thus the maximum dose this patient should receive is approximately 1.5 g.

30. c. Pop-off valves are not recommended during resuscitation attempts because higher-than-usual airway pressures are often needed to ventilate patients in cardiac arrest. Pop-off valves may prevent the creation of airway pressures sufficient to overcome the increase in airway resistance.

31. True. The "periarrest" period includes the interval preceding a cardiac arrest and the immediate postresuscitation interval.

32. b. The AVPU acronym is used to quickly assess a patient's level of responsiveness. AVPU: **A**lert, responds to **v**erbal stimuli, responds to **p**ainful stimuli, **u**nresponsive. ABCD are components of the primary and secondary surveys. OPQRST is an acronym used when evaluating a patient's complaint of pain. ALONE is an acronym used to recall medications that may be administered via an endotracheal tube (atropine, lidocaine, oxygen, naloxone, epinephrine).

33. The four critical tasks performed in a resuscitation effort are (1) airway management, (2) chest compressions, (3) monitoring and defibrillation, and (4) IV access and medication administration.

34. c. The "D" in the Primary ABCD Survey stands for *defibrillation*. If the Primary ABCD Survey reveals the patient has no pulse, an automated external defibrillator (AED) should be attached to the patient (or a monitor/defibrillator) when available.

35. True. An *advance directive* is a written document recording an individual's decisions concerning medical treatment that is to be applied (or not applied) in the event of physical or mental inability to communicate these wishes. A living will is a type of advance directive in which the patient puts in writing his or her wishes about medical treatment should he or she become terminally ill and incapable of making decisions regarding his or her medical care. A *durable power of attorney* for health care is another type of advance directive that is a written document that identifies a legal guardian to make health care decisions for a patient when the patient can no longer make such decisions for himself or herself.

36. c. Ischemic strokes account for the majority of all strokes. They rarely lead to death within the first hour of symptom onset. Hemorrhagic strokes can be fatal at onset. AV malformations account for approximately 5% of all subarachnoid hemorrhages. Hypertension is the most common cause of intracerebral hemorrhage.

37. False. Endotracheal intubation should always be *preceded* by some other form of ventilation (mouth-to-mask, bag-valve-mask).

38. c. In complete AV block, the ventricular rhythm is essentially regular. There are more P waves than QRS complexes, and the P waves occur regularly. The QRS may be wide or narrow, depending on the origin of the escape pacemaker. The PR intervals are completely variable because the atria and ventricles beat independently of each other.

39. d. With second-degree AV block type I, the PR interval becomes progressively longer until a P wave is no longer conducted. The PR intervals in second-degree AV block type II remain constant for each conducted QRS.

40. Acute coronary syndromes (ACS) include unstable angina, non–Q-wave myocardial infarction, and Q-wave myocardial infarction. These syndromes represent a physiologic continuum of clinical disease and share the common pathophysiology of atherosclerotic plaque rupture and intracoronary thrombosis. Sudden cardiac death may occur with each of these syndromes.

41. a. Immediate general treatment of this patient should include oxygen, sublingual nitroglycerin, aspirin 162 to 325 mg (if not already administered and no contraindications), and then morphine sulfate 2 to 4 mg IV if pain unrelieved with nitroglycerin.

42. Questions that should be asked of a patient to determine if he/she may be experiencing an acute coronary syndrome include age, signs and symptoms (including pain presentation: location of pain, duration, quality, relation to effort, time of symptom onset), history of coronary artery disease, and the presence of CAD risk factors, and history of viagra use.

43. False. The most common cause of an anterior or lateral wall myocardial infarction is occlusion of a branch of the *left* coronary artery.

44. c. If breath sounds were present bilaterally with bag-valve-mask ventilation before placement of an ETT, the presence of breath sounds on only one side of the chest after placement of the tube suggests right mainstem bronchus intubation. An absence of chest wall expansion and gurgling heard over the epigastrium indicate misplacement of the ETT into the esophagus.

45. d. Calcium is indicated in cases of hyperkalemia, calcium channel blocker toxicity, and hypocalcemia. It is *not* indicated in the management of a symptomatic bradycardia.

46. True. A transient ischemic attack (TIA) is a significant indicator of stroke risk. Approximately one fourth of patients presenting with stroke have had a previous TIA. Approximately 5% of patients with a TIA will develop a completed stroke within 1 month if untreated. A TIA should be treated with the same urgency as a completed stroke.

47. a. The three areas evaluated with the Glasgow Coma Scale are eye opening, best motor response, and best verbal response.

48. d. A transient ischemic attack (TIA) may last for several minutes or hours but resolves within 24 hours.

49. d. Susceptibility to dysrhythmias is greatest during the early hours of infarction.

50. c. The venodilating effects of furosemide begin approximately 5 min after administration.

[1]Cummins RO, Graves JR: *ACLS scenarios: core concepts for case-based learning*, St Louis, 1996, Mosby.

Glossary

Aberrant Abnormal.

Absolute refractory period Corresponds with the onset of the QRS complex to approximately the peak of the T wave; cardiac cells cannot be stimulated to conduct an electrical impulse, no matter how strong the stimulus.

Accelerated idioventricular rhythm (AIVR) A dysrhythmia originating in the ventricles with a rate between 40 and 100 bpm.

Accelerated junctional rhythm A dysrhythmia originating in the AV junction with a rate between 60 and 100 bpm.

Accessory pathway An extra muscle bundle consisting of working myocardial tissue that forms a connection between the atria and ventricles outside the normal conduction system.

ACRONYM A Contrived Reduction Of Nouns, Yielding Mnemonics.

Action potential A reflection of the difference in the concentration of ions across a cell membrane at any given time.

Acute coronary syndromes A term used to refer to patients presenting with ischemic chest pain. Acute coronary syndromes consist of three major syndromes—unstable angina, non–ST-segment elevation MI, and ST-segment elevation MI.

Adrenergic Having the characteristics of the sympathetic division of the autonomic nervous system.

Advance directive A written document recording an individual's decisions concerning medical treatment that is to be applied (or not applied) in the event of physical or mental inability to communicate these wishes.

AED Automated External Defibrillator.

Afterload The pressure or resistance against which the ventricles must pump to eject blood.

Agonal rhythm A dysrhythmia similar in appearance to an idioventricular rhythm but occurring at a rate of less than 20 bpm; dying heart.

ALS Advanced Life Support.

Amplitude The height (voltage) of a waveform on the ECG.

Angina Chest pain of sudden onset that may occur because the increased oxygen demand of the heart temporarily exceeds the blood supply.

Arrhythmia Term often used interchangeably with "dysrhythmia"; any disturbance or abnormality in a normal rhythmic pattern; any cardiac rhythm other than a sinus rhythm.

Arteriosclerosis A chronic disease of the arterial system characterized by abnormal thickening and hardening of the vessel walls.

Artifact Distortion of an ECG tracing by electrical activity that is noncardiac in origin (e.g., electrical interference, poor electrical conduction, patient movement).

Asystole Absence of cardiac electrical activity viewed as a straight (isoelectric) line on the ECG.

Atherosclerosis An accumulation of fatty deposits in the innermost layer of the large and middle-sized muscular arteries.

Atria The two upper chambers of the heart (singular = atrium).

Atrial kick Blood pushed into the ventricles because of atrial contraction.

Atrial tachycardia Three or more sequential premature atrial complexes (PACs) occurring at a rate of more than 100 per minute.

Augmented lead Leads aVR, aVL, and aVF are augmented limb leads. These leads record the difference in electrical potential at one location relative to zero potential rather than relative to the electrical potential of another extremity, as in the bipolar leads.

Automaticity The ability of cardiac pacemaker cells to spontaneously initiate an electrical impulse without being stimulated from another source (such as a nerve).

Autonomy In medical ethics, the principle of autonomy dictates that the patient has the right to choose among offered therapies and the right to refuse any treatment (including CPR) even though this decision may result in the patient's death.

AV dissociation Any dysrhythmia in which the atria and ventricles beat independently (e.g., VT, complete AV block).

A-V interval In dual-chamber pacing, the length of time between an atrial sensed or atrial paced event and the delivery of a ventricular pacing stimulus; analogous to the P-R interval of intrinsic waveforms.

AV junction The AV node and the bundle of His.

AV node Specialized cells located in the lower portion of the right atrium; delays the electrical impulse in order to allow the atria to contract and complete filling of the ventricles.

AV sequential pacemaker (A type of dual-chamber pacemaker) Pacemaker that stimulates first the atrium, then the ventricle, mimicking normal cardiac physiology.

Axis An imaginary line joining the positive and negative electrodes of a lead.

Baseline Straight line recorded on ECG graph paper when no electrical activity is detected.

BBB Bundle branch block.

Beneficence Doing good to others.

Bigeminy A dysrhythmia in which every other beat is a premature ectopic beat.

Bipolar limb lead An ECG lead consisting of a positive and negative electrode; a pacing lead with two electrical poles that are external from the pulse generator. The negative pole is located at the extreme distal tip of the pacing lead. The positive pole is located several millimeters proximal to the negative electrode. The stimulating pulse is delivered through the negative electrode.

Biphasic A waveform that is partly positive and partly negative.

Blocked PAC (Nonconducted PAC) A premature atrial complex that is not followed by a QRS complex.

bpm Abbreviation for beats per minute. The abbreviation bpm usually refers to an intrinsic heart rate, while pulses per minute (ppm) usually refers to a paced rate.

Bradyasystolic rhythm A cardiac rhythm in which the ventricular rate is less than 60 beats/minute and/or there are periods of asystole.

Bradycardia A heart rate slower than 60 beats per minute; brady = slow.

Bundle branch block Abnormal conduction of an electrical impulse through either the right or left bundle branches.

Bundle of His Cardiac fibers located in the upper portion of the interventricular septum; connects the AV node with the two bundle branches.

Burst   Three or more sequential ectopic beats; also referred to as a "salvo" or "run."

Bypass tract   A term used when one end of an accessory pathway is attached to normal conductive tissue.

Capacitor   A device for storing an electrical charge.

Capnography   The continuous analysis and recording of carbon dioxide concentrations in respiratory gases.

Capnometer   A device that measures the concentration of carbon dioxide at the end of exhalation.

Capnometry   The measurement of CO_2 concentrations without a continuous written record or waveform.

Cardiac arrest   The cessation of cardiac mechanical activity, confirmed by the absence of a detectable pulse, unresponsiveness, and apnea or agonal, gasping respiration.

Cardiac output   The amount of blood pumped into the aorta each minute by the heart. It is defined as the stroke volume (amount of blood ejected from a ventricle with each heart beat) × the heart rate.

Carina   The point where the trachea bifurcates into the right and left mainstem bronchi (approximately the level of the 5th or 6th thoracic vertebra).

Cerebral resuscitation   A term used to emphasize the need to preserve the cerebral viability of the cardiac arrest victim.

Compliance   The resistance of the patient's lung tissue to ventilation.

Coronary artery disease   Heart disease caused by impaired coronary blood flow; also called coronary heart disease.

Countershock   The delivery of an electrical current through the myocardium over a very brief period to terminate a cardiac dysrhythmia. There are two types of countershock: defibrillation and cardioversion.

Cricothyroid membrane   A fibrous membrane located between the cricoid and thyroid cartilage; site for surgical and alternative airway placement.

Critical incident   A situation that causes a healthcare provider to experience unusually strong emotions and may interfere with the provider's ability to function immediately or later.

Critical incident stress debriefing (CISD)   A group meeting led by a mental health professional and peer support personnel to allow caregivers to share thoughts, emotions, and other reactions to a critical event.

Crowing   Abnormal respiratory sound that suggests narrowing of the tracheal opening and laryngeal spasm.

Defibrillation   The therapeutic delivery of unsynchronized electrical current through the myocardium over a very brief period to terminate a cardiac dysrhythmia.

Defibrillation threshold   The least amount of energy in joules or volts delivered to the heart that reproducibly reverts VF to a normal rhythm.

Defibrillator   A device used to administer an electrical shock at a preset voltage to terminate a cardiac dysrhythmia.

Defusing   Shorter, less structured version of a critical incident stress debriefing for caregivers held shortly after a critical event.

Delta wave   Slurring of the beginning portion of the QRS complex cause by preexcitation.

Demand (synchronous) pacemaker   A pacemaker that discharges only when the patient's heart rate drops below the pacemaker's preset (base) rate.

Dual-chamber pacemaker   Pacemaker that stimulates the atrium and ventricle.

Durable power of attorney for health care   A type of advance directive that identifies a legal guardian to make health care decisions for a patient when the patient can no longer make such decisions for himself or herself; also called a "health care proxy" or "appointment of a health care agent."

Early defibrillation   The delivery of a shock within five minutes of the time EMS receives the call.

Ejection fraction   The percentage of total ventricular volume ejected during each myocardial contraction; used as a measure of ventricular function; normal approximately 65%.

Electrical storm   Recurrent, hemodynamically destabilizing VT or VF occurring two or more times in a 24-hour period, usually requiring electrical cardioversion or defibrillation.

Endotracheal   Within or through the trachea.

Endotracheal intubation   An advanced airway procedure in which a tube is placed directly into the trachea.

Epiglottis   A small, leaf-shaped cartilage located at the top of the larynx that prevents food from entering the respiratory tract during swallowing.

ET   Endotracheal.

ETT   Endotracheal tube.

Expiratory reserve volume   The amount of air that can be forcefully exhaled after normal exhalation.

Extravasation   The actual (unintentional) escape or leakage of an agent that is irritating and causes blistering (a vesicant) from a vessel into the surrounding tissue.

Fibrinolysis   Dissolving of a blood clot; occurs naturally by plasmin or by a class of medications called fibrinolytics.

Fixed-rate (asynchronous) pacemaker   A device that continuously discharges at a preset rate (usually 70-80 per minute) regardless of the patient's heart rate.

Functional residual capacity   The amount of air remaining in the lungs at the end of a normal expiration; the sum of expiratory reserve volume and the residual volume; normally about 2300 mL.

Ganglion   One of a group of nerve cell bodies usually located in the peripheral nervous system (pl. ganglia).

Glottis   The true vocal cords and the space between them.

Gurgling   Abnormal respiratory sound associated with collection of liquid or semi-solid material in the patient's upper airway.

Hard palate   The bony portion of the roof of the mouth that forms the floor of the nasal cavity.

His-Purkinje system   The portion of the conduction system consisting of the bundle of His, bundle branches, and Purkinje fibers.

Hypoxemia   In adults, children, and infants older than 28 days, hypoxemia is defined as an arterial oxygen tension (PaO_2) of less than 60 torr or arterial oxygen saturation (SaO_2) of less than 90% in an individual breathing room air or with a PaO_2 and/or SaO_2 below the desirable range for a specific clinical situation.

Hypoxia   A deficiency of oxygen reaching the tissues of the body.

Impedance   Resistance to the flow of current. Transthoracic impedance (resistance) refers to the resistance of the chest wall to current.

Incomplete compensatory pause   A pause is termed incomplete (or noncompensatory) if the normal beat following the premature complex occurs before it was expected.

Infarction   Necrosis of tissue due to an inadequate blood supply.

Infiltration   The intentional or unintentional process in which a substance enters or infuses into another substance or a surrounding area.

Inherent   Natural, intrinsic.

Inotropic effect   Refers to a change in myocardial contractility.

Inspiratory reserve volume   The amount of air that can be forcefully inhaled after normal inhalation. This amount is usually 3000 mL.

Interpolated PVC   PVC that occurs between two normal QRS complexes and does not interrupt the underlying rhythm.

Interval   A waveform and a segment; in pacing, the period, measured in milliseconds, between any two designated cardiac events.

Intraosseous infusion   The infusion of fluids, medications, or blood directly into the bone marrow cavity.

Intravenous cannulation   The placement of a catheter into a vein to gain access to the body's venous circulation.

Intrinsic rate   Rate at which a pacemaker of the heart normally generates impulses.

Intubation   Passing a tube into an opening of the body.

Ischemia   A decreased supply of oxygenated blood to a body part or organ.

Isoelectric line   An absence of electrical activity observed on the ECG as a straight line.

J point   The point where the QRS complex and ST segment meet.

Joule   The basic unit of energy; equivalent to watt-seconds.

Junctional escape rhythm   A dysrhythmia originating in the AV junction that occurs when the sinoatrial node fails to pace the heart or AV conduction fails; characterized by a rhythmic rate of 40-60 bpm.

Junctional tachycardia   A dysrhythmia originating in the AV junction with a ventricular response greater than 100 bpm.

Justice   In healthcare ethics, a principle that refers to fairness in the allocation of resources concerning the delivery of healthcare.

KVO   Abbreviation meaning, "keep the vein open." Also known as TKO, "to keep open."

Lacunar stroke   Small area of infarction and necrosis associated with thrombosis of small arteries of the deep white matter in the brain.

Laryngoscope   An instrument used to examine the interior of the larynx. During endotracheal intubation, the device is used to visualize the glottic opening.

Lead   An electrical connection attached to the body to record electrical activity.

Left anterior descending artery   A division of the left coronary artery.

Living will   A type of advance directive in which the patient puts in writing his or her wishes about medical treatment should he or she become terminally ill and incapable of making decisions regarding his or her medical care.

Lown-Ganong-Levine syndrome (LGL)   A type of preexcitation syndrome in which part or all of the AV conduction system is bypassed by an abnormal AV connection from the atrial muscle to the bundle of His; characterized by a short PR interval (usually less than 0.12 sec) and a normal QRS duration.

Lung capacity   The sum of two or more pulmonary volumes.

Membrane potential   A difference in electrical charge across the cell membrane.

Milliampere (mA)   The unit of measure of electrical current needed to elicit depolarization of the myocardium.

Minute volume   The amount of air moved in and out of the lungs in one minute; determined by multiplying the tidal volume by the respiratory rate.

Monomorphic   Having the same shape.

Multiformed atrial rhythm   A cardiac dysrhythmia that occurs because of impulses originating from various sites including the sinoatrial node, the atria, and/or the AV junction; requires at least three different P waves, seen in the same lead, for proper diagnosis.

mV   Abbreviation for millivolt.

Myocardial cells   Working cells of the myocardium that contain contractile filaments and form the muscular layer of the atrial walls and the thicker muscular layer of the ventricular walls.

Myocardial infarction (MI)   Necrosis of some mass of the heart muscle due to an inadequate blood supply.

Myocardium   The middle and thickest layer of the heart; contains the cardiac muscle fibers that cause contraction of the heart and contains the conduction system and blood supply.

Neurotransmitter   A chemical responsible for transmission of an impulse across a synapse.

Noncompensatory pause   A pause is termed noncompensatory (or incomplete) if the normal beat following the premature complex occurs before it was expected.

Nonconducted PAC (blocked PAC)   A premature atrial complex that is not followed by a QRS complex.

Nonmaleficence   An ethical principle embodied by the phrase, "Above all, do no harm." Harm is understood in terms of wrongfully injuring a patient, whether deliberately or negligently.

Nontransmural infarction   A myocardial infarction that is classified as either subendocardial, involving the endocardium and the myocardium, or subepicardial, involving the myocardium and the epicardium.

Ohm   The basic unit of measurement of resistance.

Overdrive pacing   Pacing the heart at a rate (usually 20% to 30%) faster than the rate of the tachycardia.

Oversensing   A pacemaker malfunction that results from inappropriate sensing of extraneous electrical signals.

PAC   Abbreviation for premature atrial complex.

Pacing interval   Period, expressed in milliseconds, between two consecutive paced events in the same cardiac chamber without an intervening sensed event (e.g., AA interval, VV interval). Also known as the demand interval or basic interval.

Pacemaker   Artificial pulse generator that delivers an electrical current to the heart to stimulate depolarization.

Pacemaker cells   Specialized cells of the heart's electrical conduction system capable of spontaneously generating and conducting electrical impulses.

Pacemaker generator (pulse generator)   The power source that houses the battery and controls for regulating a pacemaker.

Pacemaker spike   A vertical line on the ECG that indicates the pacemaker has discharged.

Pacemaker syndrome   Adverse clinical signs and symptoms that limit a patient's everyday functioning that occur in the setting of an electrically normal pacing system. Pacemaker syndrome is most commonly associated with a loss of AV synchrony (e.g., VVI pacing), but may also occur because of an inappropriate AV interval or inappropriate rate modulation.

Paired beats   Two consecutive premature complexes.

Paroxysmal   A term used to describe the sudden onset or cessation of a dysrhythmia.

Paroxysmal atrial tachycardia (PAT)   Atrial tachycardia that starts or ends suddenly.

Periarrest period   The interval preceding a cardiac arrest and the immediate postresuscitation interval, specifically, one hour before and one hour after a cardiac arrest.

Peripheral resistance   Resistance to the flow of blood determined by blood vessel diameter and the tone of the vascular musculature.

Physiologic futility   An ethical principle that applies when a treatment cannot achieve its expected effect on physiologic function.

PJC   Abbreviation for premature junctional complex.

Pocket mask   A transparent semi-rigid mask designed for mouth-to-mask ventilation of a nonbreathing adult, child, or infant.

Polarized state   The period of time following repolarization of a myocardial cell (also called the "resting state") when the outside of the cell is positive and the interior of the cell is negative.

Polymorphic   Varying in shape.

Postresuscitation period   The interval between restoration of spontaneous circulation and transfer to the intensive care unit.

ppm   Abbreviation for pulses per minute. The abbreviation ppm usually refers to a paced rate, while beats per minute (bpm) refers to an intrinsic heart rate.

Prearrest period   The interval preceding a cardiac arrest.

Precordial thump   A forceful blow delivered to the center of the sternum to terminate VT or VF.

Preexcitation   A term used to describe rhythms that originate from above the ventricles but in which the impulse travels via a pathway other than the AV node and bundle of His—thus the supraventricular impulse excites the ventricles earlier than normal.

Preload   The force exerted by the blood on the walls of the ventricles at the end of diastole.

Premature complex   An early beat occurring before the next expected beat.

Proarrhythmia   A new or worsened rhythm disturbance paradoxically precipitated by treatment with antiarrhythmic medications.

Prophylaxis   Preventive treatment.

PSVT   Paroxysmal supraventricular tachycardia; a term used to describe supraventricular tachycardia that starts and ends suddenly.

Pulmonary edema   An excessive accumulation of serous or serosanguineous fluid in the interstitial spaces and alveoli of the lungs, inhibiting oxygen and carbon dioxide exchange at the alveolar-capillary interface.

Pulseless electrical activity (PEA)   Organized electrical activity observed on a cardiac monitor (other than VT) without a palpable pulse.

Pulse generator   The power source that houses the battery and controls for regulating a pacemaker.

Purkinje fibers   An elaborate web of fibers distributed throughout the ventricular myocardium.

PVC   Abbreviation for premature ventricular complex.

Qualitatively futile Description for any treatment that preserves permanent unconsciousness or fails to end total dependence on intensive medical care.

Quantitatively futile An action with a desired outcome that is highly improbable and not systematically predictive and that if useless in the last one hundred cases can be considered futile.

Quadrigeminy A dysrhythmia in which every fourth beat is a premature ectopic beat.

R wave On an EGG, the first positive deflection in the QRS complex, representing ventricular depolarization. In pacing, R wave refers to the entire QRS complex denoting an intrinsic ventricular event.

Reentry The propagation of an impulse through tissue already activated by that same impulse.

Refractoriness A term used to describe the extent to which a cell is able to respond to a stimulus.

Relative refractory period Corresponds with the downslope of the T wave; cardiac cells can be stimulated to depolarize if the stimulus is strong enough.

Repolarization Movement of ions across a cell membrane in which the inside of the cell is restored to its negative charge.

Residual volume The amount of air that remains in the lungs after a forceful exhalation.

Retrograde Moving backward; moving in the opposite direction to that which is considered normal.

Reversible ischemic neurologic deficit (RIND) A neurological deficit that last more than 24 hours but leaves little or no neurologic deficit.

Run Three or more sequential ectopic beats; also referred to as a "salvo" or "burst."

Salvo Three or more sequential ectopic beats; also referred to as a "run" or "burst".

Segment A line between waveforms; named by the waveform that precedes or follows it.

Sellick maneuver Technique used to compress the cricoid cartilage causing occlusion of the esophagus, thereby reducing the risk of aspiration.

Sequence of survival A concept that represents the ideal sequence of events that should take place immediately following the recognition of an injury or the onset of sudden illness; early access to care, early CPR, early defibrillation, and early advanced care.

Sinoatrial node The normal pacemaker of the heart that normally discharges at a rhythmic rate of 60-100 beats per minute.

Sinus arrhythmia A dysrhythmia originating in the sinoatrial node that occurs when the SA node discharges irregularly. Sinus arrhythmia is a normal phenomenon associated with the phases of respiration and changes in intrathoracic pressure.

Sinus bradycardia A dysrhythmia originating in the sinoatrial node with a ventricular response of less than 60 bpm.

Sinus tachycardia A dysrhythmia originating in the sinoatrial node with a ventricular response between 101 and 180 bpm.

Snoring Usually indicates a partial obstruction of the pharynx by the tongue.

Soft palate Composed of mucous membrane, muscular fibers, and mucous glands and is suspended from the posterior border of the hard palate, forming the roof of the mouth.

Speed shock As systemic reaction to the rapid or excessive infusion of medication or solution into the circulation.

Splanchnic Pertaining to internal organs; visceral.

ST segment   The portion of the ECG representing the end of ventricular depolarization (end of the R wave) and the beginning of ventricular repolarization (T wave).

Stridor   A harsh, high-pitched sound heard on inspiration associated with upper airway obstruction. It is frequently described as a high-pitched crowing or "seal bark" sound.

Stroke   Any acute clinical event related to diseases of the cerebral circulation that lasts more than 24 hours.

Stroke volume   The amount of blood ejected by either ventricle during one contraction; can be calculated as cardiac output divided by heart rate.

Stylet   A malleable plastic-covered wire used for molding and maintaining the shape of an endotracheal tube.

Subendocardial infarction   A myocardial infarction involving the endocardium and myocardium.

Subepicardial infarction   A myocardial infarction involving the myocardium and epicardium

Sudden death   An unexpected death of cardiac etiology occurring either immediately or within one hour of onset of symptoms.

Supraventricular   Originating from a site above the bundle branches such as the sinoatrial node, atria, or AV junction.

Synapse   The junction between two neurons.

Tachycardia   A heart rate greater than 100 beats per minute; tachy = fast.

Threshold   The membrane potential at which the cell membrane will depolarize and generate an action potential.

Tidal volume   The volume of air moved into or out of the lungs during a normal breath. The average tidal volume for an adult male at rest is about 500 mL (5-7 mL/kg).

TKO   Abbreviation meaning "to keep open." Also known as KVO, "keep the vein open."

Torsade de Pointes (TdP)   A type of polymorphic VT associated with a prolonged QT interval. The QRS changes in shape, amplitude, and width and appears to "twist" around the isoelectric line, resembling a spindle.

Total lung capacity   The amount of air in the lungs following a maximal inhalation; the sum of the vital capacity and the residual volume; normally about 5800 mL.

Tragus   The cartilaginous area of the ear anterior to the external auditory canal.

Transient ischemic attack (TIA)   A reversible episode of focal neurological dysfunction that typically lasts a few minutes to a few hours, resolving within 24 hours.

Transmural infarction   A myocardial infarction in which the entire thickness of the ventricular wall (endocardium to epicardium) is involved.

Transthoracic impedance (resistance)   The resistance of the chest wall to current.

Trigeminy   A dysrhythmia in which every third beat is a premature ectopic beat.

Trismus   Spasm of the muscles used to grind, crush, and chew food.

Uvula   A pendulous structure that hangs suspended from the midpoint of the posterior border of the soft palate.

Vagal maneuver   Methods used to stimulate the vagus nerve in an attempt to slow conduction through the AV node, resulting in slowing of the heart rate.

Vallecula   The space (or "pocket") between the base of the tongue and the epiglottis; an important landmark when performing endotracheal intubation with a curved laryngoscope blade.

Vital capacity   The maximum volume of air that can be exhaled at the normal rate of exhalation after a maximum inhalation; the sum of the inspiratory reserve volume, tidal volume, and expiratory reserve volume; normally about 4600 mL.

Watt-second   A unit of energy equivalent to the joule.

Waveform   Movement away from the baseline in either a positive or negative direction.

Wheezes   High-pitched "whistling" sounds produced by air moving through narrowed airway passages.

Witnessed resuscitation   The process of active medical resuscitation in the presence of family members.

Wolff-Parkinson-White syndrome   A type of preexcitation syndrome characterized by a slurred upstroke of the QRS complex (delta wave) and wide QRS.

Index

575